Politics, Health, and Health Care

POLITICS, HEALTH, AND HEALTH CARE

Selected Essays

Theodore R. Marmor
and Rudolf Klein

Yale
UNIVERSITY
PRESS

New Haven & London

Published with assistance from the foundation established in memory of Amasa Stone Mather of the Class of 1907, Yale College.

Yale University Press books may be purchased in quantity for educational, business, or promotional use. For information, please e-mail sales.press@yale.edu (U.S. office) or sales@yaleup.co.uk (U.K. office).

Set in Electra type by Newgen North America.
Printed in the United States of America.

Library of Congress Cataloging-in-Publication Data

Marmor, Theodore R.
Politics, health, and health care : selected essays / Theodore R. Marmor and Rudolf Klein.
p. ; cm.
Includes bibliographical references and index.
Summary: "Two towering figures in the field of health care policy analysis, Theodore R. Marmor and Rudolf Klein, reflect on a lifetime of thought in this wide-ranging collection of essays published in the wake of President Obama's health care reform. Presented as a kind of dialogue between the two, the book offers their recent writings on the future of Medicare; universal health insurance; conflicts of interest among physicians, regulators, and patients; and many other topics"—Provided by publisher.
ISBN 978-0-300-11087-6 (alk. paper : hardback)
I. Klein, Rudolf, 1930– II. Title.
[DNLM: 1. United States—Great Britain—Essays. 2. Health Policy—Great Britain—Essays. 3. Delivery of Health Care—Great Britain—Essays. 4. Politics—Great Britain—Essays.WA 540 AA1]
362.1—dc23
2011048886

A catalogue record for this book is available from the British Library.

This paper meets the requirements of ANSI/NISO z39.48–1992 (Permanence of Paper).

10 9 8 7 6 5 4 3 2 1

CONTENTS

PREFACE

This is a book about the various issues, arguments, and conflicts that take place in one of the most important industries in the world: health care. This is an arena characterized by its heterogeneity and complexity, by the multiplicity of interests involved, and by the bitterness of the emotions that can be aroused. It is also an arena where competition among different academic disciplines in offering both analysis and prescription may compound confusion. Our intention in this book is therefore to map the territory and to provide the reader with the analytic tools required to navigate it, synthesizing insights drawn from a variety of perspectives. In this exercise, we aim to contribute to three outcomes: (1) a better understanding of the political dynamics of policy making in health care, (2) a more informed discussion of policy options, and (3) fewer cycles of naïve enthusiasm leading to disillusion.

The structure of the book is shaped by our analytic framework. Here our starting point is that the challenge of resolving issues, arguments, and conflicts—whether about resources or about values—is common to all policy arenas. An understanding of the politics of policy making is therefore prior to an understanding of what is happening in the health policy arena. Accordingly, Chapter 1 provides a general review of the dynamics of public policy, organized around the trinity of ideas, institutions, and interests. Then, and only then, Chapter 2 turns to health care. Here the argument is that the heterogeneity of the health care policy arena means that any analysis of policy and politics must be specific to particular issues or fields within that arena. In short, our assertion is that there is no such thing as the "politics of health care," as distinct from a variety of political struggles in health care. The health care arena illustrates how specific issues—as defined by changing ideas and shifting coalitions of interests—play out over time in specific national or jurisdictional contexts.

The chapters that follow reflect this organizing assumption of the first two. They fall into two overlapping categories. Some are predominantly about the play of politics and policy making in different situations at different times. So, for example, the macro politics of reforming health care systems are different from the micro politics of changing the way doctors are paid, and both may differ over time. Others illustrate more cross-cutting themes. So, one chapter examines one particularly important aspect of the time dimension: how the ideas that shape decisions—the assumptive worlds of policy makers—change over time, altering their perceptions of what is desirable and feasible. Another concentrates on the comparative study of health care systems, reflecting our contention that it is not possible to draw conclusions about what drives policy in any one country without testing that assertion against the experience of other countries with a different configuration of institutions, interests, or ideas.

These chapters are different in kind from the first two. They provide illustrative readings, or case studies, prefaced by a short introduction. These texts are drawn from our previously published papers; a painful exercise in selection that meant discarding many papers prized by their authors. This may strike some readers as an act of septuagenarian self-indulgence or even arrogance. Many others have written, and written well, about health policy and politics. It would not have been difficult to organize a book drawing on this larger literature, a book that moreover would be more comprehensive than this one. So a justification is in order.

The first, and most important, point to make in defense of our strategy is that the purpose is to set out for inspection the key ideas that informed our work over the decades in a form that would allow readers to judge their usefulness in understanding politics, policy, and health care. Our ideas have emerged over decades in a wide variety of books, journals, monographs, and reports. Indeed, the process of selection, and writing the chapter introductions, crystallized those ideas. The first two chapters (see above) set out our approach and provide the conceptual framework for what follows. The writing throughout reflects our shared intellectual style. First, we both started life as historians and take it for granted that there can be no social understanding without history, so we make no apology for using "historical studies," some dating back thirty years or more. In selecting these our test was whether or not such studies remained particularly good illustrations of our analytic approach and remained relevant for that reason. Second, we both became interested in health policy at a time when the pressure on academics to publish exclusively in specialized disciplinary journals was much less than it is today. So we felt free to use ideas drawn from a variety of disciplines, from political science to economics, via political philosophy, legal studies, and sociology.

It is this intellectual style—an unapologetic eclecticism—that is reflected in the publications included in this book. And it is this consistency of style that, in our view, justifies our exclusive reliance on them. Had we drawn on the wider academic literature we might well have gained much but would have lost that coherence, so readers anxious to know about the latest theoretical battles about path dependency or discourse analysis will be disappointed. And there are some obviously important issues, such as the emergence of regulation as a policy instrument, to which we do not do justice. Our claim in launching this book is therefore not so much that we provide an insight into every approach to (and instance of) health policy and politics, but that we do equip the reader with analytic insights and the confidence to take on the wider literature and issues for themselves.

One other feature of the book perhaps requires explanatory justification. This is the predominance of American and British experience. This reflects the balance in our work over the decades and the length of our collegial exchanges during those years. But there is a retrospective logic about it as well. The sharp contrasts between the two countries shaped our understanding of how different institutions and interests reshape similar ideas. This approach proved illuminating for us and, we hope, will be helpful to readers as well.

Acknowledgments

This book is the product of the generosity of two foundations. The Robert Wood Johnson Foundation granted us an Investigator's Award in 2003, which allowed us to lay the intellectual foundations of this volume. During the three years of the award we wrote a number of essays but never completed the promised book. The Rockefeller Foundation allowed us to spend four weeks in 2008 at Bellagio, its writers' paradise in northern Italy. During those weeks we drafted Chapter 2 and the introductions to our illustrative essays. We are grateful to our colleagues at RWJ for their courteous patience in the face of delay and to the staff of Bellagio for providing a welcoming and protective environment. Many thanks to them all.

This book uses, reflects on, and develops ideas from a variety of sources across a long period of time. In the course of our scholarly careers, we have had the benefit of numerous seminars, stimulating co-authors, and any number of influences. Some of these sources and influences are noted in the text that follows. In particular, we owe much to the co-authors of the essays in this book. Others, however, simply reflect the separate if converging intellectual trajectories of the two authors. Noting them all would require a separate essay: a review, in effect, of developments in a variety of disciplines in the anglophone scholarly world over the past fifty years.

The acknowledgments that follow are therefore inevitably—and apologetically—selective, if only because we have no doubt forgotten the sources of some of our ideas. But we are conscious of our intellectual debts to the following, some of whom have been our co-workers, while others have influenced us through their writings. In alphabetical order, they are the late Brian Barry, Morris Barer, Sam Brittan, Pat Day, Anthony Downs, Bob Evans, Jacob Hacker,

Tom Heagy, Richard Freeman, Tony King, Ed Lindblom, Jerry Mashaw, Jim Morone, Richard Nelson, Jon Oberlander, Kieke Okma, Mancur Olson, Richard Rose, Carolyn Tuohy, Albert Weale, Burt Weisbrod, Aaron Wildavsky, and Joe White.

Finally, we thank Camille Costelli, Ted's longtime assistant, without whose reliable work the organization of life and this book would have foundered. The final revisions of the book benefitted as well from the comments of two of Yale Press's anonymous readers. We wish we could thank them directly for such a high quality of appraisal and useful critical observations. They will recognize the impact of their commentary—if and when they read the book.

When reflecting on the question of a dedication, we both took note of the central importance of family in our history as writers. We wish to dedicate this volume to three generations of women: past: Jan and Jo; present: Ans, Kieke, and our daughters, Laura, Leonora, and Sarah; future, our granddaughters, Ava, Freya, Martha, and Nina.

POLITICS AND POLICY ANALYSIS

Fundamentals

Rudolf Klein and Theodore R. Marmor

There are many competing ways of analyzing the politics of public policy, of which the politics of health policy are only an example. Different disciplines, and different sects within disciplines, have all fought over the body of public policy, all seeking to impose their own definitions of the subject and to patent their own analytic methodology. To have set out the varied perspectives on offer might, in itself, have been a valuable pedagogic exercise but would have risked analyzing the subject out of existence. Instead, our aim in this chapter is to be clear about what we regard as the fundamental elements of political and policy analysis and to illustrate how we employ them in practice. We do not imagine that setting out our conception of fundamentals—a conceptual trinity—will reverse generations of heterodox view of how to make sense of the subject. But we hope that the chapters that follow will demonstrate the usefulness of our analytic framework and strategy. The test, as we see it, is not whether our approach contributes to elaborating theory but whether it helps us (and the reader) to gain a fuller understanding of the complex world of public policy making.

We define public policy quite simply. It is what governments do and neglect to do. It is about politics, resolving (or at least attenuating) conflicts about resources, rights, and values. We sideline the issue of whether the aim of analysis should be about understanding or prescribing by claiming that no prescription is worth the paper it is written on if it is not based on an understanding of how the world of policy making works. If prescription (or advice to policy makers) is not based on such a foundation, it will either mislead or fall on deaf ears. In turn, understanding depends on seeing policy making not just as a strange form of theater—with the analyst in the first row of the stalls—but on trying to capture the intentions of the authors of the drama, the techniques of the actors, and the workings of the stage machinery. Empathy, in the sense of capturing what drives policy actors and entering into their assumptive worlds, is a crucial foundation. In adopting this view we place ourselves unapologetically in the tradition of those who see policy analysis as an art and craft, not as a science (to use Wildavsky's 1979 terminology).

By assumptive worlds (Vickers 1965) we mean the "mental models" that "provide both an interpretation of the environment and a prescription as to how that environment should be structured" (Denzau and North 1994, p. 4). Policy actors have theories about the causes of the problems that confront them. They have theories about the appropriate solutions. To take an obvious example: poverty can be seen as reflecting social factors outside the control of individuals or the result of individual failings, and very different policy responses follow depending on the initial diagnosis made. There is an obvious normative component to such mental models. What counts as a problem depends once again on fundamental assumptions about the nature of society and the proper role of government. Problems are not givens but "framed": the product of social and political perceptions. If AIDS is seen as a judgment of God punishing sinful behavior, then governments will see this as a matter for the preacher, not for the politician. When such mental models or assumptive worlds are tightly organized, and internally consistent, then traditionally we tend to call them ideologies. Ideas, as identified as ideologies, fundamental beliefs, or social norms, give shape to the issues that come into the conflicts we call politics.

Ideas are therefore the first element in our trinity of conceptual building blocks. The other two are institutions and interests. In contrast to much of the literature, we define "institutions" narrowly: the constitutional arrangements within which governments operate, the rules of the game and the bureaucratic machinery at their disposal. Self-evidently the process of producing public policy will be very different in a country with a Westminster-type constitution and one with a U.S.-type constitution, with its multiple veto points.

The third element, the interests operating in the political arena, is much invoked in analysis but risks conceptual confusion unless carefully unpackaged. First, there is the distinction between material (and self-regarding) and nonmaterial (or other-regarding) interests; the former involve financial stakes, the latter are organized around notions of right or wrong or moral convictions about appropriate or inappropriate action. Second, there is the distinction between concentrated and diffuse interests. Securing a salary rise matters greatly to public employees; the cost to individual taxpayers is, however, virtually invisible. The scale of the interests also matters: whether a majority or a minority of the population are involved self-evidently makes a difference. So, too, does the intensity with which convictions are held. Using these coordinates, it is then possible to construct a conceptual map of majoritarian or minority stakeholders, material or nonmaterial stakes, and either balanced or imbalanced political settings. The configuration of interests may of course change over time, as issues are redefined or new actors enter the policy arena.

Subsequent chapters build on this conceptual trinity. This chapter, however, now turns to other dimensions of the policy process in the sections that follow. The first section's starting point is the uncontentious proposition that what (democratic) governments do—that is, the policies they advance and implement as well as reject—reflect their larger concerns about gaining (and maintaining) office and doing so legitimately. Uncontentious, even banal, though this proposition may appear to be, it is much ignored in the more rationalistic conceptions of policy analysis. The second section argues that individual policy outputs need to be interpreted in the context of the overall policy portfolio. That is, governments are almost always engaged in a complex balancing act, given that the demands for policy action usually exceed the supply of the administrative, financial, and political resources required to meet them. The third section explores the importance of taking the historical dimension into account when analyzing the fate of any particular policy episode. As a final coda, we briefly restate the case for eclecticism in public policy analysis.

THE DOUBLE IMPERATIVE

To define public policy as what governments do may seem a rather simple-minded opening gambit. In fact, much follows from it. It suggests that before analyzing the genesis and life cycle of specific policies—the focus of most of the public policy literature—we should first consider some of the larger concerns of governments: the context in which specific policy decisions are taken and which help to shape those decisions. Two such concerns, we would suggest, underlie the actions of all governments (at least in Western-style liberal democracies). The first is to gain office and, having done so, to maintain their own authority and the legitimacy of the political system within which they operate. The second is to stay in office. We explore each of these points in turn.

The authority of governments, and the legitimacy of political systems, tends to be taken for granted in much of the public policy literature. The centuries-old debate among political philosophers about the nature of, and justification for, the exercise of political power is left largely to another branch of the academic industry. And even the more recent political science literature expressing worries about the decline of active support for democratic regimes and engagement in civic participation (Putnam 2001)—as shown, for example, by the fall in voter turnout at election times—has taken a long time to percolate into the academic analysis of public policies, particularly the economistic variety, with some notable exceptions.

Do they, however, figure in the concerns of policy makers? It would be absurd to suggest that presidents and prime ministers spend sleepless nights worrying explicitly about how to maintain their authority and the legitimacy of the political system, though occasionally there are spasms of interest in such notions as social capital. Indeed it can be argued that it may be in their self-interest to gain short-term advantages for themselves—by deception or concealment—at the price of undermining confidence in the system in the long term. Nevertheless, balancing such considerations, concerns about legitimacy and authority are woven into the fabric of policy making. If they are largely invisible, it is precisely because they are so much part of normal routine. Before governments decide to act, they must consider whether they are "entitled" to do so. In short, does a proposed course of action conform to what governments are supposed to do? The fact that any such interpretation is contestable does not detract from the importance of this policy filter. And when governments decide to act, they must establish that they are doing so in the right way: whether the proposed policy conforms to contemporary understandings of the requirements of the constitution and the law and whether their implementation has followed the appropriate processes of consultation and legislation.

In short, policy making takes place in a context of established conventions and normative rules. Governments may at times attempt to stretch those conventions and to sidestep those rules. But governments that are judged to act in an arbitrary fashion, or that threaten the private sphere of the citizen, are rightly seen as undermining the basis of their authority—whose maintenance depends on its exercise conforming to the established rules and conventions. The point is obvious enough. It is emphasized here only because it is so often forgotten—because taken as "read"—in a good deal of the public policy literature.

There is a further point to note. The legitimacy of any political system depends on its ability to ensure the stability of the social order. Not only must governments, if they are to justify their authority, be able to defend the state against external enemies. They must also be able to maintain social cohesion, at least in the minimal sense of maintaining law and order and protecting the vulnerable. How best to maintain law and order is, of course, another contested topic, involving disputes about the criteria to be used in framing and judging policies (to which we return later). For example, does it simply require efficient policing and capacious prisons, or does it mean social engineering designed to deal with the sources of crime, disorder, or disaffection? Governments with different assumptive worlds will answer such questions differently. But, however interpreted, the maintenance of social cohesion is surely a fundamental concern of all governments that shapes not only individual policies but also the priorities within any list of candidate policies. And, what is more, the apparent responsiveness to these concerns is electorally important in all liberal democracies. Governments face evaluation not only for what they in fact deliver, but whether they do so in ways various publics regard as legitimate.

The other obvious concern of governments, once in office, is to keep themselves there: to secure their own reelection. From this perspective, the production of public policy can be seen as an exercise in maximizing their chances of winning office (Downs 1957). This raises both analytical and normative issues. The notion that politicians design their policies (and, more often still, the presentation of those policies) to win votes prompts criticism on normative grounds. It is often seen as an abuse of politics: a misuse of political authority and power. It can suggest bad faith, manipulative cynicism, and the deceptive use of power (Goodin 1980). Far be it for us to suggest that politicians do not engage in manipulation: there is no shortage of examples of "spin," of misrepresentation of the evidence, and of the selective use of data by governments. Indeed, there are few better examples in recent history than the case made in 2003 by the United States and British governments for invading Iraq. Subsequently no evidence was found to justify the claim that Iraq had the capacity to use weapons of mass destruction (R. Butler 2004; Woodward 2004). The story also provides a warning: whatever the motives that drove George Bush and Tony Blair, their policies were not simple exercises in vote maximization (and, to the extent viewed as such, they turned out to be a massive miscalculation). But, if we change the wording—if, instead of talking about vote chasing, we substitute the assertion that in a democracy politicians should be sensitive and responsive to public concerns—we will get approving nods. Politicians are not necessarily or exclusively vote maximizers. They may, for example, be maximizers of moral rectitude (or history book reputation).

Moving one step further, let us take a slightly weaker but more realistic definition of the political imperative from which somewhat different normative conclusions follow. If we assume that one of the tests applied to the production of public policies by governments is their acceptability, then we may conclude that this is a perfectly legitimate concern. Not only are governments that produce policies unacceptable to the public less likely to be reelected. They will also be condemned as foolish or authoritarian, on the grounds that unacceptable policies will either not be implementable or violate the conventions that delineate the proper role of government (or both). The introduction in the 1980s of the poll tax by Margaret Thatcher's government in Britain would be one example of producing an unacceptable policy that was roundly (and plausibly) condemned and subsequently abandoned;[1] the U.S. example of the repeal of catastrophic coverage for Medicare in the late 1980s is more complicated. It was in fact a perfectly sensible policy that was widely misunderstood as unfair (Oberlander 2003).[2]

There is a fine borderline between, on the one hand, the investment of political capital and the use of rhetoric in persuading the public of the necessity and desirability of policies—in rallying support and making them acceptable, in other words—and, on the other hand, manipulative cynicism in their presentation. We praise the former as political leadership—only consider Churchill's use of rhetoric in rallying the British people in the dark days of 1940 or Roosevelt's defense of the Lend-Lease policy—while condemning the latter. Modeling governments as prudential, self-regarding actors does not, therefore, capture the complexity of the real world of public policy. It leaves unexplained, for example, why governments take policy decisions that will benefit only their successors. It also creates a puzzle: why do governments address moral or ethical issues that at best are neutral in their impact on voting behavior or at worst may turn out to be stirring up an angry hornet's nest of opposition?

The case of pension policy in the opening years of the twenty-first century illustrates the first point. Across most OECD (Organisation for Economic Cooperation and Development) countries governments were anxiously addressing the problem of aging populations and the expected (and often exaggerated) burden of meeting the consequent pensions bill. In doing so, they were looking twenty and more years ahead. Why did they do so when, on the face of it, they appeared to have had little to gain by such a strategy? After all, no government in office in 2000 would have to answer to the electorate of 2030. One reason may of course be that they were using the future as a pretext for pursuing present reform proposals (such as further pension privatization) that otherwise might be regarded as unacceptable.[3] Ideology was at work for sure, but so was serving the interests of allies in the finance community. This is a defensible interpretation of the Bush administration's embrace of Social Security pension reform as "required" by the feared insolvency that population aging foreshadows. The argumentative structure and rhetoric is familiar: actuarial forecasts project increasing pension claims and, assuming no change in benefits or contributions, "bankruptcy" at some future date is a mathematical certainty. The fact that "trust fund" language originally was meant to communicate political commitment is lost. Instead, the analogy to private trust funds, which can go broke, becomes a contemporary source of public fearfulness (Marmor 2004).

However, even conceding this explanation, invoking the interests of yet-to-be-born voters can be seen (like hypocrisy) as the tribute paid by vice to virtue. Governments rightly presume that they are expected to take a long-term view, and the fact that policy makers feel obliged to invoke this justification for their policies illustrates the extent to which public policy is shaped by such normative considerations. Which is not to argue, of course, that governments invariably (or even usually) examine the long-term implications of their policies: witness, for example, the problem of nuclear waste that will remain radioactive for generations. Rhetorical long-sightedness can sit alongside policy myopia.

Again, the self-image of policy actors—who want to be seen to be following certain ideal types of behavior—seems to be at least as important as their narrow self-interest when it comes to ethical and moral issues. Only consider President Bill Clinton's ill-fated decision at the very outset of his presidency about how to treat homosexuality in the American armed services. In February 1993, his very first presidential decision on defense matters was to propose that the U.S. military change its long-standing objections to having homosexuals in the services. The presidential suggestion provoked sharp criticism within the military, enthusiastic support from the organized homosexual community, and derision among the chattering classes for its timing, content, and presumed insensitivity to military norms. In terms of self-seeking political behavior this made no sense, as quickly became apparent. But it did make sense in terms of the president's sense of what was right and appropriate in terms of his self-image as a progressive liberal. (It also made Clinton the recipient of substantial financial support from the gay community, which is comparatively rich, ready to spend, and politically active.)[4]

The same point could be made about many other governmental "policy outputs." In the case of the United Kingdom, for example, successive governments have resisted attempts to restore capital punishment, even though survey evidence suggests that bringing back the hangman would earn them applause from a majority of the population and the tabloids. However, such a move would bring them more than condemnation from the liberal establishment and the broadsheets. For many legislators opposition to the death penalty is a core value that they are prepared to put before majoritarianism. The 2003 controversy over the religious symbolism of attire in French schools—with the state forbidding the wearing of head scarves—obviously involved ideals of secular republicanism as well as prejudice against Islamic fundamentalism. In short, policy actors have moral constituencies, as well as constituencies of material interest, and follow moral imperatives. It is not unknown for policy actors to congratulate themselves on pursuing unpopular policies in pursuit of what they consider right. Invoking considerations of moral rectitude earns points in this world as well as (possibly) the next. And any convincing analysis of their assumptive worlds must take this into account.

THE POLICY PORTFOLIO: WHY THE CONTEXT MATTERS

Analyzing the genesis, development, and implementation of individual policies is misleading to the extent that it misses out on an important characteristic of public policy making. This is that demands for public action tend to exceed any government's capacity to supply policy responses. The portfolio of policies that eventually emerges therefore is the product of a complex process of bargaining, negotiation, and political calculation. On the one hand, there is competition between and among interest groups and departments pressing for action on their concerns. Governments are not unitary actors, although for convenience we refer to them as a collectivity in the text (Allison 1971; Allison and Zelikow 1999). Cabinet ministers with different and sometimes conflicting priorities jostle for space in the legislative program. On the other hand, there are judgments about where the investment of administrative capacity and political capital will yield the largest returns—judgments that are filtered through the lenses of the "mental models" of the policy actors whose interests will be affected. In short, the launch of a policy may reflect as much the desire to have a "balanced portfolio" (whether in terms of maintaining the legitimacy of the government or in terms of political expediency) as factors intrinsic to the specific policy arena.

The heterogeneity of such a policy portfolio is illustrated by both the British examples of policy promises in the first few years of the twenty-first century and American counterparts in the same period (see Appendixes A and B). The first are from the Queen's Speech delivered to the Parliament in November 2003, outlining the British government's legislative program for the next year. The U.S. examples come from the State of the Union speech given by President Bush to the Congress in January 2004. Both sets of examples should be seen as illustrative, not representative. The contents of these two speeches are time specific. Under different governments, at different stages in the life cycle of any administration, and in a different global environment, they could have been very different. Our concern here, however, is not so much with the details of the policies involved—which are discussed only to the extent that they need to be comprehensible to the reader—but with the overall style and shape of such policy portfolios at one particular historical moment.

Even the long laundry list that is the 2003 Queen's Speech greatly understates the extent and variety of British public policy "outputs" in any given year. Most importantly, it excludes fiscal policies: decisions by the chancellor of the exchequer about the level of spending on specific programs and the design of the system of taxes and benefits. And it cannot include, by definition, government policies—whether administrative, legislative, or judicial, prompted by the outbreak of an epidemic, a natural disaster, or an external threat.

Immediately striking is the prominence in this particular portfolio of what might be called social stability concerns. These included: tightening up the appeal system in asylum cases, working toward the introduction of national identity cards, and modernizing the law and system for protecting women and children. All three examples can be understood as public policy in the responsive mode, reacting to external events and, perhaps even more importantly, to public perceptions of those events. The tightening up of the appeals system and the incremental development of identity cards can both be seen as part of a strategy for reassuring the public that the government was acting to stop the United Kingdom from being flooded by fraudulent asylum seekers and illegal immigrants. These were concerns with high political salience that had attracted much attention in the media in the United Kingdom, as in many other European countries. The improvement of services for protecting children was again a response to an issue with a high public and media profile: a series of appalling cases of child abuse had revealed great shortcomings in the existing system of surveillance and protection.

All three examples also, however, underline the importance of distinguishing between *why* a particular issue makes it onto the agenda for action and *how* it is then translated into a specific public policy measure. In all three cases, the government's decision to respond to public worries could be interpreted either as (three cheers) a demonstration of its sensitivity to public concerns or (boos) as a cynical political maneuver designed to prevent the opposition from exploiting these issues. But all three cases had long histories. The U.K. system for processing asylum seekers had long been recognized as a shambles (not least because of the hardships inflicted on genuine cases). What is more, previous attempts to improve it had produced meager results. The introduction of identity cards had been debated since at least the 1960s, though the debate was given new impetus after 2000 by both developments in technology and increasing concern (whether justified or not) about illegal immigration. Child protection had been an ongoing worry, with recurring scandals despite a succession of attempts to improve the system, for at least as long. As this historical example shows, a raised sensitivity to public concerns (or, pejoratively, political expediency) opened the window for the various government agencies that had long been working on these problems to get their ideas onto the agenda for action (Kingdon 1995). The specific measures that eventually emerged reflect as much bureaucratic bargaining and negotiation, organizational routines, and notions of the administratively feasibility as political-electoral considerations. The factors that influence the timing of public policy do not necessarily determine the contents.

There are some other points to note about this particular British policy portfolio. First, little of the proposed legislation involved classic pressure group activity. Like the three examples already discussed, most of the initiatives represented a response to diffuse public concerns rather than to demands from organized interest groups (though in the case of pension reform the government was involved in tough negotiations with employers, the insurance industry, and the trade unions when it came to the details of the legislation). Second, much of it represented the incremental processes of government rather than policy innovation: for example, the proposals to make the planning system faster and to improve traffic flows—a reminder that public policy is as much drudgery as drama, a constant process of tinkering and repairing. The small print of public policy (we all care about traffic flows) matters if governments want to demonstrate their competence in dealing with the day-to-day concerns of their citizens. Most of public policy is as boring as darning old socks. Third, policy may represent a moral commitment, which has little or nothing to do with political expediency. The proposed legislation to allow the registration of civil partnerships between same-sex couples is a case in point. This was symbolism not as a substitute for action but as a signal that the government's heart was in the right place: that it was a liberal, progressive administration. In this sense, it was an important part of a balanced portfolio, a rebuttal of the charges of authoritarianism prompted by some of the Blair government's law and order policies.

Quite different in kind was one of the most contentious measures in the 2004 Queen's Speech: reform of the House of Lords. Here the fissures were as much within the governing Labor Party as between Labour and the Conservative opposition. In the case of the House of Lords, there was cross-party agreement that the hereditary element should be eliminated. But divisions existed within all parties about how the new composition of the second chamber should be determined, whether by election or nomination: a series of votes in the House of Commons on various options had failed to produce a consensus about the composition. This, then, can be seen as the attempt of a government to exploit confusion and disagreement to impose its own preferred option: a second chamber appointed by an independent commission, its party composition reflecting voting patterns. In the event, the attempt failed, but this unusual and rare form of public policy-making is worth noting because it underlines the difficulty of classifying and anatomizing the diversity of the activities that go under that label.

The State of the Union speech, given January 20, 2004, set out President Bush's legislative aims for 2004 and beyond. The contents of the list range from announcing broad policy aims to proposing legislative action: It is the breadth of the range—and the loose connection to likely legislative action—that most sharply distinguishes the American practice from that of parliamentary leaders like Blair.

Yet, the similarities of the two forms are striking. The Bush speech offered to its audience just the kind of "balanced portfolio" presented to the Commons. In other words, within the heterogeneous legislative proposals and public policy concerns there was a parallel mix of appeals. For example, all of the funding proposals were incremental, with flourishes about "doubling" efforts to encourage sexual abstinence and to make the world safer for democracy, free markets, and free speech. Evident as well were the responses to what we have characterized as diffuse concerns about social stability. So, we find aspirational gestures toward such difficult subjects as how to control medical inflation with policies as weakly connected to the purpose as tax subsidies for catastrophic plans. Likewise, there was top billing for concerns about terrorism, however uncertain the connection between means and ends. And, finally, the speech appealed for support of two very controversial legislative actions: the reenactment of the Patriot Act (and its attendant conflict with civil liberties) as well as the proposal for a temporary workers program (which excites the ire of the labor movement). Very few of the American proposals looked like simple responses to classic pressure group demands. Or, put another way, the language suggested responsiveness to diffuse rather than concentrated organizational concerns.

Institutional structures and the policy context of the moment explain much of the remaining differences between our two illustrations. The most obvious feature of the Bush laundry list is its aspirational character, not its predictive accuracy. In the U.S. system of government, the general rule is that the Administration proposes, but the Congress disposes. And what the Congress does is not usually decided by general elections, as it is in parliamentary regimes. There is no necessary policy majority in the Congress even when controlled by one party, as it was in 2004. As a result, no one could have said with any certainty in January of 2004 whether any of the actions President Bush proposed would become law that year. In the event, the worsening circumstances in Iraq during the spring and summer of 2004 rendered the president's influence in the Congress less decisive. The electoral context increasingly made the Democrats unwilling to cooperate, and fissures within the Republican congressional majority made legislative majorities harder to construct.

This brings us back to the most general conclusion of this section: namely, that it is very difficult to classify (or describe the anatomy of) public policy. The character, distribution, and alignments of stakeholders, we have seen, are not self-evident. What counts as an issue, or what similar "issues" evoke, depends, as we have argued, on context broadly construed, which in turn is filtered through the mental models of actors and audiences. So, for instance, the salience of immigration reform in the United Kingdom is not reflected in the modest reference by the Bush administration to a temporary worker program. In 2004, immigration had priority on the policy agendas of the European Union generally, reflecting domestic conflict over amnesty programs, EU worker mobility policies, and claims of foreigner "misuse" of welfare state programs. Nothing of that kind is evident in the U.S. document, and the reason is largely institutional rather than ideological. American federalism shapes welfare state disputes in the United States so that conflicts over access to medical care programs (like Medicaid) or educational expenses of newcomers (local and state funding issues) are channeled away from national debates. The same range of sentiments that excited debate in the United Kingdom during the first years of the twenty-first century did appear in the United States, but not, during those years, on the national agenda. California enacted measures limiting the access to social programs by foreign, largely Mexican workers; Texas confronted cross-border concerns in state legislation. And, at the national level, the federal Immigration and Naturalization Service increasingly used helicopters to interdict workers crossing deserts and rivers to enter the Southwest. But the "face" of immigration policy looked different across the Atlantic, which illustrates our classificatory caution.

THE HISTORICAL DIMENSION

Much is made in the literature about path dependency, variously defined. At one level this is simply another way of describing the incremental, adaptive nature of much policy making: that (as we have seen in our examples) public policy consists to a large extent of patching and repairing, building on, and learning from experience (Heclo 1974). Again, the fact that policy makers faced with a new problem tend to draw on an established repertory of tools reinforces the bias of public policy against radical innovation, as does dependence on existing organizations for delivery. More narrowly and rigorously, path dependency is seen as flowing from the structure of interests created by prior policy (Tuohy 1999; Hacker 2002). Decisions taken at point A in time entrench—sometimes indeed create—interests that come to constrain decisions at point B and beyond. Either way, what is interesting and appears to call for explanation are the rare occasions when public policy takes a new turn, whether successfully or not, rather than the sock-darning dimension of public policy.

So history matters. But, we would suggest, it matters in a more profound sense still. Not only are policy makers obliged to work within the context of inherited institutions—constitutional arrangements and conventions and the administrative machinery of government—as well as the structure of interests created by previous policies, as noted. But their world of ideas is also the product of history. This is so in a double sense. On the one hand, their notions are likely to be shaped by early experience and the culture of their time, as with all of us. On the other hand, they are likely to use history (or rather their own interpretation of it) as a quarry for policy exemplars or warnings.

From this wider perspective, history can be used to explain change and divergence from existing paths as well as continuity. Consider, for example, the generation of politicians who grew to maturity in the years of slump and mass unemployment of the 1920s and 1930s. The experience persuaded even those in the middle of the political spectrum (Roosevelt in the United States; Macmillan in the United Kingdom) to adopt radical social and economic policies. And, to underline the importance of ideas, they could draw on Keynesian theory to justify their policies. In short, there was a change not only in what was considered politically important but also in what was considered to be possible in practice. The converse applies to the next generation, who grew up in a period of unprecedented economic growth and full employment. They proved, when in power, less sensitive to unemployment statistics. And, again, they could turn for justification to the new economic paradigm (Hall 1993), which challenged Keynesian notions by arguing that there was a natural rate of unemployment about which governments could do little and only at the risk of fueling inflation.

What matters in all this, of course, is not history as written in academic text books but the interpretations put on it by policy makers: the lessons they choose to draw from the past. (Neustadt and May 1988). So, for example, the nebulous Third Way as espoused by Clinton and Blair in the 1990s—the latest in a long line of attempts to find a middle way (Macmillan 1938) — cannot be understood without taking into account their diagnosis of the mistakes made by their predecessors as party leaders. The interpretation of history need not be correct to be noteworthy. Some disastrous policy decisions have flown from the misapplication of supposed historical lessons, largely as a result of misspecifying the similarity between past and present situations. The conclusion that it never pays to appease dictators drawn from the abject surrender of the Western Powers to Hitler at Munich in 1938, plus the equation of Nasser with Hitler, was used to justify Britain's disastrous Suez adventure in 1956. And Bush's initiation of the 2003 Iraq war may, also, in part at least, have reflected a misreading of history. Bush's Iraq policy appeared to some a reaction against his father's "failure" to topple Saddam. Whatever the president's motives, the justifications offered — that weapons of mass destruction in the hands of a dictator will be used and therefore must be "taken out" preventively — relied on historical claims. In another sense, the Iraq policy was an earlier conviction searching for an occasion, a commitment to get rid of Saddam by officials from George H. W. Bush's presidency acted upon in George W. Bush's administration (Woodward 2002, 2004; Dean 2004).

Particular readings of history may also persuade policy makers to diverge from the trodden path. Policy change is not only the result of windows of opportunity suddenly opening as the result of some upheaval in the economic or political environment. Policy change itself may open such windows by demonstrating that the previously unthinkable has become doable. A case in point is the repudiation in the 1980s by Mrs. Thatcher of the assumption shaping the policies of all post-1945 British governments that they needed the cooperation of the trade-union movement to manage the economy. Instead, she was prepared to confront and fight the unions (Young 1989). The skies did not fall in. And Tony Blair, as Labour prime minister, shaped his policies accordingly, largely sidelining the unions when he took office in 1997 and making a political virtue of his independence of them.

The 2004 Bush administration's approach to old-age and retirement policy illustrated similar risk-taking. By suggesting that what Americans call social security retirement pensions should be partially privatized, President Bush repeatedly risked identification as an enemy of a public policy "sacred cow." The cliché has been that "social security is the third rail of American politics, electrocuting all those who touch it." Yet, throughout his administration's first term, Bush called for private, individual pension accounts funded by a proportion of the compulsory "contributions" that all Americans pay. This innovation, the president claimed, was the right response to the fiscal strains the aging

American society faces. Leaving aside the merits of this view—which are few if any—this bold rhetoric in presidential speeches and proposals did not provoke the public condemnation pundits anticipated on the basis of Social Security's status as a supposed "sacred cow." In turn, the rhetoric emboldened the interest groups who would gain financially if the American government required some share of social insurance taxes to be invested in the stock and bond markets. As a result, the presidential election of 2004 was replete with references to the differences between the traditional defense of social insurance (largely by Democrats) and the call for private individual accounts (largely by Republicans).

Innovation occurs, but not as commonly as appeals to its possibility (Baumgartner and Jones 1993, 2002). Nonetheless, without history there can therefore be no understanding of public policy. And without history there can also be no realistic evaluation of public policy. For if evaluation does not take into account what policy makers were trying to achieve, if the criteria used in judging the success or otherwise of policies are those of the evaluator rather than those of the originator, the result will at best yield a very partial, perhaps anachronistic verdict. By this we do not claim an historical monopoly on either the understandings or the evaluation of public policy. But we do connect our insistence on the explanatory importance of the assumptive world of policy actors with the truism that all our assumptions incorporate historical understandings, both biographical and cultural.

THE CASE FOR ECLECTICISM

One reaction to our argument so far may well be to dismiss it as an exercise in trying to have it all ways: eclecticism as a substitute for intellectual orderliness. However, we make no apology for this. In practice, no public policy analyst can use all the tools of the trade all the time: a rational choice analyst in the morning, a psycho-biographer in the afternoon, a historian in the evening, and a political theorist in the hours when sleep does not come. However, our contention throughout has been that the attempt to draw on all these disciplines is essential. Trying to understand and explain public policy as a whole—making sense of what governments do, rather than analyzing specific election results or policy outputs—has to be, in our view, an exercise in synthesis.

The point can be simply illustrated, bringing together many of the issues previously discussed. Central to most public policy analysis (including our own) is the notion of self-interest. We invoke the self-interest of politicians in getting elected and staying in office. We invoke the self-interest of lobbies in pressing for their share of pork or in pursuit of some ideology. Yet as Thomas Macaulay (cited in Wildavsky 1994, p. 155) pointed out some 150 years ago in his critique of utilitarianism: "One man cuts his father's throat to get possession of his old clothes; another hazards his own life to save that of an enemy. One man volunteers on a forlorn hope; another is drummed out of a regiment for cowardice. Each of these men has no doubt acted from self-interest. But we gain nothing from knowing this, except the pleasure, if it be one, of multiplying useless words."

In short, much of public policy analysis involves giving meaning to what, in the absence of background knowledge, is indeed an empty word. How people define their self-interest (their assumptive worlds) depends on culture and history. How people, in turn, act to further that self-interest will depend on the institutions within which they operate. And the definitions, and the way in which they are translated into practice, will vary and evolve over time as the intellectual, social, and economic environment changes. So, for example, no one can understand the evolving history of Britain's National Health Service (Klein 2001) without taking into account the changing environment in which it operates.

In summary, then, we have argued that no sensible understanding of what liberal democratic governments should do, have done, or will do is possible without attention to the realities of office-seeking and office-keeping, and how those realities are perceived by those involved. This theme—stunningly obvious in one sense—is nonetheless all too frequently ignored. The history of efforts to make the analysis of public policy more scientific, rigorous, and thereby more helpful for policy development is a fascinating (and controversial) one, but has not been our concern here. Rather, our contribution is to insist that whatever technical improvements are possible—in polling accuracy, in economic modeling, in the simulation of policy options, and so on—it remains essential to emphasize the centrality of the most basic features of governmental policy making in democratic polities. These, we suggest, include the need to maintain regime legitimacy, the competitive struggle to achieve (and keep) office, and the search for a balanced policy portfolio.

Beyond that, we have emphasized the importance of understanding the constellation of ideas, institutions and interests that converge in any policy activity. Here the focus is, as argued above, on how historical evidence—and evidence about history—shapes the options available to policy makers, their understanding of the material (and other) interests at stake, and their interpretation of what contemporary audiences will make of their ideas. Throughout we have illustrated our claims about historical understanding by citing examples that appear to tell an apt illustrative story—in line with our contention that the analysis of public policy, like policy making itself, is an exercise in persuasion (Majone 1989). Hence the importance of examining critically the rhetoric of persuasion used by both policy makers and public policy analysts.

The later discussion of comparative policy will emphasize still another essential element in the art and craft of policy analysis. Comparing formulations of policy problems across national borders illustrated the degree to which the mental worlds of actors are shaped by their distinctive historical understandings and the ideas that stakeholders in particular settings take for granted, as well as being a protection against explanatory provincialism. Finally, we note the complexities of evaluating public policymaking once the perspectives of policy makers are taken as central to understanding their options and choices. Put another way, an appreciation of what policy makers believe they are doing is a necessary—albeit far from sufficient—condition for understanding and evaluating their actions.

Exhibit A. The Queen's Speech, November 2004: The UK Government's Legislative Programme

The Queen's Speech announced the following planned legislation, for the 2004/2005 session of Parliament. The bills announced would:

- Enable young people to people to benefit from higher education and abolish up-front tuition fees.
- Encourage employers to provide good-quality pensions and individuals to save for retirement, and set up a pension protection fund to protect people when companies becomes insolvent.
- Allow registration of civil partnerships between same-sex couples
- Establish a single tier of appeal against asylum decisions.
- Take forward work on an incremental approach to a national identity cards scheme.
- Modernize the laws on domestic violence and improve services designed to protect children.
- Remove hereditary peers and set up an independent Appointments Commission.
- Enable a referendum on the single currency, subject to the government's five economic tests being met.
- Make the planning system faster and fairer with greater community participation.
- Improve traffic flows and manage road works more effectively.

- Modernize charity law and allow for the creation of Community Interest Companies.

Exhibit B. Bush's 2004 State of the Union Address Summary of Contents

- Continue support for the War on Terror; a peaceful, stable, and democratic Iraq; and homeland security.
- Renew the Patriot Act, which is set to expire in 2005.
- Put pressure on regimes that support and harbor terrorists and seek to obtain weapons of mass destruction.
- Double the budget for the National Endowment for Democracy to help it develop free elections, free markets, free press, and free labor unions in the Middle East.
- Give students the skills they need to succeed in the workplace with Jobs for the 21st Century, a series of measures that includes extra help for students falling behind in reading and math, greater access to advanced placement programs in high schools, private-sector math and science professionals teaching part-time in high schools, larger Pell grants for college students, and increased support for community colleges.
- Make the temporary tax cuts permanent to keep the economy going strong.
- Help small business owners and employees find relief from excessive federal regulation and frivolous lawsuits.
- Enact energy-related measures to modernize the electricity system, protect the environment, and make America less dependent on foreign oil.
- Create Social Security Personal Retirement Accounts.
- Cut the federal deficit in half over five years with a budget that limits growth in discretionary spending to 4 percent.
- Reform immigration laws to create a temporary worker program allowing illegal immigrants to obtain temporary legal status.
- Control medical costs and expand access to care by letting small businesses collectively bargain with insurance companies, giving refundable tax credits to low-income Americans so they can buy their own health insurance, computerizing health records to improve quality and reduce cost, reforming medical malpractice law, and making the purchase of catastrophic health care coverage 100 percent tax deductible.
- Increase funding to combat drug use through education, drug testing in schools, and asking children's role models to set a good example.
- Double federal funding for abstinence programs to reduce the incidence of sexually transmitted diseases.
- Prevent same-sex marriages, using the constitutional process if necessary.

- Codify into law the executive order allowing faith-based charities to compete for federal social service grants.
- Enact a prisoner reentry program providing better job training and placement, transitional housing, and mentoring.[5]

Notes

1. After decades of discussion about reforming Britain's system for funding local government—a mixture of property taxes and central government grants—the government of Mrs. Thatcher decided to replace the former by a poll tax, as from 1988. The decision was widely criticized, led to sometimes violent demonstrations, and prompted widespread evasion. While eight million people gained as a result of the switch from property taxes to the poll tax, twenty-seven million lost. As one of Mrs. Thatcher's ministers subsequently commented: "It was fundamentally flawed and politically incredible. I guess it was the single most unpopular policy any government has introduced since the War" (quoted in the classic account of this episode: Butler, Adonis, and Travers 1994, p. 1). The poll tax fiasco greatly weakened Mrs. Thatcher's position and contributed to her subsequent downfall. Her successor's government promptly dropped the poll tax.

2. The legislation to add catastrophic health insurance and outpatient prescription drug coverage to Medicare in 1987–88 was and is regarded as a debacle. The legislation, repealed within a year, addressed two serious problems, but was financed exclusively by increased premiums on beneficiaries, which in turn was neither explained nor justified well by the Reagan administration and the reform's defenders in the Congress. In a memorable incident, the then chairman of the House Ways and Means Committee, Congressman Dan Rostenkowski, was pelted with tomatoes by older constituents in Chicago who were outraged by this unorthodox form of financing a social insurance program. The obvious truth was that while the program had merit, the financing means were genuinely a surprise, not well defended, and especially vulnerable to the claim that they had not been legitimated by broad public discussion and understanding.

3. There is no question that President Bush was hesitant about direct criticism of the U.S. social insurance pension programs. The use of specters of an aging America was a vehicle for prompting present adjustments in the name of necessity. The change he proposed—using social insurance contributions for investments in individual risk-bearing accounts—was deeply controversial within the policy analytic community, but amplified rather than ridiculed by the media.

4. The Clinton suggestion ended up with what came to be known as the "don't ask, don't tell" policy. While not what President Clinton called for, this operational policy has no doubt changed military norms substantially.

5. Adapted from G. W. Bush, *State of the Union Address*, January 20, 2004, available at http://www .whitehouse.gov/news/releases/2004/01/ 20040120-7.html.

References

Allison, G. 1971. *Essence of Decision: Explaining the Cuban Missile Crisis*. Boston: Little Brown.

Allison, G., and P. Zelikow. 1999. *Essence of Decision: Explaining the Cuban Missile Crisis*. 2nd ed. New York: Longman.

Baumgartner, F., and B. Jones. 1993. *Agendas and Instability in American Politics*. Chicago: Chicago University Press.

Baumgartner, F., and B. Jones. 2002. *Policy Dynamics*. Chicago: Chicago University Press.

Butler, D., A. Adonis, and T. Travers. 1994. *Failure in British Government: The Politics of the Poll Tax*. Oxford: Oxford University Press.

Butler, R. 2004. *Review of Intelligence on Weapons of Mass Destruction*. London: The Stationery Office.

Dean, J. 2004. *Worse Than Watergate: The Secret Presidency of George W. Bush*. New York: Little, Brown and Co.

Denzau, A. T., and D. C. North. 1994. Shared Mental Models: Ideologies and Institutions. *Kyklos* 47:1 3–31.

Downs, A. 1957. *An Economic Theory of Democracy*. New York: Harper and Row.

Fox, D., P. Day, and R. Klein. 1989. The Power of Professionalism: Policies for AIDS in Britain, Sweden and the United States. *Daedalus* 118(2):93–112.

Goodin, R. E. 1980. *Manipulative Politics*. New Haven, CT: Yale University Press.

Goodin, R. E. 2000. Institutional Gaming. *Governance* 13(4):523–33.

Hacker, J. S. 2002. *The Divided Welfare State*. New York: Cambridge University Press.

Hall, P. A. 1993, April. Policy Paradigms, Social Learning and the State. *Comparative Politics* 25:275–96.

Heclo, H. 1974. *Modern Social Politics in Britain and Sweden*. New Haven: Yale University Press.

Hunter, D. 1995, March. A New Focus for Dialogue. *European Health Reform: The Bulletin of the European Network and Database*, no. 1.

Jacobs, A. 1998. Seeing Difference: Market Health Reform in Europe. *Journal of Health Politics, Policy and Law*. 23:1 1–33.

Jacobs, L., T. Marmor, and J. Oberlander. 1999. The Oregon Health Plan and the Political Paradox of Rationing: What Advocates and Critic Have Claimed and What Oregon Did. *Journal of Health Politics, Policy and Law* 24(1):161–80.

Jacobs, L. R., and R. Y. Shapiro. 2000. *Politicians Don't Pander: Political Manipulation and the Loss of Democratic Responsiveness*. Chicago: University of Chicago Press.

Kennedy, J. 1964. *Profiles in Courage*. New York: Harper & Row.

Kingdon, J. W. 1995. *Agendas, Alternatives and Public Policies*. 2nd.ed. New York: HarperCollins.

Klein, R. 1991. Risks and Benefits of Comparative Studies. *The Milbank Quarterly* 69(2):275–91.

Klein, R. 1995. Learning from Others: Shall the Last Be the First? In K. Okma, ed., *Four Country Conference on Health Care Reforms and Health Care Policies in the United States, Canada, Germany and the Netherlands: Report*. The Hague: Ministry of Health.

Klein, R. 2001. *The New Politics of the NHS*. 4th ed. Harlow, Essex: Prentice Hall.

Macmillan, H. 1938. *The Middle Way*. London: Macmillan.

Maioni, A. 1998. *Parting at the Crossroads: The Emergence of Health Insurance in the United States and Canada*. Princeton, NJ: Princeton University Press.

Majone, G. 1989. *Evidence, Argument and Persuasion in the Policy Process*. New Haven, CT: Yale University Press.

Marmor, T. 1999. The Rage for Reform: Sense and Nonsense in Health Policy. In D. Drache and T. Sullivan, eds., *Health Reform: Public Success, Private Failure*. London: Routledge. 260–72.

Marmor, T. 2004. The U.S. Medicare Programme in Political Flux. *British Journal of Health Care Management* 10, no. 5.

Marmor, T., and R. Freeman, and K. G. Okma, eds. 2009. *Comparative Studies in the Politics of Modern Medical Care*. New Haven, CT: Yale University Press.

Neustadt, R. E., and E. R. May. 1988. *Thinking in Time: The Uses of History for Decision Makers*. New York: Free Press.

Oberlander, J. 2003. *The Political Life of Medicare*. Chicago: University of Chicago Press.

Putnam, R. 2001. *Bowling Alone: The Collapse and Revival of American Community*. New York: Simon & Schuster.

Tuohy, C. H. 1999. *Accidental Logics*. New York: Oxford University Press.

Vickers, G. 1965. *The Art of Judgment*. London: Chapman & Hall.

White, J. 1995. *Competing Solutions: American Health Care Proposals and International Experience*. Washington, DC: Brookings Institution.

Wildavsky, A. 1979. *The Art and Craft of Policy Analysis*. London: Macmillan.

Wildavsky, A. 1994. Why Self-Interest Means Less Outside of a Social Context. *Journal of Theoretical Politics* 6(2):131–59.

Williams, A. 2001. *Science or Marketing at WHO? A Commentary on World Health 2000*. *Health Economics* 10(2):93–100.

Woodward, B. 2002. *Bush at War*. New York: Simon & Schuster.

Woodward, B. 2004. *Plan of Attack*. New York: Simon & Schuster.

World Health Organization. 2000. *The World Health Report 2000, Health Systems: Improving Performance*. Geneva: World Health Organization.

Young, H. 1989. *One of US: A Biography of Margaret Thatcher*. London: Macmillan.

WHAT'S SPECIAL ABOUT HEALTH CARE AND ITS POLITICS?

Rudolf Klein and Theodore R. Marmor

THE HEALTH CARE WORLD

From one perspective, there is no other policy area quite like health care. It is exceptional in the scale, the cost, and the sheer variety of the activities that go under the general label of "health care." It involves a huge cast of actors, ranging from people who clean floors to ground-breaking scientists in search of Nobel Prizes. It deals with issues of life and death; the emotional pitch of debate is often high. Although other policy areas share some of these characteristics, none has quite the same high-octane mix. It is therefore all too tempting to claim that politics and policy making in the health care arena should be analyzed in terms of its special characteristics. But from another perspective, the health care arena is no different from any other policy area. The concepts discussed in the previous chapter provide the analytic tools for understanding the disputes and conflicts that take place within this policy area, as in others. Ideas about what is desirable and feasible change over time. Interest groups jostle for position, as they battle over the distribution of resources and values. Governments have to decide where, and how, to use their political capital in specific institutional contexts.

Both perspectives matter, since the ways in which ideas, interests, and institutions inter-act vary with the context, nature, and timing of specific disputes. Accordingly, this chapter starts by sketching the distinctive characteristics of the health policy arena. It then moves from description to analysis, setting out taxonomy of the categories of conflicts and disputes that arise within it. Note that in all this, we do not attempt to relate either description or analysis to specific health care systems. That comes later in the chapters that compare specific types of conflict in particular national settings.

Health care is one of the fastest-expanding, as well the largest, industries in all rich, developed countries. Although dedicated in theory to improving the well-being of populations, it is also the only industry whose expansion is a cause of political concern rather than self-congratulation: a seeming paradox that suggests a certain ambiguity in perceptions of the relationships among the costs involved, methods of funding it, and benefits produced. As the largest industry, it also has the largest labor force. Its activities can thus be usefully analyzed in terms of the benefits—incomes and profits—for those working in the industry, as well as the benefits for patients. But while talking about health care as an industry accurately underlines the sheer scale of the enterprise, and is a useful corrective to a sentimental view of it as the setting for selfless doctors and nurses engaged in casualty room heroics, it is misleading in one respect. It suggests homogeneity where there is in fact only heterogeneity. So let us unpack, starting with the organizational structure of the industry in order to identify interests and players in the arena.

At one end of the spectrum, there are the big pharmaceutical companies. These are powerful international actors, able to play off the governments of different countries against each other: political pressure to cut drug prices is met by the threat to relocate research or production facilities. In the same category, if perhaps on a slightly smaller scale, are manufacturers of medical technology, such as scanning equipment, hip or knee replacement implants, and so on. In both cases there is the same set of incentives: not only to acquire a larger share of the market but to expand the market. In both cases, too, the firms concerned invest heavily in both political lobbying and promoting their products. Hence they tend to reinforce one of the characteristics of the health care arena that we will have occasion to note in other contexts as well: the itch and drive to innovate both by expanding the realm of the possible and by substituting new products for old.

At the other end of the organizational spectrum, there are solo medical practitioners, small-group practices, and free-standing specialist clinics. These, in effect, are small businesses, with an incentive to maximize their income though constrained by professional norms (about which more below) and the rules of the particular health care system within which they operate. Organized in quasi–trade unions, usually presenting themselves as professional bodies, they are active on the national political stage. Moreover, doctors, because of their intimate day-to-day contacts with patients, are well placed both to mobilize opinion and to present themselves as the voice of the public—though often equating self-interest with the public interest. Collectively they may therefore have a strong voice in national policy disputes.

Hospitals are small enterprises compared with the big pharmaceutical companies but important players in local settings. They are often the largest single employer in a town and a driving force in the local economy. Their siting, and even more the threat of closure, can unleash strong local feelings. They can appeal to, and mobilize, local constituencies. Collectively, too, they have a strong national constituency: in the second half of the twentieth century, hospital building programs were seen as vote winners by governments, both locally and nationally. For hospitals are the temples of modern medicine, whose priests carry out the high-technology ceremonies of saving lives and allowing the lame to walk again. In less picturesque language, hospitals and the specialists who work in them have a hugely symbolic role—and thus a high political profile—because of their place at the top of the hierarchy of medicine. And it is to the role of medicine and its practitioners in modern societies that this character sketch of health care now turns.

One of the defining features of health care is that while doctors represent only a small fraction of those working in it—approximately one in ten—it is their activities that dominate public perceptions and scholarly attention. Nurses account for a far greater proportion of the labor force. Their role in shaping the patient experience and contributing to successful outcomes is crucial, and they have in recent years played an increasingly important role in making treatment decisions. But in accounts of policy making in health care they are largely invisible. So too are the growing numbers of nonmedical professionals, computer experts, and skilled technicians required to deliver high-tech medicine. And the army of floor cleaners, kitchen staff, laundry workers, porters, and other ancillaries features only on rare occasions of industrial action about working conditions or wage levels. More prominent in some settings—particularly in the United States—are the management consultants, health insurance executives, lawyers, and accountants who increasingly provide costly professional services to one or another part of the health care industry.

There are many reasons why doctors mostly dominate public perceptions and scholarly analyses in the health care field. The first, and very obvious one, is that doctors do indeed make the decisions that impact directly on patients, determine what should be done for whom, and consequently largely drive health care spending. The second reason, somewhat more elusive and difficult to pin down with precision, is the investment of faith we all make in what doctors do: our expectations—inflated decade after decade by new techniques and new drugs—that they can make a difference, whether by prolonging lives, restoring failing functions, or easing pain. Much of this faith is justified; some of it is not. There is much dispute as to what contribution medicine has made to extending life expectancy, though it can claim dramatic successes in its repair and maintenance function. But it is precisely because of this element of faith that it is so tempting to reach for religious metaphors—as above—when discussing the place of the engineers of the human body in the health care arena.

Had this chapter been written a couple of decades ago, and certainly if it had been written much earlier in the twentieth century, the story could probably have ended here. Medical domination of health care could have been taken for granted and rightly so. Collectively organized as a profession, riding the crest of a wave of dramatic innovations in surgery and an expanding repertory of drugs, doctors had in the course of the first half or so of the century established themselves as the monopolists of relevant knowledge and successfully asserted the principle that only they could judge medical performance and conduct. Medical autonomy ruled without challenge.

This judgment must now be qualified. As always in analyzing policy and politics, chronology matters, and the same actors may play different roles at different points in time. Over the years medical autonomy has increasingly come under twin pressures. On the one hand, an international explosion in health care spending led from the 1970s onward to a heightened awareness by economists and policy makers of extreme variations in medical practice, with the consequent scope for saving money by identifying and implementing more cost-effective ways of working. On the other hand, and at much the same time, deviant voices within the profession itself—epidemiologists and public health specialists—were calling attention to the same phenomenon, launching what became the evidence-based medicine movement. It was a movement that drew attention to the fact that evidence about the efficacy of many—perhaps most—medical interventions was lacking and which argued the need to generate such evidence. The notion of defining treatments for specific conditions, set out in clinical guidelines based on hard evidence rather than a professional consensus, followed.

No longer could individual clinicians interpret medical autonomy to mean that they could exercise unfettered discretion, even while grumbling about being forced into practicing "cookbook" medicine. The way was open for increased external control over clinical activities. The extent to which this happened has varied from system to system; so, too, has the degree to which discretion in interpreting guidelines is allowed. But insofar as the profession itself retains control over the process of defining what counts as good evidence and appropriate treatment, as it largely does, it has managed to safeguard its collective autonomy even while sacrificing that of its individual members. This is less the case in the United States, where those who pay for care—public or private—increasingly assert their authority over what is permitted by what will be paid for. Threats to autonomy, then, come in different guises.

The position of the medical profession has come under challenge in other ways as well. Its ability to impose its own view of the world—to shape the assumptive world of policy makers and the public—has weakened. The extent to which medicine can claim credit for improving population health has, as already noted, been questioned. A counterparadigm of health policy argues that improving population health depends on collective social policies and public interventions to change personal behavior. At the same time, a combination of insistent media attention, more Web-based information than most individuals can cope with in a lifetime, and changing cultural attitudes has meant that medicine (like other professions) can no longer rely on its mystique to command automatic respect. Any pretensions to professional infallibility have long since been stripped away; automatic trust or deference can no longer be taken for granted. "Expert patients" have emerged as actors in the health care arena; usually organized around chronic diseases, these patients can define and articulate their own needs. Like the advocates of women's health needs, they repudiate medical paternalism.

There has also been a shift of power within hospitals and other health care delivery organizations. The language of efficiency, competition, and performance measurement translated into a much enlarged role for professional managers. Administrators were reincarnated as chief executives. Managerial salaries and numbers rose.

All this should not be taken to mean that the medical profession is now an overworked, overcriticized, and overmanaged group denied the respect that it deserves. This does seem to be the self-image of many doctors; lowered medical morale is an international phenomenon. The critical views of the profession—as distinct from organized medicine—appear to be concentrated among the elite chattering classes. Survey evidence shows that trust in doctors remains very high. It is certainly very much higher than trust in politicians, a not insignificant fact when it comes to explaining the role of the medical profession in the politics of policy making. A shroud-waving doctor, claiming that public policy or lack of funds is endangering the lives of his or her patients, carries more conviction on television than a politician spouting statistics. Add the fact that while awareness of the fallibility and limitations of medicine has been growing, so too have the hopes induced by the potentials of genetic engineering: visions of immortality are beckoning—a vision to be delivered by doctors.

The dramatics of high-technology medicine and the high visibility of doctors may be the most obvious characteristics of the health care scene. But concentrating on these features of the scene gives a distorted, partial view. Health care is as much about prevention and care as about cure. And in prevention and care, the role of the medical profession is at best marginal. In prevention, the emphasis is on social engineering and personal behavior. In matters of care, nurses are the leading actors, and nursing homes rather than hospitals are the most important institutional setting. And the importance of care is being reinforced by demography. The elderly are by far the heaviest consumers of health care, and as populations age, so the importance of the caring function—as well as of the repair and maintenance role—of medicine increases.

To underline the heterogeneity of the health care arena suggests two conclusions about what makes it special. The first is that it is an arena marked by an exceptionally high degree of internal competition for resources between actors: between different hospitals, between different specialists within them, between hospital- and office-based doctors, between professions, and between the claims of different patient groups, among others. In other words, the health care arena is characterized by the multiplicity of internal actors, or interests, making competing demands on a variety of policy makers. Other policy arenas share some of these characteristics, of course. In education, for example, there are a variety of institutions (schools, colleges, universities) and competition among different sectors. Defense, too, is another huge and complex policy arena, where different branches of the armed forces compete for resources. The claim being made here is simply that the degree of competition in health care is—like its organizational complexity and the heterogeneity of the interest involved—of greater order. The second, following on from this, is that just as governments have to decide how to devise a balanced portfolio, so policy makers in the health care arena have to perform a balancing act in dealing with different types of issues. And it is to the conceptual characterization of these issues—as distinct from the characterization of the arena in which they are played out—that this chapter now turns.

POLITICAL ANALYSIS OF HEALTH CARE

INTRODUCTION

The components of the medical care industry—the topic of this chapter's opening part—constitute one obvious possible grouping for political analysis. Hospitals, physicians, and nurses would provide the categories for analyzing major providers of care. The politics of provision, of payment, and of regulatory oversight could well be another basis of categorization. And so on. Equally, one might proceed as if the special features of medical care shaped the politics of every issue in this industry. This would presume a common politics of health care.

The first option—politics categorized by industry characteristics—is certainly possible. But using professional and industry categories strikes us as presuming too much about the common features of these topics, subordinating the differences in their historical and institutional contexts. The second option— presuming a common politics of the industry—we regard as empirically misleading. The undeniable politics _in_ health care do not, we contend, constitute a common politics _of_ health care.

Instead, the institutional, ideational, and interest structure of politics—Chapter 1's themes—is the starting point of our analysis. From there we arrange our chapters by the types of conflicts—their scope and structure—that regularly arise in health care. We introduce each of the chapters and locate the articles in time. We will identify the general themes illustrated by the articles and, where important, what the articles lack. Next, however, we explain broadly the analytic groupings we have employed.

The articles in Chapter 3 address disputes about how medical care should be financed, delivered, managed, and regulated. The criterion of selection is the scope of changes proposed and disputed. The particular illustrations take up the macropolitics of such conflicts over the decades. They highlight the power and relevance of dominant ideas, their changes over time amid slowly shifting institutional arrangements and always-alert interest groups. Most strikingly, these are the politics of highly salient issues. Such struggles invariably rouse the best organized and financed interest groups, and the struggles typically constitute front-page news and compel television commentary. "High politics" is a useful shorthand description for what we want to emphasize here. With that comes emphasis on how much such overt struggles differ from the quieter and largely hidden politics that attend many of the other policy issues in health care.

The articles in Chapter 4 also take on highly controversial struggles. But rather than addressing the history of such issues, the articles focus on episodes of contentious reform politics at one point in time. The U.K. illustration is of the Thatcher government's determined introduction in 1989–90 of market instruments into the management of the National Health Service (NHS) despite rampant opposition. The American episode is the famously rejected reform of American health finance proposed by the Clinton administration in 1993. Each article reviews competing explanations for these disputed developments and aims to provide a plausible and enduring account.

These episodes of "high politics" have the drama of fundamental struggles. Leaders are castigated or celebrated, news conferences abound, and journalists hunt for inside stories to complement the mind-numbing disputes about statistical claims. These are majoritarian issues in the sense that most of the population has a stake—whether as citizen, patient, worker, or partisan. And with that comes the media attention that in turn creates the opportunity for drama. Both articles emphasize the difference between explaining why an issue is on the political agenda and explaining the results of the subsequent struggle. In both cases, however, the explanatory emphasis is on governmental institutions.

The next set of articles—in Chapter 5—highlights the role of ideas, the second of our trinity of fundamental building blocks. The review essays analyze important, long-standing ideas about the basic purposes public policy should and should not serve. These articles set out how Marxian critics have construed the political economy of the welfare state and how advocates of classic liberalism and social democrats have approached the same topics. Without claiming to be a survey of political philosophy, these separate essays illustrate how ideas shape the assumptive worlds of political actors. The other illustration of the movement of ideas emphasizes dissemination across borders of rapidly changing ideas, some fundamental, some faddish. The final article in the chapter addresses the disciplinary migration of ideas. It illustrates how different social sciences understand interests and their significance for policy making. The particular topic is the collective problem of medical inflation, its causes and control. But the illustration is how using economic analyses of interests—their composition, intensity, and distribution—can contribute to the political analysis of topics like inflation.

Chapter 6 addresses the role values play in understanding political behavior and policy results. The two articles in the chapter share three themes. Both acknowledge the important role values play both in the origins of major programs of health care reform and in ruling out some types of subsequent adjustment. Each is somewhat skeptical about how central values are in explaining policy changes over time, which explains their claiming a fundamental, but restricted scope for values as explanatory tools. And both articles also call attention to how the appeal to values—particularly those touted as fundamental—has become a familiar, popular feature of health care debates, in part because of their malleability.

From here on, each grouping of writings illustrates a somewhat different type of political conflict. Within each chapter, the illustrative cases exhibit a distinctive configuration of interests, institutions, and competing ideas. So, Chapter 7 is about politics and the medical professions. It describes the historical prominence of doctors in many areas of health policy, but notes the limits on their power in the high politics of large-scale policy changes. As suggested earlier, the political influence of physicians has altered considerably over time, which means that our illustrative analyses, to be useful, have to provide the basis for understanding those changes as well.

Chapter 8 introduces the comparative, cross-national dimension to this book of essays. The first article reviews the purposes comparative policy analysis can serve: providing perspective, checking the validity of national explanations, and discovering unexpected generalizations. It also notes the perils of such work done superficially, a particular risk in the modern world of instant communication by fax, telephone, radio, and television. From this broad article we turn to a commentary on the challenges to cross-national policy learning, including the sharp distinction between understanding other health care arrangements and learning from them. These articles draw from comparative investigations of five industrial democracies, but their implications are not restricted to Germany, Holland, Canada, Britain, and the United States. The purpose of this chapter is to illustrate the promise and limits of the comparative approach to politics and policy analysis and, in so doing, to set the stage for a number of the following chapters.

Chapter 9 addresses a topic that has undeniably excited much comparative interest: the role of rationing and resource allocation in health care. The chapter begins with a critical discussion of a prior topic—the belief that if only wasteful care could be reduced, rationing could be avoided. Having rejected that contention, the chapter turns to two essays on the rationing experience of the state of Oregon. That state's innovative attempt to ration relatively expensive care so as to make affordable wider coverage of basic health insurance drew an extraordinary amount of cross-national attention. But that attention brought neither clear understanding of Oregon's reality nor a transplantable model. A further article on strategies takes for granted that rationing must take place. But it differs from the previous articles by describing the many different forms of restricting access to all that is possible in modern health care. The chapter presents finally a detailed comparative study of how different countries handled the demands for including Viagra in the package of publicly financed medical services. That discussion, along with the other articles in this chapter, illustrates the importance of context, how the same general issue can play substantially different roles in diverse settings and how important that difference is when policy transfer is at stake.

Chapter 10 brings together two examples of how the demand for representing lay interests in health care emerged and operated in the United States and the United Kingdom during the 1970s. The issues raised by both articles remain relevant, with the representation of patient, taxpayer, and citizen interests always a subject of dispute. The explosion of information about health has changed the balance between professional and lay persons, but the distribution of stakeholder power in such matters—and their legitimacy—remains problematic. The appeals to giving voice to underrepresented (or unrepresented) interests reflect two other enduring elements as well: opposition to the dominant role of doctors in many areas of health care policy and a suspicion that bureaucratic elites are too much influenced by organized interest groups and pay too little attention to citizens and their other concerns. These issues, we are certain, will reappear again and again on the policy agenda.

The articles we have included in Chapter 11 describe at length public health episodes that were frightening. We have characterized the genre as the political analysis of panics. There are many sources of panics, and our review might just as easily have taken severe acute respiratory syndrome (SARS)—the bird flu scare—as the illustrative example. But, our greater interest in the category of analysis—rather than its timeliness—led us to use examples we had studied in some detail and that illustrated our comparative perspective as well. So, we chose articles on the various national responses to acquired immune deficiency syndrome (AIDS) in the 1980s, including the contaminated blood scandal that devastated the hemophiliac community in the same decade. Both episodes excited widespread dispute and fear, though with particular victims bearing the brunt of medical injury. Both illustrated intense scientific disputes about causation, fights about appropriate intervention, and deep conflicts about remedies and compensation. But, most of all, these examples reveal both the obvious importance of these panics to governments and the heterogeneity of their responses. The same health threat, in different institutional contexts, prompts variable responses. That conclusion, in turn, suggests that whether one is concerned about threats like bovine spongiform encephalopathy (BSE), nuclear accidents, contaminated water, or asbestos exposure—threatening devastating loss amid considerable uncertainty—such threats produce distinctive political stories. The details of the timing and consequences—the results of the configuration of threat and particular context—will, as the articles suggest, be neither random nor universal.

Chapter 12's topic has similarities to the politics of panics. The politics of crusades is our label, but the distinguishing feature of the category is the link between health threats and scandal. Among possible illustrations, the range goes from the restrictions on alcohol to restrictions on smoking, from the control of sexual conduct to campaigns against obesity, from environmental cleanup campaigns to disputes over nuclear energy. The comparative politics of tobacco control is the illustration we use, but many others come to mind. The tobacco story reflects on the experiences of eight industrial democracies, the same nations in the blood scandal analysis in the previous chapter. As a topic of comparative investigation, it is ideal, with the analysis drawing from detailed national studies.

Tobacco control is a useful illustration in another important respect. It calls attention to two separate questions about any public health campaign. What is the explanation when a number of countries—over a long period of time—move in the same direction on public health, as was the case with tobacco? Where direction is common, the question remaining is what explains the timing and character of particular national reforms. On the one hand, tobacco control became a common object of reform across the world of industrial democracies in the 1970s and beyond. But, as with panics, the country findings reveal just how much the distinctive mix of institutions, ideas, and the distribution of interests affects the ways tobacco has been controlled over time and at any one time. Finally, the tobacco story, like many other political crusades, reveals the relevance of nonmaterial stakes in health controversies. No one can miss the anger at tobacco firms for misrepresenting scientific findings and the parallels with scandalous conduct in other controversial areas. Libertarians had their moral claims as well, insisting that the right to smoke was one no one had a right to take away unless they were hurt too. And so it was that secondhand smoke—an important element in the tobacco wars—provided the critics of smoking with an argument John Stuart Mill would have recognized as legitimate.

The articles in Chapter 13 shift the subject matter from health care to health and present different perspectives on what determines the health status of entire populations. From the 1970s on, the notion spread across borders that modern societies with ample access to health care had populations whose health profiles were the product largely of nonmedical forces. On the one side were those stressing the physical environment, the conditions of work, and healthy habits. This understanding is the subject of the article on the 1974 Lalonde Report in Canada, whose cross-national influence continues to this day. On the other side, there was emphasis—especially in the United Kingdom—on the distribution of income and opportunity as determinants of health status. The presumption, illustrated by the article on the United Kingdom's experience, was that a fairer society would be a healthier one. The articles in this chapter emphasize shifting ideas over time. They emphasize the gap between the skepticism about modern medicine's impact and action based on it.

The final chapter is a brief coda. It reflects on both what we have not addressed and what we have learned. It looks back on our four decades of analysis and wonders what purchase those understandings might give to future analysts. We leave to readers to decide whether our way of describing, explaining, and evaluating health and health care policy will be helpful in the decades ahead.

THE HIGH POLITICS OF SYSTEMS
CHANGE OVER TIME

For different reasons, and with different outcomes, debate about how to finance and organize health care has helped to define politics both in the United States and in Britain over the decades. Come presidential elections in the United States or general elections in Britain, health care issues are invariably high on the agenda of party confrontation and on the acrimony scale. The articles in this chapter describe and analyze the changing nature of this debate, and the evolution of policy over time.

The explanatory challenge of the two cases is, of course, not the same. The case of health care in the United States offers an example of conflict without consensus. Policies have indeed changed over time, but without agreement about what would constitute a solution that reasonably satisfies the requirements for a stable and workable system. American exceptionalism, in its failure to develop anything that looks like the kind of comprehensive health care system found in all other rich countries, marked the whole period under review. The case of Britain's National Health Service, in contrast, offers an example of conflict contained by consensus. Policies have changed over time, but the political parties continue to compete to proclaim their total commitment to the NHS. Measures designed to change the system's internal dynamics did indeed provoke political controversy and professional opposition, but there was no questioning of the NHS as a tax-funded, comprehensive service.

There is a common element to both cases, though. While there was indeed a series of policy lurches in both the United States and Britain, in neither country did the institutions of government change. Throughout the period in question the United States offered the model of a country whose constitution allows great scope to opposition, whereas Britain's winner-takes-all majoritarian system allows prime ministers to ride roughshod over opposition. Institutional factors do indeed explain the outcome of specific legislative initiatives, as the next chapter shows. But unchanging institutions do not provide much explanatory leverage for changing policies over time. Similarly, there is no little or no evidence that the policy changes were prompted by shifts in the configuration of interests, though they were certainly consistent with the rise of consumer and patient activism (in both countries) and the expansion (in the United States) of capital-intensive firms in the health care arena.

So we come to the third of our explanatory trinity: ideas. The assumptive world of policy makers changed over time, as both articles document, as new ideas about how to run large-scale human services took hold. This change in the intellectual climate and its policy implications is explored in detail in Chapter 5, as well as its birth in the disillusionment of the 1970s when global stagflation called into question the economic and social policies followed in the post-1945 period. Here some specific features of the change, crucial to an understanding of the pattern of policy making over time in the two countries, must be noted.

In simple terms, the switch in ideas represented a reaction against bureaucratic regulatory bodies (in the United States) and hierarchic bureaucratic control (in Britain), anchored in a shared faith in the benefits of competition. The inspiration for this, in both cases, lay outside the health care arena. And the health care arena became the laboratory, as it were, for trying out notions generated in other fields. In the case of the United States, a notable example for the new direction in health care was the deregulation of the airline industry. In the case of Britain, the NHS became a proving ground for what was called the New Public Management, as the language of economics crept into the language of public policy and hands-on managers replaced traditional civil servants in the Department of Health.

In these respects, the similarities are remarkable, not least because Britain was hugely influenced by American ideas. But there are also some striking differences. In the United States, the motor of the drive to innovate in health care policy—whatever the direction—was, and continues to be, alarm about the ever upward, seemingly unstoppable rise in costs. In Britain this was not the case. When Margaret Thatcher, as prime minister, in 1989 first introduced an internal market—based on the notion that health care providers should compete for custom and income—the NHS was a model of successful cost containment. But while the economic costs of the NHS were low, the political costs of successful cost containment were high: long waiting lists lost votes. Hence Britain adopted American-style ideas about competition in order to pursue a very different political agenda from that of the United States: in order to promote greater efficiency within a capped budget system (see next chapter).

There is a further twist, however, to the British story of how its political institutions enable governments to drive through their policy proposals. The same
institutional system also makes it easy to reverse policy. When Tony Blair came
into office in 1997, his Labour government abolished the internal market with
great rhetorical flourish, even while quietly preserving some of its features.
There followed a period of increasingly intrusive central bureaucratic control
in the NHS. Policy changed yet again in the new millennium, however, with
the reinvention of the internal market, and the language of consumer choice,
competition, and payment by results came back into good currency. Strong
governments do not necessarily mean consistent or stable policies.

If the British political system is a model of concentrated authority, the United
States is characterized by the fragmentation of authority. The institutions of
financing, regulating, and providing health care are dispersed. Policy initiatives
may come from a variety of sources, whether at the state or federal level, but
none can be assured of implementation. While the focus of the two articles
dealing with policy change over time in the United States differs, both give a
picture of piecemeal, incremental tinkering (or sock darning, to revert to the
image offered in Chapter 1). Providing an overview of the health care policy
field over the decades, the first article documents the births and deaths of a variety of policy initiatives, all of which fell short of providing the building blocks
for the emergence of a comprehensive or coherent health care system. Concentrating on Medicare, the central example of the social insurance principle
at work in American health care, the other article shows how the ambitions to
scale up this program for the most worthy section of the population had to be
scaled back, yielding once again to step-by-step tinkering.

The articles in this chapter all end on a note of uncertainty about the future,
but the nature of the uncertainty is different in kind in the two countries. In
the United States, the question left open at the time of writing is what kind of
health care system—if any—will emerge in response to the demand to expand
coverage while at the same time controlling costs at a time of economic distress.
In Britain, the nature of the health care system is a political given, with no party
challenging the structure of the NHS, but it is far from clear which of two contradictory streams of policy—central, bureaucratic control or funds and power
to the periphery—will emerge victorious.

American Health Care Policy and Politics

The Promise and Perils of Reform

Theodore R. Marmor

2007–8: LOOKING BACK, LOOKING NOW

The continuities of American medical politics, despite the surges of reform enthusiasm, are impressive. As the presidential election of 2008 draws closer, all the candidates feel compelled to offer plans for universal health insurance. That was the case in the buildup to the presidential election of 1992, and what followed was the birth and death of the Clinton reform plan. Now, as then, huge majorities of Americans claim they want reform—universal insurance coverage—and disagree about what that would be. Then, as now, interest groups mobilize for battle, trading sound bites and horror stories attacking and defending particular reforms. At the same time, the more quiet politics in health care continue to unfold off the front page and the evening television news: the moral disputes over abortion, euthanasia, and stem-cell research, the distributive, intense local politics of hospital closures and clinic openings, the Washington and state capital fights in hearing rooms over the rules governing the practices of nurses, chiropractors, and physicians, let alone the armies of lobbyists struggling to start or stop health insurance reforms in the states. The cost of health insurance—public and private—dominates the surface of discussion, but the distributive realities of who bears those costs continue to bewilder commentators. To understand all these variables in the American medical political agenda, it is essential to shift from the details of medical care to the ordinary categories of policy and political conflict.

The broad history of American medical care from the 1970s to the first decade of the twenty-first century is one of diverse conflicts, turbulent change, and a persistent sense that the vast health expenditures of these decades failed to provide good value for money.[1] Senator Edward Kennedy's 1972 book, *In Critical Condition: The Crisis in America's Health Care*,[2] reflected in its title the atmosphere of urgency at the time. Indeed, this sense of trouble—of seemingly continuous inflation, a complex and fragmented organization of care, and both under-insurance and lack of coverage for many millions—was so widespread that Republicans and Democrats, liberals and conservatives, competed over which form of national health insurance to offer in response. The regulations that emerged, however, were dispersed bureaucratically, disconnected from the major public programs financing care and celebrated with visions of eventual success that no reasonable analyst should have accepted. Professional Standards Review Organizations (PSROS), for instance—established by the federal government to monitor quality of care—were relegated in 1972 to a different set of agencies, dominated by physicians and disconnected in practice from the payment systems of Medicare, Medicaid, or private health insurance plans. Medicare and Medicaid, once separate organizationally, were technically joined in an agency known as the Health Care Financing Administration (HCFA). But this new organization (now the Center for Medical Services) failed to unify Medicare and Medicaid administrations, much less have an impact on health planning. In all these cases, the political struggles were intense, dominated by groups with financial and professional interests in the policies and reported in the trade press and professional medical journals. But they all fell short of the national attention that debates over universal health insurance always prompt.

All through the 1970s, commentators complained about the uneven distribution of care and the high rates of inflation in medicine, but few fundamental changes were made. The Nixon administration tried wage and price controls, but gave up on them. The Carter administration supported legislation to contain hospital costs, but was defeated by opposition from hospitals and general skepticism that the federal government could accomplish what it promised. Inflation continued unabated amid naïve rhetoric about a "voluntary effort" to control costs by the health industry. It all seems very long ago, looking back from the perspective of 2008 to this earlier flurry of proposals and stalemate over universal, government-financed health insurance.[3]

In the 1980s the picture was different, politically, economically, and intellectually. Few prominent figures promoted government-financed universal health insurance, either for the nation or for a particular state. The deficits of the Reagan and Bush years continued to dominate political discourse, and reformers turned first to bureaucratic realignments as a means to rationalize medical care provision and then to financing through such policies as diagnostic-related group payments (DRGs) to hospitals. When those strategies failed, many reformers looked to competition and privatization as their panacea, appealing both to the ideology of market competition and to the grief caused by the persistent relative inflation in the costs of health care.

The earlier attention to national health insurance gave way to a wide variety of other initiatives. At the state level, there were earnest but unsuccessful efforts to expand insurance coverage. At the business level, there were noteworthy attempts to broaden the benefits in employment-related health insurance. And there were innovative experiments in financing second opinions, wellness programs, pre-paid group practice plans, and exercise facilities at the workplace. Medicare and Medicaid tried a variety of payment reforms, including the diagnosis-related group method of paying hospitals and complex formulas to adjust physician fees to standards of relative value.

But the fundamental reform of the rules of the American medical game was off the political agenda, and the major changes that were attempted were basically private initiatives. Attracted by the gold mine of funds flowing through a system of retrospective, cost-based reimbursement, the captains of American capitalism came to see opportunity where the politicians had found causes for complaint. In the hospital world, small chains of for-profit hospitals—the Humanas and Hospital Corporations of America, to name but one—grew into large companies. "Health maintenance organizations" (HMOs)—a Republican-backed variant of the pre-paid group practice model of American liberals that increasingly reorganized the delivery and financing of care for Americans—were soon dominated by for-profit firms and expanded rapidly. Industrial giants like Baxter-Travenol and American Hospital Supply took their conventional dreams of competitive growth and extended them to vertical and horizontal integration.[4] A glut of physicians started to come into practice, weakening the traditional market power of doctors to determine their terms of work.

All of these changes in the structure of American medicine took place within the context of increasingly anti-regulatory and anti-Washington rhetoric. Democrats and Republicans alike had been influenced by a generation of academic policy analysts—mostly economists—who ridiculed the costliness and captured quality of the decisions taken by supposedly independent regulatory agencies in Washington. The Civil Aeronautics Board and the airlines industry came to represent the distortions likely when government regulates industry and, with time, the convention of describing any set of related activities with economic significance as an "industry" demythologized medicine as well. So, even before the Reagan administration came into office, the time was ripe for celebrating "competition" in medicine, getting government off the industry's back, and letting the fresh air of deregulation solve the problems of access, cost, quality, fragmentation, and the sheer complexity of health care. The irony is that the most consequential health initiative of the 1980s—Medicare's prospective payment system by diagnosis-related groups—was an exceedingly sophisticated, highly regulatory form of administered prices.

THE CONTEMPORARY SCENE

After more than 30 years of talk about an American medical world in critical condition, little progress has been made in the search for a major policy change. The United States is now the only major industrial nation without a universal or near-universal health care program. Rather, Americans get health insurance from a mix of private and public sources—employers (60%), private individual plans (9%), and various governmental financing programs (27%). The largest government plans are Medicare (the federal social insurance program financing more than 40 million elderly and disabled Americans) and Medicaid (the state-administered, means-tested program covering 38 million low-income Americans). The public share of financing, however, is more than half of the 2.1 trillion dollars Americans spent on healthcare in 2006; this includes not only the major programs noted above, but the Veterans Administration network of hospitals and clinics, special programs for Native Americans and the Armed Services, and the tax expenditures that help to finance the employment based coverage that insures most working Americans (and is fraying).

At any one time, some 46 million Americans are without health insurance, though emergency care at hospitals is legally available to all, whether they can pay or not. Still, medical bills remain the second major cause of personal bankruptcy. The problems of access have worsened, and the list of the uninsured and the under-insured has grown. (The number of those who are uninsured within a two-year period, it is estimated, is nearly twice the 46 million noted above.) The relative rate of medical inflation has continued, and its relentless rise shows no signs of slowing, despite the extraordinary changes that have been made in the rules of the professional medical game: America spent about 7 percent of its national income, or GNP, on health in 1970, over 9 percent by 1980, more than 11 percent by 1990, and something close to 16 percent in 2008. With the highest health cost per capita of any country in the world, the United States was ranked 37th in overall performance by the World Health Organization (WHO). (The WHO did evaluate American health care first in the world in level of responsiveness and 72nd in general health. Since Canada was 33rd in overall performance, and Oman was 8th, one should use these figures with caution.) It is simpler to say that Americans spend the most and feel among the worst about their value for money.

Before elaborating on this contemporary portrait of American medical care and its politics, there are some analytical preliminaries to address. First, there is no such thing as a common politics of American medicine. One can rightly emphasize the politics *in* the nation's medical care, but not a politics *of* American medical care. In practice, that requires distinguishing among the most prominent varieties of political dispute and resolution:

- System reform: ideologically controversial disputes about whether and how to change the major features of a medical care system—whether financing, quality, costs, or delivery. The struggles over state insurance reform in Massachusetts and California in 2007–8 exemplify these politics.
- Rationing: disputes about the extent to which and the explicitness with which medical care is apportioned at any one time—a topic of differential intensity across national borders and within them. These struggles are usually dominated by professional medical care groups but find expression in the mass media, as with the denial of access to organ transplantation.
- Prevention: disputes about the effectiveness and cost implications of efforts to prevent illness, disease, and injury, as well as conflicts over the benefits and costs of so-called healthy public policies. There is great variability over time and space in the salience of these disputes, with current attention in the United States focused on wasteful treatment as compared to possible improvements in preventive care.
- Professional accountability, autonomy, and power: the extent to which the medical profession is being subjected to external scrutiny and losing control over its own activities. These issues are obviously of greatest interest to the affected professional parties.
- Panics: issues where public anxiety and governmental action are generated by unexpected or unpredicted epidemics or health crises (e.g., AIDS, BSE, contaminated blood, SARS). These episodes result initially in a period of strict order, followed by intense politics, and struggles that dominate the mass media for a time before they disappear.
- Consumer empowerment: disputes over efforts to increase the role of ordinary citizens, whether patients, taxpayers, or caregivers, in the making or implementation of policies in health care. While highly variable in salience over time and space, this topic has emerged in the Bush administration under the rubric of "consumer-directed healthcare." In practice, that euphemistic phrase refers to high-deductible health insurance plans

with or without the tax incentives represented by medical savings accounts (MSAs).

- Moral crusades: disputes about abortion, stem-cell research, euthanasia, smoking bans, alcohol control, and other contentious issues of individual versus social choice.

These categories should help us to explore the distinctive configurations of interests, institutions, and processes shaping current debates about specific health care issues.

COMPETITION VERSUS REGULATION

Is the idea of complete government control over and administration of medical care financing the answer to the continuing debate over containing health care expenditures? Some Americans—policy-makers and medical care professionals as well as ordinary citizens—think that the only way to get the problems of America's health care system under control is to follow the model of the British National Health Service.[5] That model, however, invokes the unhappy image of severe rationing of care and long waits for all but the most pressing medical problems. It also conjures up images of "socialized" medicine, with all the loss of individual control and freedom of choice for both practitioner and patient that the slogan implies. The widely acknowledged seriousness of American medicine's present problems has not produced clear public support for the British policy. By contrast, considerable support has been expressed at various times for versions of national health insurance modeled on Medicare, the Canadian national health insurance program. Interestingly, that is less so in 2008 than in either the early 1970s or the period leading up to the Clinton reform struggle of 1991–94.

Alternatively, at the other extreme in American health policy, is the answer a set of ideas known as the "competitive health strategy"?[6] Though their arguments vary, advocates of competition believe that restructuring financial incentives is crucial to restraining medical inflation and controlling both public and private health expenditures. Their central policy prescription is the introduction of greater price competition in the delivery of care. In the presence of widespread health insurance, these advocates argue, there is scope for price competition in premiums. They also argue that substantially increased cost-sharing by patients is helpful on the demand side of the market.

The eventual outcome of any thoroughgoing competitive health care strategy was and remains uncertain. The strategy has not been implemented on a wide scale anywhere in the postwar period. For all these reasons, the reality of health politics from the 1980s on has been incremental steps of both a regulatory and a competitive variety—what we might call "agitated incrementalism."[7] There was little coherent public concern about the rising costs of health care in the United States, though polls revealed continuing public anxiety. The concerns that mattered were the costs of care to individuals (in premiums or cost sharing when ill), to firms (in increased expenditures for employee health insurance), and to governments (in rising outlays for particular programs—Medicare for federal officials; Medicaid for state and federal officials). Concern about relative inflation in medical care—the concern that the society is spending more for care in the aggregate than its citizens receive in benefits—is an academic's problem. America may well be, as Brian Abel-Smith wrote some years ago, a country where we receive insufficient "value for money."[8] But, where medical care is concerned, the public worries more about access, financial protection, and quality than about value for money. And that is why, at this point, the concern about the dismantling of employer-related health insurance has prompted so much national attention.

Cost containment, when seriously attempted, arises from actions to control the rising burden of medical care to particular payers, most prominently the federal government and hardly less so to particular states and corporations.[9] The problems with that approach are all related to the obvious fact that actions that save federal (or state or corporate) dollars do not necessarily constitute anti-inflationary successes. Indeed, actions that have substantially shifted costs among payers have had little or no effect on total health care expenditures.

Turning now to delivery, the dispensing of American medical care "can be simultaneously described as a system on the brink of crisis and as a strong and growing industry, with seemingly equal accuracy."[10] In attempting to explain this situation, we need first to emphasize the enormous influence of providers in the imbalanced political marketplace of many of the health policy struggles. And worsening that imbalance is the lack of sustained public opinion marshaled around any one of the various formulations of the problems of cost, access, and quality of American medicine. A large part of the explanation for the U.S.'s current health situation is the pluralism of American politics and the parallel dispersion of countervailing power in both the political and the economic marketplaces. Our federalism has spread the authority for regulating medical care between the national government and the many states. Our financing splits private and public payers, with considerable discrepancies among them in each sector.

Two explanatory factors for the cost pressures in American medicine become central. Medical care is widely regarded as a merit good, still widely insured through work, and a part of the American private and public welfare state. The fragmentation of finance has meant that, once payers are aroused, the problem they separately address is that of their own costs, not of American medicine. Pluralistic finance, combined with extensive third-party coverage, is a predictable recipe for inflation. Only those regimes that have concentrated the stakes of medical payers—Great Britain, Canada, Germany, for instance—have been better able to restrain the forces of medical inflation. And such countervailing power is but the necessary condition for restraint. Political will is also essential. In some instances, as in Sweden, the governments with concentrated authority have chosen to spend more on medical care—as governments have, too, in recent years, in Canada. Those countries made these choices through balancing the gains and losses of increasing expenditures. In the United States, in contrast, we have discovered our inflating health outlays, not chosen them.

Rapidly inflating medical care costs are not only a central problem that reformers must address but also a major barrier to sensible reform debate in the United States. The controversies over the American Medicare program in the period after the Clinton reform failure (1995 to the present) illustrate clearly this feature of contemporary health politics. Budget politics provided the setting, but the themes were much broader. They help us to understand the context facing the United States in the presidential battles of 2008.

MEDICARE: AFFORDABILITY, FAIRNESS, AND MODERNIZATION

Medicare, largely ignored in the battle over health care reform in the early 1990s, returned to center stage following the Republican congressional victories of 1994. Given bipartisan calls for reductions in the nation's budget deficits and hostility among some Republicans to Medicare's social insurance roots, it was almost certain that this program would again generate intense and very public debate and conflict. Moreover, like Social Security pensions, long-term projections of Medicare spending prompt worries about unsustainable budget outlays—especially in light of the aging population and the hugely expensive medical technologies and prescription drugs increasingly becoming available.[11] The public commentary about Medicare in the 1990s incorporated arguments that were to reappear in vivid language over the next decade and more. Unaffordability, unfairness, and somewhat masked ideological objections—operating under the banner of "modernization"—all these terms were applied to social insurance itself and, by extension, to "government medicine."[12]

AFFORDABILITY

The truth is that fearful projections of Medicare's fiscal future reflect a problem of U.S. medicine, not a crisis caused by Medicare's structure. In fact, for most of Medicare's history, program spending grew about as rapidly as outlays in the private medical economy. Table 1 shows a number of temporal shifts, which help explain particular episodes of fearfulness. From the early 1990s, per capita medical costs grew much faster than per capita gross domestic product (GDP) in both the private sector and Medicare. But from about 1993 through 1997, private health outlays grew far less rapidly than Medicare outlays. This discrepancy itself prompted many cries of alarm. Since then, however, the relationship has shifted back and forth. The important reality in the period after 1997 is rapid inflation in U.S. medical care generally, not just, or even particularly, in Medicare. Over the long run—from 1970 to 2001, for instance—Medicare spending per enrollee grew less rapidly (9.6 percent per year) than spending for the privately insured (11 percent). Over the period 1990–2003, spending rose at similar rates for both Medicare and private insurance.[13] These data give no reason to be complacent about the costs of U.S. medical care. But nor do they support the claim of Medicare's incapacity to control medical inflation.

Table 1: Trends in Health Care Costs per Capita, United States, 1991–2003

| | *Percent change by spending category* | | | |
	GDP per capita	*Non-Medicare health services*	*Large employer premiums*	*Medicare per enrollee*
1991–1993	3.3	6.2	10.1	–*
1994–1997	4.4	2.4	2.4	–*
1998–2000	4.6	6.7	5.0	0.3
2001–2003	2.8	9.0	13.3	7.2
1990–1996	3.7	(4.5)	(7.4)	(8.7)
1995–1997	4.8	(2.6)	(1.3)	(6.5)

Source: J. White, "Transformations of the American Health Care System: Risks for Americans and Lessons from Abroad" (Unpublished manuscript, 2006).
Note: GDP is gross domestic product.
*Not available.

Yet, whenever there has been a more rapid rate of increase in Medicare spending in combination with projected deficits in the Medicare Part A Trust Fund, critics use projections of Medicare's future outlays to suggest that the program must be fundamentally reformed now. Suggestions for reform are often fabulously complex, but they tend to have these common features: the explicit or implicit claims that the "common pool," or social insurance features, of Medicare are the cost-control culprit; and the idea that adding choice, competition, and individual responsibility ("consumer-driven health care" now) will solve the problem.

The common pool feature of Medicare cannot plausibly be a cause for fiscal concern. In other developed countries, experience has repeatedly demonstrated the superior capacity of more universal social insurance programs to restrain growth in overall medical spending. As noted earlier, any comparison of growth in health spending of the United States and social-insurance nations like Germany, the Netherlands, and France would show U.S. spending growing more rapidly in recent decades. And these other countries have older populations and more widespread use of health care than is the case in the United States.[14]

One might argue more plausibly that fiscal restraint is difficult because Medicare does not cover everyone. Medicare has indeed few instruments to control capital spending. But its powerful constraints on payments to hospitals and doctors spill over onto pressures on private payers. The latter fight back by adapting some of Medicare's techniques, which then increases political pressures from providers to ease up on cost control. The experience of the past 30 or more years demonstrates that fragmented U.S. arrangements for financing medical care are comparatively weak instruments for controlling spending growth. That does not indict Medicare, but it does highlight a serious problem that Medicare (and the rest of the medical economy) will have to confront.

Critics—especially those concentrated in the pro-market wing of the Republican Party—have increasingly appealed to individual responsibility, choice, and competition as the "solution" to the problems of both U.S. medicine generally and Medicare's fiscal problems in particular.[15] One response is the broad proposal for health savings accounts (HSAs). Instead of participating in group insurance at the place of employment or paying the health insurance portion of *Federal Insurance Contributions Act* taxes, Americans are urged to contribute, tax free, to health savings accounts to cover their medical care needs. A version of such accounts was included in the 2003 *Medicare Prescription Drug, Improvement, and Modernization Act (MMA)*. The buildup in these accounts, along with an inexpensive "high-deductible" or "catastrophic" insurance policy, would, it is claimed, provide sufficient reserves for medical care both while employed and during old age.

There are major transitional problems with this scheme, but those need not distract from the main line of argument. For the young, the healthy, and the affluent, a health savings account approach is a great deal, particularly so if, as is virtually certain, these tax-free savings could be tapped for other purposes once a sufficient cushion was achieved. What happens to the rest of the population is only slightly less clear but broadly predictable. With "good risks" now not in the insurance pool, bad risks must be "insured" by general taxation. In short, instead of medical care as a part of a national pool of social insurance financing (or its Canadian equivalent), the system would move rapidly toward segmentation: private insurance for the young, healthy, and relatively well-off; welfare medicine for everyone else.

An alternative "privatization" approach retains Medicare's social insurance coverage for the elderly but attempts to save public funds by having privately managed care plans compete for Medicare patients. This alternative poses no direct threat to social insurance. Rather, the worrisome issue is whether managed care can both save money and deliver decent medical care at the same time to the elderly, or to anyone else. These are crucial questions for the whole of U.S. medicine, not just Medicare.

FAIRNESS

A more fundamental issue then is financial fairness in medical care. Should the insurance risks of ill health be dealt with in a universal, contributory, or tax-financed "public insurance" program or left to a patchwork system of private payment, private insurance, and diverse public subsidies for veterans, the aged, the poor, participants in employment-based health insurance, and so on?

The place of Medicare in this more fundamental discussion is, in 2008, odd. From the standpoint of universal protection, Medicare was and remains conceptually divided. It separates retired workers from those still on the job, thus breaching one version of social solidarity and giving rise to concerns about unfair special treatment for one segment of society. And because Medicare covers only three groups of the population—those "retired" because of age, disability, or renal failure—it can all too easily take on the coloration of interest-group politics. These politics are not the vitriolic struggles of us-them welfare policy. But it is quite easy to claim as "unfair" the relatively generous treatment of Medicare beneficiaries compared with the circumstances of ordinary American families flailing in the sea of either uncertain insurance coverage or added constraints on their choices within insurance coverage. The question is whether the rest of the population shares this vision of unfairness, as opposed to wanting Medicare's security and choices in their own coverage.

Developments during the past two decades have undermined a common experience of health insurance coverage. Traditional private, non-profit Blue Cross, Blue Shield plans have largely disappeared. Where they exist, they mostly use commercial health insurance practices.

There is no evidence that any substantial number of Americans accepts "unfairness" claims or favors moves to align Medicare's coverage with what has emerged in the private market. Nor, as the discussion of affordability reveals, is there any reason to believe that competition yields cost savings that will permit a "fairer" distribution of coverage. Indeed, the only "modernization" movement that has gained traction was the complaint about Medicare's failure to respond to changes in the nature of medical care, not changes in insurance plans. There the critics had obvious grounds for their charge. In 1965 drugs used outside the hospital were a modest part of the medical budget, and, in any case, Medicare reformers assumed that there would be persistent expansions of populations and services covered. Neither development took place according to plan. As pharmaceuticals came to play a larger role in medical care and as the world of private U.S. health financing diverged from the older Blue Cross, Blue Shield model, Medicare became an outlier in form and, in substance, fell short of the breadth of services covered by many private plans. Medicare beneficiaries were not getting the drug coverage that had become standard for other insured Americans.

MODERNIZATION

As of 2003, Medicare could be perceived as unfair in two ways: Medicare beneficiaries had more comprehensive coverage and choice of providers than many insured non-retired people had, but less coverage of increasingly important and expensive prescription drugs. Enter the *Medicare Prescription Drug, Improvement, and Modernization Act* of 2003, a fantastically complex piece of legislation designed to combat both "unfairnesses" by rolling them into a common call for "modernization." Medicare beneficiaries would obtain drug coverage, but in a "choice of plans" form that relied on private insurance provision, competition, and consumer choice. Moreover, the statute went beyond drug coverage to pursue the "modernization" of other health insurance areas. These included a complex set of incentives and financing arrangements intended to promote movement out of traditional Medicare into private plans more like those available to most other insured Americans. "Modernization" in this form implicitly promised cost containment through competition. Indeed, the statute went so far as to prohibit the one proven cost-constraint mechanism in Medicare's arsenal: use of its market power to bargain down prices, a technique too close to government price setting to satisfy the Bush administration and its allies in the 2003 Congress.

This Act was, in many respects, legislation by stealth. Here, and elsewhere, "modernization" has become a code word that masks ideological hostility to the public social insurance structure with which Social Security and Medicare began. It holds out the hope that truly modern systems of social provision will be both more affordable and fairer than "relics" of our New Deal and Great Society past that have outlived their usefulness. And in the current U.S. political context, to be modern means to hold a distinctive ideological position—at least to every one of the Republicans who sought their party's nomination in 2007–8. It is the power of individual choice, market competition, and personal responsibility to remake social policy to fit the demands of the 21st century.

I believe these "hopes" to be profoundly misguided. Fragmenting risk pools will not increase the fairness of American medical care. And choice and competition have no proven record of cost control in medical care in either the United States or elsewhere. Modernization in this guise is a Trojan horse. Inside is a complex set of devices that increase individual risk bearing and decrease the economic security traditionally provided by government health insurance in its social insurance or tax-financed form. Nonetheless, the contemporary debate has been profoundly influenced by the struggle over Medicare in the period after the Clinton reform failure. What appears sensible to promote is constrained by the interpretations of affordability, fairness, and modernity just discussed.

HEALTH REFORM IN 2007–8

Americans are not well served by their current medical care arrangements. Compared to our major trading partners and competitors, we are less likely to be insured for the cost of care, and the care that we receive is almost certain to be more costly. Though the leader in expenditures for medical research, U.S. medicine is not the undisputed leader in medical innovation except in the costliness and ubiquity of high-technology medicine. Most Americans "covered" by some form of health insurance still worry about its continuation when they or a close family member become seriously ill. Some are locked into employment they would gladly leave but for the potential catastrophic loss of existing insurance coverage. Something needs to be done, as the presidential candidates all acknowledge.

One fact remains obvious, however. Americans have long been dissatisfied with the nation's medical arrangements, but our political system has been unable to come up with a solution that satisfies enough of the public to overwhelm the institutional and interest group barriers to reform.[16] There is now, to be sure, once again a remarkable consensus that American medical care, particularly its financing and insurance coverage, needs a major overhaul. The critical unanimity on this point bridges almost all the usual cleavages in American politics: between old and young, Democrats and Republicans, management and labor, the well paid and the low paid. The overwhelming majority of Americans (including Fortune 500 executives) tell pollsters that the medical system requires substantial change. This level of public discontent was good news for medical reformers in 1993, just as it is again.[17]

The bad news for reformers, then and now, is that, for ideological and institutional reasons, American politics makes it very difficult to coalesce around a solution that reasonably satisfies the requirements for a stable and workable system of financing and delivering modern medical care. Agreement on the seriousness of the nation's medical ills will not necessarily generate the legislative support required for a substantively adequate and administratively workable program. That is as true in 2007–8 as it was in 1948, 1971, 1993, and 2000.

The most obvious point is that the presidential competition for 2007–8 has already recapitulated the run-up to its parallels in earlier struggles. Contenders —particularly among the Democratic hopefuls—feel compelled to propose detailed plans or are put on the defensive for not doing so. To date, the result has been depressingly familiar in a number of ways. Not one candidate has stated straightforwardly the core values health reform should express. Rather, the enumeration of complaints has dominated. The result is a pattern of problem identification and gestures toward complicated steps to broader health insurance coverage. The differences in values between a plan presented by Governor Schwarzenegger and any of the Democratic contenders are not easy to identify. None of the plans discussed—whether the expansions of child health insurance mentioned by Senator Clinton, the appeal to mandated coverage by Clinton and John Edwards (and incorporated in the California and Massachusetts plans), the Obama proposal of incentives for health insurance expansion, or the Bush administration's embrace of medical savings accounts and changes in the tax code's treatment of employer-arranged health insurance celebrated by Republican policy experts—seriously address persistent medical inflation. Yet it is the contemporary costs (16 percent of national income) and the rate of increase (1.5 to 2 times the growth of American incomes) that is at the core of the coverage problems the United States faces.

The gap between diagnosis and remedy is not an oversight, however. Candidates understandably are wary of announcing who the losers would be if their favored approach were actually to become a program fact. After all, if our medical arrangements are to become more affordable, some of those whose incomes constitute health expenditures must get less in the future than they might like. But so far, the presidential campaign of 2007–8 shows no sign of improvement over the Clinton period and has less clarity, about values or program structure, than the campaign of the early 1970s. That is not a healthy sign, but it is a good reason to reconsider the serious values debate: over values at stake, international experience, and a sober review of the United States' own history with public and private financing of medical care.

Notes

1. The sketch of American medical politics and policy is drawn from my previous work: "Commentary," on Kenneth R. Wing, "American Health Policy in the 1980s," *Case Western Reserve Law Review* 36, no. 4 (1985–86): 608–85, at 686–92; and a review of Robert G. Evans, *Strained Mercy: The Economics of Canadian Health Care* (Toronto: Butterworths, 1984), in *Journal of Health Politics, Policy, and Law* 11, no. 1 (1986): 163–66 (for an expanded version, see *Perspectives in Biology and Medicine* 30, no. 4 [1987]: 590–96).

2. Edward M. Kennedy, *In Critical Condition: The Crisis in America's Health Care* (New York: Simon and Schuster, 1972).

3. In 1974, for instance, the now forgotten Kennedy-Mills proposal received extended consideration in the finance committees of the Congress, as did the Nixon CHIP plan and the catastrophic health insurance bill of Senators Long and Ribicoff. The politics of this period are reviewed in Lawrence D. Brown, *Politics and Health Care Organizations: HMOs as Federal Policy* (Washington, DC: Brookings, 1984); and T. R. Marmor, *Political Analysis and American Medical Care* (New York: Cambridge University Press, 1983).

4. For a varied discussion of these new elements in American medicine, see Jeffrey Goldsmith, "Death of a Paradigm: The Challenge of Competition," *Health Affairs* 3 (1984): 7–19; Paul Starr, *The Social Transformation of American Medicine* (New York: Basic Books, 1984); and T. R. Marmor, Mark Schlesinger, and Richard W. Smithey, "A New Look at Nonprofits: Health Care Policy in a Competitive Age," *Yale Journal of Regulation* 3 (1986): 313–49.

5. See, for instance, Henry J. Aaron and William B. Schwartz, *The Painful Prescription: Rationing Health Care* (Washington, DC: Brookings, 1983).

6. See Alain C. Enthoven, *Health Plan: The Only Practical Solution to Soaring Health Care Costs* (Reading, Mass.: Addison-Wesley, 1980); Clark C. Havighurst, "Competition in Health Services: Overview, Issues, and Answers," *Vanderbilt Law Review* 34 (May 1981): 1115–78; and T. R. Marmor, Richard Boyer, and Julie Greenberg, "Medical Care and Procompetitive Reform," *Vanderbilt Law Review* 34 (May 1981): 1003–28.

7. These ideas are drawn from T. R. Marmor and Jon B. Christianson, *Health Care Policy: A Political Economy Approach* (Los Angeles: Sage Publications, 1982).

8. Brian Abel-Smith, *Value for Money in Health Services* (London: Heinemann Educational Books, 1976).

9. For an extended presentation of the politics of medical inflation, see Wing, "American Health Policy in the 1980s."

10. Ibid., 612.

11. Boards of Trustees of the Federal Hospital Insurance and Federal Supplemental Health Insurance Trust Funds, 2005 Annual Report, March 23, 2005, http://new.cms.hhs.gov/ReportsTrust Funds/downloads/tr2005.pdf (accessed February 27, 2006).

12. J. Oberlander, *The Political Life of Medicare* (Chicago: University of Chicago Press, 2003); and Marmor, *The Politics of Medicare* (New York: A. de Gruyter, 2000, 2nd edition).

13. C. Boccuti and M. Moon, "Comparing Medicare and Private Insurers: Growth Rates in Spending over Three Decades," *Health Affairs* 22, no. 2 (2003): 235.

14. T. R. Marmor, "From the United States," in E. de Gier, A. de Swaan, and M. Ooijens, eds., *Dutch Welfare Reform in an Expanding Europe: The Neighbours' View* (Amsterdam: Het Spinhuis, 2004), 111–34.

15. For some illustrations, see S. Butler and D. B. Kendall, "Expanding Access and Choice for Health Care Consumers through Tax Reform," *Health Affairs* 18, no. 6 (1999): 45–57; and H. J. Aaron and R. D. Reischauer, "The Medicare Reform Debate: What Is the Next Step?" *Health Affairs* 14, no. 4 (1995): 8–30.

16. While substantial change took place in the United States in the decades from 1980 to 2000, most of it was privately generated. What is called the "managed care" movement altered the way most American physicians practice and get paid, and it had a lot to do with the changing ownership and shape of American hospitals. These changes stand in contrast to the publicly organized reforms in the United Kingdom (internal markets in the 1990s) or Canada (national health insurance in the period 1957–71). For more on health reforms, especially "nonpublic change," see Carolyn H. Tuohy, *Accidental Logics: The Dynamics of Change in the Health Care Arena in the United States, Britain, and Canada* (Oxford: Oxford University Press, 1999).

17. For more on the public desire for substantial change in health care, see Robert J. Blendon and John M. Benson, "American's Views on Health Policy: A Fifty-Year Historical Perspective," *Health Affairs* 20, no. 2 (March/April 2001): 33–46. A New York Times/CBS news survey in February 2007 confirmed this historical pattern, with "an overwhelming majority" saying that "the healthcare system needs fundamental change or total reorganization." Robin Toner, "U.S. Guarantee of Care for All, Poll Finds," *New York Times*, March 2, 2007.

Medicare's Future

Fact, Fiction and Folly

Theodore R. Marmor and Gary J. McKissick

INTRODUCTION

This article seeks to clarify the contemporary Medicare debate by providing, first, an historical perspective on Medicare's origin and development and, second, an understanding of the particular damage done by an all-too-common style of Medicare policy analysis.

We have two central claims. First, we argue that the contemporary debate over Medicare reflects the program's distinctive political development, its generally low salience among the public, and the partisan rhetoric of politicians engaged in broader ideological battles. Born of a political more than a programmatic logic, Medicare's guiding social insurance philosophy was never fully articulated to the broader public. Moreover, its social insurance rationale has eroded over time, in part through piecemeal changes to the program. The public seems to have embraced Medicare with only a modest understanding of its functional form and remains largely ignorant of the program's real status or likely future. Moreover, the typically remote position Medicare occupies in public discourse feeds into the recurring atmosphere of crisis so easily stoked and exploited by partisans hoping to frame debate over Medicare to their ideological and electoral advantage.

Our second point is that the debate's confusions have been magnified by the lack of rigor with which many policy analysts have characterized the political context of Medicare reform. Because many policy analysts pay only cursory attention to the political analysis of Medicare's origins and recent developments, the fundamental issues at stake in the debate over Medicare's future are regularly obscured.

I. THE RECURRING FLAP OVER MEDICARE

Perhaps no single policy topic better illustrates the tensions within American politics at the beginning of a new millennium than does Medicare, the nation's thirty-five year commitment to ensuring senior citizens' financial protection against the costs of acute medical care. Our politics seems nearly overwhelmed by conflicting promises to balance the budget and pay down the national debt, enact tax cuts and protect broadly popular "entitlements." Medicare, one of the largest of such entitlement programs, has become a lightning rod for conflicts over how to resolve these competing goals. As a result, the nation finds itself in the midst of a bewildering mix of crisis talk, fact throwing and ideological name calling, with all the confusion and distortion one would expect from such a mix.[1]

Sadder still, this confusing debate is all too familiar. Electoral campaigns during the last half of the 1990s highlighted conflicts over Medicare policy. The budget politics of the decade also spurred debates over the program's structure and financing. When electoral and budget forces interacted, as they did most notably in the aftermath of the Republicans' congressional gains in the 1994 elections and the 1996 presidential race, the conflict over Medicare was particularly intense and visible.[2] But if the confluence of electoral dynamics and budget politics raised the decibel level of the debate over Medicare, they have done little to reduce and much to amplify the muddle of that debate.[3]

As a new century begins, therefore, we are left with a public battle over one of the nation's largest domestic programs that paradoxically is as familiar as it is confusing. This Article seeks to clarify the contemporary Medicare debate by providing, first, an historical perspective on Medicare's origin and development and, second, an understanding of the particular damage done by an all-too-common style of Medicare policy analysis.

We have two central claims. First, we argue that the contemporary debate over Medicare reflects the program's distinctive political development, its generally low salience among the public, and the partisan rhetoric of politicians engaged in broader ideological battles. Born of a political, more than a programmatic logic, Medicare's guiding social insurance philosophy never was fully articulated to the public. Moreover, its social insurance rationale eroded over time, in part through piecemeal changes to the program. The public seems to have embraced Medicare with only a modest understanding of its functional form, and remains largely ignorant of the program's real status or likely future. Moreover, the typically remote position Medicare occupies in public discourse feeds into the recurring atmosphere of crisis so easily stoked and exploited by partisans hoping to frame debate over Medicare to their ideological and electoral advantage.

Our second point is that the debate's confusions have been magnified by the lack of rigor with which many policy analysts have characterized the political context of Medicare reform. Because many policy analysts pay only cursory attention to the political analysis of Medicare's origins and recent developments, the fundamental issues at stake in the debate over Medicare's future are regularly obscured.

In the sections that follow we more fully articulate these two basic claims. The first task is to highlight the features of the program's history that most directly bear on contemporary debates about its future. This historical overview involves a discussion of Medicare's origins in Part II of this Article and subsequent evolution in Part III. The historical overview is followed by Part IV, which provides a critical review of common modes of analysis that generate dismay over both Medicare's status and the prospects for maintaining its historical social insurance roots. Finally, in the conclusion to this Article we examine the implications for policymakers and analysts of adopting an analytical framework that incorporates careful political analysis.

II. THE ORIGINS OF MEDICARE

Medicare, enacted in 1965[4] and fully operational in 1966, has complicated historical origins that are difficult to understand in the political environment at the dawn of the twenty-first century.[5] Perhaps the best way to understand Medicare's origins is to appreciate how peculiar it is from an international perspective. The United States is the only industrial democracy that initiated compulsory health insurance only for its elderly citizens.[6] Even those countries that started national health insurance programs with one group of beneficiaries did not start with the elderly.[7] Almost all other Organization for Economic Cooperation and Development (OECD) nations began with coverage of parts of their work force[8] or, in the case of Canada, with special programs for the poor.[9] In a later stage the programs expanded coverage to include other segments of the population. This cross-national pattern means that peculiarly American circumstances, rather than some common feature of modern societies, account for the reasons why compulsory government health insurance in the U.S. began with the recipients of Social Security cash pensions.

The roots of this particular history lie in the U.S.'s distinctive rejection of national health insurance in the twentieth century. First discussed in the years before World War I, national health insurance fell out of favor in the 1920s.[10]

When the Great Depression made economic insecurity a pressing concern, the Social Security blueprint of 1935 broached both health and disability insurance as controversial items of social insurance[11] that should be included in a more complete scheme of income protection. From 1936 to the late 1940s, liberals recurrently called for incorporating universal health insurance within America's emerging welfare state.[12] However, the conservative coalition in Congress defeated this attempt at expansion, despite its great public popularity.[13]

The original leaders of Social Security, well aware of this frustrating opposition, reassessed their reform strategy during President Truman's second term of office. By 1952, they had formulated a plan for incremental expansion of government health insurance.[14] Looking back to a failed 1942 proposal that medical insurance be extended to Social Security contributors, the proponents of what became known as Medicare shifted the category of beneficiaries to elderly retirees while retaining the link to social insurance.[15]

Medicare thus became a proposal to provide retirees with limited hospitalization insurance. It was a partial plan for the segment of the population whose financial fears of illness were as well grounded as their difficulty in purchasing health insurance at modest cost. With this, the long battle to turn a proposal acceptable to the nation into one passable in Congress began, stretching from its strategic birth in the early 1950s to a fully developed legislative plan by 1958.[16]

This initial design of Medicare has much to do with expectations of how it was to develop over time. The incrementalist strategy assumed that hospitalization coverage was the first step in benefits and that broader entitlements would follow under a common pattern of Social Security financing.[17] Likewise, the strategy's proponents presumed that eligibility would gradually expand.[18] They believed that it would take in most, if not all, of the population, perhaps extending first to children and pregnant women.[19]

All the Medicare enthusiasts took for granted that the rhetoric of enactment should emphasize the expansion of access, not the regulation and reform of American medical practice. The clear aim was to reduce the risks of financial disaster for the elderly and their families, and the clear understanding was that Congress would demand a largely hands-off posture toward the doctors and hospitals providing the care that Medicare would finance.[20] Thirty-five years later, that vision seems odd. It is now taken for granted that how one pays for medical care affects the care given. But in the buildup to enactment in 1965, no such presumption existed.

The incrementalist strategy of the 1950s and early 1960s assumed that most citizens supported efforts to address the health insurance problems of the aged. It also took for granted that social insurance programs enjoyed vastly greater public acceptance than did means-tested assistance programs.[21] Social insurance in the U.S. was acceptable to the extent that it sharply distinguished its programs from the demeaning world of public assistance. "On welfare," in American parlance, is largely a term of failure, and the leaders within the Social Security administration made sure that Medicare fell firmly within the tradition of benefits that are "earned," not given.[22] The elderly, consisting largely of retirees, could be presumed to be both needy and deserving. Through no fault of their own, they had lower earning capacities, and on average, higher medical expenses than any other age group. The Medicare proposal avoided a means test by restricting eligibility to persons over age sixty-five, and their spouses, who had contributed to the Social Security system during their working life.[23] The initial plan limited benefits to sixty days of hospital care while it excluded physician services in hopes of softening the medical profession's hostility to the program.[24]

The hybrid form adopted, Social Security financing and eligibility for hospital care and premiums plus general revenues for physician expenses, had a political explanation, but no clear philosophical rationale. The very structure of the benefits, providing acute hospital care (Part A of the legislation)[25] and physician treatment (Part B) as an unexpected afterthought,[26] was not tightly linked to the special circumstances of the elderly. Left out were provisions that addressed the problems of the chronically sick elderly, those whose medical conditions would not dramatically improve and who needed to maintain independent function more than triumph over discrete illness and injury.

There is another problem beyond the mismatch between Medicare's benefits and the health circumstances of the elderly. Medicare's social insurance rationale provided a statutory basis for the "right" to insurance coverage, but the character of that right and the extent of its protection has never been clarified. Here the absence of a clearly articulated guiding philosophy becomes most apparent. One interpretation of the right to medical care emphasizes equality of access.[27] Protection from medical care expenses, from this point of view, would simply mean that equally ill elderly would receive the same treatment and that their ability to pay for care would be irrelevant to the care they would justly receive. The right to such treatment would place a corresponding obligation on the guarantors of the right to make other considerations, such as race, class, or region, irrelevant to the treatment deemed appropriate. Note that this conception does not logically imply anything about the costs or quality of treatment provided. Equal opportunity in this context simply means *equal* treatment, not luxurious treatment, heroic treatment or unlimited treatment. Ascetic equality is justified just as luxurious equality of treatment might be. Considerations other than equality of opportunity, such as society's ability and willingness to bear and share the costs of illness and injury, would affect the extent of treatment that would be equally available.

Medicare's programmatic form reflected a set of specific policy choices and underlying assumptions about what was obtainable politically in the 1960s and likely to develop in the future. The pragmatism that counseled an incremental approach to achieving national health insurance necessarily stripped the program of an easily understood and fully articulated public philosophy. The last-minute addition of physician insurance and its separate financing mechanism further blurred the social insurance rationale at the heart of proponents' efforts. Viewed as a first step, the initial Medicare program made strategic sense. But the risk-averse decisions of the 1960s, however comprehensible, were consequential. They rested on presumptions about Medicare's incremental expansion that simply did not turn out to be the case. Instead, the next thirty-five years saw neither a serious restructuring of the benefits nor any dramatic expansion towards Medicare for all. We now turn to this subsequent operational history of Medicare.

III. MEDICARE'S OPERATION: A SKETCH OF THIRTY YEARS OF EXPERIENCE

As with any substantial program, the history of Medicare's operational experience is full of complexity. The main outline of that experience, however, can be easily summarized in four chronological periods.

A. 1966–1971: A HALF DECADE OF ACCOMMODATION

The period from 1966 to 1971 was more one of accommodation to American medicine than of efforts to change it. To ease the program's implementation in the face of heated resistance from organized medicine, Medicare's first administrators resisted radical changes. They adopted benefits and payment arrangements that exerted inflationary pressure and hindered the government's ability to control increases in program costs over time.[28] For example, the decision that hospitals should be paid their "reasonable costs" and that physicians should be paid their "customary charges" created significant loopholes that prompted energetic gaming strategies on the part of American doctors and hospitals.[29] Unusually generous allowances for depreciation and capital costs were a further built-in inflationary impetus.[30] The use of private insurance companies as financial intermediaries provided a buffer between the government and American physicians and hospitals, but it weakened the capacity of government to control reimbursement.[31] It was left to these intermediaries, like Blue Cross/ Blue Shield and private health insurers, to determine the reasonableness of hospital costs under Part A and physician charges under Part B.[32]

The truth is that in the early years of Medicare's implementation, the program's leaders were not disposed to confront the necessity of restraining costs.[33] They felt they needed the cooperation of all parties for Medicare's implementation to proceed smoothly and vigorous efforts at cost control would have threatened this relationship.[34] Medicare's administrators, fully aware of the need for cost control, were initially reluctant to make strong efforts for fear of enraging Medicare's providers.[35]

With the benefit of hindsight, it is easy to criticize this accommodationist posture. At the time of the program's enactment, however, Medicare's legislative mandate was not just to protect the nation's elderly from the economic burdens of illness, but *to do so without interfering significantly with the traditional organization of American medicine.*[36] It was with this aim in mind that Medicare's leaders were accommodating so as to ensure a smooth, speedy start to the program. It was not until the 1980s that Medicare was seen as a powerful means to control the costs and delivery of medical care.[37]

The results of accommodation were quite predictable: efficient implementation of the Medicare program with inflation built in.[38] Between 1967 and 1971, the daily charges of American hospitals rose by an average of thirteen percent per year.[39] Medicare's definition of reasonable charges paved the way for steep increases in physicians' fees.[40] In the first five years of operation, total expenditures rose over 70%, from $4.6 billion in 1967 to $7.9 billion in 1971.[41] Over the same period, the number insured by Medicare rose only 6%, from 19.5 to 20.7 million people.[42]

B. THE 1970S: MEDICARE AND FAILED ATTEMPTS TO REFORM AMERICAN MEDICINE

By 1970, there was a very broad agreement among students of American politics and medicine that health inflation had become a serious problem.[43] For some, Medicare was the cause of what became a pattern of medical prices rising at twice the rate of general consumer prices.[44] Throughout most of the 1970s, however, adjustments to Medicare took a subordinate political position to nationwide medical reform.[45] That does not mean Medicare was inert. Rather, major program changes to the program, such as experimentation with different reimbursement techniques in the early 1970s;[46] the expansion of Medicare to the disabled and those suffering from kidney failure in 1972,[47] and administrative reorganization in the late 1970s that took Medicare out of Social Security into the newly created Health Care Financing Administration (HCFA),[48] all became the subject of intense but low visibility interest group politics.[49] These politics were closely watched by the nation's burgeoning medical care industry, elderly pressure groups and specialized Congressional committees, but they were not the dramatic stuff of Medicare's original legislative fight or the continuing ideological battle over national health insurance.

The narrower, less public politics that characterized Medicare during this period ensured that its attenuated philosophical rationale would fade even further from public consciousness. The creation of HCFA further weakened these social insurance connections. The reorganization not only severed Medicare's administrative link to Social Security, America's benchmark social insurance program, but it also placed Medicare within the same government agency as Medicaid, the means-tested health insurance program for the poor.[50]

By the end of the 1970s, alarm had grown over both the troubles of American medical care generally and the costs of Medicare specifically.[51] The struggle over national health insurance ended in stalemate by 1975,[52] and the effort to enact national cost controls over hospitals also had failed by 1979.[53] All the while, Medicare, like American medicine as a whole, was consuming a larger and larger slice of the nation's economic pie, crowding out spending on other goods and services.[54] National health expenditures in 1980 represented 9.4% of gross domestic product, up from 7.6% in 1970.[55] Medicare alone amounted to 15% of the total health bill in 1980, up from 10% a decade earlier.[56] With costs on a steep upward trajectory and Medicare's programmatic principles increasingly obscured, the decade ended with signs that Medicare's politics were about to change.[57]

C. 1980–1992: BUDGET DEFICIT POLITICS AND THE CONTROL OF MEDICARE'S COSTS: ACHIEVEMENT, IGNORANCE AND CONTROVERSY

Since 1980, the politics of the federal deficit have largely driven Medicare policymaking.[58] This has had two consequences. The first is that Medicare is no longer an intermittent subject of policymakers' attention, but a constant target in the annual battles over the federal budget.[59] Second, concerns over Medicare's effect on the deficit facilitated far-reaching changes in the ways the program pays medical providers. In contrast to the accommodationist policies of the early years, federal policymakers implemented aggressive measures to hold down Medicare expenditures in the 1980s.[60] In pursuing measures such as paying hospitals fixed sums per diagnosis in 1983[61] and restricting fee increases to physicians in 1989,[62] they gave priority to the government's budgetary problems over the interests of hospitals and physicians. The result of these changes was a considerable slowdown in the rate of growth in Medicare expenditures that did not compromise the program's universality.[63]

Table 1: Medicare Expenditures as Percentage of Total National Health
Expenditures, Selected Calendar Years, 1967–1984

Year	Health Expenditures ($ billion)	Health Expenditures as Percent of GNP	Medicare[a] ($ billion)	Medicare[a] Percentage of National Health Expenditures
1967	51.1	6.4	4.7	9.2
1970	75.0	7.6	7.5	10.0
1975	132.7	8.6	16.3	12.3
1980	247.5	9.4	36.8	14.9
1981	285.2	9.6	44.7	15.7
1982	321.2	10.5	52.4	16.3
1983	355.1	10.7	58.8	16.6
1984	387.4	10.6	64.6	16.7
ACRG[b]	12.6	—	16.7	—

Source: T. R. Marmor and J. L. Mashaw, *Social Security: Beyond the Rhetoric of Crisis* (1988),
Table 7.2, p. 190.
[a] Includes administrative expenses.
[b] Annual compound rate of growth 1967–1984.

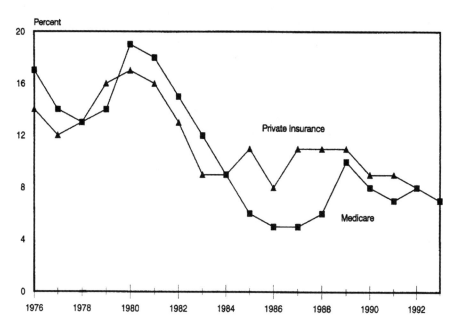

Figure 1. Per Capita Growth Rates of Services Covered by
Both Medicare and Private Insurance

Source: M. Moon, *Medicare Now and in the Future*, 2nd ed. (1996).

As effective as these changes in Medicare payment policy appear to have been in holding down the rate of growth in the program's expenditures, their impact on Medicare politics extended beyond these simple expenditure effects. First, and most obviously, less accommodation of medical providers necessarily made the politics of Medicare more explicitly conflictual. The rate of increase in Medicare's expenditures fell. But the "cost" of that was an increasingly transparent zero-sum politics, with doctors and hospitals as the most identifiable "losers." The reforms of the 1980s guaranteed that, from the perspective of those shouldering the burden, the program could be seen as restraining Medicare's costs "on the backs of" hospitals and physicians. Policymakers could hardly have welcomed this development, given the conflict that comes with zero-sum games and the enduring public support for Medicare. There are few recipes more distasteful to politicians than the mix of zero-sum politics with broadly popular programs.[64]

A second noteworthy feature of the 1980s reimbursement reforms was their limited effect on the broader public. The relative success of these reforms in restraining Medicare's costs received almost no public attention. As a result, most Americans have a distorted sense of Medicare's record of inflation, viewing it as rapid, unchanging and apparently uncontrollable. In fact, the experience of the 1980s and early 1990s demonstrated that Medicare *could* restrain its costs with changes in policy and political will. These savings, as the historical record shows, did not require a departure from Medicare's basic design as a social insurance program open to beneficiaries regardless of income.[65]

While the changes in Medicare payment policy during this decade received little public attention, a concurrent expansion of benefits did.[66] For a brief period in the late 1980s, the addition of so-called catastrophic protection to Medicare coverage became a major topic of media interest.[67] The passage and repeal of the catastrophic health insurance bill was a searing experience for Washington insiders, many of whom came away from the aptly named catastrophic insurance experience with a vivid reminder of the risks of awakening a powerfully organized constituency like America's senior citizens.[68]

The lessons drawn from the catastrophic insurance battle received further reinforcement during the 1992 presidential campaign, when there was a brief, but heated, flap over a Bush Administration proposal to reduce federal spending on Medicare and Medicaid by some $260 billion between 1993 and 1997.[69] That policy, charged then-candidate Clinton, would eviscerate Medicare,[70] increase the shifting of medical costs to employment-based health insurance and lead to millions of lost jobs.[71] The Bush campaign, while charging the Democrats with familiar scare tactics, nonetheless distanced President Bush from the flare-up.[72]

Bush called the proposal, which was publicly linked to Budget Director Richard Darman, merely one "option."[73] As a result, Medicare politics faded from public view, blocked for the next three years by the larger debate over "comprehensive" health care reform.

These experiences in the late 1980s and early 1990s left lasting impressions on Washington policymakers. But the interest-group politics that fed politicians' fears of changing Medicare were the stuff of highly attentive, well-organized constituencies and their predictable reactions to perceived cuts. These conflicts, however, only momentarily reached the public at large. What remained from this period, and what did have an eventually important impact on the public, was a very large federal deficit. Medicare, central to the budget fights of the Reagan and Bush administrations, would become a hostage to budget deficit politics in the years ahead.

D.1993–1999: PARTISANSHIP, PANIC AND PREMIUM SUPPORT

The discussion of Medicare and its problems practically disappeared from the national public agenda during the Clinton health reform struggle. But that did not remain so for very long. A combination of events transpired to thrust Medicare back into the center of national politics. The conflicts that emerged, however, might strike observers as difficult to reconcile with the battle over Clinton's failed initiative.[74] One could imagine, for instance, a visitor from Canada, having observed the fight over the Clinton health reform proposal in the early 1990s, reacting with surprise upon returning to the U.S. in 1995 to witness the advocacy of Republican legislative leaders for a system of vouchers in Medicare.[75] Had the visitor stayed on to observe the struggle over the terms of the Balanced Budget Amendments of 1997[76] and the subsequent deliberations of the National Bipartisan Commission on the Future of Medicare,[77] the puzzle would have deepened. How did the criticism of "managed competition" that helped sink the Clinton health care plan give way so quickly to a newfound enthusiasm for "managed care" prescriptions when the object of reform changed from universal health insurance to Medicare? In brief, the story of Medicare's politics over these last few years is very much one of explaining the puzzle of this apparent flip-flop.

A full account of what happened to Medicare in the last half of the 1990s will require considerable scholarly investigation in the years to come. The main features of the story, however, are relevant to understanding the past, present and future of Medicare's politics. Media attention returned to Medicare as soon as the trustees' 1995 report forecasted fiscal trouble.[78] The trustees projected that the hospital insurance trust fund would be bankrupt by 2002 if revenues and outlays behaved as currently estimated.[79] The Republicans, fresh from their historic victories in the 1994 elections and happy to capitalize on the trustees' report, promoted vouchers for Medicare in 1995 in an effort to remake American social policy.[80] President Clinton took the bait, vetoing the bill and running his 1996 re-election campaign in part as a defender of what later came to be called "traditional Medicare."[81] Convinced sometime after the election that a balanced budget was a desirable legacy for his presidency, Clinton made common cause with this longstanding Republican article of faith. But with balancing the budget came the need to sharply reduce Medicare's forecasted general revenue expenditures, and that in turn required congressional-presidential cooperation. The price of that cooperation was acceptance of some of the Republican's Medicare reforms along with those already favored by congressional Democrats.[82]

What happened next was fateful, but largely unanticipated. The 1997 Balanced Budget Act authorized a Bipartisan Commission on the Future of Medicare.[83] While the bipartisan title implied the prospect of consensual and careful deliberation, the reality was a group of ideological opposites. The Commission's leaders, Senator John Breaux (D-LA) and Congressman Bill Thomas (R-CA), were both well-known critics of the growth of entitlements generally and social insurance programs like Medicare particularly. For the most part, they used the Commission's work to advance their own vision of Medicare reform—the voucher plan of 1995 revised and relabeled as "premium support."[84] Predictably, their approach met with the fierce opposition by the Commission's liberal Democrats, and the whole effort came to a close in March of 1999 without a formal recommendation.[85] Though the Commission disbanded in March, the battle over Medicare reform was hardly over. The Commission chairmen introduced their proposal in Congress in May, 1999, and their bill prompted weeks of hearings and substantial media coverage.[86] They did not, however, produce any greater consensus, as the hearings that ensued re-enacted the very disputes that had stalemated their earlier efforts.

This sketch of the developments over the late 1990s makes clear that the transformation of Medicare reform proposals into a version of Clinton's once maligned managed competition, while puzzling at first blush, does not constitute an inexplicable anomaly. To understand Republican leaders' conversion to a managed competition plan for Medicare, with vouchers renamed "premium support," requires distinguishing Republican distaste for "big government" initiatives, such as the Clinton health reform plan, from Republican pragmatism about how to control existing government programs like Medicare. Combining a promise of cost control with the image of consumer choice, vouchers appear consonant with traditional Republican ideology.[87] In the case of Medicare, vouchers seemed an acceptable way to reduce federal expenditures in the future and thus to secure the balanced budget that fiscal policy conservatives had long sought.[88] The use of "premium support" as a synonym for vouchers illustrated the search for euphemisms that excited less controversy. Voucher proposals are notoriously conflictual in the world of public education, and the language of supporting premiums seemed more neutral.[89]

Pro-competitive proposals like the Breaux-Thomas plan were among the available reform options in part because of the tireless work of policy entrepreneurs inside and outside the medical care community.[90] It also helped that industry groups such as the American Medical Association and Federation of American Health Systems came to view vouchers as a preferred reform alternative to protect their economic interests.[91]

Finally, the Republican domination of Congress after 1994 sharply limited what a Democratic President could accomplish without bipartisan support. As long as the fight was over whether to balance the budget, Democrats could rail against Republican proposals to "cut" Medicare severely and they did so successfully in the 1996 presidential race.[92] However, in order to enact a balanced budget bill, the President and the Republican majority would have to find common ground. There would have to be political credit for both parties and the balanced budget would require substantial reductions in Medicare's projected expenditures that both parties could accept. Those budgetary reductions took place in 1997 through a combination of traditional and innovative policy adjustments in Medicare, an amalgam of what Democrats traditionally had used for cost control and what appealed to Republican advocates of competition.[93]

Understood this way, the widely touted competitive strategy for Medicare reform of 1995 through 1999 was the result of the broader electoral and partisan developments during the first half of the decade. In hindsight, this lineage is clear, even if the outcome would not have been expected at the beginning of the decade. Once the Clinton Administration embraced "competition" as the right answer to America's medical woes in 1993 with the Managed Competition Act of 1993,[94] the President could not easily reject that "solution" for Medicare when Republican and conservative Democratic legislators embraced it again in 1999.[95] To do so would be to discredit his New Democrat conviction that big government was no longer required and market devices were generally the most effective instruments of public policy. Republican control of Congress after 1994 meant, moreover, that their leaders could be counted on to advance such market solutions. Just as with the birth of Medicare, the changing partisan composition of Congress during the 1990s made the crucial difference in what was treated as plausible reform.[96] Once again, the framework for debating

Medicare's future was substantially altered by shifts in the distribution of congressional power.[97] This altered framework, it should be emphasized, still left the country well short of consensus.[98] As the decade closed, Medicare remained high on the public fiscal agenda, but with nothing approaching agreement about either the seriousness of its future problems or the right remedies for them.

IV. THE CONFUSING DEBATE: WHAT NEEDS TO CHANGE AND WHY

The current discussion of Medicare, like its history, includes considerable disagreement, with frustrating gaps between claims and evidence. Here, we emphasize an especially important source of distortion, namely policy commentary that reflects careless and misleading political analysis. This problem is unmistakable in the arguments voucher proponents made in the debate over Medicare's future during the late 1990s.[99] In this section, we address three aspects of what we regard as myth-ridden debate: (1) the unsubstantiated invocation of public opinion to justify policy judgments; (2) misplaced confidence in long-term forecasts and inattention to the interaction of economic and political factors in forecasting; and (3) contestable claims presented as "conventional wisdom." We rely on arguments for vouchers to illustrate the problematic use of public opinion and the limits of political forecasting. Addressing misconceptions in the conventional wisdom broadens our focus beyond vouchers. But throughout, we aim to clarify the Medicare debate by approaching these topics as political scientists, a perspective too often absent from the larger national debate.

A. VOUCHER PLANS REVISITED: HOW NOT TO USE PUBLIC OPINION

Enthusiasm for converting Medicare into a system of voucher payments culminated, as noted, in the majority-supported proposal of the Breaux-Thomas Commission and its subsequent introduction as legislation.[100] To see how voucher advocates have justified these plans analytically, we turn to the work of economists Henry Aaron and Robert Reischauer, whose writings on vouchers have been especially extensive, if in the end still disappointing. The reputation for thoughtfulness of these scholars makes the imprecision of their Medicare political analysis all the more troubling. Their 1995 *Health Affairs* article, "The Medicare Reform Debate: What Is the Next Step?"[101] is a particularly revealing illustration of misleading political analysis.[102]

The scope of their article is quite broad: the proposal to convert Medicare "from a 'service reimbursement' system into a 'premium support' system."[103] They liken this proposal to "many that are now reshaping private employer-based insurance."[104] They purport not only to describe the technical issues that "cannot be solved quickly" and "preclude quick budget savings," but also to provide a brief history of Medicare and why it is unsustainable in its present form.[105] In short, they engage in historical characterization, political analysis, policy evaluation and program forecasting. They also take pains to caution readers that "[t]he history of reforms in U.S. social policy is replete with exaggerated claims of the benefits the reform will produce. To muster enthusiasm, supporters of reform paint rosy pictures of the marvelous benefits that will ensue if only their recommendations are adopted."[106] They could have added that reform advocates regularly invent political analysis to bolster their claims of expertise. Aaron and Reischauer have many sensible things to say about how Medicare has operated and why cost savings are difficult under any implementable reform. However, their characterization of Medicare's political history and contemporary political circumstances is simply misleading.

The most striking feature of this kind of analysis is misplaced analytical confidence. Consider, for example, two of the opening paragraphs of their examination of the Medicare reform debate in 1995.[107] "Five central facts," the reader is told, "will shape the debate on the future of Medicare."[108]

First, Medicare enjoys overwhelming support among the American electorate, a popularity that is well deserved because the program has achieved all of its designers' major objectives. Second, the cost of providing Medicare benefits is projected to rise very rapidly and will exceed projected revenues by ever larger amounts. Third, legislative reform of the entire health care system is now off the political agenda and likely will remain so for years to come. Fourth, there exists a strong and broad consensus against raising taxes. Fifth, dramatic changes are taking place in the way health care is financed and delivered for the non-Medicare population.[109]

The implications of these facts are straightforward. First, before changes are made in Medicare, policymakers will have to assure the general population and beneficiaries alike that the reforms will not compromise the attributes of the program that the public values so much. Second, Congress will have to act soon to restore Medicare's financial viability. Third, the measures that Congress adopts will not be part of any major legislative effort to reform the overall health care system. Fourth, most, if not all, of the budgetary savings on Medicare will come from reducing federal payments to providers and raising costs to beneficiaries, not from raising Medicare payroll taxes. Fifth, congressional reforms will—and should—bring Medicare more in line with the structure of health care financing and delivery that is evolving to serve the non-Medicare population.[110]

To the scholar of Medicare, these are truly stunning claims. They are a mix of plausible surmises with historical inaccuracy, possible scenarios presented as certain fact, facts set out as if they were open to only one interpretation, and forecasts of the distant future that are not rooted in the indeterminacy of political and economic predictions. Here we focus on a subset of the factual claims and their supposedly obvious "implications" to illustrate the weaknesses of this sort of political analysis.

The claim that Medicare's "popularity" is not only "overwhelming" but "well deserved because the program has achieved all its designers' major objectives"[111] is clearly contestable. The authors cite no evidence to support their claims about the breadth and depth of the public's views.[112] While the work of Larry Jacobs and other public opinion scholars establishes that Medicare is broadly approved, that same work undercuts the easy connection between knowledge of the program (especially the extent to which objectives are understood to have been satisfied) and the support for the program.[113] To the extent Medicare is broadly popular, that support mostly reflects relatively superficial understanding of Medicare's role in helping America's elderly with large medical expenses. Other than that, the public is largely uninformed.[114]

Nor can it be the case that the public is satisfied because the major objectives of Medicare's designers have all been achieved. That, of course, is one of the major conclusions of the program's history we have sketched: the key objective of expansion has not been achieved.[115] The original hope was that Medicare would grow into universal health insurance, not coverage only for the elderly, the disabled, and those suffering from renal failure.[116] Moreover, the reformers anticipated that Medicare would largely remove financial fearfulness from the lives of older Americans facing sickness, injury and other medical burdens.[117] That, as Marilyn Moon and others have amply demonstrated, has not been accomplished and for a variety of reasons.[118] Since the claims are factually false, so are the causal connections.

Moreover, if the factual claims about politically relevant factors are questionable, the "implications" drawn are equally suspect. None of them are "straightforward" in the sense that reasonable analysts could not find grounds for questioning their normative plausibility or predictive accuracy. Consider one claim where the grounds for objection are quite obvious: the assertion that "congressional reforms will—and should—bring Medicare more in line with the structure of health care financing and delivery that is evolving to serve the non-Medicare population."[119]

Underlying this claim is the view, later made explicit, that Medicare should be adapted to what itself is "evolving" as a practical matter of avoiding resentment.[120] It is difficult to argue with the contention that resentment, should it materialize, would be a real threat to the program's viability. But before resentment can serve as a convincing justification for policy change, one ought to at least pause to consider the evidence that a groundswell of resentment is on the horizon. How likely is this alleged resentment? What might be its source?

Aaron and Reischauer have only one possible source of the alleged resentment: the fact that Medicare does not "look like"—in form more so than content—the health insurance most commonly available in the private market. That fact, we hasten to note, has always been true in one important way: Medicare's status as an entitlement has *always* distinguished it from the health insurance privately available to the rest of the population. But we take Aaron and Reischauer to mean something different. Their claim, as we read it, rests on the presumption that the greater freedom of choice available to Medicare recipients than to the non-Medicare population is the source of resentment. This assumes but does not substantiate the belief that Medicare's operation should resemble the health insurance practices other Americans confront, *irrespective of any demonstrated superiority of the "evolving" practices and public support of them.* That assumption ought to invite skepticism on normative grounds, but the more important point for present purposes is an empirical one. Simply put, there is no credible evidence for the prediction that voucher enthusiasm will arise from resentment about the elderly having a broader set of choices than younger Americans. By our reading, what evidence there is actually suggests just the opposite.

To understand the public's likely response to such ideas, one must recognize that Medicare vouchers presume a large shift to managed care organizations.[121] The interpretation of resentment by voucher enthusiasts thus requires a groundswell of support for moving the elderly into managed care. But therein lies an immediate puzzle. How can that be reconciled with the evidence about the public's critical views of the managed care industry? A managed care backlash has by now become a well-established finding in research on the public's views on healthcare.[122] Table 2 and Figure 2,[123] for instance, give just a small sampling of the accumulated evidence of this backlash. If anything, views about the managed care industry only became worse over the latter half of the 1990s.[124] The evidence of a backlash against managed care reflects considerable frustration with constraints on patient choice.[125] But, it

Table 2: Evidence of a Backlash in Attitudes About Managed Care
(a) Given what you know, on the whole do you think this trend away from traditional
fee-for-service coverage and toward managed care is a good thing or a bad thing?

	7/95[a]	8/96	8/97	7/98
	(%)	(%)	(%)	(%)
Good Thing	59	44	44	40
Bad Thing	28	37	44	47
Neither (vol.)	1	4	6	6
Not Sure	11	15	6	6
N	605	1,008	1,007	1,011

[a] "Overall do you think this trend toward more managed care is a good thing or a bad thing?"

(b) Do you think the trend toward more managed care—with more people belonging
to HMOs, PPOs and other managed care plans—will improve or harm the quality of
medical care people like you receive?

	7/95[a]	8/96	8/97	7/98
	(%)	(%)	(%)	(%)
Improve	48	38	33	31
Harm	39	43	54	58
No Effect	4	7	7	4
N	605	1,008	1,007	1,011

Source: Kaiser Family Foundation/Harvard University, Public Opinion
Update: Managed Care, September 17, 1998. Taken from: L. R. Jacobs and R. S. Shapiro, The
American Public's Pragmatic Liberalism Meets Its Philosophical Conservatism. *Journal of Health
Politics, Policy and Law* 24(5), Tables 2 and 3, pp. 1024–5 (1999).

is not at all obvious that such frustration has led to any resentment of Medicare's benefits. Indeed, the opposite seems more plausible. If the reactions
embodied by the efforts to legislate a "patient's bill of rights" are any indication, the general public's dissatisfaction with "choice" will more likely produce more vigorous efforts to make private health care more like "traditional"
Medicare.[126]

What explains such ill-supported claims of resentment? Two accounts come
to mind. The first (and, we hope, least likely) possibility is that voucher proponents, as trained economists, see little value in the systematic study of public

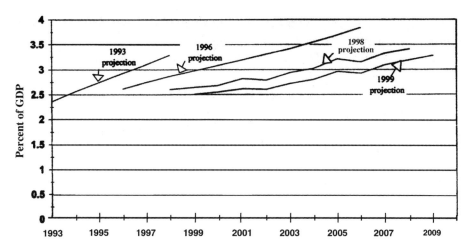

Figure 2. Medicare and Medicaid Spending, Congressional
Budget Office Projections (Selected Years)

Source: Henry J. Aaron, *Thinking About Aging: What We Know, What
We Can't Know, and Why It Matters* (unpublished manuscript, on file with the author).

opinion. In this view, appealing to public opinion is often little more than sto-rytelling, a sort of fanciful speculation about what sorts of attitudes might exist that would justify a particular overhaul of Medicare. Casual speculation is not, however, a basis for credible policy analysis. The second, more generous inter-pretation, then, is that these claims rest on a distinctive reading of the available data. It is true, for instance, that younger cohorts typically express less support for Medicare and greater skepticism about the program's future than do older cohorts.[127] To note these differences is one thing. To interpret them as evidence of generational resentment is quite another.[128] In this case, the inferential leaps do not withstand serious scrutiny. In the first place, they require stability in cohort-specific preferences over time that is unlikely. Second, they disregard the likelihood that the preferences of younger cohorts may largely reflect their relative ignorance of Medicare's operation.

Differences across age groups at any one time say nothing about the evolution of preferences within any given cohort *over time*. This point is true of all inter-generational claims about social insurance programs for the elderly.[129] Even if we assume that the differences among cohorts reflect (narrowly) self-interested responses to the differential incidence of costs and benefits,[130] it remains likely that the "self-interest" of current eighteen- through thirty-year-olds will be quite different when that cohort approaches retirement age. But if the preferences of current young adults are sufficient grounds for drastically changing Medicare,

are we then supposed to shift course again when, thirty years down the road, this same cohort suddenly discovers the merits of social insurance protections against the costs of health care? What, exactly, privileges the claims of these particular individuals?

The claim of festering resentment becomes even harder to sustain once one recognizes that support for and confidence in the program are not the only differences in cohort-specific public opinion.[131] For instance, public opinion data regularly show that younger cohorts are less knowledgeable about the specifics of current Medicare policy.[132] Younger citizens' greater skepticism about Medicare is surely a function of their relative ignorance of the program's operations and their inexperience with how the threat of near-term crises in popular programs tends to focus elected leaders' minds in constructive ways.[133] If so, the prudent course would seem to be some combination of discounting the alleged "resentment" implied in the (mis)reading of their views of the program and proactive education about its structure and politics. From this perspective, drastic restructuring of Medicare is an odd response to the available data.

If the problems with Aaron and Reischauer's treatment of public opinion were idiosyncratic, there would be no point belaboring them. Unhappily, the weakness of their approach is representative of many Medicare analysts. The failure to attend seriously to public opinion research on Medicare reflects a troubling tendency in much health services scholarship. In this sense, Aaron and Reischauer exemplify a broader problem. Economists, in particular, all too frequently practice a strain of policy analysis that treats the "political" part of political economy as barely more than an afterthought.[134] To be sure, one might expect a tilt toward a scholar's home discipline.[135] In our view, however, the emphasis on economic analysis at the expense of politics needs rebalancing.

That rebalancing requires eliminating casual appeals to mass attitudes and substituting attention to the existing research on public opinion. This research makes clear that the mapping of attitudes expressed in public opinion surveys onto specific policy proposals is rarely straightforward.[136] Substantial uncertainty and unclear preferences can be masked in responses to questions about policies as removed from public understanding as is Medicare.[137] Moreover, as Jon Oberlander has argued, public opinion has, at moments, stopped Medicare reform, but it has never driven it.[138] It typically has a more negative impact on policy-making, serving to constrain policy options rather than create them. To the extent it has been influential, it has set limits on efforts to transform Medicare, particularly serving to constrain program cutbacks.[139] In so far as voucher proposals can be seen as an attempt to cut back public benefits indirectly, there is no demand for them from the public.[140] As congressional Republicans learned during the 104th Congress, Medicare cutbacks are extremely difficult to achieve in the absence of clear public mandates for change.[141]

Public opinion, properly understood, may doom voucher reforms. But it did not produce them, and it provides little support for making Medicare into a system of vouchers. There may well be a defensible rationale for vouchers, but it can not be found in the evidence available from research on American public opinion.[142]

B. VOUCHERS REDUX: THE PERILS OF PREDICTION

Aaron and Reischauer provide a second reminder of the importance of prudent political analysis with the boldness of their claims about the future. Recall, for instance, the assertion that "the cost of providing Medicare benefits is projected to rise very rapidly and will exceed projected revenues by ever larger amounts."[143] It was obvious in 1995 that Medicare's projected costs were rising and that the revenues were expected to rise less rapidly than the forecasted costs. But that merely illustrates a truism: forecasts are not so much serious predictions as conditional claims whose truth depends entirely on the accuracy of the premises.[144] By 2000, the view that Medicare's costs would continue to rise at ten percent per year into the indefinite future[145] seemed odd indeed.

Likewise, the prediction that comprehensive health care reform would remain off the "political agenda . . . for years to come"[146] illustrates easy extrapolation rather than serious forecasting. In 1995, Washington insiders, reeling from the Clinton reform debacle, were surely predisposed to think health care reform was over for as far as the eye could see.[147] But they turned out to be wrong, as healthcare issues returned to the agenda in limited form.[148] Moreover, at the time of this writing (March 2000), these issues arose again in connection with the 2000 election. Both candidates seeking the Democratic presidential nomination had unveiled serious proposals for healthcare reform—this on top of months of congressional attention to reforms of the health insurance industry embodied in the so-called "Patients' Bill of Rights."[149] According to a November 1999 poll by the New York Times and CBS News, health care topped the list of issues the public most wanted the Congress and president to address.[150]

The reappearance of health care reforms on the national agenda is a reminder that political forecasting is always an exercise fraught with uncertainty. Scholars of agenda-setting have established that the ebbs and flows of political agendas are a complex product of many forces. Each of these forces is subject to considerable uncertainty at any given time, and their combination is even more difficult to predict.[151] Periods of continuity can coexist with sudden and large changes in policy agendas.[152] While agenda scholars understand the families of factors that affect both the incremental and dramatic dynamics of policy debates, we are incapable of anticipating the precise timing and consequences of these factors as they interact. As a result, point predictions of future political agendas should be viewed with great skepticism.[153]

The futurology of Aaron and Reischauer, as with their use of public opinion, is important because it conforms to wider practices that have long plagued Medicare policy analysis. Medicare's harshest critics have regularly engaged in a form of "future dread," where projections of Medicare's financial status decades into the future are dressed up with a certainty that cannot be justified.[154] Such long-range projections are notoriously sensitive to even slight changes in their underlying components. Witness, for example, the difference between HCFA's 1995 projection that kick-started the current debate over massive changes and its report just four years later that projected an additional thirteen years of "solvency."[155] For good reason, analysts, at least sensible ones, approach long range forecasts with caution. But the same logic that recommends caution in projecting a program's financial future also requires restraint in using those very same projections to make the case for major changes from current policy. To do otherwise, as when proponents of restructuring Medicare forecast a future of certain crisis, is to misuse such long-range projections. The need for an honest recognition of the limits of forecasting increases in the case of Medicare, where the environment is marked by frequent technological change and is embedded in a larger and changing world of private and public health care.[156] Of course, this point is not lost on analysts as experienced as Aaron and Reischauer. Indeed, Aaron himself recently issued similar cautions, going so far as to assert "a fog of fundamental unknowability shrouds projections of Medicare costs beyond just a few years."[157]

The uncertainty about Medicare's future costs is but one limitation on confident forecasting. It is compounded by the dependence on such forecasts in the service of promoting current proposals for reform. Too often, the inherent risks of long-range forecasts are subordinated to the desire to rationalize policy prescriptions — a danger that even the most thoughtful analysts face. When such impulses are combined with a failure to recognize the even greater difficulty in forecasting politics (as opposed to demographics or economics), the dangers of what we have described as unfounded futurology are maximized. The result is all too often fear-mongering masquerading as forecasting, a practice that distorts one's understanding of Medicare's current problems and future possibilities.[158]

C. CONFUSIONS OF CONVENTIONAL WISDOM

Another source of confusion in the Medicare debate arises from claims reported as current conventional wisdom about the program's future. One is the mistaken view that because Medicare faces financial strain, the program requires dramatic transformation.[159] The experience of the 1980s and much of the 1990s showed that Medicare's administrators, when willing and able, could limit the pace of increase in the program's costs.[160] Consider, also, that Medicare controlled its outlays more tightly than did private health insurance during most of the last two decades[161]—this even though private insurance was undergoing massive changes aimed at controlling costs during this period.[162] To be sure, controlling the program's future costs poses undeniable challenges to policymakers, just as it has before. Mustering the political will to implement cost-control measures is no small feat. But it is worth remembering that policymakers have managed the task in the past without having to reshape Medicare radically.[163]

The very language used to define the financial problems Medicare undoubtedly faces is another source of distortion. Republican as well as a number of Democratic critics continue to use the fearful language of insolvency to describe Medicare's future.[164] That future, according to this group, is a dreaded one in which the program's trust fund will be literally "out of money."[165] This language represents the unfortunate triumph of metaphor over thought.[166] Thinking that the trust fund is the crucial fiscal variable is analogous to thinking that a thermometer's reading constitutes a heat wave or a freeze.[167] The program's hospital "trust fund" refers to an accounting term, a conventional way to describe earmarked revenue and spending. The very notion of a public trust fund combines the language of trust with the funding-source reality of payroll taxes to underscore the solidity of commitment to finance promised benefits in social insurance programs.[168] The appeal to "insolvency" as a danger needs to be recognized for its symbolic and strategic value in framing the debate over Medicare. Such symbolic framing can be politically consequential.[169] For that very reason, though, policy analysts should guard against misleading symbols. Whatever its psychological and political importance, the trust associated with the fund is a fiscally neutral element in the goods and services Medicare finances. Congress can change the taxes that finance Medicare if it has the will. Likewise, it can change the benefits and reimbursement provisions of the program. Or it can do some of both, as it has at different times in Medicare's operational history. Channeling the program's revenues through something called a "trust fund" changes nothing in the real political economy. Thinking so is the cause of much muddle, unwarranted fearfulness, and misdirected energy.[170]

D. MEDICARE REFORM: PUTTING POLITICAL ANALYSIS BACK IN

Our commentary has been sharply critical of a particular type of thinking about Medicare's politics and policies. Casual political analysis undermines the authority of careful policy analysis. The remedy for it is a mix of self-restraint and more serious attention to what political science can (and cannot) tell us about Medicare's likely future.[171] It hurts rather than helps public understanding of what should and can be done in American policymaking to substantiate program evaluation with politically superficial judgements. This is particularly important where the political analysis is presented as scholarship, but not bolstered by evidentiary support or defensible inferences. We do not argue that scholars should hide their normative preferences. They should state them clearly. Nor do we suggest that political scientists have a monopoly on commentary about American political realities (or Medicare's). Rather, our claim is that scholarly standards should apply to claims about politics by those invoking analytical authority for their policy conclusions.

To view the debate over Medicare's finances as distorted is not, of course, to suggest the program is free of problems. But it is important to understand that Medicare can be adjusted in ways that fully preserve the national commitment to health insurance for America's elderly and disabled. In our view, the task for futurologists is not so much to concentrate on Medicare's uncertain level of future expenditures or the obvious demographic pressures, but to anticipate the varying political contexts that may face policymakers in the first decades of the twenty-first century.

V. CONCLUSION

There is ample justification for a debate over how Medicare should be "reformed." What is not needed is a debate that scares the country about Medicare's future by false claims about the program's unsustainability. It would indeed be a crisis if the legitimate medical costs of America's aged and disabled were unaffordable. From our perspective, though, the more immediate and real problem is the misleading nature of the debate over Medicare's current status and its future.

Making sense of Medicare's contemporary condition and meeting the challenges of the future requires a clear understanding of where we have been. The program's early implementation stressed accommodation to the medical world of the 1960s. Its objective was to keep the economic burden of illness from overwhelming the aged or their children. Medicare's initial leaders proceeded from the premise that the program required a smooth start and that Congress demanded accommodation to American medicine's rules.

Thirty-five years later, the setting is radically different. The difficulties of Medicare are similar to those of American medicine generally, not just the program's administration. We pay too much for some procedures and we do too many things that either do some harm or do little good in relation to their costs. In the world of American private health insurance, cost control has now arrived with a vengeance. Medicare is unsettled and is likely to remain so in the context of budget politics unless it is understood that bordering what Medicare spends need not require transforming the program. It *will* require that the costs of cost control be borne, though. And decisions about such issues should link political understanding to the ordinary practice of policy analysis. It is, in fact, a sobering commentary on the nature of American politics that this argument even needs to be made. Isn't politics, after all, about just such things—the well-worn who gets what, when and how?

Such questions remain at the heart of Medicare's politics. Indeed, one of the most striking features of Medicare's political evolution is how the ideological cleavage that attended its birth reappeared, in a different guise, more than three decades later. Although few political actors claim anything other than the aim of "saving Medicare," the obvious truth is that the program still excites fundamental differences about the proper role of government in health insurance. No program can remain static as conditions change. But there is no necessary reason why Medicare, with incremental adaptations, could not be maintained into the indefinite future. For those who embrace its social insurance purposes, this would be satisfaction. For those who reject those principles as inappropriate, the fight over "reforming" Medicare is in fact about changing it fundamentally. The scholarship on Medicare, from whatever discipline, cannot afford to ignore this central feature of the program. Medicare's future, like its past, remains a fundamentally political matter.

Notes

1. *See* Theodore Marmor & Jerry L. Mashaw, *The Future of Entitlements: How "Future Dread" Distorts the Debate over Social Security Pensions and Medicare, in* THE OXFORD COMPANION TO POLITICS OF THE WORLD (2d ed., 2001) (arguing that the claim that American social policy is unaffordable, unmanageable and undesirable is factually questionable, interpretively misleading and widely disseminated).

2. *See* Thomas B. Edsall, *The GOP's Flawed Fable: The Miracle of Michigan Traps the Party's Thinking*, WASH. POST, Jan. 21, 1996, at C1; Norman Ornstein, *Dems, Beware of Medicare: Seizing on GOP Quandary Could Backfire in the Long-Term*, USA TODAY, June 1, 1995, at 11A.

3. The muddle encompasses different perceptions of Medicare's problems and proposed solutions to them. For some policymakers, the main problem is a shortage of future revenues. As Health and Human Services Secretary Donna Shalala put it, "There is simply no substitute for more money to come into the system." Stephen Nohlgren, *Lawmakers Lobby for Reform of Medicare at USF Forum*, ST. PETERSBURG TIMES, Oct. 12, 1999, at 1B. For others, the problem is more fundamental. "I think putting surplus dollars into the Part A Trust Fund doesn't fix Medicare's underlying problem. I've likened it to putting more gas in an old car — it still runs like an old car and doesn't have any of the features of a new car." John Breaux, *Opening Statement: Medicare Commission* (visited May 12, 2000), http://rs9.loc.gov/medicare/breaux31699.html. Similarly, reforms such as proposals to introduce "competition" into the program provoke widely divergent reactions. A *New York Times* story about one such proposal, a bill introduced by Senator John Breaux (D-LA), illustrates such competing perspectives: "The goal, proponents say, is to harness competition to drive down costs, encourage innovation and improve quality. . . . [But former administrator of the Health Care Financing Administration Bruce] Vladeck disagreed, saying that the 'notion that competition in health care for the elderly will cut costs and improve quality is a fantasy.' He predicted that the Breaux plan would 'segment the market,' steering the poor into low-cost, poor-quality H.M.O.'s while 'the rich will flock to fee-for-service.'"

   Michael M. Weinstein, *For Medicare, a Rocky Road to Competition*, N.Y. TIMES, Feb. 21, 1999, at § 3, 1. Even the basic premises of proposed reforms are contested. Representative John D. Dingell (D-MI) worries that Senator Breaux's proposal "would convert Medicare from a universal guarantee to a government voucher for private insurance." Robert Pear, *Medicare Panel, Sharply Divided, Submits No Plan*, N.Y. TIMES, Mar. 16, at A1. This view was flatly denied by the plan's sponsor. "This proposal is not a voucher program," he said. "It is not an end to Medicare as an entitlement." *Id.*

4. The narrative history sketched in Sections II and III of this Article draws upon the more extensive analysis of Medicare's origins and operations detailed in THEODORE R. MARMOR, THE POLITICS OF MEDICARE (2d ed., 2000).

5. Medicare is the federal health insurance program for the aged and disabled established by Congress as Title XVIII of the Social Security Act. 42 U.S.C. § 1395 (1994).

6. *See* Theodore R. Marmor, *Coping with a Creeping Crisis: Medicare at Twenty*, in SOCIAL SECURITY: BEYOND THE RHETORIC OF CRISIS 177, 178 (Theodore R. Marmor & Jerry L. Mashaw eds., 1988).

7. *See id.*

8. For example, in both Germany and England, government-sponsored health insurance began in the late 19th and early 20th centuries as a government mandated membership in preexisting mutual benefit funds. Seen as a way to maintain the incomes and productivity of the working class, it was originally limited to wage earners. *See* PAUL STARR, THE SOCIAL TRANSFORMATION OF AMERICAN MEDICINE 237–40 (1982).

9. From this starting point, Canada went to universal programs for one service (hospitals) and then shifted to another (physicians). *See* Theodore R. Marmor, *Can the U.S. Learn from Canada?*, in NATIONAL HEALTH INSURANCE: CAN WE LEARN FROM CANADA? 231, 233–41 (Spyros Andreopoulos ed., 1975).

10. There were a number of reasons why health insurance failed to be enacted during this period, including the fact that national health insurance was portrayed by opponents as a German concept inconsistent with American values. *See* STARR, *supra* note 8, at 253 (quoting a pamphlet written in 1917 by a group of California physicians that describes compulsory social health insur-

ance as "a dangerous device, invented in Germany, announced by the German Emperor from the throne the same year he started plotting and preparing to conquer the world").

11. *See id.* at 266–69.

12. *See id.* at 282–84.

13. *See* MARMOR, *supra* note 4, at 6–10.

14. *See id.* at 23.

15. *See id.* at 10–11.

16. *See id.* at 17.

17. *See id.* at 10; *see also* Marmor, *supra* note 6, at 179.

18. *See* MARMOR, *supra* note 4, at 95–96.

19. For a more detailed discussion of the Congressional fight over the enactment of Medicare and the expansionist aspirations of its supporters, see generally SHERI DAVID, WITH DIGNITY: THE SEARCH FOR MEDICARE AND MEDICAID (1985), LAWRENCE JACOBS, THE HEALTH OF NATIONS: PUBLIC OPINION AND THE MAKING OF AMERICAN AND BRITISH HEALTH POLICY (1993), and MARMOR, *supra* note 4. The basis for the presumption of Medicare's architects' views about future expansion is largely Marmor's service as Wilbur Cohen's special assistant the summer of Medicare's operational start in 1966.

20. Indeed, the first section of the Medicare statute is entitled "Prohibition Against any Federal Interference," and states: "Nothing in this subchapter shall be construed to authorize any Federal officer or employee to exercise any supervision or control over the practice of medicine or the manner in which medical services are provided, or over the selection, tenure, or compensation of any officer or employee of any institution, agency, or person providing health services; or to exercise any supervision or control over the administration or operation of any such institution, agency, or person."

42 U.S.C. § 1395 (1994).

21. *See* JACOBS, *supra* note 19, at 94, 148.

22. *See id.* at 94.

23. *See id.* at 90.

24. *See id.* at 152–53, 206–07.

25. *See* 42 U.S.C. § 1395d (1998).

26. *See id.* § 1395k.

27. *See* MARMOR, *supra* note 4, at 12–13.

28. *See id.* at 97.

29. *See id.*

30. *See id.*

31. Although Medicare is a federal program administered by the Health Care Financing Administration (HCFA), within the federal Department of Health and Human Services, much of the day-to-day running of Medicare is carried out by private insurance companies under contract to HCFA. These companies, known as "fiscal intermediaries" (Part A) or "carriers" (Part B), process claims, and make coverage and payment decisions. For a more extended discussion see MARMOR, *supra* note 4, at 95–99.

32. *See id.*

33. *See* STARR, *supra* note 8, at 375–76.

34. *See id.*

35. *See id.*

36. *See supra* note 20 and accompanying text.

37. *See infra* notes 65–68 and accompanying text.

38. *See* MARMOR, *supra* note 4, at 97–99.

39. *See id.* at 98.

40. *See id.* (noting that the rate of physician fees more than doubled in the year between enactment of Medicare and its original operation).

41. *See* Marian Gornick et al., *Twenty Years of Medicare and Medicaid: Covered Populations, Use of Benefits, and Program Expenditures, in* HEALTH CARE FIN. REV. 13, 43 (Ann. Supp. 1985).

42. *See id.* at 36.

43. *See, e.g.,* THEODORE R. MARMOR ET AL., AMERICA'S MISUNDERSTOOD WELFARE STATE: PERSIS-TENT MYTHS, ENDURING REALITIES 178–85 (1990) (describing the change from the 1960s, where the lack of access to health care for portions of the population was viewed as the major concern of the American health care system, to the 1970s, where dramatically spiraling health care costs became the major concern).

44. *See id.* at 180.

45. *See id.* at 182–83 (discussing actions indicating the government's movement toward universal health insurance coverage).

46. *See id.* at 186–87 (explaining various reimbursement schemes such as increasing deductibles, co-insurance and cost sharing between employer and patient-employee, as well as increased use of health maintenance organizations (HMOs) and Preferred Provider plans to contain costs).

47. *See* 42 U.S.C. § 426(b) (1994) (extending Medicare coverage to certain people with disabilities who are under age 65); *Id.* § 426–1 (1994) (extending Medicare coverage to people under age 65 who suffer from end-stage renal disease).

48. Medicare was initially administered by the Bureau of Health Insurance within the Social Security Administration of the Department of Health, Education and Welfare. *See* Timothy S. Jost, *Governing Medicare,* 51 ADMIN. L. REV. 39, 86 (1999). In 1977, Congress created HCFA as a separate agency to administer Medicare. *See id.*

49. *See* MARMOR, *supra* note 4, at 17–21, 77–78 (discussing the growth of special interest groups arising from early cleavages within the Medicare debate).

50. *See* David S. Broder, *Major Reorganization Announced for HEW,* WASH. POST, Mar. 9, 1977, at A1.

51. *See* Matt Clark et al., *Health Care Battle,* NEWSWEEK, May 28, 1979, at 28, 29.

52. *See* James A. Morone & Theodore R. Marmor, *Representing Consumer Interests: The Case of American Health Planning, in* POLITICAL ANALYSIS AND AMERICAN MEDICAL CARE 76, 77 (Theodore R. Marmor ed., 1983); Theodore R. Marmor & Morris Barer, *The Politics of Universal Health Insurance: Lessons for and from the 1990s, in* HEALTH POLITICS AND POLICY, at 306, 309–10 (Theodor J. Litmar & Leonard S. Robins eds., 3d ed., 1997).

53. After the Carter administration's attempts to secure passage of legislation that explicitly regulated hospital costs was blocked, the hospital industry adopted a "voluntary effort" to control spending. This voluntary effort, however, was a disappointment in practice. *See* Mark A. Peterson, Interest Groups as Allies and Antagonists: Their Role in the Politics of Health Care Reform (1995) (unpublished manuscript, on file with author).

54. *See* Clark, *supra* note 51, at 29.

55. *See* Table 1, *infra* at 250.

56. *See id.*

57. *See* THEODORE R. MARMOR & JERRY L. MASHAW, SOCIAL SECURITY: BEYOND THE RHETORIC OF CRISIS 190 (1988).

58. *See* Jost, *supra* note 48, at 67–70.

59. *See id.*

60. *See id.*

61. With the enactment of the Social Security Amendments of 1983, Pub. L. No. 98–21, 97 Stat. 65 (1983), the manner in which hospitals were to be paid for providing services to Medicare beneficiaries was changed from a "reasonable cost" basis to a "prospective payment" system,

where the hospital would be paid a fixed amount depending upon the patient's diagnosis. For a detailed discussion of this change see generally David M. Frankford, *The Medicare DRGs: Efficiency and Organizational Rationality*, 10 YALE J. ON REG. 273 (1993).

62. *See* 42 U.S.C. § 1395w-4 (1988 & Supp. 1989).

63. *See* Figure 1, *infra* at 252; MARYLIN MOON, MEDICARE NOW AND IN THE FUTURE 19 (2d ed. 1996).

64. The point here is not that these measures were necessarily misguided or should have been avoided because of the increasingly zero-sum nature of the conflict they helped foster. Rather, it is simply that the heightened zero-sum politics created different, if quite predictable, conflicts than had been the case in the earlier period of accommodation.

65. *See* Henry J. Aaron & Robert D. Reischauer, *"Rethinking Medicare Reform" Needs Rethinking*, HEALTH AFF., Feb. 1998, at 69, 69.

66. *See* MARMOR, *supra* note 4, at 123.

67. *See generally* Lawrence R. Jacobs et al., *The Polls—Poll Trends: Medical Care in the United States—An Update*, 57 PUB. OPINION Q. 394 (1993) (giving the results of public opinion polls regarding health care issues in the 1992 presidential campaign).

68. The Medicare Catastrophic Coverage Act of 1988, Pub. L. No. 100-360, 102 Stat. 683, was enacted in June 1988, became effective on January 1, 1989, and was terminated on November 30, 1989, by the Medicare Catastrophic Repeal Act of 1989, Pub. L. No. 101-234, 103 Stat. 1979. For a discussion of this process and its effect on Washington policymakers, see generally RICHARD HIMELFARB, CATASTROPHIC POLITICS: THE RISE AND FALL OF THE MEDICARE CATASTROPHIC COVERAGE ACT OF 1988 (1995); PAUL LIGHT, STILL ARTFUL WORK (2d ed., 1995).

69. *See Point Counterpoint, At Issue: Would Bush Plan Gut Medicare Benefits?*, L.A. TIMES, Sept. 3, 1992, at A19.

70. Clinton said, "President Bush's budget would gut Medicare benefits, making 'elderly people and their children pay more for basic health care.'" *Id.*

71. *See* MARMOR, *supra* note 4, at 124.

72. *See* Cathleen Decker, *Bush's Cuts Aimed at Sick, Elderly, Clinton Charges*, L.A. TIMES, Sept. 2, 1992, at A6.

73. *See id.*

74. *See generally* JACOB HACKER, THE ROAD TO NOWHERE (1997) (discussing the development and policy choices of President Clinton's health reform proposal); THEDA SKOCPOL, BOOMERANG (1996) (analyzing the battle over the Clinton Health Security Act); Marmor & Barer, *supra* note 52, at 310–15.

75. Under the Republican proposal, Medicare beneficiaries would receive a voucher to purchase health insurance from the private insurance market, and this would replace the government-organized insurance Medicare currently provides. *See* Theodore Marmor & Jonathan Oberlander, *Rethinking Medicare Reform*, HEALTH AFF., Jan.–Feb. 1998, at 52, 53.

76. Balanced Budget Act of 1997, Pub. L. No. 105-33 § 4021, 111 Stat. 251, 347 (1997) (establishing a bipartisan commission charged with examining the Medicare program and making recommendations to strengthen and improve it for the future).

77. *See National Bipartisan Commission on the Future of Medicare* (visited May 12, 2000), http://thomas.loc.gov./medicare/index/transcripts.html [hereinafter *Medicare Comm'n Web Site*].

78. *See 1995 Annual Report to the Board of Trustees of the Federal Old-Age and Survivors Insurance and Disability Insurance Trust Funds* (visited May 12, 2000), http://www.ssa.gov/history/reports/trust/1995/trdoc.html. As described more fully *infra* at note 170, Part A of Medicare, like the Social Security program on which its financing was modeled, is funded through payroll taxes earmarked for an accounting trust fund. There are six "Medicare Trustees" who review that trust fund, and make annual reports to Congress.

79. In the language of the actuaries, that would take place when trust fund reserves would no longer be sufficient to pay the program's promised benefits. Projections by the trustees of impending trust fund insolvency have regularly triggered Medicare "crisis" talk. For an analysis of the regularity with which looming shortages in the Part A trust fund have translated into crisis responses by Medicare policymakers, see Jon Oberlander, Medicare and the American State (unpublished Ph.D. dissertation, Yale University 1995) (on file with UMI Dissertation Services, University of Michigan).

80. *See* Kenneth J. Cooper, *GOP's Medicare Pitch Faces a Tough Crowd on the Road*, WASH. POST, Aug. 15, 1995, at A1.

81. *See* Robert Dodge, *Republicans Push Vote on Senate Budget Plan, Democrats Force Delays*, DALLAS MORNING NEWS, Oct. 28, 1995, at 1A.

82. *See GOP Response Signals Bipartisan Cooperation*, ORLANDO SENTINEL, Dec. 29, 1996, at A1.

83. *See* Balanced Budget Act of 1997, Pub. L. No. 105–33, 111 Stat. 251.

84. *See* Bill Walsh, *Lott Endorses Market-Oriented Medicare Reform; Breaux Drops Push to Raise Eligibility Age*, TIMES-PICAYUNE, May 27, 1999, at A1.

85. *See* Robert Rosenblatt, *Medicare Panel Fails to Adopt Rescue Plan*, L.A. TIMES, Mar. 17, 1999 at A1. *See generally Medicare Comm'n Web Site, supra* note 77 (providing the Commission's final recommendations and transcripts of its hearings). Stalemate was made more likely by the Commission's ground rules requiring a super-majority (at least 11 of 17 members) to transmit a formal proposal to the Congress and the President. *See id.* With seven of the Democrats firmly opposed to the Breaux-Thomas plan, no such supporting coalition could be crafted. *See* Rosenblatt, *supra* at A1.

86. *See Editorial, Breaux Plan a Threat to Medicare*, OMAHA WORLD-HERALD, June 7, 1999, at 7.

87. *See id.*

88. *See* Joseph White, *"Saving" Medicare—From What?, in* UNDERSTANDING LONG-TERM MEDICARE COST ESTIMATES (2000).

89. *See* Marmor & Oberlander, *supra* note 75, at 54 (describing the politics and policy implications of voucher proposals); *see also* Aaron & Reischauer, *supra* note 65, at 69; Stuart M. Butler, *Medicare Price Controls: The Wrong Prescription*, HEALTH AFF., Jan.–Feb. 1998, at 72, 73.

90. *See* National Bipartisan Commission on the Future of Medicare, *Building a Better Medicare for Today and Tomorrow* (visited May 12, 2000), http://medicare.commission.gov/medicare/bbmtt31599.html; *see generally* Thomas Richard Oliver, *Conceptualizing the Challenges of Public Entrepreneurship, in* THE INTEGRATION OF PSYCHOLOGICAL PRINCIPLES IN POLICY DEVELOPMENT 5 (Chris E. Stout ed., 1996) (providing a comprehensive discussion of the role entrepreneurship has played in recent health care and Medicare reforms such as the Oregon Health Plan, the growth and expansion of HMOs and the growth and development of grass roots organizations).

91. *See* Ramón Castellblanch, *Medicare's Critical Condition*, IN THESE TIMES, May 2, 1999, at 12, 12.

92. *See* John F. Hams & Eric Pianin, *Parties Swap Fire on Medicare: Details of Plans Remain Hidden*, WASH. POST, July 26, 1995, at A4; Robert Pear, *Democrats Storm Out of Medicare Session*, N.Y. TIMES, Oct. 3, 1995, at A20; Eric Pianin & Judith Havemann, *Gingrich, Dole Attack Clinton Over Medicare Salvage Effort*, WASH. POST, May 3, 1995, at A6.

93. *See* Mark A. Peterson, *The Politics of Health Care Policy: Overreaching in an Age of Polarization, in* THE SOCIAL DIVIDE 181, 219 (Margaret Weir ed., 1998).

94. *See id.* at 190–91.

95. *See* Roger Hickey & Thomas Bodenheimer, *Vouchers Would Raise Costs: Breaux and Thomas May Argue that Competition Among Private Health Plans Will Control Costs. The Facts do not Support that Belief*, FT. LAUDERDALE SUN- SENTINEL, June 22, 1999, at 13A.

96. *See* Peterson, *supra* note 93, at 192–214 (discussing at length the Medicare reform debate between President Clinton and the GOP).

97. *See id.*

98. *See id.*

99. *See* Marmor & Oberlander, *supra* note 75, at 52.

100. *See* National Bipartisan Commission on the Future of Medicare, *Building a Better Medicare for Today and Tomorrow* (visited May 14, 2000), http://thomas.loc.gov/medicare/bbmtt31599.html.

101. Henry Aaron & Robert Reischauer, *The Medicare Reform Debate: What Is the Next Step?*, HEALTH AFF., Winter 1995, at 8.

102. *See id.*

103. *Id.* at 20.

104. *Id.* at 8.

105. *See id.*

106. *Id. at* 27–28.

107. *See id.* at 8.

108. *Id.*

109. *Id*

110. *Id. at* 8–9.

110. *Id.* at 8.

112. Public finance economists are well known for not consulting public opinion findings or qualitative work on social beliefs from anthropology or social psychology. *See* Theodore Marmor, *How We Got to Where We Are: American Health Care Politics, 1970 to 1990, in* UNDERSTANDING HEALTH CARE REFORM 28, 28–30 (Theodore Marmor ed., 1994).

113. *See* JACOBS, *supra* note 19, at 192–200; Jacobs et al., *supra* note 67, at 394–427. *See generally* Karlyn Bowman, *Public Opinion and Medicare Restructuring: Three Views, in* MEDICARE: PREPARING FOR THE CHALLENGES OF THE 21ST CENTURY 281 (Robert D. Reischauer et al. eds., 1998) (examining the significance of public support and public opposition to Medicare reforms).

114. Indeed, the public is remarkably willing to admit its lack of knowledge. For instance, a 1997 Washington Post/Kaiser Family Foundation/Harvard University poll found a full 53% of respondents willing to say they knew "very little" about Medicare. *See Public Agenda, Medicare: Red Flags* (visited Jan. 14, 1999), http://www.publicagenda.org/issues/red_flags_detail.cfm?issue_type=medicare&list=1&area=2.

115. *See* Section II of this Article.

116. *See* MARMOR, *supra* note 4, at 4–8.

117. *See id.* at 10–15.

118. *See* MARILYN MOON & JANEMARIE MULVEY, ENTITLEMENTS AND THE ELDERLY: PROTECTING PROMISES, RECOGNIZING REALITY 35, 89–127 (1996).

119. Aaron & Reischauer, *supra* note 101, at 9.

120. *See* Aaron & Reischauer, *supra* note 65, at 69.

121. *See* Marmor & Oberlander, *supra* note 75, at 59.

122. In fact, the *Journal of Health Policy, Politics and Law* devoted its entire October 1999 issue to the reasons for and implications of the managed care backlash. Readers interested in a wide range of scholarship devoted to the question of this backlash should read this issue. *See generally* 24 J. HEALTH POL., POL'Y & L. 860 (1999).

123. *See* Table 2 *infra* at 251, and Figure 2 *infra* at 253.

124. Another illustration of the ill-regard with which the public views the managed care industry comes from a 1998 Harris poll. In that poll, managed care firms ranked second from the bottom

in terms of the public's positive feelings about them. Who was the bottom-dweller in that survey? Tobacco companies. *See* Robert J. Blendon et al., *Understanding the Managed Care Backlash*, HEALTH AFF., July–Aug. 1998, at 80, 85; *see also* Lawrence R. Jacobs & Robert S. Shapiro, *The American Public's Pragmatic Liberalism Meets Its Philosophical Conservatism*, J. HEALTH POL., POL'Y & L. 1021, 1024–25 (1999); Kaiser Family Foundation, *National Survey on Medicare: The Next Big Policy Debate?* (visited May 16, 2000), http://www.kff.org/content/archive/1442/reform_cp.pdf [hereinafter *National Survey on Medicare*].

125. For further analysis, see generally the October 1999 issue of the *Journal of Health Politics, Policy and Law, supra* note 122. In particular, see the following articles in that issue: Mark A. Peterson, *Introduction: Politics, Misperception, or Apropos?*; Gail R. Wilensky, *What's Behind the Public's Backlash?*; and Lawrence R. Jacobs & Robert Y. Shapiro, *The American Public's Pragmatic Liberalism Meets Its Philosophical Conservatism. See also* Blendon et al., *supra* note 124, at 81.

126. *See* Table 2, *infra* at 251. When one considers the character of some of the other policy changes that the managed care backlash has helped produce, such as restrictions on insurers' ability to limit hospital stays after routine births, the odds increase that this alternative reaction will occur. *See* Eli Ginzberg & Miriam Ostrow, *Managed Care—A Look Back and a Look Ahead*, 336 NEW ENG. J. MED. 1018, 1018–20 (1997). Combine a general antipathy toward managed care firms with sympathetic target groups (new mothers, vulnerable patients) and the impulse toward restricting the practices of insurers fits with our general understanding of the ways in which lawmakers respond to public opinion. *See generally* R. DOUGLAS ARNOLD, THE LOGIC OF CONGRESSIONAL ACTION (1990) (discussing ways in which politicians anticipate and respond to the preferences of constituents and worry about the incidence of costs and benefits distributed across groups of voters). Despite the efforts of generational equity enthusiasts to paint the elderly as "greedy geezers," senior citizens remain, as a group, closer to the new mothers/vulnerable patients end of the scale than to the greedy insurers end. *See* Jacobs & Shapiro, *supra* note 124, at 1024–25; *National Survey on Medicare, supra* note 124.

127. Note that Medicare is still quite popular among even the youngest cohorts. To say that younger voters are *less* supportive of Medicare is not to say that they are *unsupportive* of it. Solid majorities remain for the program, even among young adults. As for the measures of skepticism about the program's future, it is harder to say what such expressions of doubt mean. After all, one may like a program and still have doubts about its future. In that sense, expressions of skepticism do not provide meaningful direction for policy-making in the way that expressions of support and opposition do. As Bowman has argued, concern about a program's future and talk of crisis may be "simply a way for people to say to their elected legislators: 'Pay attention. This issue is important to me.'" Bowman, *supra* note 113, at 283. With these caveats in mind, we simply note that young adults show up as *more* skeptical than older adults. But skepticism among the latter age group is easy to find in the survey data as well. What the skepticism means remains open to debate, a debate that in our view is unlikely to be resolved without richer data. For a recent study that reports greater skepticism among other younger cohorts, see generally Robert J. Blendon, *Public Opinion and Medicare Restructuring: Three Views, in* MEDICARE: PREPARING FOR THE CHALLENGES OF THE 21ST CENTURY, *supra* note 113, at 288, 288. He found, for instance, that the under 30 cohort was the only one in which a majority of individuals predicted bankruptcy for Medicare. *See id.* at 290.

128. It is also the case that neither the size nor the direction of the differences has operated in the past as the resentment advocates would claim. According to one scholar of public opinion and the elderly, based on survey data from the National Election Study through 1988, "the nonelderly were consistently more likely to say the federal government spends too little on Social Security and health care, Medicare, or care for the elderly." Laurie A. Rhodebeck, *The*

Politics of Greed? Political Preferences Among the Elderly, 55 J. POL. 342, 350 (1993). Given the increased conservatism of younger cohorts in recent years, we do not want to make too much of the patterns found by Rhodebeck. *See* Alan I. Abramowitz & Kyle L. Saunders, *Ideological Realignment in the U.S. Electorate*, 60 J. POL. 634, 634 (1998). It is enough for our purposes simply to note that, in the not too distant past, younger cohorts seemed perfectly willing to support programs for the elderly.

129. This is a common criticism of the "generational equity" arguments popularized by advocates such as the Concord Coalition. Norman Daniels has put the argument succinctly:

> Justice between age groups . . . is a problem best solved if we stop thinking of the old and the young as distinct groups. We age. The young become the old. As we age, we pass through institutions that affect our well-being at each stage of life, from infancy to very old age.

NORMAN DANIELS, AM I MY PARENTS' KEEPER? AN ESSAY ON JUSTICE BETWEEN THE YOUNG AND THE OLD 18 (1988). On the need to realize that social insurance systems simultaneously distribute income among particular age cohorts *and* over the life cycle of given individuals, see generally Theodore R. Marmor et al., *Social Security Politics and the Conflict Between Generations: Are We Asking the Right Questions?*, *in* SOCIAL SECURITY IN THE 21ST CENTURY 195 (Eric R. Kingson & James H. Schultz, eds., 1997).

130. "Narrow" in the sense that younger voters are taking into account only the Medicare taxes they pay and the non-existent Medicare benefits they currently receive, without factoring into their assessment the burden they might bear to meet their aged parents' medical care costs in the absence of Medicare. For an interesting examination of the degree to which preferences across generations fit with such self-interested expectations, see generally Susan A. MacManus, *Taxing and Spending Politics: A Generational Perspective*, 57 J. POL. 607 (1995).

131. For more detailed discussions of the differences between younger and older individuals, see generally CHRISTINE L. DAY, WHAT OLDER AMERICANS THINK: INTEREST GROUPS AND AGING POLICY (1990); Christine L. Day, *Older Americans' Attitudes Toward the Medicare Catastrophic Coverage Act of 1988*, 55 J. POL. 167 (1993); Rhodebeck, *supra* note 128.

132. *See* Kaiser Family Foundation, *National Survey on Medicare: The Next Big Health Policy Debate?* (visited Jan. 13, 2000), http://www.kff.org/content/archive/1442/reform_pr.html. The 1998 poll by the Kaiser Family Foundation/Harvard School of Public Health found consistent gaps in knowledge about specific aspects of Medicare when respondents were divided by age. *See id.* Individuals age 65 and above knew more about Medicare's details than did those under age 65. *See id.* The most dramatic difference concerned knowledge about Medicare's non-coverage of prescription drugs: 63% of those 65 and older knew that Medicare generally does not cover prescription drugs, while only 22% of the younger cohort knew this. *See id.* On other specifics, the differences between age groups were less dramatic, generally in the range of 10 points or so. *See id.*

133. On the tendency for elected leaders to take action in the face of "action forcing crises" in social insurance programs, see generally R. Douglas Arnold, *The Political Feasibility of Social Security Reform*, *in* FRAMING THE SOCIAL SECURITY DEBATE: VALUES, POLITICS, AND ECONOMICS 389–417 (R. Douglas Arnold et al., eds., 1998).

134. *See* Anthony Beilenson, *Leadership and Politics: Four Views*, *in* MEDICARE: PREPARING FOR THE CHALLENGES OF THE 21ST CENTURY, *supra* note 113, at 280, 285.

135. Given the benefits of specialization it is hardly surprising—and may even do some good—that economists tend to approach these questions by putting economics front and center. For a more extended discussion, see MARMOR, *supra* note 4, at 185–91.

136. *See* Marmor, *supra* note 112, at 28–30.

137. *See* Jacobs & Shapiro, *supra* note 125, at 1021; *see generally* Lawrence R. Jacobs & Robert Y. Shapiro, Politicians Don't Pander: Political Manipulations and the Loss of Democratic Responsiveness (2000) (arguing that politicians often produce—rather than respond to—public opinion, strategically manipulating polls and question wording to, in effect, create mass "preferences" consistent with their policy objectives).

138. *See* Oberlander, *supra* note 79.

139. *See id.*

140. One experienced public opinion analyst characterizes the available evidence on the public's support for vouchers this way: "A voucher system described in various ways in various polls seems to attract the support of about 30 percent of the population. It is not clear from the data I have seen exactly how firm that support is. Do these respondents reject the system we have now? Is the response simply a message to do something to save the system? Or is the 30 percent a measure of actual support for a voucher system or some alternative? I am not sure that we know the answers judging from the current questions in the public domain."
Bowman, *supra* note 113, at 285.

141. *See* Peterson, *supra* note 93, at 201–19.

142. *See generally* Marmor & Oberlander, *supra* note 75 (providing a fuller discussion of the many reasons not to support voucher plans); *see also* Aaron & Reischauer, *supra* note 101; Butler, *supra* note 89 (providing responses to Marmor and Oberlander's arguments and a defense of vouchers).

143. *See* Aaron & Reischauer, *supra* note 101, at 8.

144. *See* Marmor, *supra* note 43, at 216–18.

145. *See* Aaron & Reischauer, *supra* note 101, at 10.

146. *Id.* at 8.

147. *See* Robin Toner, *Health Care Autopsy: Plenty of Targets to Blame for Failure*, Phoenix Gazette, Sept. 27, 1994, at A1.

148. *See* Robin Toner, *The Hard Lessons of Health Reform*, N.Y. Times, July 4, 1999, at § 4, 1.S.

149. 1256, 105th Cong. (1999).

150. *See* Sean Wilentz, *For Voters, the 60's Never Died*, N.Y. Times, Nov. 16, 1999, at A27.

151. *See generally* John W. Kingdon, Agendas, Alternatives, and Public Policies (1984) (discussing how political agendas depend on a confluence of problem recognition, policy solutions and political conditions); Frank R. Baumgartner & Bryan D. Jones, Agendas and Instability in American Politics (1993) (proposing a punctuated equilibrium model of policy change, tracing the history of policy change in 20th century America, and analyzing the long-term changes in the structures and context of American political institutions).

152. *See* Baumgartner & Jones, *supra* note 151, at 57.

153. *See generally* Theodore R. Marmor, *Forecasting American Health Care: How We Got Here and Where We Might be Going*, 23 J. Health Pol., Pol'y & L. 551 (1998) (providing a more extensive discussion of the dangers of forecasting).

154. *See* Marmor, *supra* note 43, at 136–38.

155. *See* Figure 2, *infra* at 253; Henry J. Aaron, Thinking About Aging: What We Know, What We Can't Know, and Why It Matters (Feb. 15, 1999) (unpublished manuscript, on file with author).

156. For similar points about the consequences of Medicare's complex environment, see Jerome P. Kassirer, *Managing Managed Care's Tarnished Image*, 337 New Eng. J. Med. 338–39 (1997), and Aaron, *supra* note 155.

157. Aaron, *supra* note 155, at 16; *see also id.* at 20–21.

158. For a similar point about the misuse of long-range projections, *see id.* at 7–10, 15–17.

159. *See* Marmor, *supra* note 4, at 189–91.

160. *See* Moon, *supra* note 63, at 19.

161. See Marilyn Moon, Beneath the Averages: An Analysis of Medicare and Private Expenditures (visited Mar. 13, 2000), http://www.kff.org/content/1999/1505/Moonbeneath.pdf.
162. *See* MOON, *supra* note 63, at 19.
163. Doubts about policymakers mustering the political will required to impose fiscal discipline on the program through marginal adjustments stand curiously at odds with radical reformers' strong faith in these same policymakers' willingness to summon the political courage to make fundamental changes to the program's design.
164. *See* Remarks on Returning without Approval to the House of Representatives the "Taxpayer Refund and Relief Act of 1999," 35 WEEKLY COMP. PRES. DOC. 1793 (Sept. 23, 1999).
165. *See President Touts Successes in Remarks to LR Chamber*, ARK. DEMOCRAT-GAZETTE, Dec. 12, at A21.
166. There is an irony to this development. The same social-insurance financing of hospital services that was so critical to gaining political support for Medicare in the first place has, through its artifact, the trust fund, become one of its greatest political vulnerabilities and the nominal foundation to support the attacks of the program's harshest critics. *See generally* MARMOR, *supra* note 4 (describing further the ironies of the political evolution of Medicare's trust fund); *see also* Oberlander, *supra* note 79. *But see* Eric Patashnik & Julian Zelizer, Paying for Medicare: Benefits, Budgets, and Wilbur Mills's Policy Legacy (1999) (unpublished manuscript, on file with author) (disputing the view that this development is an ironic legacy of the trust fund device). Patashnik and Zelizer argue instead that fiscal conservatives understood the implications of the trust fund mechanism from inception, and its ability to impose discipline on Medicare's budget was crucial to their willingness to support the program. *See id.*
167. Another analogy is useful here. When the U.S. declares war, no one shouts that the Department of Defense is going to run out of money. There is, of course, debate over the wisdom of the military engagement and disputes over the willingness of Congress to pay for the additional war-related expenses. However, no one would contend that the increased expenses due to a new military engagement will "cause" the Department of Defense to become bankrupt.
168. *See* ERIC M. PATASHNIK, PUTTING TRUST IN THE FEDERAL BUDGET: TRUST FUNDS, TAXES, AND THE EVOLUTION OF POLICY INHERITANCES (2000).
169. *See, e.g.,* MURRAY EDELMAN, THE SYMBOLIC USES OF POLITICS (1964) (exploring the symbolic processes underlying political claims); CHARLES ELDER & ROGER COBB, THE POLITICAL USES OF SYMBOLS (1983) (examining the importance of symbols as a basis for political activity); Gary J. McKissick, Defining Choices: Interest Group Lobbying and the Framing of Policy Alternatives (2000) (unpublished manuscript, on file with author).
170. The oddity of worrying about a Medicare bankruptcy is also apparent when one considers the different political responses to the funding shortfalls for Medicare's hospitalization coverage (Part A), on the one hand, and the shortfalls for its coverage for physician services (Part B), on the other. Hospitalization insurance alone is financed by payroll taxes earmarked for Medicare's Part A trust fund. This is a mechanism designed explicitly to echo the same social-insurance principles as Social Security pensions. In contrast, when physician services were tacked on as Part B of the 1965 Medicare bill, physician expenses were to be financed by premium payments from current beneficiaries and by general federal tax revenues. Because general tax revenues can only run *short*, but not *out*, projected shortfalls in paying for physician services have simply been covered by additional general revenues, by increased premiums, or by cutbacks in expenditures. As a consequence, there have never been Medicare-Part-B crises of the form associated with Part A. It is only the projected shortfalls in the hospital trust fund that have triggered the recurrent crises over Medicare and the use of bankruptcy language. Thus, the experience with the trust fund demonstrates how important the funding mechanisms can be for the politics of a program. In that sense, the use of a trust fund is more than an accounting term of art. It has very real political implications and consequences. *See* Oberlander, *supra*

note 79, for a cogent discussion of the different "crisis" politics of Medicare's component parts, and PATASHNIK *supra* note 168, for an insightful analysis of the politics of government trust funds.

171. What should one expect from those expert on the details of Medicare's programmatic operation who commit the conceptually distinct sin of leaving out political analysis altogether? For this sin of omission, the answer is this: a clear acknowledgement of the limitations of such assessments for the purposes of either predicting Medicare's future or prescribing reforms at any particular time. Such work makes a valuable contribution in providing such careful attention to the programmatic details of Medicare's history. Nevertheless, the caution about limits remains.

From Church to Garage

Rudolf Klein

The world into which the National Health Service was born in 1948 no longer exists. The half century that separated the installation of Clement Attlee and Tony Blair as Labour Prime Ministers, in 1945 and 1997 respectively, witnessed a transformation in the social, economic and political environment of the NHS. The industries nationalised in the Attlee years have been sold off. Britain's class and industrial structure has changed dramatically; the new economy is based not on digging coal or building cars or ships but on services and information technology. Real incomes per head have more than doubled: the era of post-war austerity has given way to a flamboyant consumerism. The credit card culture has replaced the piggy-bank culture. Although Britain has not become a more egalitarian society, as many hoped in the flush of post-war optimism, its people have become much better housed, better educated and better able to make their own life-style decision. With greater resources, and infinitely greater access to information, the sphere of personal autonomy has expanded for most (though by no means all) of the population: the ability to make choices has, to an extent which would have astonished in 1945 or 1950, been democratised. In turn, there has been a transformation in the assumptive world of policy makers. The commitment to collectivism and faith in central planning that marked the Attlee epoch—and shaped the NHS—have both gone. A new public philosophy—certainly more sceptical about the role of the State and perhaps more individualistic—has emerged.

Not only has the environment of the NHS altered dramatically. So has the role of the NHS itself, for reasons that have little or nothing to do with decisions of Ministers about its funding, organisation or structure. The pattern of demand for health care and the technology of medicine have both changed.[1] On the one hand, coronary heart disease and cancer have become the new epidemics, largely displacing infectious diseases, while chronic degenerative conditions like arthritis and dementia have become ever more significant in an ageing population. On the other hand, new drugs and innovations in surgery and diagnostic equipment have not only revolutionised medical practice but have also created possibilities of treatment where there were none before. Long hospital stays belong to the past while drop-in repairs are the new reality: 80 per cent of operations are done as day cases. The point is obvious enough. But it has been stressed because it underlines the fact that much government policy making is a response to challenges or opportunities created by the process of continuously evolving practice at the coal face of the NHS. Like other health care systems, the NHS has its own momentum and rhythm: Ministers waving their conductor's baton can exhort the brass to blare out more loudly or tell the strings to make the *allegro* more *furioso*, but they don't write the score when it comes to medical practice.

Nor does the importance of changes endogenous to the NHS end there. More than half the graduates from medical school are women and, whether as a result or not, attitudes within the medical profession are changing. The rising generation of doctors see medicine as a career rather than a vocation, are more inclined than their elders to regard medicine as a job like any other and believe that work should be organised to balance career and family life.[2] They also accept corporate responsibility for their colleagues and are ready to share responsibility for patient care with other health professionals.[3] At the same time the balance between different health professionals is shifting, in recognition that the delivery of health care is a team effort. In the emergent health care system, it has been argued, "nursing is the key profession."[4] While nurses have been significant absentees on the scene of high politics, they are key players in the micro-politics of day to day life in hospitals and community care. If government sponsored changes in professional regulation over the past 20 or so years have encountered less opposition than might have been expected from the early history of the NHS, it is at least in part because the professions themselves have changed.

To emphasise the transformation in the NHS's environment, and within it, is also to suggest that what needs explaining is less the series of radical changes introduced first by the Conservative Government of Mrs. Thatcher and then by Tony Blair than the fact that its defining features have survived unscathed in the process. It remains a tax-financed, universal service where health care is available free to all at the point of delivery. The waves of change have swirled around the NHS but have not swept it away. An institution that often seemed to be a national problem—its history punctuated by crises and prophecies of impending collapse—has survived as a national treasure. Public support remains rock solid: political parties compete to proclaim their faith in the service and their role as guardians of its future.

For Old Labour believers in Creationism this is not, of course, a puzzle. The NHS's survival, and its unique place in the hearts of the British people, is seen as testimony to the wisdom of the founding fathers. Institutions not only reflect the values of the time that gave birth to them but also shape the values of the future. In symbolising the commitment to social solidarity of the post-war era, the NHS has helped to perpetuate that commitment. If the NHS often failed to deliver the goods—if long since it ceased to be the envy of the world—it was simply because it had been under-funded over the decades:[5] an argument which, however, begs the question of why the founding fathers had devised a funding system which institutionalised parsimony for most of the NHS's existence. For New Labour (and other) believers in Evolution, this is at best a partial truth. For them the survival of the NHS is contingent on adaptation to a changing external and internal environment: the battle for public support is a continuing one. The believers in Intelligent Design see the NHS as a church; the believers in Evolution see it as a garage.[6] The different elements, and characteristics, of the two models of the NHS are summed up in Table 1.

The model of the health care as a secular church represents the tradition maintained and carefully tended over the decades by the disciples of Aneurin Bevan, the Minister responsible for the 1948 design of the NHS: indeed it was one of those disciples, Barbara Castle, who explicitly invoked the religious metaphor. Creating the NHS was seen as an act of social communion, celebrating the fact that all citizens were equal in the sight of a doctor.[7] But it was also a model based on the assumption that it would be the doctor who would

Table 1: The Competing Models

Model 1: health care as church	Model 11: health care as garage
Paternalism	Consumerism
Planning	Responsiveness
Need	Demand
Priorities	Choice
Trust	Contract
Universalistic	Pluralistic
Stability	Adaptability

determine who should get what. The vision informing the design of the NHS was as much one of technocratic rationality as one of social justice. Indeed technocratic rationality was equated with social justice. It was the experts who would determine needs, frame priorities accordingly and implement their policies universalistically throughout the NHS. The model was based on trust: the professionals working in the NHS would, it was assumed, put the interests of patients before their own and quality would be assured by the dedication of doctors, nurses and others.

The alternative model of health care as a garage has never been articulated as clearly or explicitly. It is implicit, however, in the invocation of a patient-driven NHS and the design of a mimic market for health care. In this model decisions are driven not by experts but by consumer preferences: the body is taken in for repair by its owner who retains control over what happens to it. The ability to choose between garages becomes crucial, as does access to information about how the garages perform. Given the multiple preferences of consumers, diversity of provision is to be encouraged. Choice and competition will, in turn, lead to greater responsiveness (as well as efficiency). Professional providers cannot be trusted to be selfless altruists, so appropriate incentives and quality tests are required.[8] Consumer sovereignty, however, is also seen as carrying consumer responsibilities: the garage model implies a responsibility for looking after our bodies, in the same way as we look after our cars—hence an emphasis on self-care and the importance of leading healthier lives.

Like all models, these over-simplify a complex reality. The evolution of model 1 into model 11 has not only been gradual but also partial. The NHS's centre of gravity has indeed shifted from paternalism to consumerism, from need to demand, from planning to choice. Equally, the decision-making system of the NHS has shifted over the decades from relying primarily on collegial control by professionals to one based on bureaucratic, hierarchic control, which in turn has yielded to a more market-orientated approach.[9] But in no case has the shift been complete. National priorities continue to be proclaimed; hierarchic control has not ceased. Paternalism has migrated from the health service to health promotion: there may be more choice about where to go for treatment but there is less choice about where to smoke. Above all, policies are still shaped by the values that gave birth to the NHS as an instrument of social justice. The policies of the Blair Government can therefore best be described as an attempt to combine the best features of the church with the most attractive characteristics of a garage: to design, as it were, a drive-in church.

The next section briefly sets out the evolution of policy under the Blair Government. The following section asks to what extent New Labour policies reflected the special circumstances of the NHS—and British politics—as distinct from trends common to all health care systems in rich countries.

THE DRIVE-IN CHURCH MODEL

A dispassionate analysis of the Conservative legacy to Labour in 1997 might have suggested that the main lesson to be drawn was that implementing radical change in an organisation as complex as the NHS was invariably much more difficult than anticipated. The internal market model for the NHS—as set out in Mrs. Thatcher's 1989 White Paper, *Working for Patients*[10]—involved the separation of the purchaser and provider roles, the introduction of competition between providers and was critically contingent on radical improvements in the NHS's financial information system as well as in its managerial culture and capacities. In the event, therefore, implementation was both cautious and partial. An analysis of the (somewhat limited) evidence about the impact of the new model suggested that both its advocates and its critics had over-stated their case.[11] The changes were neither as transformative as the advocates of change had hoped nor as perverse in their impact as the prophets of disaster had predicted. Nevertheless, Labour's first impulse on coming into office was, in line with the party's uncompromising denunciation of Mrs. Thatcher's proposals, to kill the internal market.

The obituary took the shape of a new White Paper, *The New NHS: Modern-Dependable*,[12] published in 1997. Some of the changes introduced by the Conservatives—such as the purchaser/provider split—were indeed retained. But co-operation, not competition, was to mark the NHS in future. In an unconscious echo of the paternalist language of the founding fathers, the White Paper proclaimed that "Local doctors and nurses who are in the best position to know what patients need will be in the driving seat in shaping services." That was not to be, however. The NHS church was not going to be run by the parish priests, far less the congregation, but from the centre. The next few years were marked by the creation of a command and control structure, unprecedented in the history of the NHS, based on centrally determined targets and rigorous performance management. Old Labour hearts could rejoice: the faith of the 1940s in central planning and technocratic rationality still appeared to be alive.

Come the next century, however, and New Labour pragmatics replaced Old Labour faith. A commitment to increasing spending on the NHS dramatically led, in turn, to a search for ways of ensuring that the extra money would be spent efficiently and effectively. It was a search that led the Government to re-invent, step by step, the internal market.[13] Only this time it was to be a far more sophisticated, far more completely thought-through system. And it would, moreover, be a system driven by consumers. The patient, not the doctor, was to be in the driving seat. If there was to be real competition, there had to be more capacity in the system: so the extra funds pouring into the NHS were used to attract new, for-profit providers. If providers were to be sensitive to what purchasers wanted, then money had to follow patients: so a new system of payment by results, using a modified DRG formula, was introduced. If consumer preferences were to shape the NHS, then patients had to be free to choose where to be treated: so patients would not only be free to choose between competing providers but would also be provided with information about their performance. Not only had Mrs. Thatcher's model been resurrected but it was being implemented in more radical and rigorous way, even though policy practice as always often lags behind policy rhetoric and unresolved tensions remain.

No longer will the NHS be unique among European health care systems in the degree of its centralisation. Instead, Ministers will be insulated from responsibility for the day to day operations of the service by a battery of regulators, while still setting national priorities. No longer will the collective funding of health care require the collective ownership of provision. Instead, there is to be a plurality of diverse providers, with choice and competition providing the dynamic of what remains a universal system providing comprehensive care. Technocratic paternalism has given way to consumerism in a mimic market. The objectives of policy have not changed. The emphasis on seeing the health care system as an instrument of social justice, with much emphasis on tackling inequalities in health outcomes, remains. But the means for achieving them have changed radically. A halting process of policy improvisation and discovery has seemingly produced a new model with a compelling logic of its own: a transformation of the NHS mirroring the transformation of society noted at the beginning of this chapter and mirroring also New Labour policies in other policy areas, notably education.

POLICY MAKING IN AN INTERNATIONAL CONTEXT

Explaining the evolution of health care policy in England in terms of the special characteristics of the NHS and the national political system carries a danger. It is that the account will fall into the trap of ethnocentric over-explanation. What if all health care systems in rich countries are moving in the same direction? Would this not suggest that policy is being driven by the dynamics of health care—the effects of the ever expanding technology of medicine, compounded by demography as populations everywhere age—rather than country specific institutional or political factors? To address these questions, this article therefore looks briefly at the international experience.

There are indeed common themes, just as there are common pressures, across most if not all the rich countries of the West. With ever increasing levels of spending on health care, the preoccupation with making the system more efficient and effective is universal. The twin concepts of choice and competition, "the master myth of modern societies,"[14] appear to be guiding policy makers in Europe and the United States, pushing them in the same direction. Reform of health care systems has become an international phenomenon. For example, Germany, the Netherlands and Sweden are among the countries to have adapted their systems to widen choice and competition since the 1990s.[15] Other themes, too, have crossed frontiers. There has been a trend towards devolution, as in the case of Italy and Spain. There has been increasing emphasis almost everywhere on putting primary care in the driver's seat.[16] Many of the same policy instruments, too, have been introduced: for instance, systems of payments to hospitals adapted from the American DRG (diagnostically related groups) model have spread through Europe. So what, if anything, is different about Britain?

In answering this question, the most important to note is that the convergence of countries towards a common, market-like model is more apparent than real.[17] The vocabulary of policy discussion may be much the same, but the meaning of the words depends on national context.[18] For example, the Dutch and the Germans (like most other West European nations) have long enjoyed free choice of doctors and hospitals under their social insurance models of health care. The new element introduced in those countries was choice of insurer. The expectation was that insurance funds competing for subscribers would have an incentive to keep their subscription rates down and to exert pressure on health care providers to cut costs, as well as tailoring the packages on offer to the preferences of consumers. The case of Sweden is rather different. Its publicly funded, universal system is first cousin to Britain's NHS, albeit based on local government. In Sweden, in contrast to the Netherlands and Germany, choice of doctor was conspicuous by its absence until the 1990s when patients were given the right to choose their primary care physician and some county councils gave patients the option of seeking care from public or private providers outside their area if their local hospital could not offer treatment within three months, with money following the patient. Nor has change been a one-way street.[19] In France, where traditionally there has been almost unlimited choice of both primary care physicians and specialists, policy has switched to introducing financial incentives designed to encourage patients to sign up with a specific GP and to limit their choice of specialists.

So the notion that Britain is simply being swept along by an irresistible, universal wave of change does not stand up to scrutiny. Shared concerns do not necessarily mean shared solutions; the march of medical technology and the geriatrification of society do not compel the adoption of a particular model of health care. Even within Britain, following devolution, health care policy-making in Scotland and Wales has followed a divergent path from that pursued in England despite the shared framework of the NHS.[20] Local politics and local culture clearly matter, a point further explored below. But so do the ideas in good currency—the assumptive world of Ministers and civil servants—that feed into policy-making. And in this respect there is indeed good reason to think that the policies pursued by successive British Governments reflect international trends. No account of the evolution of NHS policy in Britain can ignore the globalisation of ideas that has taken place over the past decades, a phenomenon which has little or nothing to do with the specific circumstances of health care systems. The consequent transformation of the world of ideas is at least as important as the transformation in the social, economic and political context of the NHS in explaining the direction of change if not the precise form of that change.

The new, international language of policy discourse is heavily accented by economic theory. Its vocabulary is that of incentives, choice and competition. It is the language of international institutions like the World Bank and the Organisation for Economic Co-operation and Development (OECD), whose analyses and recommendations span the whole range of government activity— from economic management to health care. It is also a language with a strong American accent. To the extent that many of its leading exponents are American economists (or European economists trained in the United States), so it is an instrument for exporting American-style analysis and prescription: the role of Alain Enthoven, who introduced the notion of an internal market to British audiences, is a case in point. But, as the example of Alain Enthoven also shows, intellectual influence does not necessarily translate into policy output: the internal market that actually evolved under Mrs. Thatcher was very different from that which he had envisaged and bore the imprint of a wide range of institutional and political factors. Again, therefore, it must be stressed that none of the international trends identified—whether demography, medical technology or intellectual change—*determine* policy. The new language of discourse certainly enlarged the repertory of options and instruments for policy makers, probably affected the way in which they interpret the world around them and perhaps also imparted a bias towards economistic, market-style solutions, but it did not dictate their decisions: free will still reigned, as the variations in national policies underline.

How to explain those variations? The role of ideology, and competition between parties of the Left and Right, was much invoked to explain differences in the original design of health care systems. However, change (or its absence) in mature systems calls for a somewhat different explanatory strategy. Here an ever expanding academic industry provides a number of competing tools of understanding.[21] Dominating much analysis is the notion of path dependency,[22] the notion that the structure of institutions—in the widest sense to include the norms of policy making—and interests created at one point in time will constrain future policy choices. History matters. The difficulty is that this theory is better at explaining policy inertia than at helping us to understand policy change. Enter the notion of "windows of opportunity."[23] These open when Governments with a new policy agenda, forged perhaps under economic pressure, come into office. Mrs. Thatcher's reform of the NHS provides a neat example; Tony Blair's commanding parliamentary majority provides another, less neat, case since he could have used the size of that majority to maintain the *status quo*. When the windows open, the entrepreneurs of new ideas can seize the opportunity. Other institutional factors may still frustrate them. In countries such as France or Germany where the legislative system has many veto points or where there is a tradition of policy making through consensus—so allowing interest groups like the medical profession to block or modify initiatives— change may be more difficult, and certainly slower, to achieve.[24] Conversely, countries with a Westminster-style constitution, where Governments can use their majorities to ram legislation through the legislature, offer fewer obstacles: Britain and New Zealand are cases in point, both offering examples of a rapid cycle of change.

But there is an all-important difference between explaining why change does or does not take place and explaining the actual nature of the policies that are or are not adopted. Here the model of policy as a learning process is helpful.[25] This sees policy making as puzzle solving: a quasi-experimental strategy, with policy makers learning from both success and failure. Inherited institutions define the landscape within which those policy experiments take place: perceived problems and possible solutions will be different in a tax-funded, centralised system like the NHS from those in a social-insurance based, pluralistic system like Germany's, in a system which is considered to be under-funded from one which is seen as over spending. But while institutions may constrain policy choices, they leave space for autonomous decision making by policy makers: were it not so, there would be no scope for political debate about the course of action to be taken and policy would be on automatic pilot. What policy makers learn, and the implications they draw, depends on who they are: the lenses through which they see the world. Thus the lessons which Frank Dobson, the first Secretary of State for Health in the Blair Administration, drew from his experience of running the NHS were very different from those of his successor, Alan Milburn, as Old Labour lenses were replaced by New Labour ones.

The learning process also has an international dimension.[26] An explosion in the availability of comparative information about health care systems has meant that "learning about other countries is rather like breathing—only the brain dead are likely to avoid the experience."[27] But until the 1980s the experience of other countries tended to reinforce complacency about the NHS: no other country appeared to have a health care system which delivered universal, comprehensive health care as parsimoniously as the NHS. While other countries appeared to be on an unstoppable escalator of rising spending, the NHS was a model of successful cost-containment. When civil servants were sent to look at alternative systems of funding health care in Europe, as they were from time to time, they brought back the reassuring message that the disadvantages of social insurance outweighed the claimed advantages. So what was there to be learnt, apart from the fact that the British system was the best? From the 1980s onward, however, the Department of Health became "much more willing to learn from others," in the words of its former Chief Economic Adviser.[28] By the turn of the millennium, international comparisons were used not for self-congratulation but for self-criticism, as we have seen. In making the case for investing more in the NHS, the Wanless Inquiry (set up by the Treasury to review the spending level) asked the question of 'How does the UK match up to other countries?" The answer was that, in important respects, the standards of the NHS—as measured by outcomes—were below those achieved in many European countries.[29] International comparisons had helped to turn the NHS's fabled virtue—parsimony—into a vice: "A new mechanism for the upward ratcheting of health expenditure had been born."[30]

Not only did the experience of other countries provide benchmarks against which the performance of the NHS would be measured. It also fed into the process of developing new policy instruments. When the Department of Health set about devising its payment by results scheme, it looked to the lessons to be drawn from those countries which were already operating such a system. Similarly, when it was designing its Performance Assessment Framework—a set of indicators and targets against which providers could be scored—it looked at the methods developed in the United States to compare the performance of health plans. And there were many other such examples. Further, international experience widened the menu of policy options. For example, from Sweden came the notion of NHS trusts imposing financial penalties on local government social services if the latter were responsible for late discharges from hospital. Such direct transplants were very much the exception, however. More usually, and perhaps more importantly, knowledge of other health care systems served to underline the singularity of the NHS and to extend the range of ministerial thinking about alternative futures. So when Milburn announced his conversion to devolution, and the launch of Foundation Trusts—a new organisational form which gave providers a semi autonomous status—he invoked the example of other European countries, pointing out that the NHS was unique in the degree of centralisation and the uniformity of its ownership of providers: plurality of provision was the norm.[31]

Interpreting the experience of other countries was not, of course, a straightforward matter. For example, there was much interest in the performance of Kaiser Permanente, a United States health maintenance organisation, following the publication of an analysis in 2002 which showed that it had hospital admission and utilisation rates well below those of the NHS and thus appeared to provide better value for money.[32] In turn, this prompted a rush of policy makers to California to dig in the statistics and investigate how this had been achieved. The Director of the Department of Health's Strategy Unit concluded that the NHS could indeed learn much from "Kaiser's integrated approach . . . and the leadership provided by doctors in developing and supporting this model of care."[33] But it was less than self-evident precisely *how* the Kaiser model could be translated into the very different context of the NHS or indeed what lessons should be drawn from it. Was the lesson that primary and secondary care should be integrated—and, if so, did this mean that Primary Care Trusts should take over hospitals or that hospitals should expand into primary care?[34] Or did the key to Kaiser's success lie in its organisational structure, and the sense of ownership this gave doctors?[35]

International experience thus rarely spoke without ambiguity, all the more so since few of the reforms and models had been rigorously evaluated in their countries of origin. It was used selectively by Ministers and other policy makers. It influenced the design of policy instruments, not policy goals. It provided not so much lessons—i.e. clear messages about what ought to be done—as prompts to the policy imagination. Its influence was mostly indirect and perhaps all the more powerful as a result: it helped to shape the lessons which Ministers drew from their own experience of running the NHS by challenging the assumption that everything that was unique about the NHS was also necessarily desirable.

Notes

1. For a history of the NHS which analyses the impact of changes in medical practice and technology, see Geoffrey Rivett, *From Cradle to Grave*, King's Fund: London 1998.
2. Isobel Allen, *Committed but Critical: An Examination of Young Doctors' Views of Their Core Values*, British Medical Association: London 1997.
3. *Health Policy and Economic Research Unit, Professional Values*, British Medical Association: London 1995.
4. Nick Black, "Rise and Demise of the Hospital: A Reappraisal of Nursing," *British Medical Journal*, Vol. 331, 10 December 2005, pp. 1394–1396.
5. This is roughly the view taken by Charles Webster, *The Health Service Since the War*, vols. 1 and 2. The Stationery Office: London 1988 and 1996.
6. Rudolf Klein, *The Goals of Health Policy: Church or Garage* in Anthony Harrison (ed.), *Health Care UK, 1992/93*, King's Fund Institute: London 1993.
7. For the most eloquent exposition of this view, see Richard M. Titmuss, *The Gift Relationship*, Allen & Unwin: London 1970.
8. For an analysis of the challenge to the Titmuss view, see Rudolf Klein, "The great transformation," *Health Economics, Policy & Law*, Vol. 1, No. 1, 2006, pp. 91–98.
9. Carolyn Tuohy, *Accidental Logics*, Oxford University Press: New York 1999.
10. Secretaries of State for Health, Wales, Northern Ireland and Scotland, *Working for Patients*, HMSO: London 1989, Cm. 555.
11. Julian Le Grand, Nicholas Mays and Jo-Ann Mulligan eds., *Learning from the NHS Internal Market: A Review of the Evidence*, King's Fund: London 1998.
12. Secretary of State for Health, *The New NHS: Modern-Dependable*, The Stationery Office: London 1997, Cm. 3807.
13. Rudolf Klein, "The Troubled Transformation of Britain's National Health Service," *New England Journal of Medicine*, Vol. 355, 4 July 2006, 27 July 2006, pp. 409–415.
14. Donald Light, "Sociological Perspectives on Competition in Health Care," *Journal of Health Politics, Policy and Law*, Vol. 25, No. 5, October 2000, pp. 969–974.
15. For surveys of recent developments across a clutch of countries, on which this account draws, see the special issues of *Health Economics*, Vol. 14, No. S1, September 2005, and *Journal of Health Politics, Policy and Law*, Vol. 30, Nos. 1/2, February/April 2005.
16. Richard Saltman, Anna Rico and Wienke Boerma, eds., *Primary Care in the Driver's Seat*, Open University Press: Buckingham 2005.
17. Alan Jacobs, "Seeing Difference: Market Health Reform in Europe," *Journal of Health Politics, Policy and Law*, Vol. 23, No. 1, February 1998, pp. 1–33.
18. Ted Marmor, Kieke Okma and Richard Freeman eds., *Comparative Studies and the Politics of Modern Medical Care*, Yale University Press: New Haven, 2009.
19. Adam Oliver, "Inconsistent Objectives—Random Reflections on Health Care Policy Developments in Europe," Mimeo, London School of Economics: London, February 2006.
20. Scott L. Greer, *Territorial Politics and Health Policy*, Manchester University Press: Manchester 2005.
21. For an excellent analysis of the competing theories of explanation, and their application to the NHS, see Ian Greener, "Understanding NHS Reform: The Policy-Transfer, Social Learning and Path-Dependency Perspectives," *Governance*, Vol. 15, No. 2, April 2002, pp. 161–183.

22. The notion of path dependency, or historical institutionalism as it is styled in one of its forms, has many interpretations: see Adam Oliver and Elias Mossialos, "European Health Systems Reforms: Looking Backward to See Forward?" *Journal of Health Politics, Policy and Law*, Vol. 30, Nos. 1/2, February/April 2005, pp. 7–28. My use of the terms follows Carolyn Tuohy, *Accidental Logics*, Oxford University Press: New York, 1999.

23. John W. Kingdon, *Agendas, Alternatives and Public Policies*, Little, Brown: Boston, 1984.

24. Ellen M. Immergut, *Health Politics: Interests and Institutions in Western Europe*, Cambridge University Press: Cambridge, 1992.

25. Hugh Heclo, *Modern Social Politics in Britain and Sweden*, Yale University Press: New Haven, 1974.

26. For an authoritative survey of this topic, see Ted Marmor, Richard Freeman and Kieke Okma, "Comparative perspectives and Policy Learning in the World of Health Care," *Journal of Comparative Policy Analysis*, Vol. 7, No. 4, December 2005, pp. 331–348.

27. Rudolf Klein, "Learning from Others: Shall the Last Be the First?" *Journal of Health Politics, Policy and Law*, Vol. 22, No. 5, October 1997, pp. 1267–1278.

28. Clive Smee, *Speaking Truth to Power*, Radcliffe Publishing: Oxford, 2005. See Chapter 11. My analysis draws heavily on this insider account. See also M. Exworthy and R. Freeman, "The United Kingdom: Health Policy Learning in the NHS," chapter in Marmor, Okma and Freeman, 2007, *op.cit.*

29. Derek Wanless, *Securing our Future Health: Taking a Long-Term View, Interim Report*, HM. Treasury: London, November 2001. See Chapter 5.

30. Smee, 2005, *op.cit.*, p. 178.

31. Secretary of State for Health, *Redefining the National Health Service*, Speech to the New Health Network, Department of Health: London, 15 January 2002.

32. Richard G. A. Feachem, Neelam K.Sekhri and Karen L. White, "Getting More for Their Dollars: A Comparison of the NHS with California's Kaiser Permanente," *British Medical Journal*, Vol. 324, 19 January 2002, pp. 135–141.

33. Chris Ham, Nick York, Steve Sutch and Rob Shaw, "Hospital Bed Utilisation in the NHS, Kaiser Permanente and the US Medicare Programme: Analysis of Routine Data," *British Medical Journal*, Vol. 327, 29 November 2003, pp. 1257–1260.

34. Richard G. A. Feachem and Neelam K.Sekhri, "Moving Towards True Integration?" *British Medical Journal*, Vol. 330, 2 April 2005, pp. 787–788.

35. Donald Light and Michael Dixon, "Making the NHS More Like Kaiser Permanente," *British Medical Journal*, Vol. 763, 27 March 2004, pp. 763–765.

4

HIGH POLITICS, OR EXPLANATIONS OF GREAT CONFLICTS IN THE WORLD OF HEALTH CARE

The two articles in this chapter address conflicts of great intensity in the worlds of American and British health care. The first describes and offers an explanation of how, and why, the Thatcher government of 1989 precipitated a dramatic political conflict with its proposals for introducing radical change in the National Health Service. The story of the defeat of the Clinton health reform plan of 1993 is a parallel study in a number of respects. In both instances, what was proposed became front-page news and the subject of extended television commentary. Both proposals excited enormous opposition, from the medical profession, the trade unions, and the Labour Party in Britain, and from the private health insurance industry and its ideological allies within the business community and organized medicine in the United States.

The stakeholders in these battles had both material and ideological grounds for objection or celebration. Trade unions, doctors, and defenders of the traditional NHS order regarded the Thatcher reforms as a fundamental assault on the proper way of running an iconic institution that publicly financed health care and provided most of it in state-owned and -regulated settings. While fundamental in some senses, the NHS dispute did not involve a change in citizen entitlement to care; it was about changing the way that care was managed. In the American case, the stakes were even broader, a proposed reworking of how medical care was to be governed altogether: its entitlement, its financing, its regulation, its mix of private and public provision.

The two stories, then, represent one of the major types of political struggles in health care: the highly salient clash of ideas, interests, and institutional models. In such struggles, there is no mistaking who the stakeholders are. There is much investment in manipulating public perceptions of what is at stake. The fights are public, the interests of the major groups are clearly represented, and institutional settings advantage some and disadvantage others.

The most parsimonious explanation for the outcomes of the two political battles is institutional. There is no need to look farther than the institutional setting of both reforms to understand why Thatcher was able to overcome great objection and Clinton's reform died of political asphyxiation. Other analysts have offered somewhat different or more complex explanations, but both articles in this chapter point unambiguously to this straightforward conclusion.

A British prime minister who commands the support of her or his party can impose her or his will on the legislature, independently of whether or not the party was elected by a majority of voters. Only in exceptional circumstances can the House of Lords put obstacles in the government's way. So once Mrs. Thatcher had decided on her program of reform, there was no legislative obstacle to its introduction in the NHS. No such institutional portrait characterizes American national politics when large-scale change is at stake. If British politics is majoritarian within its party structure, American politics disperses authority and power, as noted previously. Elections do not settle whether the legislature has a policy majority on any topic; party platforms are banal wish lists and appeals to values that have an uncertain relation to an intense partisan struggle. The president proposes—as indeed Clinton did in his scheme for "managed competition" in September 1993. But a year later, the game was up, with neither that reform enacted nor, indeed, any other.

So, the question is why. In both articles, the explanatory approach taken insists on a configuration of factors that make the results explicable. And, in both instances, while institutional factors provide a crucial element, the stories are richer for separating policy genesis and policy outcomes. This approach—the explicit arraying of different ways to present and explain a story—is evident in both these articles, though independently written.

The Politics of the Big Bang

Rudolf Klein

There are a number of different ways of telling the story of how, in January 1989, the Government came to precipitate the most serious conflict in the history of the National Health Service by publishing its manifesto for change, *Working for Patients*.[1] First, there is the Cleopatra's nose version.[2] If Mrs. Thatcher's temper had been on a longer leash, and if it had not been tried so severely by a sustained barrage of criticism about her Government's management of the NHS, she might not suddenly have surprised television viewers of *Panorama* (and some of her Cabinet colleagues) by announcing her Review while appearing on that program in January 1988. Second, there is the economic determinism version. Caught between the imperative of containing public expenditure and the pressure to expand the NHS's activities, the Government had no option but to consider ever more radical ideas for the financing and organisation of health care. Third, there is the ideological "outing" version. The Government, its confidence boosted by a third election victory, finally felt strong enough openly to pursue its ideological commitment to the market, having previously only been able to do so by stealth. Fourth, there is the policy-learning version.[3] From its own experience both in the health policy arena and in other policy fields like education, the Government could draw the lesson that it was possible to overcome obstacles to change previously considered to be insurmountable: the horizons of the possible had widened out. Fifth, there is the policy soup version.[4] By the end of the 1980s, the Government was able to draw on a rich mix of ideas, home grown and imported, which allowed it to choose from a wider policy menu than when it had first come into office: the clear (if thin) consommé of ideas that had shaped the NHS in 1948 had become a thick (if confusing) minestrone. Lastly, there is the organisational predestination version. Nothing that the Government did should have surprised anyone aware of the changes in theory and practice, largely made possible by information technology that was transforming large organisations everywhere.

All these interpretations contribute to an understanding of the circumstances that led to the Review and to the publication of *Working for Patients,* if with varying degrees of plausibility. They are complementary rather than competitive, in that they help us to understand different aspects of the policy-making process. Some help to identify the factors that precipitated action and led to the decision to set up the Review; some help to identify the factors that predisposed Ministers to adopt particular policy options during the course of the Review; others help to identify the factors that enabled the Government to implement particular policy solutions. None can claim any exclusive explanatory monopoly. In what follows, therefore, this article will draw on the different modes of explanation, as appropriate, in tracing the evolution of policy from the decision to set up the Review to the implementation of the proposals set out in *Working for Patients.*

Consider, first, the circumstances that precipitated Mrs. Thatcher's decision to overcome her own reluctance to address the reform of the NHS head-on. The 1987 General Election had been "a bruising experience so far as the NHS was concerned" for the Conservatives.[5] Subsequently every Tuesday and Thursday, at Prime Minister's Question Time in the House of Commons, Mrs. Thatcher "had thrown at her case after case of ward closures, interminably postponed operations and allegedly avoidable infant deaths, all of them attributed to Government parsimony."[6] The newspapers and television programs, too, served up "horror stories about the NHS on an almost daily basis" and Mrs. Thatcher's irritation was further compounded by the failure (as she saw it) of the Department of Health and Social Security to come up with effective replies to criticisms.[7] Finally, bringing her exasperation to the boiling point, she felt outraged when the Presidents of the Royal Colleges publicly denounced the Government's policies. This represented, in her view, a repudiation of the implicit concordat between the State and the medical profession forged by the creation of the NHS, whereby the former accepted the autonomy of the medical profession in decisions about the use of resources while the latter accepted the right of the State to set the budgetary constraints within which it worked.[8] The basis of the accommodation between the State and the medical profession had been betrayed.

But if the media pressures and the *pronunciamento* of the Presidents of the Royal Colleges all helped to push Mrs. Thatcher over the precipice, she had already been moving towards the edge for other reasons. Her Chancellor of the Exchequer, Nigel Lawson, took the view that "we had reached the point where the pressures to spend more money on the Health Service were almost impossible to resist." But the Treasury was reluctant to agree to more money for the NHS without an assurance that this would yield "real value for money in terms of improved patient care." Hence, Lawson argued over dinner with the Prime Minister, the case for a review of the NHS.[9] However, according to Mrs. Thatcher's own account, she did not need prompting from her Chancellor. She had started discussions about how to ensure better value for money from the existing system with her new Secretary of State for the Social Services, John Moore, soon after the General Election.[10] It seemed to her that "the NHS had become a bottomless financial pit," where the providers blamed the Government for all that went wrong. It was thus a political liability and, with her thoughts turning to a fourth General Election victory, she saw advantages in quick action that would put any reforms in place before the time came to face the voters again.

The proximate cause for the decision to set up the Review can therefore be seen as the Prime Minister's resolve to escape from what was becoming an ever more embarrassing political situation. But what created that situation was the failure of the Government's policies to resolve the tension between constrained budgets and expanding demands. Despite the Government's value-for-money crusade, despite the statistics about the increasing number of doctors and nurses employed and the rising number of patients treated which the Prime Minister reeled out whenever challenged about the NHS, the public obstinately continued to see the Health Service as a casualty of the Thatcher administration's parsimony. Given the crucial importance of the issue, the next section therefore examines in more detail the debate about NHS funding.

A DIALOGUE OF THE DEAF

The increasingly fierce political debate about NHS funding that characterized the 1980s was revealing not so much for any conclusions reached about the adequacy or otherwise of its budget but for its demonstration that it was impossible to come to anything like an agreed verdict. It was a reminder—if a reminder was needed—of the view taken by the 1979 Royal Commission that "There is no objective or universally acceptable method of establishing what the 'right' level of expenditure on the NHS should be."[11] But failing such a formula for resolving argument, or any set of agreed criteria or benchmarks against which the level of funding could be assessed, the political dispute inevitably turned into a dialogue of the deaf. In these circumstances, the medical profession—as so often before in the history of the NHS—was able to impose its interpretation on the situation. If there was no agreed way of using statistics to give an accurate picture of the adequacy or otherwise of funding, if there was no authoritative evidence that would command general assent, doctors (and, to a lesser extent, nurses) were the obvious witnesses. Who, after all, was better placed than they to provide testimony based on their own day-to-day experience? If they declared the NHS to be on the point of collapse—as they did with increasing stridency as the decade went on—who could question their authority? In short, the ambiguity of the evidence available—and the lack of consensus about how to assess it—reinforced the power of those able to impose their interpretation of reality: unsurprisingly the proportion of the public declaring themselves to be dissatisfied with the NHS rose from 25 per cent in 1983 to 46 per cent in 1.989.[12]

But why was it so difficult to assess the evidence? The simplest way of answering this question is to examine further the debate between the "inputters" and the "outputters," between the Government's critics and successive Secretaries of State, already briefly referred to in the previous chapter. The criticism of the Government's expenditure plans, as articulated by the all-party Social Services Committee of the House of Commons in a succession of reports, drew attention to a widening gulf between the inputs of resources and what was deemed to be required. To define what was required the Committee used a formula first devised in the 1970s in order to extract money from the Treasury: an exercise in ingenuity by civil servants which came to haunt their departmental colleagues in the 1980s. The formula suggested an annual growth in the NHS budget of about 2 per cent in real terms. As one much quoted Ministerial statement[13] put it:

> One per cent is needed to keep pace with the increasing number of elderly people; medical advance takes an additional 0.5 per cent and a further 0.5 per cent is needed to make progress towards meeting the Government's policy objectives (for example to improve renal services and to develop community care).

Comparing actual spending levels with the expenditure needed to produce an annual growth of 2 per cent, it was then a simple arithmetical exercise to calculate the deficit. Using this method, the Social Services Committee in 1986 produced a figure of £1.325 billion as the cumulative under-funding of the hospital and community services. It was a figure which was to reverberate throughout the entire debate, feeding alike the sense of grievance within the NHS and the indignation of Opposition politicians.

The Government, in contrast, put the emphasis on outputs, i.e. on what the NHS was actually producing. This, of course, was the logic of a value-for-money approach, hinged on the *relationship* between inputs and outputs, which defined performance in terms of activity rather than the level of resources. Already in 1983 the Government's preparation for the General Election included the publication of a document setting out the increase in activity.[14] And this remained the Government's response to criticisms of inadequacy throughout the 1980s and into the 1990s. In its evidence to the 1988 Social Services Committee inquiry,[15] the DHSS provided figures showing the increase in the number of patients treated and specific operations carried out, arguing that rising productivity had allowed the NHS to provide more and better services despite tight budget constraints.

The arguments proved impossible to resolve. The Government's logic in directing attention to the outputs of the NHS was impeccable. The level of inputs tells us nothing of itself; the adequacy or otherwise of any given bundle of resources depends on how they are used. However, the Government's line of reasoning was vulnerable on two counts. First, its story about increasing activity and improved productivity could say nothing about the adequacy of what was being produced. Given the lack of any measure of demand—let alone need—increasing activity could still be compatible with a shortfall in what was required. Moreover, the persistence of waiting lists—and the growth of the private sector—seemed eloquent evidence of the NHS's failure to meet demand. Second, the Government was vulnerable to the criticism that quantity was being achieved at the expense of quality, as lengths of stay in hospitals fell and as the proportion of operations carried out on a day care basis rose. It was an argument which could neither be proved nor refuted: the required benchmarks of quality simply did not exist.

The case for the prosecution was also flawed. The demonstration of underfunding by the Social Services Committee depended crucially on the baseline chosen.[16] Yet there was no particular logic about choosing 1980 as the starting point for the exercise; there was no conceivable way of telling whether the NHS was over- or under-funded in that year. So the deficit could just as easily have been twice as large as claimed or non-existent: given the Social Services Committee's methodology, there was no way of telling. Moreover, the method extrapolated into the future costs based on past practices at a time when it was public policy to change those patterns of service delivery. Lastly, the calculations ignored some significant inputs into health care. They did not include either the growing primary health care budget or the billions flowing into the long-stay sector via the social security system. And no one even raised the question of whether or not the extra spending on private health care should be brought into the reckoning.

Nor could appeal to comparisons with other countries settle the matter. By international standards Britain was indeed a low spender on health care.[17] Expenditure on health care in the mid-1980s was, at 6 per cent of the Gross Domestic Product, significantly lower than in France (9 per cent) or Germany (8 per cent)—let alone the United States (10 per cent). Such comparisons were indeed much invoked by the Government's critics, political and professional. But, again, the figures did not speak for themselves. It was quite possible to mount a counter-attack. Britain's apparent parsimony could be seen as a tribute to the ability of the NHS to keep down costs and to stretch the available resources to better effect than other health care systems. By successfully containing salary and wage increases, by avoiding the excesses of American medicine, the NHS was able to deliver more care for each unit of input than other systems. There was no way of resolving this clash of views on the basis of the available evidence.

So if the 1980s debate was a dialogue of the deaf, it was because there was no agreement about the currency of argument and no consensus about how to define key terms like adequacy, need or quality. Lacking such an agreed vocabulary and generally accepted measuring rods, no resolution was possible. There was little that the technicians—whether statisticians or epidemiologists, economists or social policy experts—could do to resolve the dispute. It was inevitably politicised. And therein precisely lay the real significance of the debate. Its nature was defined less by the issues involved than by the characteristics of the policy arena.

The characteristic of the health care policy arena that determined the nature of the debate about NHS funding in the 1980s—as in previous decades—was the central role of the health service professionals. It was they who largely orchestrated and shaped the perception of crisis. There was nothing new in this. What needs explaining about the 1980s—and, in particular, the confrontation between the medical and nursing professions and the Government that precipitated Mrs. Thatcher's decision to set up the Review of the NHS—is the scale and ferocity of that conflict.[18] It was marked by a concerted and determined attempt by the professions to demonstrate that the NHS was (yet again) on the point of collapse and thus to mobilise public opinion in a campaign for extra funding.[19] It was, moreover, an extremely successful campaign: as previously noted, the evidence of public opinion surveys during this period shows an increase in the proportion of people declaring themselves to be dissatisfied with the NHS *and* supporting an increase in spending on the service.

It was, in retrospect, a battle that the Government was bound to lose. While Ministers depended on abstract statistics, the critics could translate their concerns into human terms and concrete images. In so doing, they could exploit the bias of the media towards the dramatic. The extent and intensity of the media coverage were, indeed, unprecedented in the history of the NHS. There was a succession of reports about hospital wards which had to be closed because of cash crises. There was a procession of consultants complaining about being unable to carry out life-saving operations because of inadequate resources. The picture that emerged forcibly and vividly from all these accounts was that of a Health Service where the staff felt themselves unable to deliver care of adequate quality, where patients were being turned away and where morale and standards were both plunging.

But the NHS balance sheet offers—at best—only a partial explanation of the conflict between the Government and the medical profession. The pressures on the NHS in the 1980s were not different in kind—though perhaps more intense and certainly more sustained—from those in previous decades. It was the willingness of the medical and nursing profession to accept those pressures which appears to have diminished drastically. If doctors and nurses perceived the NHS to be in a state of crisis, it was largely if not exclusively because they saw themselves threatened by the Government's policies for solving that crisis. On first taking office in 1979 Mrs. Thatcher's administration had quite deliberately decided to avoid any kind of radical reform of the health care system—as we have seen—because of the political risks involved. Instead, it had introduced a series of organisational changes inspired by a report written by Sir Roy Griffiths, managing director of one of Britain's largest chains of grocery supermarkets.[20] The changes antagonised the NHS professionals who saw their power and autonomy diminished by the strengthened managerial structure that emerged. By 1988, therefore, the Government appeared to have little to lose—and perhaps much to gain—from taking the step it had so long tried to avoid: the stage was set for Mrs. Thatcher's announcement of her Review of the NHS. Far from marking the triumphalism fulfillment of a long-standing ideological ambition, the announcement was in effect a confession of failure: the Government had been driven to adopt a posture of radicalism which it had strenuously sought to avoid. And reluctant radicalism was to characterise—as we shall see in the next section—the Review itself.

REVIEWING THE OPTIONS

The central paradox of the Review of the NHS was that, although prompted by the widespread perception of financial crisis, no proposals for change in the method of funding emerged from it. The 1948 model was preserved: the NHS remained a universal, tax-financed health care system. Instead, the aim of *Working for Patients* was to change the dynamics of the 1948 model. Specifically, it introduced two major—and highly contentious—reforms. First, there was the separation of the purchaser and the provider roles: health authorities would in future be responsible only for buying health care from the providers. The providers, both hospitals and community services, would be transformed into autonomous trusts, whose budgets would depend on their competitive efficiency in getting contracts from purchasers. Second, general practitioners were given the option of becoming fundholders, i.e. of getting a budget from which to purchase the services required by their patients, excluding only the most expensive or long-term treatment. Thus was created the notion of the internal or mimic market: the NHS was to mimic those characteristics of the market that would promote greater efficiency within the framework of a public service committed to the non-market value of distributing access to resources according to need. Financial incentives would be used not to generate profits, as in the marketplace, but to sharpen the incentives of everyone working in the NHS to make more efficient use of public funds. *Working for Patients* introduced a number of other changes as well but it was precisely this central thrust of its proposals, the attempt to introduce financial incentives into the NHS, that colored perceptions of the reform package as a whole and led to it being denounced both by the medical profession and the political opposition as a betrayal of the principles of 1948.

There is a real puzzle, therefore. Why were reforms that preserved the basic constitution and commitments of the NHS widely seen as destructive of its ethos and a threat to its principles? The best way to start answering this question—before moving on to consider the options on offer—is to look at the form that Mrs. Thatcher's Review took, since this largely determined the reactions to its outcome. In its style, though not in its outcome, the Review marked a brutal break with the past. Whereas the history of the NHS up to 1979 can be largely written as an attempt to maintain a consensus, however fragile at times, about the main elements of health care policy, Mrs. Thatcher explicitly repudiated the notion that consensus-seeking was a desirable form of political activity. In doing so, she also repudiated the traditional instruments of consensus-engineering: Royal Commissions. None were appointed during her tenure in office. The Review of the NHS was carried out by a Cabinet Committee of five: the Prime Minister, Nigel Lawson and John Major from the Treasury, John Moore and Tony Newton from the DHSS (the latter two being replaced by Kenneth Clarke and David Mellor halfway through the review, following John Moore's resignation and the decision to hive off Social Security from the Department of Health, as it then became). Sir Roy Griffiths and John O'Sullivan, a member of the Prime Minister's Policy Unit, were also regular attenders.[21]

The very notion of setting up a Cabinet Committee was, of course, an affront to the tradition embodied in the Royal Commission approach. The membership of Royal Commissions invariably incorporated representatives of the main interests. In contrast, a Cabinet Committee excluded precisely those—notably the medical profession—who had come to think of themselves as participating in the policy-making process as of right. It was this sense of exclusion, the feeling of being denied their proper place at the top policy-making table, that shaped the medical profession's perceptions of the whole process. In this respect, there is a close parallel with the bitter confrontation between the Government and the medical profession that led up to the creation of the NHS: much of the hostility to Aneurin Bevan reflected as much resentment of his style as disagreement over substance. In short, the way in which Mrs. Thatcher set up her Review was a direct challenge to the medical profession's view of its own position in the constellation of power.[22] Nor was the style of conducting the Review likely to smooth down resentment. As part of the exercise, there were two meetings at Chequers with NHS doctors and managers respectively. However, those invited to these meetings were selected not because they were representative of the professional interests involved (the Royal Commission model) but precisely because they were unrepresentative in their sympathy for ideas of radical reform.

Everyone could, of course, contribute to the policy soup of ideas from which the Cabinet Committee itself was drawing. And many did so: the announcement of the Review precipitated a variety of policy cooks into action, each ready with his or her own recipe for what needed doing about the NHS.[23] Analysing the various contributions does not necessarily establish the paternity of the proposals in *Working for Patients*: ideas often become politically acceptable only when they have become part of the common intellectual currency, their precise origins long since forgotten. But it does illustrate the extent to which the debate about the NHS widened out in the course of the 1980s to embrace ideas not even considered by the 1979 Royal Commission. And it thus allows the reforms that finally emerged from the Review to be placed in the spectrum of options— from the conservative to the radical—available to Ministers.

The medical profession, speaking through the voice of the British Medical Association (BMA), stood firmly at the conservative end. Having raised the spectre of radical reform, it took fright. In its evidence to the Government Review, the BMA argued that only "a relatively small percentage increase in funding" was needed and that it would be "a serious mistake to embark on any major restructuring of the funding and delivery of health care in order to resolve the present difficulties"[24] though some form of hypothecated taxation might be desirable.

In making the case against radical reform, the BMA provided an eloquent testimonial to the NHS, 40 years after having fought its introduction:

> While many of the alternative systems have shown superficially attractive features, we have always been led to the inescapable conclusion that the principles on which the NHS is based represent the most efficient way of providing a truly comprehensive health service, while at the same time ensuring the best value for money in terms of the quality of health care. They also enable the cost of health care to be controlled to a much greater extent than has been achieved with other systems, as has been shown by the experience of other countries.

At the radical extreme were a number of proposals for privatising the finance of health care, and giving the consumer the ability to choose between competing schemes, by increasing the role of private insurance. The role of the State should be limited, it was argued, to ensuring that everyone had the resources required to buy health care. Decisions about the appropriate level of spending on health care would be largely de-politicised because diffused among consumers, the NHS's budget would depend on its ability to attract customers in the face of competition from other providers.[25] It was a model which had first been put forward 25 years previously by the Institute of Economic Affairs, an independent research organisation set up to propagate libertarian market doctrines, and generally dismissed as one more example of the IEA's eccentricity in trying to revive nineteenth-century ideas. By the 1980s, however, the IEA's championship of market liberalism seemed to have triumphed.[26] Its ideology appeared to be the Prime Minister's. In practice, Mrs. Thatcher was a somewhat wayward disciple—all too ready to listen to the seductive voices of Think Tanks more prepared to bend their notions to political expediency. But the IEA remained the voice of ideological conscience: the home of the Old Believers in the doctrines of market liberalism. Its ideas therefore provided a touchstone for testing the Government's policies for ideological purity: a test which (as in the case of health care reform) the Government frequently failed.

If some of the policy recipes were primarily designed to change the method of financing health care, others were more concerned with changing the dynamics of the existing health care system drawing largely on American ideas. This import of American ideas was, in many ways, surprising: it was very much a case of experts on obesity advising a patient suffering from anorexia. American experience in trying to contain (unsuccessfully) a health care cost explosion was not self-evidently relevant to the British debate about under-funding. Perhaps, however, it was the frustrating failure of American policy which prompted the development of a highly sophisticated body of theory that proved to be highly contagious, as transmitted by globe-trotting economists, and influenced opinion in Britain and elsewhere. Two different types of policy approach, derived from this body of theory, must be distinguished. There were those who saw change as being driven by consumers while others saw it as being driven by managers. In the former (arguably more radical) category were proposals for allowing citizens to choose their own health care providers, who would then be reimbursed on a capitation basis by a central funding agency. The appropriate health care providers might be either GPs or specially formed Health Maintenance Organisations (HMOs) on the American model. In the latter category came the proposal for giving district health authorities a budget with which to buy the health services required by their populations from independent providers, thus leaving health authority managers (rather than consumers) to make the choices. Again, the American inspiration was evident: the notion of such an internal market had been first put forward by a visiting American academic, Alain Enthoven, in 1985.[27] It was a quite deliberate compromise between what Enthoven himself perceived as the greater advantages of the more radical, consumer-driven HMO approach—known, in the American context, as managed competition—and what he considered to be politically feasible in Britain. But it did address the central weakness of the NHS, as perceived by most policy cooks and by Ministers, which was that money did not follow patients.

It was a diagnosis with which the all-party House of Commons Social Services Committee—which in 1988 conducted its own review of the various options in parallel with the Cabinet Committee—largely agreed. The Committee rejected the more radical proposals for change in the funding or organisation of health care. But it gave a qualified welcome to the notion of an internal market as an idea which deserved further exploration and development. Specifically, it proposed "limited experiments" to test its practicability, urging that "it should not be introduced nationally before a thorough piloting had been done."[28] Given the need to maintain consensus on the all-party Committee, in order to produce a unanimous report on a politically explosive topic, even such a degree of cautious interest was perhaps somewhat surprising. Certainly it would have been difficult to predict, on the basis of this Parliamentary report, the denunciations of the Government that followed its decision to adopt the internal market option in *Working for Patients* six months later.

The decision came only after the Cabinet Committee had wasted some months, in the view of some of those involved, exploring a series of policy deadends. For contrary to the view that the contents of *Working for Patients* were predetermined by the Government's ideological agenda, the Review of the

NHS appears to have been a singularly rudderless operation. Far from steering a pre-set course, the Review tacked rather erratically between different options, only settling down to developing something approaching a coherent package towards the end of its existence. There certainly was an ideological *bias* among many of those taking part, in that they tended to share a belief in the merits of markets and competition. But there was nothing like an ideological *programme*. One of the most striking characteristics of the Review was that no one—not even the Prime Minister—appears to have had a clear agenda, apart from wishing to find some formula that would bring peace and prosperity to the NHS. There were lots of problems in the NHS; there was a long list of possible solutions. But matching problems and solutions turned out to be a fumbling process.

There were a variety of reasons for the Review's uncertain start. The Department of Health, which might have been expected to take the lead in shaping the agenda of any Review of the NHS, turned out to the ineffective in this role. Although John Moore, the Secretary of State, was anxious to demonstrate his credentials as an aspiring Dauphin by demonstrating his ideological radicalism, his health broke down; it was not until the much more pragmatic Kenneth Clarke replaced him that there was an effective Department of Health voice and that the Review moved towards developing a more coherent approach. Furthermore, the memoranda submitted by the DHSS civil servants were felt, by most of the Review's members, to be inadequate in their analysis and timid in their prescriptions. Instead, they tended to rely on the advice pouring in from other sources: the Treasury, Mrs. Thatcher's No. 10 Policy Unit and various Conservative Think Tanks.

But perhaps the most important reason for the meandering start of the inquiry had nothing to do with the characteristics of the Review or of the actors involved. This is that there is no magic formula for health care reform[29] and that any attempt to devise one inevitably turns into a conflict between competing claims and interests. This became clear early in the life of the Review when, in a somewhat half-hearted way, it examined alternative ways of funding health care, looking at the experience of other countries. It quickly became apparent that the weakness of the funding system for the NHS in the eyes of its critics (the fact that it kept health care on short rations) was precisely its strength in the eyes of the Treasury (the fact that it could not be bettered as an instrument of public expenditure control). "It did not take long to conclude that there was surprisingly little that we could learn from any of the other systems," Nigel Lawson noted,[30] "To try to change to any of the sorts of systems in use overseas would simply be out of the frying pan into the fire." In turn, when the DHSS sought to argue the case for funding health care by means of a hypothecated

tax—which would have guaranteed the NHS a stable and increasing income—
this was strenuously resisted, after an initial show of flirtatious interest, by the
Treasury, whose control would have been threatened by any such move. Accordingly, the Prime Minister soon decided that the Review should concentrate
"on changing the structure of the NHS rather than its finance."[31] This did not
stop her from grinding her own favorite axe—tax reliefs for those taking out private insurance—throughout the rest of the Review. Nor did it stop the Treasury
from resurrecting the case for increasing and extending charges throughout the
NHS, as it had done regularly for the previous 40 years: a proposal on which
the Prime Minister firmly stamped, as she records, as threatening to discredit
any reforms. But it did mean that the most radical options—i.e. those designed
to transform the way in which the health care system in Britain was funded and
organised—had been ruled out of court.

The rejection of changes in the methods for funding health care—and the
veto on further discussion of moving towards either the European social insurance model or a voucher-based market model—did not lead to the instant
adoption of the internal market notion. The internal market emerged as the
by-product of policies designed to change the NHS's dynamics, by giving more
autonomy to the providers and introducing more incentives to efficiency. In
this respect, the White Paper that emerged from the Review—*Working for
Patients*—accurately mirrored its proceedings. All the emphasis is on specific
measures, like splitting the purchaser and provider functions and giving hospitals independence, not on the abstract notion of creating a market. Specifically, the measures followed from the Review's diagnosis of the NHS's central
weakness: that money did not follow the patient, thereby penalising rather than
encouraging productivity. Increasing activity sent up costs in a hospital, operating under a budget fixed by the health authority, without increasing its income.
There were no incentives to be sensitive to demands, particularly those coming
from outside the authority's administrative boundaries. The logic of the analysis
suggested devising a system of internal NHS finance that would relate hospital
incomes more directly to their activities and giving hospitals more freedom to
behave entrepreneurially in responding to new opportunities.

The idea of giving more independence to hospitals, and allowing them to
emancipate themselves from bureaucratic control, was in itself calculated to
appeal to a Conservative administration.[32] The model had already begun to be
tested in the case of education where the Government had earlier given schools
the right to opt out of control by the local education authorities and to become
self-managing institutions whose budgets would depend on the number of pu-
pils they managed to attract. So here there was a ready-made example, and

there is no doubt that it influenced Kenneth Clarke and other Review members. There were significant differences between health and education, not least that in the case of schools the rationale behind the changes was that they would transfer power to parents by giving them the ability to choose between schools. But education was, in a sense, the laboratory in which Conservative Ministers first invented internal or mimic markets, subsequently drawing what they perceived to be the appropriate lessons for health.

It was not at all self-evident how the general principle of giving hospitals more independence or autonomy should be translated into practice. Who would own them? Who should run them? A Treasury paper, which caught the Prime Minister's fancy, suggested that hospitals should be contracted out: staff consortia, private companies and charities would all be able to bid. Again, as so often with the Review, a more cautious option prevailed. There was to be no competition for the right to manage hospitals; the final solution adopted was that of self-governing Trusts, with the Secretary of State nominating the board and retaining the ultimate power of control. Similarly, there were various ways in which the principle of money following patients could be translated into practice. One was the solution finally adopted: the purchaser–provider split, with hospitals dependent on the contracts obtained in a competitive market in which private providers could also compete. For once the Review chose the bolder option. The Treasury had argued for a less radical solution. Under its scheme hospitals would have continued to receive their basic budget from health authorities, but there would additionally have been a central funding pool from which they would have been paid for meeting, or exceeding, performance targets set by central government. This, the Treasury argued, would give them an incentive to greater activity while yet retaining the capacity to plan the NHS's strategic direction and maintaining expenditure control.

Overall, however, Mrs. Thatcher worried that "we were losing our way" and "moving away from, rather than towards, radical reform."[33] Accordingly she seized upon the idea of GP budgets[34] with some enthusiasm, when this surfaced halfway through the life of the Review. The idea had been urged upon her by the No. 10 Policy Unit; Kenneth Clarke independently had also come to embrace this option, which he came to see as very much his own contribution to the reform cocktail. There was some opposition. Many of the Review members, the Treasury Ministers in particular, thought that their inquiry should concentrate on the hospital sector. But the notion of GP budget holding appeared to offer something which none of the other contemplated reforms could do: it brought the choice of what was to be purchased nearer to the consumer. The general practitioner would be the consumer's voice and consumers would be free to change their GP if they did not approve of his or her use of resources on their behalf. GP budget holding was thus much nearer the education model than any of the other reforms introduced by the Review. There were objections. The Treasury questioned whether GPs would be able to manage large budgets and worried about the creation of a powerful new lobby for extra health spending. However, the objections were over-ruled and GP fundholding became one of the most contentious parts of *Working for Patients*.

A number of other matters were settled as well, before the Cabinet Committee completed its labours after 24 meetings. The White Paper put forward managerial and organisational changes that were to prove almost as contentious as its introduction of the internal market and GP budgets. But there was also a private, internal battle to be settled. Pressed hard by the Prime Minister to introduce tax relief for private health care, the Chancellor of the Exchequer overcame his objections of principle to any such concession and offered a compromise: no change in the tax treatment of the benefit of company health insurance schemes but tax relief for policies taken out by the over-60s. It was a concession that Nigel Lawson subsequently came to regret, even though its financial implications were insignificant. Nevertheless the Treasury felt satisfied enough with the outcome of the Review to announce, as an overture to the publication of the White Paper, a 4.5 per cent increase in real terms in spending on the NHS, the first in a series of similar announcements over the next three years. The Review may have done nothing to change the system of financing health care that had provoked the "under-funding" crisis but, ironically, the Government's determination to ensure the success of its reforms brought about a rare period of rapid growth in the NHS's budget.[35] But, as if to underline that the "under-funding" crisis had been as much about the changing balance of power within the NHS as about the money, the generous financial settlement did nothing to ease the acceptability of the Government's plans. The antagonisms aroused by those plans ran too deep, as the reception of *Working for Patients* and the subsequent months were to show, to be assuaged by money alone.

AN EXPLOSION OF OPPOSITION

When launching their White Paper—an exercise carried out with a fanfare of publicity, at considerable cost to the public purse—Ministers faced a dilemma. Should they stress the radicalism of their proposals and thus claim credit for their boldness in changing the health care system? Or should they emphasize the strong element of continuity and thus claim credit for their determination to preserve the NHS? In the event, the strategy adopted in *Working for Patients* was to present the specific policy proposals as building on the achievements of the past: as a way of releasing the full potential of the NHS. There was a re-affirmation of the 1948 settlement and a celebration of the success of the NHS: "The principles which have guided it for the last 40 years will continue to guide it into the twenty-first century. The NHS is, and will continue to be, open to all, regardless of income, and financed mainly out of general taxation." Echoing Bevan, the White Paper further proclaimed: "The Government wants to raise the performance of all hospitals and GP practices to that of the best." The twin aims of the proposals were to give patients "greater choice of the services available" and to secure "greater satisfaction and rewards for those working in the NHS who successfully respond to local needs and preferences." Who could possibly disagree with such general, benevolent aims?

The answer came quickly: almost everyone. The Labour Party position as enunciated by Robin Cook, its front-bench spokesman, was simple. The Government's strategy, he argued, was "to destabilise the National Health Service and replace it with a commercial one." The logic of the changes would lead inexorably to the ultimate horror: "market medicine as it is practised across the Atlantic." The conclusion was clear: "We are in danger of losing a Health Service that is motivated by dedication and replacing it with one that is driven by financial targets."[36] Much the same charges were made by the BMA—which throughout worked in a curious, unspoken alliance with the Labour Party—in an advertisement campaign that more than matched the Government's own expenditure on publicity. On the hoardings a poster picturing a giant steam-roller carried the legend: "Mrs. Thatcher's Plans for the NHS." In the newspapers, full-page advertisements carried the message: "The NHS. Underfunded, Undermined, Under Threat." In GP surgeries, a BMA pamphlet—designed to be handed out to those waiting—asked, among other questions, "Do you want the cheapest treatment or what is best for you?" The BMA's indictment of the Government's proposals was comprehensive.[37] The proposals, argued the BMA, ignored the issue of under-funding. They would "lead to a fragmented service," "destroy the comprehensive nature of the existing NHS" and "cause serious damage to patient care." Instead of increasing patient choice, the changes would limit it. Political and professional voices spoke with a rare unanimity and with the same intent: to induce terror and apprehension at the thought that the Government was planning to replace the primacy of the patient with the primacy of the pound, forcing doctors to subordinate the search for health to the search for solvency.

Nothing like it had been seen in the NHS policy arena since the opposition provoked by Nye Bevan 40-odd years before. Nor was the intensity of the conflict the only similarity. In both cases, the degree of hostility appears—in retrospect, at least—disproportionate to the causes. In both cases, too, the ostensible pretexts for the conflict concealed other motives. Disentangling the reasons for the extreme reaction to the White Paper reforms is therefore complex. Some were not specific to the NHS. A generalised hostility to Mrs. Thatcher—who by 1989 was widely seen as a domineering autocrat intent on imposing her own vision on the world—spilled over into the health care arena. Any proposal which carried her stamp of approval was therefore automatically tainted in the eyes of many. More directly, the circumstances in which the Review had been set up and carried out tended to condition the response to it. If the Royal Commission procedure was a device for creating consensus, the Review method was designed to provoke schism. The British style of adversarial politics was further calculated to amplify disagreement. So, too, was the combative style of the two leading political protagonists—Kenneth Clarke and Robin Cook—whose verbal violence seemed to escalate with each encounter. The Government's insistence that it would drive through its reforms, whatever the criticisms, strengthened in turn the root-and-branch opposition to the principles that shaped the plans.

Thus was created a cycle of mutual and mounting antagonism. Ministers were strengthened in their conviction that engaging in discussion was futile. The Government's critics, conversely, were confirmed in their belief in a conspiracy to undermine the NHS. It was not a situation calculated to encourage discussion of how the reforms might best be introduced, even though it was clear that the impact of the Government's somewhat sketchy outline proposals would largely depend on the way in which they were implemented.

Opposition to the Government's plans cannot, however, be dismissed as an artefact of the political situation. The fact that the Opposition saw an opportunity for further exploiting public reservations about the Thatcher administration's record on the NHS and the medical profession's sense of outrage at its exclusion from the policy process both explain much. But the reasons for the hostility go deeper. Some were specific to particular policy areas: the special case of the reform of primary health care is examined separately in the next section. Others revolved around fundamental questions about the nature of the NHS. Was it possible to maintain the historic facade while gutting the building behind it without also destroying those characteristics of the NHS which made it special? Would not the reforms destroy the web of assumptions, loyalties and relationships, built up over the decades, which had sustained the NHS and allowed it to perform better than might have been expected from the size of its budget?

There was an irony in the evocation, by the Government's critics, of the traditions of the NHS: a Burkean defence of an existing institution on the grounds that the introduction of changes based on a priori ideas would threaten to unravel the delicate fabric woven by history. For this appeal to history as embodied in an existing institution was very much at odds with the origins of the NHS. The NHS was the product of faith in scientific rationalism. It was designed as a machine for making generally available the benefits of scientific medicine[38] using the tools of planning as an instrument for doing so. Services were to be free at the point of delivery precisely in order to ensure that treatment would be determined by scientific judgements about need, not by the financial resources of the patient. But by the 1980s, most of the assumptions built into this design were under challenge. There was increasing scepticism about the scientific basis of much of medicine and increasing resistance to accepting the judgement of doctors about need. Planning, as an instrument of public policy, was discredited. Feminism joined consumerism to question the medical determination of how patients should be treated.

Conversely, a new form of rationalism was in the ascendant: that of the econocrats.[39] The rise of the economists in the policy arena in the 1970s has already been noted. By the 1980s they had become the Savonarolas of public policy, denouncing inefficiency and ignorance as the ultimate sins. Efficiency in health care, it was argued,[40] was not just desirable: it was an ethical imperative, since wasting resources meant losing the opportunity to provide beneficial treatment to someone. It was this new-style rationalism—the Benthamite streak in Thatcherism—that helped to shape the Government's proposals.[41] And the proposals were seen as threatening—rightly—to many of the assumptions on which the NHS rested. The real threat came not from ideology conceived in the narrow and limited sense of the Conservative Party's belief in markets and privatisation but from ideology seen as a way of defining problems and devising solutions.

Perhaps the most important founding myth of the NHS was that it divorced the practice of medicine from money. It did no such thing, of course. The NHS's great achievement was rather different: it largely cut the links between the practice of medicine and the income of doctors, thus removing any perverse incentives for either the selection or treatment of patients. Money remained, as the whole history of the NHS demonstrated, the great constraint on medical practice: hence the events leading up to the Review. However, the Government's internal market proposals rested on the assumption that doctors (like everyone else) would be responsive to financial incentives, even if these did not touch their personal incomes. The internal market thus raised the spectre that medical practice would be corrupted by a competitive drive to attract custom, setting doctor against doctor, with treatment being determined by financial considerations rather than need. The criticism betrayed a certain lack of faith in the moral fibre of doctors and their dedication to the code of medical ethics. Equally, it ignored the fact that competition between consultants for funds, beds and merit awards had characterised the NHS throughout its entire history. But suspicions of a deep-laid plot to subvert the values of medicine, as embodied in the NHS, were further fuelled by GP fundholding. For here undeniably there appeared to be perverse financial incentives. If GPs were to stick within their budgets—or to make a surplus, which they could then plough back into improving their surgeries—they might be tempted either to deny their patients expensive treatment or to recruit only the healthiest patients to their list.

So, for anyone with ideological hackles to raise, there was plenty of provocation in the White Paper. There might well be ways of dealing with the potential threats to the NHS's values posed by the reforms. Everything, it could be argued, would depend on their implementation: in the event, as we shall see, few—if any—of the prophesied disasters happened. But in 1989 one of the casualties of the political situation was precisely any willingness to discuss the nuts and bolts of implementation; the Government's insistence on driving through its proposals, without much attention to the mechanics of change, meant that all debate tended to be framed in apocalyptic terms. Discussion revolved around a mythologised past (an NHS in which money did not matter) and a demonised future (an NHS in which medical practice was driven by money).

The 1989 reform package could also be seen as a challenge to the traditions of the NHS in another respect. It marked the transformation of an organisation based on trust into an organisation based on contract.[42] Symbolic of this transformation were the changes proposed by the White Paper in contracts for consultants. Previously, such contracts had been held at the regional level, so in effect insulating consultants from the managers of their institutions. Now, however, the Government took the view that "it is unacceptable for local management to have little authority or influence over those who are in practice responsible for committing most of the hospital service's resources." In future, therefore, local management (which soon came to mean the management of the provider Trusts) would negotiate and monitor contracts. These would include "a fuller job description than is commonly the case at present" and specify the responsibilities of consultants "for the quality of their work, their use of resources, the extent of the service they provide for NHS patients and the time they devote to the NHS." Further, the quality of professional practice would in future have to be demonstrated, rather than being taken for granted: all consultants would be expected to take part in medical audit, reviewing their own practices, the use of resources and the outcome for patients.

Medical audit turned out to be one of many examples of the profession's ability to modify—if not to subvert—the Government's intentions during the process of implementation. Consultants displayed only a fitful and erratic interest in audit, despite generous financial subsidies.[43] But there were plenty of other reasons for the apprehensions of doctors and others about the shift from trust to contract, from professional to managerial values, implied by the White Paper. The logic of market competition reinforced the logic of many of the managerial changes introduced before the Review. If there was to be market competition, there would have to be more and better information about activities and costs. It would therefore mean giving visibility to, and putting a price on, what the professionals were doing. Moving from a culture based on trust to one based on contract was therefore inevitably threatening to those working in the NHS in so far as it represented a switch of emphasis from autonomy to accountability: the books of the NHS were to be opened, literally as well as metaphorically, with the activities of both purchasers and providers being made subject to the scrutiny of the Audit Commission, an independent financial inspection agency. It was an opportunity which the Audit Commission was to exploit with enthusiasm, issuing a series of reports that questioned medical practices.[44]

The question of how and at what pace the White Paper proposals should be implemented was almost as contentious as its substance. The Government presented its reforms as a remedy for the NHS's ills which had to be swallowed whole and at a gulp. Ministers made few concessions of substance during the passage of the National Health Service and Community Care Act, which gave effect to *Working for Patients*, and the new legislation came into effect on 1 April 1991. The time between conception and birth was short. Yet the White Paper's proposals were little more than outline sketches, even when supplemented by a series of Working Papers put out by the Department of Health that sought to put some administrative flesh on the skeleton of ministerial ideas.[45] No one really knew how an internal market would work; almost everyone (including the Prime Minister) agreed that the NHS's existing information system was incapable of meeting the new demands that would be made on it. It was a timetable which, the Government's critics argued, was driven more by political expediency—a desire to get the NHS reforms in place before the next General Election—than by any regard for the good of the service: a brutal assault on the fragile fabric of the NHS, calculated to lower morale even further. Instead of gambling with the future of the NHS by introducing untested ideas wholesale,

it was argued, the Government should have first experimented with pilot projects. The refusal of Ministers to do so was widely seen as the victory of political
brute force over rationality in policy-making.

However, given that even a study carried out four years after the introduction
of the internal market found it extraordinarily difficult to evaluate its effects,[46] it
seems implausible to assume that any firm conclusions could have been drawn
from pilot schemes restricted to a politically realistic time-table. The rational
model of policy-making—first experiment, then evaluate, finally decide—may
thus be based, the case of the NHS suggests, on a series of irrational assumptions
about the feasibility of applying it. In contrast, ministerial strategy seems to have
been based—no doubt unconsciously—on a very different model of rationality
in policy-making.[47] This sees policy-making itself as an experiment—the testing of theory by putting it into practice. From this perspective, no apology was
needed for using the NHS as a laboratory for testing the Government's ideas,
since there was no other way of finding out what would or would not work—
and what adaptations were required to improve the design. If the 1948 NHS
reflected the period's certain confidence in its ability to design institutions that
would mould the future, the 1989 model reflected the loss of this confidence
and decreasing certainty about what the future would bring. The Government
had created—whether by intention or by inadvertence—an institution which
would invent its own future in a process of trial and error.[48]

Notes

1. Secretaries of State for Health, Wales, Northern Ireland and Scotland, *Working for Patients*,
   HMSO: London 1989, Cm. 555.
2. Pascal, *Pensees*, Flammarion: Paris 1976, p. 95: "Le nez de Cleopatre: s'il eut at' plus court, toute
   la face de la terre aurait change."
3. Hugh Heclo, *Modern Social Politics in Britain and Sweden*, Yale UP: New Haven 1974.
4. John W. Kingdon, *Agendas, Alternatives and Public Policies*, Little, Brown and Company: Boston 1984.
5. Nicholas Ridley, *My Style of Government*, Hutchinson: London 1991.
6. Nigel Lawson, *The View from No. 11*, Corgi Books: London 1993, p. 612.
7. Margaret Thatcher, *The Downing Street Years*, HarperCollins: London 1993, p. 608.
8. The notion of the implicit concordat between the State and the medical profession was originally put forward in the first (1983) edition of this book. However, it is said that the Prime
   Minister—who doubtlessly had not actually read this book and relied on garbled, second-hand
   versions—sent her civil servants scurrying in search of the contract in her anger with the Presidents of the Royal Colleges. It was, alas, not to be found.
9. Lawson, op. cit., p. 614.
10. Thatcher, op. cit., p. 608.
11. Sir Alec Merrison (chairman), *Royal Commission on the National Health Service: Report*,
    HMSO: London 1979, Cmnd. 7615.

12. Ken Judge and Michael Solomon, "Public Opinion and the National Health Service: Patterns and Perspectives in Consumer Satisfaction," *Journal of Social Policy*, vol. 22, no. 3, 1993, pp. 299–327.

13. Social Services Committee Fourth Report, Session 1985–86, *Public Expenditure on the Social Services*, HMSO: London 1986, HC 387. The Minister concerned, Mr. Barney Hayhoe, did not survive long in office.

14. Department of Health and Social Security, *Health Care and Its Costs*, HMSO: London 1983.

15. Social Services Committee First Report, Session 1987–88, vol. 11, *Minutes of Evidence*, pp. 96–108.

16. Organisation for Economic Co-operation and Development, *Financing and Delivering Health Care*, OECD: Paris 1987.

17. For an excellent contemporary record, see Nicholas Timmins, *Cash, Crisis and Cure*, The Independent: London 1988.

18. For an academic retrospective on events, see John Butler, *Patients, Policies and Politics*, Open University Press: Buckingham 1992.

19. Central Committee for Hospital Medical Services, *NHS Funding: The Crisis in the Acute Hospital Sector*, BMA: London 1988.

20. For analyses of the Griffiths report and its impact on management in the NHS, see Patricia Day and Rudolf Klein, "The Mobilization of Consent versus the Management of Conflict: Decoding the Griffiths Report," *British Medical Journal*, vol. 287, 10 December 1983, pp. 1813–1816, and Stephen Harrison, *Managing the National Health Service*, Chapman and Hall: London 1988.

21. The analysis of the Review is based on the accounts, rather different but not contradictory, given in Thatcher and Lawson, op. cit., supplemented by interviews with some of the participants in the process.

22. Patricia Day and Rudolf Klein, "Constitutional and Distributional Conflict in British Medical Politics: The Case of General Practice, 1911–1991," *Political Studies*, vol. XL, no. 3, September 1992, pp. 462–78.

23. For an excellent review of the various proposals, on which this account draws, see John Brazier, John Hutton and Richard Jeavons (eds.), *Reforming the UK Health Care System*, Centre for Health Economics: York 1988, Discussion Paper 47.

24. "Evidence to the Government Internal Review of the National Health Service," *British Medical Journal*, vol. 296, 14 May 1988, pp. 1411–13.

25. David Green, *Everyone a Private Patient*, Institute of Economic Affairs: London 1986.

26. Richard Cockett, *Thinking the Unthinkable*, HarperCollins: London 1994.

27. Alain C. Enthoven, *Reflections on the Management of the National Health Service*, Nuffield Provincial Hospitals Trust: London 1985.

28. Social Services Committee, Fifth Report, Session 1987–88, *The Future of the National Health Service*, HMSO: London, HC 613.

29. Rudolf Klein, "Health Care Reform: The Global Search for Utopia," *British Medical Journal*, vol. 397, 27 September 1993, p. 752.

30. Lawson, op. cit., p. 616.

31. Thatcher, op. cit., p. 609.

32. In this stress on independence, an important—if indirect—influence appears to have been a book published several years earlier: John Vaizey, *National Health*, Oxford: Martin Robertson 1984.

33. Thatcher, op. cit., p. 614.

34. The paternity of the notion of GP fundholding is much in dispute. A strong candidate is Alan Maynard. See, for example, "Performance Incentives in General Practice" in George Teeling

Smith (ed.), *Health, Education and General Practice*, Office of Health Economics: London 1986.

35. In the three years from 1985–6 to 1988–9, the NHS budget rose by a total of 1.8 per cent in volume terms. In contrast, in the years from 1989–90 to 1991–2, the increase was 10.4 per cent. Karen Bloor and Alan Maynard, *Expenditure on the NHS During and After the Thatcher Years*, Centre for Health Economics: York 1993, Discussion Paper 113, Table 1, p.3.

36. Parliamentary Debates, vol. 152, no. 103, 11 May 1989, col. 1035.

37. "BMA Launches Campaign against White Paper," *British Medical Journal*, vol. 298, 11 March 1989, pp. 676–9.

38. Daniel M. Fox, *Health, Policies, Health Politics*, Princeton UP: Princeton 1986.

39. Peter Self, *Econocrats and the Policy Process*, Macmillan: Basingstoke 1975. See also Daniel M. Fox, *Economists and Health Care*, Prodist: New York 1979.

40. Alan Williams, "Health Economics: The End of Clinical Freedom?," *British Medical Journal*, vol. 297, 5 November 1988, pp. 1183–6.

41. For an acute analysis of the new "ideology" of managerialism and economism, and its impact on policy, see Peter Self, *Government by the Market?*, Macmillan: Basingstoke 1993.

42. Rudolf Klein, "From Status to Contract: The Transformation of the British Medical Profession" in Hugh L'Etang (ed.), *Health Care Provision Under Financial Constraint*, Royal Society of Medicine: London 1990.

43. Susan Kerrison, Tim Packwood and Martin Buxton, *Medical Audit: Taking Stock*, King's Fund Centre: London 1993.

44. Audit Commission, *A Short Cut to Better Services: Day Surgery in England and Wales*, HMSO: London 1990; *Lying in Wait: The Use of Medical Beds in Acute Hospitals*, HMSO: London 1992; *A Prescription for Improvement: Towards More Rational Prescribing in General Practice*, HMSO: London 1994.

45. Eleven Working Papers were published by the Department of Health. These included No. 1, *Self-Governing Hospitals*, and No. 2, *Funding and Contracts for Hospital Services*, HMSO: London 1989.

46. Ray Robinson and Julian Le Grand, *Evaluating the NHS Reforms*, King's Fund Institute: London 1994.

47. Giandomenico Majone, *Evidence, Argument and Persuasion in the Policy Process*, Yale UP: New Haven 1989. The argument that policy-making should be seen as the experimental testing of theories is also very much associated with Aaron Wildaysky.

48. Patricia Day and Rudolf Klein, "The Politics of Modernization," *The Milbank Quarterly*, vol. 67, no. 1, 1989, pp. 1–34.

The Politics of Universal Health Insurance

Lessons for and from the 1990s

Theodore R. Marmor and Morris L. Barer

For a brief period in the early 1990s (from roughly 1991 to early 1993) the enactment of national health insurance once again appeared imminent in American politics. Public opinion seemed supportive, a new President had campaigned on the promise, and interest groups of all stripes claimed that the medical status quo was unsustainable. To understand how fundamental reform rose to the top of the public agenda and almost as quickly disappeared is the major topic of this chapter. To do so it helps to understand not only the behavior of the Clinton Administration but the history of comparable reform efforts in twentieth century American politics. That background makes possible educated projections of what will happen to medical care issues in the politics of the next decade and beyond.

In 1990, national health insurance was hardly mentioned by pundits, politicians, or the press. The November 1991 election of the largely unknown Democrat Harris Wofford to fill the senatorial seat opened by the unexpected death of Republican Senator John Heinz changed all that. In an instant, Wofford's upset victory, widely attributed to his advocacy of national health insurance, suddenly and dramatically turned the attention of the nation's political commentators to the troubled state of American medicine.[1] Yet, the very fact of Wofford's groundswell indicated how misleading conventional wisdom's earlier dismissal of national health insurance had been.

The nation's reporters—and many of its politicians—discovered what students of American politics had known for a decade or more. A remarkable consensus had emerged over the 1980s that American medical care—particularly its financing and insurance coverage, needed a major overhaul.

The critical unanimity on this point—what political sociologist Paul Starr rightly termed a "negative consensus"—bridged almost all the usual cleavages in American politics—between old and young, Democrats and Republicans, management and labor, the well-paid and the low-paid. Americans had come to spend more on and feel worse about medical care than our economic competitors, with nine out of ten (including Fortune 500 executives) telling pollsters that American medical care required substantial change. That was the good news for medical reformers, whether in Congress, among interest groups or in what would become the Clinton Administration.

The bad news for reformers was, as had been the case in earlier decades, a bitter truth. A consensus on the seriousness of American medical care problems did not signify agreement on the shape, magnitude or priority of those problems. Nor did a negative consensus bring with it agreement on remedies. For a variety of ideological and institutional reasons, American politics makes it very difficult to coalesce around any acceptable policy solution. And this applies all the more particularly to a policy that would satisfy the requirements for a stable and workable system of financing and delivering modern medical care. No one has assurance that agreement on the seriousness of the nation's medical ills can generate the legislative support required for a substantively adequate and administratively workable program of reform. That understanding, however, was not apparent to the enthusiasts President Clinton brought to the White House in January of 1993.

The precise shape of the plan President Clinton proposed in October of 1993 could not have been anticipated from his campaign promises. As a campaigner, he had understandably avoided the details of health reform or its implementation. As President, he had different obligations, opportunities, and risks. The product of his unprecedented Health Task Force was but the beginning of a furious debate that concentrated more on ideological name calling and mind-numbing claims than clarification of the substantive policy and political choices. Whether the President's plan, or adjustments to it, could have commanded a majority of the Congress was made moot by the proposal's slow death in September 1994. This humiliating policy defeat has prompted a furious and continuing round of blaming, exculpatory rhetoric, and scholarly inquiry (including Fallows, 1995; Hacker, 1996; Mashaw and Marmor, 1996; Starr, 1995; Steinmo and Watts, 1995; White, 1995; and Yankelovich, 1995). What is far less clear is the meaning of this defeat for the future of American health policy.

HISTORY: LESSON OR LAMENTATION?

The task of substantially changing the rules of American medical care is one of the most difficult any set of reformers faces. At four other moments in twentieth century American politics, advocates of national health insurance and their presidential backers tried. In the Progressive era, during the New Deal, under President Truman, and during the early 1970s, many advocates thought universal health insurance was imminent only to be ultimately disappointed. In the 1990s, as earlier, entrenched interests helped block national health insurance by skillfully manipulating Americans' deepest fears to protect what they regarded as their interests. In 1993, to be sure, those interest groups seemed to be on the defensive; the time for sweeping reform appeared to have arrived. The President's speech of September 22, 1993, put the issue squarely on the legislative agenda and the initial public response to the call for "comprehensive" reform was favorable. But before the Clinton administration and Congress could meet the challenges of workable reform, they had to resolve—or at least cope with—some of the nastiest ideological and budgetary conflicts available in American politics. And that proved impossible.

What might be learned by reviewing this and earlier efforts by presidents committed to reform, but faced with seemingly intractable problems of substance, symbol, and support? Those who do not learn the lessons of history, academics regularly say, are doomed to repeat past mistakes.

PROGRESSIVE FRUSTRATION: 1912–1920

Early in this century, reformers of the Progressive era were convinced that broadened medical insurance, financed and administered as social insurance, held the key to improved health, medical, and economic security. But theirs was an elite consensus, helped in the pre–World War I period by the apparent, but momentary acquiescence of the American Medical Association. Yet, it turned out, there was nothing like a massive popular consensus on the need for change and, when the AMA turned against the idea, the reform movement withered. The transition during this period—from academic reform plans to Progressive state plans to political oblivion—was, as a number of historians[2] have made plain, bitterly disappointing to the reformers. A negative consensus on the need for change may be necessary in American politics. But it has not been a sufficient condition for the enactment of major reform programs in medical care—or most other areas of American politics and policy.

THE LOST REFORM: COMPULSORY HEALTH INSURANCE IN THE NEW DEAL

The agony of the Great Depression opened up enormous opportunities for change in American domestic politics. President Franklin D. Roosevelt led the way, commissioning expert group after expert group to take up reforms proposed for welfare, unemployment, agricultural failure, banking collapse, and the institutions of economic security more generally.

The opening for universal health insurance came in 1935 with the famous Committee of Economic Security (CES). A Cabinet-level special committee, the CES took a year to review the circumstances of welfare, unemployment, child health, and old age poverty and to arrive at a package of programmatic suggestions. They did their work with admirable skill and timeliness, fashioning workable ideas from a far-flung research investigation of various methods to resolve these difficult problems. Unemployment and welfare were the most pressing and obvious problems. Retirement benefits, though they have loomed much larger in subsequent decades, did not dominate their deliberations. With compulsory health insurance, President Roosevelt hesitated, worried that the presumed opposition of the American Medical Association and their ideological allies might jeopardize the success of the bulk of his social insurance reform package. So it was that the Committee refrained from even formally studying health insurance reform, leaving that to congressional advocates. Over the next decade, those advocates, under the banner of successive Wagner-Murray-Dingell bills, would repeatedly but unsuccessfully attempt to generate majority support in Congress for national health insurance.[3]

FROM NHI TO MEDICARE: THE DOGGED RETREAT

President Truman's experience with national health insurance was no less frustrating. He fought the election battle of 1948 with national health insurance prominent among his proposals for a Fair Deal. But he faced, during the election and after, a barrage of ideological criticism that demonized national health insurance by linking it with socialism, communism, and the Soviet Union. After years of facing certain defeat in Congress, Truman turned his executive advisors to a more modest goal: a health insurance program for Social Security recipients that would in time (14 years) become the Medicare program of 1965. During Truman's presidency, the general public was, according to the polls, always supportive of government health insurance. But this support was neither deep nor informed; socialized medicine was a tag that scared many, enough so that no amount of presidential enthusiasm seemed adequate to generate majority support in Congress. Opposition from the conservative coalition of powerful Southern Democrats and their ideological counterparts among the Republicans was enough to defeat every attempt at universal coverage—whether for all Americans or just those 65 and over.[4]

The fight over Medicare illustrates the conditions required for successful reform, even partial reform. Before the election of 1964, the conservative coalition remained formidable. The Democratic landslide of that year, however, swept away their key institutional bases of power: dilatory tactics symbolically represented by the Rules Committee, control of other key committees without threat from the Democratic caucus, and an ideological balance in the Congress as a whole less liberal than Presidents Kennedy or Johnson. But the massive electoral shift of 1964 held a lesson for future reformers. A sufficient condition for reform proved to be the two-to-one Democratic majority in the House of Representatives. This was a margin large enough to contain within it an issue majority on Medicare. In retrospect, a Medicare majority might well have emerged incrementally from the narrow defeats of the early 1960s. The election of 1964 prevents us from ever knowing for sure whether such a development might have taken place at some later date.

THE NIXON YEARS: SEEMING CONSENSUS, UNDENIABLE DISAPPOINTMENT

By 1970, the controversial topic of health reform had shifted back from Medicare to national health insurance once again. Though it is difficult for many to remember, the striking feature of the 1970–74 period was the intense competition among proponents of different forms of universal health insurance. There was the catastrophic coverage proposal Senators Russell Long (D-LA) and Abraham Ribicoff (D-CT) advocated, the Kennedy-Corman bill that closely resembled Canada's universal health insurance program, and the Nixon Administration's plan for mandated health insurance for employed Americans known then as the Comprehensive Health Insurance Plan (CHIP).[5]

The lessons of this period were surely relevant to American circumstances in the early 1990s. There was stalemate over the reform proposals of the 1970s because shifting coalitions defeated every attempt at compromise—cycling negative majorities we might say in political science. The majority that agreed on the need for reform consisted of factions committed to different proposals. The more modest proposals, like the Long-Ribicoff bill, seemed too limited to those who wanted to translate the negative consensus into universal, broad coverage. The proposal for employer-mandated insurance—similar in financing to what President Clinton in fact proposed later—seemed too indirect, incomplete, and incapable of cost control to those favoring more straightforward forms of national health insurance. Even Senator Kennedy, who moved away from his more ambitious version of national health insurance (the Kennedy-Corman bill) to a compromise plan that he and the powerful Ways and Means Committee Chairman Wilbur Mills could accept, was incapable of generating majority support among a coalition of liberal and conservative Democrats.

It is no wonder that many congressional figures from the 1970s were anxious to act once Clinton became president. They had come so close once—and with a Republican president (Nixon) in the White House. However, the cautionary point here is that the lessons of the 1970s are multiple and complicated, not single and simple. What might well have made sense then—namely, mandated, employment-based coverage—need not define the limit of what would be possible twenty years later. Indeed, sensibly sorting out the implications of more than two decades of frustration with partial reform was a major task facing advocates of universal health insurance in the early 1990s.

THE REFORM TASK IN 1992–94: DAUNTING BUT DO-ABLE?

The lessons of history are never simple. What worked once may not, in changed circumstances, work again. What failed earlier may succeed later. And some constants in American politics are always relevant to lesson drawing. Consider the following regularities.

First, compulsory health insurance—whatever the details—is an ideologically controversial proposal that involves enormous symbolic, financial and professional stakes. Such legislation does not emerge quietly or with broad bipartisan support, either here or elsewhere. Legislative success requires active Presidential leadership, the commitment of an administration's political capital, and the exercise of all manner of persuasion and arm twisting. This President Roosevelt was unwilling to do in the New Deal and President Nixon refrained from doing in the early 1970s. President Johnson was fully willing to use all his legendary legislative energy in 1965, but the composition of Congress then hardly made it necessary. Giving priority to the Medicare bill (with H.R.1 and S.1 as the numerical symbols) represented President Johnson's determination as well as his concentration on Medicare as the legislative centerpiece of his administration's first year.

Second, the limits of political feasibility are far less distinct than Beltway commentators seem to recognize. Political constraints are real, but they do not submit to estimates as precise as the budgetary work of the Congressional Budget Office. For example, the Johnson Administration, anxious to make sure its first step would be overwhelmingly acceptable in 1965, requested hospital benefits under Medicare only. But the oddest thing happened. A combination of liberals anxious to make the Medicare program broader and conservative Democrats wishing to head off step-by-step expansion later produced a wider reform than Johnson requested. Not only was physician insurance (what is now known as Part B) added to Medicare by the Ways and Means Committee, but Medicaid emerged as part of an unexpected "three-layer cake." Accordingly, no one should assume that the substantive and ideological packages sent to Congress as health reform are fixed in stone. And no one should treat legislative outcomes—whether enactment or stalemate, as the purposeful achievements of skillful entrepreneurs. Such outcomes—or resultants—emerge from very complicated bargaining and are a challenge to explain or to predict. The lesson is not that anything is possible but rather that feasibility estimates must acknowledge considerable uncertainty (see Marmor, 1973, chapter 6).

Third, the role of language and emotive symbols in this policy world cannot be overestimated. How a President reaches out to the public, what counts in the evening news and the morning newspapers as the central reform (or anti-reform) themes, and whether Congress faces a determined grass-roots movement—all shape the legislative outcome and, even more important, whether the resultant is sufficiently coherent and implementable to satisfy the expectations for reform. Pressure groups that can prevail in quiet politics are far weaker in contexts of mass attention, as the American Medical Association learned to its regret in the Medicare battle of 1965.

But the central lesson of the past—of both defeats and victories like Medicare—is cautionary in a different sense. It is wise to wait if what is acceptable is not workable. It is foolish to hesitate if what is workable can be made acceptable. If the central elements of a workable plan are acceptable, the pace of implementation can be staggered. But American political history in this area shows that the opportunities for substantial reform are few and far between, precious enough to make their squandering close to a sin.

THE CLINTON REFORM EFFORT REVISITED

It all began with such marvelous intentions, back in the late 1992 U.S. post election-victory glow of the Clinton Administration's agenda for the first 90 days. A federally crafted health care reform was finally going to lay to rest the ghosts of health-care-reform-efforts-past, along with the dual bugaboos of out-of-control costs and a large, growing, and embarrassing un- and under-insured population.

But as everyone who cares to know now knows, this road to reform was filled with potholes and poorly-concealed land mines as all efforts past; in September 1994 those travelling along it came to the precipice and turned back (Clymer, 1994). What went wrong, and what is likely to happen next?

To understand the failure of this particular initiative, one must first recall its origins and objectives. Two political imperatives justified the Clinton campaign's promise of reform and the White House's mounting a serious effort to deliver it. The first was that the nation's health care costs were predicted, prior to Clinton's election, to reach 18% of GDP by the turn of the century (Burner et al., 1992). With the U.S. already spending far more than all other advanced industrialized countries (Schieber et al., 1993), and the gap between it and the rest of its economic competitors getting larger, there was increasing concern

about the (economic or opportunity) cost of health care costs. Additional resources going into health care meant less competitive American goods and services, lower exchange rates and more expensive imports, or lower American
worker wages (Reinhardt, 1989; United States Congressional Budget Office,
1992). Health care had become, or at least seemed to be, a burden on general
economic growth and prosperity.

The second imperative was the growing insecurity of middle-class America
about the adequacy and stability of their health insurance. At any given point in
time, approximately 15% of the population is without health insurance coverage
(with many more having inadequate coverage) (Employee Benefits Research
Institute, 1993). But that is a static, and incomplete view of the extent of the
predicament. Over any recent two-year period, as many as 50 million to 60 million Americans will have had the pleasure of experiencing life without health
care coverage.

It was those *with* coverage, who wanted some assurance that they would be
able to keep it and that it would be there when they needed it, who represented
the potent political force. As the costs of coverage rose, more and more employers were eliminating or modifying the options they offered to their employees,
and the private insurance sector was becoming increasingly adept at risk selecting, and payment avoidance (Light, 1992). Not only could middle-class working
families not be sure that their current coverage would still be there next year,
or even next week, but they could be relatively sure that, if they had any health
problems, switching jobs was likely to be a costly venture (insurance coverage
is rarely, if ever, portable across carriers in the U.S.).

With these problems widely (if superficially) understood, Clinton's vision of
reform expressed two key initial objectives: cost control, and "health security"
(or guaranteed lifetime insurance coverage for all Americans). The details of
the Clinton's strategy for achieving these objectives are now well known, and
will not be repeated here. There has also been no shortage of blow-by-blow
descriptions of the demise of this reform initiative. But there have been few
attempts to date to sift the sense from the nonsense, the plausible from the im-
probable in those many pages of hand-wringing and second-guessing that have
fed the "Theory of the Month" club (*New York Times*, September 27, 1994). It
is surely worth considering the claims and counterclaims about the size and
placement of the most critical potholes, because such reflection holds the key
to understanding what is likely to come next in the U.S. health reform soap
opera.

One can usefully group the proffered reasons for failure into six categories:
external events; timing; the policy itself; politics; communication/media cover-

age; and interests. These are not independent, as we will see. But in considering each, it is important to ask ourselves, "Absent this reason, or category of reasons, would we have new federal health care legislation in place today in the United States?" If the answer is "No," or "Probably not," then such individual elements may have been interesting sideshows, but *on their own* they were clearly not decisive. Of course it is possible that a *collection* of individually unimportant reasons could, nevertheless, be critical. In the analysis that follows, we attempt to do some grouping of elements that appear to be intertwined in this way.

EXTERNAL EVENTS

Closely tied to the "timing" reason is the argument that events beyond the control of the Clinton administration (e.g. the fiasco in Somalia, the ongoing distraction of Bosnia) intervened at politically inopportune moments to suck the administration's (and the American public's) energy and attention from the health care reform effort.

TIMING

There are two quite separate components to this argument—external and internal. The external version is simply that the recession (and the public concern about jobs, incomes, and employment-related health insurance) ended too soon. This in turn undermined a key source of reform pressure. It was this "premature" recovery that underpinned the Republican challenge to the very need for comprehensive reform. The "What Crisis?" campaign by the Republican leadership, on this view, cast doubt on the case for system overhaul at a critical juncture.

The internal version has to do with the policy development process itself. This argument has included many sub themes. But the dominant version characterizes the administration as squandering its "window of opportunity" by becoming mired in a complex, consultative, time-consuming development process. Why should careful policy development work against the chances of enactment? It is because such policy development takes time, thus giving opponents plenty of opportunity to mobilize their constituencies, refine their rebuttals, and search for allies.

THE POLICY ITSELF AND THE LEGISLATIVE PROCESS

The *Health Security Act*, 1,342 pages long, was, arguably, too complex and bureaucratically cumbersome to have any hope of being understood, let alone embraced, by the general public. The proposal tried to find some middle ground that would satisfy both those who would have preferred a single-payer model of national health insurance with no role for the private insurance sector, and those who would have preferred nothing more than "lite insurance reform." This strategy satisfied neither group and so, on this argument, was doomed to failure.

In the many arcane details of the American political process, the one legislative feature that some have presented as the key determinant of stalemate over reform is the necessity to obtain at least sixty votes in the Senate in order to overcome a possible filibuster. Had the health reform initiative been piggybacked onto the budget-reconciliation bill, it would have required only a simple majority vote for passage. But the Administration was unable to get the political support for this approach because of the opposition of a few key members of the Senate

ELECTORAL POLITICS

With Clinton's victory in 1992, and Democratic party control of Congress, was supposed to come the end of policy gridlock in Washington (looking back, one might be excused for not having noticed any difference). The early version of this position was straightforward: the party seen as blocking health care reform would be doomed at the midterm (fall 1994) elections. However, as the process dragged on, as the Democrats failed to reach consensus on their own reform proposal (Rosenthal, 1994), and as the special interests made their influence felt on Congress and on public opinion, the Republicans realized they could afford to drag their heels. By the summer of 1994, the official unofficial Republican Party position was that *no* Democratic proposal would see the light of day. And the Republicans had the votes to ensure that this was the case.

To be fair, the Republicans could not have carried out their agenda had it not been for divisions within the Democratic party. One of the structural realities of American politics is that a partisan majority does not guarantee a *policy* majority. Democrats in Congress rarely stand united on a key policy issue, and this was particularly true during the health care reform debate. Policy solidarity takes a back seat in this process.

COMMUNICATIONS/MEDIA COVERAGE

There are two arguments here that initially appear to be in conflict. One is that the media did an abysmal job of providing informed, balanced analysis of the implications of the administration's plan to the public. Instead, the media treated the reform process as political theater in which who said what today was more important than a careful determination of the likely effects of the reforms on different subsets of real American people (Hamburger et al., 1994).

The second view is that the Administration failed to recognize the critical importance of communication in "selling" its policy, and so gave short shrift to involving the press, particularly its Washington corps, in getting the message out. There was no "elevator speech," that could be delivered during the trip up to the fifth floor, and which captured the essence of the plan in a way easily understandable, and attractive to the (wo)man on the street.

There is the temptation to argue that these cannot possibly both be true. After all, if the administration was unwilling to involve the press in the early stages of policy evolution, how could the press be taken to task for simply reporting on the congressional and committee mudslinging? Or, turning it around, if the administration knew how the media was likely to report on health care reform, how could it possibly entrust the same media with the inner details of the plan's logic and analysis?

In fact, our view is that both are to a large measure correct and that both could (and did) exist. The Administration did make some early strategic errors in its failure to hone an "elevator speech" and in its interaction with the Washington press in particular (Fallows, 1995). But once details of the plan were public, there was in fact a dearth of informative reporting and analysis by the media. It is likely that the latter was a more critical determinant of the outcome.

INTERESTS

While the media may not have done its job in sorting out for the public who would gain and who would lose as a result of the Clinton reform plan, those in the latter category were quick to recognize themselves and to mobilize. And the Clinton administration appears to have made some rather egregious errors in sizing up which interests could be counted on as allies, and which were likely to be opposed (Silver, 1995). What resulted may, in retrospect, turn out to have been one of the most effective public influence campaigns ever waged, even in America. It was clear from the outset who the winners and losers were likely to be. The uninsured and underinsured would be better off, at least in terms of insurance security, but also likely in terms of overall cost per family.

Despite the fact that the administration's plan left private insurance as the central player in providing coverage, it was likely that many smaller insurance companies (and those insurers unable to make the transition from fee-for-service to managed care) would have been "shaken out" of the market. Managed care was likely to take a big bite out of pharmaceutical company bottom lines, and to put downward pressure on (at least specialist) physician incomes. And malpractice reform would be a direct hit on the bottom line of many of the country's trial lawyers.

It was no surprise, then, that the Health Insurance Association of America (HIAA), the American Medical Association, and the Pharmaceutical Manufacturers' Association, jumped into the fray, early and often, and that, behind the scenes, lobbyists for associations such as the Trial Lawyers of America, the Life Underwriters, and the Health Underwriters were hard at work doing what they do best (and succeeding) (Franklin, 1995). The overall strategy appears to have been best captured by a line in the famous "Harry and Louise" ads sponsored by the HIAA. After anguished discussion about how the plan was going to remove their choice of physician and benefits, they conclude that "There has to be a better way." If the objective of the campaigns, littered in inaccuracies and half truths (*Consumer Reports*, 1994), was to sow seeds of doubt in the minds of the public, then it was wildly successful. And doubt was really all that was needed to scuttle the plan, because there was a dearth of easily digestible, and personally relevant, information being provided by the administration (Lefebvre, 1994). This made it relatively easy for powerful congressional factions to succumb to the pressures of the lobbyists, knowing full well that doing so would not alienate their increasingly doubtful constituencies. There was also a ready political ear for those targeted campaigns. What the Republicans did not want, most of all, was a made-in-Democrat-country health reform bill (see *"Politics"* above).

Of course the media was largely complicitous because of the virtual absence of balanced, critical discussion, both of the issues, and of the claims (see, e.g., Silver, 1995). In stark contrast to the media coverage of the O. J. Simpson murder case, the media (with few exceptions) did nothing to clear up the confusion created by the paid advertisements (Marmor, 1995).

THE CRITICAL FACTORS OF DEMISE

As we noted above, it is helpful in sifting through the various claims about the reasons for the failure of the Clinton plan (or even of any of the alternatives that came with a rush toward the end), to ask ourselves whether the absence of a particular reason would have meant a different outcome. In some cases, the answer seems relatively simple. For example, we believe that the first three categories—external events, the policy itself and timing—were secondary at best. If there had not been these particular external events, there would have been others. The nature of politics (as with life itself) is that one never has the luxury of focusing on only one thing, and it would be naive of anyone to believe that the Clintons thought this would be possible or desirable.

As for the policy and the legislative process, despite its length and apparent complexity, one must recall that the details of the act were never meant for public consumption. The details of the *American Social Security Act*, or the *Environmental Protection Act* are no less complex—little more than the titles are understood by the public—yet they became law. More important by far was the failure to communicate the key features (see below), and to effectively counter the vested interests' clever use of the media.

To sustain the external timing argument, one would have to believe that, had the U.S. remained in recession, the plan, or a modification, would by now have been passed into law. There is no evidence of which we are aware that would support such a view. The internal timing arguments are equally difficult to support, requiring that quicker introduction, or introduction as part of the budget bill, would have resulted in passage. In this case possible, but unlikely.

But why unlikely? Because of the three other categories—politics, communication/media coverage, and interests. The American constitutional dispersion of power and authority, and the resulting labyrinthian political process, makes passage of much less complex and far-reaching initiatives exceedingly difficult. It is no surprise that American policy is shaped by incrementalism (Morone, 1986). Desperate times may call for desperate measures, but if such are not possible, well, maybe the times are not quite that desperate after all.

It may be, however, that the greatest single impediment to passage of this, or any other significant reform proposal, is the insidious interplay among the special interests, the public and their elected politicians, through the media. Any major reform involves intent to change the distribution of costs and benefits; if it did not, it would not be reform. In health care, change invariably involves diffuse benefits, and concentrated costs—a bit better insurance coverage for a whole lot of people, at the expense of lost or reduced incomes for those involved in the health insurance business; more integrated patient care (and perhaps even better patient outcomes) through managed care, at the expense of reduced pharmaceutical company revenues, fewer (and lower) specialist physician incomes, and fewer hospital-based incomes; less unnecessary defensive medicine and lower medical and legal costs, at the expense of the incomes of malpractice lawyers; and so on.

Those concentrated interests with the most to lose have far more powerful incentives to get their case across, than does anyone to make the case for the effect of reform on the average American. And the calamities that are just around the corner if reform X is passed tend to fit much more closely with the sort of story that every editor of every daily newspaper or television news magazine admonishes his/her staff to seek out, than do careful analyses or dull interviews with pointy-headed experts. Most of the latter have already been done, at least once. They are no longer "fresh material," even if they are no less true today than when first run.

Furthermore, the vested interests have at their disposal resources that far outstrip the resources available to (or likely to be committed to) a "voice on the other side." Not only do those interests represent important sources of campaign funding in an environment where election (and re-election) is prohibitively costly (Silver, 1995), but they are also able to support academics promoting "friendly" proposals (*The Lancet,* 1993), and to engage high-priced and obviously quite effective help in the "media influence" game.

In sum, from where we sit, it appears that politics, the media coverage, and interests were the critical factors in undermining this particular effort at significant reform, but these are not separable elements, and it is their interaction that produced the mix of discourse to which the American public was subjected. By November 1994, the American public, which had earlier been so supportive of health care system reform, was now "rejecting a major overhaul of the system" (Henry J. Kaiser Family Foundation, 1994). In the final analysis, disinformation and the spin-doctors, won out again.

WOULD IT HAVE MATTERED ANYWAY?

But we lose ourselves in such debates over the key reasons for policy development failure at our peril, for there is something more fundamental of which we should not lose sight. As we noted at the outset, two political imperatives drove the Clinton reform initiative—cost control, and security of benefits—which leads us to a fundamental question: Would any plan passed in this latest round of health care reform frenzy have achieved either or both of these overarching objectives?

The administration understood that leaving the cost control piece to market forces, whether through managed competition or other mechanisms, was likely to fail (Aaron and Schwartz, 1993). That is why they built limits on premium increases into their proposal, as an explicit attempt to limit the rate of growth of funding, and thus expenditures. Yet very early in the debate, the interest in cost control simply disappeared. The "untouchable" piece of the Clinton plan was universal and lifelong coverage for some basic package of health care benefits; everything else was on the table.

And then even the untouchable became vulnerable. By the summer of 1994, universal coverage had given way to a willingness to accept coverage for 95% of Americans as "universal" (Goldberg et al., 1994). By early September, that number had slipped even further, until it looked not a whole lot different from the unsatisfactory *status quo* (about 85% of the population covered) (Starr, 1994).

And therein lies a continuing and fundamental dilemma for U.S. health reform. The rest of the developed world figured out some time ago that providing universal coverage did not have to mean uncontrolled costs, and that controlling costs did not have to mean foregoing universal coverage. Those simple facts are still largely seen (or at least promoted) within U.S. health policy circles as fundamental contradictions, and for good reason. Those with the most to lose (see above) have compelling reasons (controlled costs = lower/controlled incomes) to keep the confusion levels high.

In fact there are a small number of beliefs, promoted by a small number of powerful special interests, and embraced for political/ideological reasons by key members of Congress and the Senate, which seem to us to stand in the way of any health reform initiative that is likely to achieve cost control and universal coverage in the United States (Barer, 1995). The first of these, as noted above, is the firmly held belief that universal coverage will require additional revenue. There are good reasons to question this belief (Barer et al., 1994; Wolfe, 1993). The international evidence provides striking proof that the opposite can be true. Where the "made in America" analyses fall down is in their failure to take a population-based approach to estimating the impact of extending coverage to those presently without it.[6]

A second fundamental, perhaps even more deeply held, belief that stands as an impediment to successful reform is the notion that "big government" will mishandle it, or, taken the other way, that the private sector is more efficient at providing health insurance coverage than the public sector. This view continues to be promoted heavily by the private insurance sector, for obvious reasons. But that promotion is given weight by many American health economists, who seem (have) to believe fervently that private markets (the invisible guiding hand) must (by assumption) be able to respond to the preferences of a population far better than any government or public sector structures.

Of course this view conveniently ignores the litany of evidence to the contrary (Friedman, 1991; Light, 1994), largely on the grounds that some additional private market reforms are all that stand between the current problems and health insurance nirvana. Yet it seems obvious to most interested observers outside the United States that much of the activity in which the U.S. private insurance sector engages is little more than waste motion—necessary only because of the peculiar ideological need (powerfully promoted, of course) to cling to the private market and support many corporate players. Risk pooling and community rating would eliminate the need for much of this busy work, but would, by definition, also eliminate many jobs and a lot of insurance company black ink.

Add to these the strong and enduring beliefs in the need to incorporate significant user fees in any reform package (presumably to control costs, but again in the face of compelling evidence to the contrary), and to hitch the funding of the system to place of employment (despite the complications and additional opposition from the small business community so created), and one has a formidable set of structural impediments to any attempt at health care system reform. In the face of such a collection of strongly held beliefs, there seems to us to be little prospect of seeing either universal coverage or (even less likely) cost control in the U.S. any decade soon.

SO, WHAT WILL HAPPEN NEXT?

In keeping with the American approach to reform, there is a lot of incremental reform activity either in place, or being actively considered. This is of three types: federal; state-initiated; or self-propelled (e.g. reform initiated by payers and providers).

FEDERAL ACTIVITY

With the 1994 mid-term elections, the Republican agenda came to the fore. The Republicans have all along had far less interest in extending coverage, and have argued (even if rhetorically, at times) that costs were not really a problem. Their major thrust in their first few months was to develop an agenda structured around downsizing the role of government. Given the prominence of government programs such as Social Security, Medicare and Medicaid, we are far more likely to see efforts to shrink coverage (or at least the depth and breadth of benefits) than to expand those programs or create new ones (Iglehart, 1995).

With Clinton's re-election, he might be or may be expected to do what he has done throughout his political career—learn from his mistakes. He has invested considerable political capital in the health care reform effort; it seems unlikely that he will simply turn his back on that. However, any new Clinton-initiated federal reform plan would be far more incremental than the *Health Security Act*, and would involve key concessions to the major players noted above. In the end, any reform that can be supported by all the key interest groups is likely to be tepid at best, with its publicity value far exceeding any real benefits to the average American and most likely leaving the original two driving forces—rising costs and spotty and unreliable coverage—largely intact. For as Steinmo and Watts (1995) have noted, "America cannot pass major comprehensive health care reform that will control costs and offer complete coverage to all Americans because here political institutions are designed to prevent this kind of reform." (For a somewhat less pessimistic emphasis on the same structural barriers to action, see Mashaw and Marmor, 1996.)

STATE REFORM: SPINNING GOLD FROM STRAW?

Many political observers in the U.S. now feel that the best hope for significant reform lies at the state level, and that a few successes there will motivate a bandwagon effect. More than 20 years ago, Hawaii went out on a limb and implemented an employment-based health care system built around an employer mandate. Since then, many of the coverage gaps have been filled by supplemental programs, so that virtually all Hawaiians have health care coverage, and at a cost lower than, or comparable, to states with far less extensive coverage.

More recently, a few states have passed legislation that promises to increase coverage and control costs. However, these states, and any that follow in their path, face formidable obstacles (Mashaw and Marmor, 1996), of which the following are but a few:

(a) ERISA exemption: any state wishing to mandate all employers to provide health insurance to their employees require a federal exemption from the *Employment Retirement Income Security Act* (ERISA) of 1974. No state has been granted an exemption in the past 20 years, and multistate businesses stand firmly behind ERISA because it allows self-insured employers freedom from state mandates.

(b) fiscal reality: state coffers are notoriously the first to feel the effects of a recession, and the last to recover from one. Only now are they beginning to recover from the 1991 recession; in the meantime, the costs of education, justice and Medicaid, which provides health care coverage for America's most indigent have all continued to expand. Because of the widespread perception that further health care coverage extension will increase costs (see earlier discussion), this will be an extremely hard sell.

(c) interest group reality: all of the pressures to retain the *status quo* at the federal level also reside in the states, albeit unevenly distributed. New Jersey, for example, has a high concentration of pharmaceutical companies; Massachusetts and Texas are homes to major academic medical center complexes; Illinois is home to the American Medical Association and the national Blue Cross and Blue Shield Associations, and several major world-class teaching hospitals; and so on. The accounting reality, that cost control must imply income control or job loss, will be even more difficult to hide at the state than at the federal level.

(d) the limits of state policy: many of the key drivers of health care costs are not likely to come under state jurisdiction any time soon. For example, health care professionals are free to cross state borders, irrespective of where they were trained. Even if California chose to get really serious about cost control, and decided to reduce the intake of medical students to state schools, it would have no control over the size of the schools in Massachusetts, or Texas. Similarly, the diffusion of expensive technology into clinical sites within a state are largely beyond the direct control of that state. Yet in the absence of control over those cost drivers, there is little hope for long-term cost control unless states are prepared to preside over forceful prices and incomes control policies.

MARKET, HEAL THYSELF: PAYERS, PROVIDERS AND PIPE DREAMS

And so we come to the last great hope: market reform through capitated health care, total integration, and cost control. Faithful followers of this approach claim that requiring physicians or physician groups to accept financial risk for their clinical decisions will bring both better quality care and lower costs.

Although it is true that some health maintenance organizations and long-standing large physician group practices have been successful in reducing unnecessary care and hospital utilization rates while increasing access to primary and preventive care services, the potential to replicate these successes tends to be grossly over-estimated. The environmental and organizational forces required to extend the reach of such truly integrated health care minisystems quite simply do not exist in much of the United States. Many areas continue to be served by rural, solo, fee-for-service physicians, with no logical reason to change their circumstances, and in no position to be able to take on any significant level of financial risk-bearing.

Furthermore, even moderate expansion of the reach of such integrated systems would still leave intact a largely patchwork system of coverage, with many opportunities for cost-shifting and cream skimming. Where such opportunities exist, they will be taken. The route from individual mini- or microsystem cost control, to macrosystem-level cost control is neither obvious nor simple. But movements such as this need pay little heed to such mundane matters as aggregation fallacies. Nor is it in the interests of many of their disciples to promote such hidden truths.

At the same time, the insurance sector is becoming more vertically integrated by absorbing the managed care sector; this allows large insurers to be better positioned to benefit from a wider range of possible reform initiatives. This may not, in and of itself, be a bad thing. But will it bring cost control or universal coverage? We think not. What seems far more likely is that an increasing share of a still increasing health care pot will be channeled to nonclinical activity, and this in a country that is already top-heavy in health care administration costs.

That is not to say that the bottom-up process of reform which has begun and is gaining speed in some jurisdictions, such as California, cannot succeed in achieving coverage extension and cost control. The route from here to there is simply not obvious, at least to these observers. So long as the vested interest groups control the political agenda and can continue so effectively and without opposition to sow the seeds of doubt that support the *status quo*, and so long as the "market metaphor" (Annas, 1995) with its "invisible hand" dominates thinking about health care, it will be virtually impossible to mobilize change.

In sum, while there are opportunities for incremental reform within both the public and private health care sectors, there are realistically now no opportunities in sight for major and meaningful advances in providing health care coverage to all Americans, or in reining in their runaway health care costs. Where glimmerings of success appear to emerge—where the market may actually be doing what proponents argue it can do, as exemplified in the recent slowing in pharmaceutical cost escalation relative to other sectors of the health care economy (Levit et al., 1994)—one can expect increasingly intense lobbying intended to undermine free market forces. Advocates of markets will be advocates only so long as the stylized, and often highly regulated markets in which they are accustomed to prospering continue to serve their bottom lines.

REFORM AND UNDERSTANDING: THE ROLE OF POLITICAL SCIENCE

The role of political scientists (and political science) in the twentieth century battles over universal health insurance is not a subject to which much attention has been paid. That, of course, is no reason to ignore it.

Until the Truman period political scientists did not play a prominent intellectual role in the debate over what form, if any, government health insurance should play in the American version of a welfare state. The social insurance reformers of the Progressive era took their cues from Europe, especially Germany, and included in their numbers lawyers, public health figures, insurance experts, and what were then known as political economists. By the time of the New Deal, there were two major streams of intellectual commentary: those like I. S. Falk from public health and those like Witte, Perlman, and Epstein from the specialized arena of social insurance. At that time, many American universities, particularly land-grant ones, had within their economics, sociology and history departments experts in social insurance. At the University of Wisconsin particularly, this expertise was transferred to state reform action (in unemployment insurance, for example) and to the New Deal reforms, where Witte was the executive director of the Committee on Economic Security.

The persistent clash over the Wagner-Murray-Dingell proposal for national health insurance between 1939 and 1948 brought health politics to country-wide media attention. And, in the wake of that, political scientists concerned with public opinion and the operation of pressure groups in American politics came to address national health insurance more directly. The American Medical Association, then the leading critic of "government medicine," expended considerable resources trying to defeat the Truman reform plan and became a prominent example of interest group exertion of power in America's fragmented political system. Stanley Kelley's *Professional Public Relations and Political Power* (1966) addressed this phenomenon directly, supplementing what had become the conventional explanation by journalists for why the United States, unlike most other industrial democracies, had rejected national health insurance.

Kelley's interest in the battles of the 1940s was supplemented by considerable attention to the long struggle over Medicare. Books by political scientists Eugene Feingold (1966), Judith Feder (1977), and Marmor (1973) addressed the origins, enactment, and early implementation in this controversial program of the Johnson years. But, for all the attention Medicare's legislative struggle generated, political scientists have largely ignored the administrative experience of that program and left the analysis of subsequent disputes over America's so-called health crisis to other fields. There are exceptions to be sure: Larry Brown's (1983) writing on the politics of the HMO movement, Jim Morone's work on health planning (1990), Mark Peterson's (1993) focus on the health politics of the 1970s and 1980s, as well as Larry Jacobs' recent book (1993) comparing the political struggle over the NHS and Medicare. But the general point remains.

Economists particularly expanded into the health arena in the 1960s, following not surprisingly the expanded market for research on this growing industry. Whether this market development has illuminated our policy issues is a controversial matter, but it would be surprising to find an essay, like Dan Fox's (1979) critique of modern health economics, written on the role of political science in the past twenty years of health policy disputes.

The irony, however, is this. As we try to understand the fate of health reform in the 1990s, assumptions about political feasibility are central to the policymaking arguments made and their fate. Those who most regularly voice opinions about this matter tend not to be professional political scientists. Economists like Henry Aaron, Uwe Reinhardt, and Eli Ginzberg,[7] among many others, claim confidently that they know what American politics will and will not permit.

What is striking about such commentary is the thinness of the evidence on which such judgements are made. None of the economists cited have themselves studied the changing constraints of American politics. None of them have systematically investigated the role of public opinion in policymaking in ways, for example, illustrated by the work of Benjamin Page, Robert Shapiro, or Larry Jacobs. Yet the economist commentators appear to have no doubt that their judgements are more than conventional wisdom applied to an arena of politics that has confused even the most searching of scholars. I leave it to historians to wonder about why this should be the case.

There is, however, another side to the fate of health reform in the 1990s. A number of political scientists joined forces to comment on the claims and counterclaims about reform. Organized in reaction to the Jackson Hole Group and known informally as the "No Holes Group," these policy commentators are in fact largely political scientists. Their names will be familiar to those interested in the place of medical care in American political studies: Larry Brown of Columbia, Tom Oliver of Maryland, Jim Morone of Brown, Mark Peterson of Pittsburgh, Larry Jacobs of Minnesota, Christa Altenstetter of CUNY, David Wilsford of Georgia Tech, Deborah Stone of Brandeis, and myself. This group, augmented by a number of other sociologists, economists, and lawyers, represents the culmination of a development dating back to the late 1960s: the initiation of a Committee on Health Politics. From that beginning emerged *The Journal of Health Politics, Policy, and Law* and a considerable amount of scholarship. What the No Holes Group illustrates is the movement from academic inquiry to a politically more active role, one illustrated not simply by published work, but congressional testimony, media appearances, and other forms of policy participation. Whether that shift in effort will be influential is something no one can be sure about at the time of this writing (summer 1995).

CONCLUSION

The American politics of universal health insurance was anomalous from the perspective of industrial democracies in the 1990s. Everywhere, it appeared, health reform, with different priorities, was on the agenda, but nowhere was the question of universal coverage in dispute. Cost control, concern about the quality of care, worry about responsiveness to citizen wishes, and the possibility of more efficient delivery and organization of care—all had the attention of national political elites in Japan, France, Holland, Sweden, Britain, Australia, and elsewhere. Because the entitlement to health insurance coverage had been settled earlier, these political battles differed from what took place in the United States even though the rhetoric of common problems typically obscured this fact.

National health insurance as the reform objective suffered a crushing defeat in the summer of 1994. A kind of political amnesia came over the reporting of the subject. Where it had been one of the two or three most prominent topics on the Clinton administration's agenda during the 1993 and 1994 legislative sessions, universal health insurance disappeared from the president's messages and, with that, from much Washington commentary. But the reform of American medical care hardly died. Indeed, unprecedented change has taken place in the wake of the president's initial reform efforts and only more so since their demise.

In this respect, the stalemated politics of national health insurance had consequences far wider than those initially expected from the legislative battle. The Clinton administration sought to find common ground between liberal and conservative advocates of health reform. It adopted the language of market reform—"managed competition" was its initial slogan—and explicitly rejected universal health insurance on the model of Canada or as an expansion of Medicare (which was very close to the same thing). Instead, it sought the results of traditional health insurance while extolling the virtues of competitive plans vying for customers and bargaining hard with the providers of care. The result is that we have declining insurance coverage, enormous pressure to reduce costs from payers, and enormous uncertainty about what American medical care—or its public policy—will look like by the end of the twentieth century.

The lessons from this experience go beyond national health insurance, however. American politics are fragmented and the opportunities for substantial change are few and far between. What seems striking about the fate of the Clinton reform effort, in retrospect, was the strategy chosen and its unexpected consequences. The very window of opportunity opened up by the conjunction of presidential leadership, a negative elite and public consensus on the need for change, and the presence of energetic advocates let in surprising changes. In prospect, actors tried to adjust to the presumption that the Clinton plan would pass and did so by trying to adapt to its design features. In the wake of defeat, these very same actors had a headstart on change without an organized opposition. The states that tried to anticipate the Clinton program—like Kentucky,

Florida, Minnesota and Vermont—generated changes in the rules of medical organization and finance, but not the funds for universal coverage. The health insurance industry, particularly its largest firms, accelerated its departure from traditional, indemnity plans into the role of "health management" companies. Even drug firms took up the banner of management, touting themselves as in the business of disease management. In this respect, the marketing and managerial ethos that dominated the Clinton administration's approach to selling national health insurance survived as the undeniable commitment to universal coverage collapsed. There have been few more ironic episodes in American politics in this or any other century.

Notes

This article was first published as Chapter 14 in *Health Politics and Policy*, 3rd ed., ed. Theodor J. Litman and Leonard S. Robins (Albany: Delmar, 1997). Morris L. Barer is Director, Centre for Health Services & Policy Research, Professor, Department of Health Care & Epidemiology, University of British Columbia. This commentary expresses some views published elsewhere. See especially Marmor (1994a). Some of the historical commentary appeared in the introductory chapter of Marmor (1994b) and is reprinted here by permission of Yale University Press. The analysis of the failure of the Clinton health plan was previously published by Barer with Marmor and Morrison (1995). Reprinted from Morris L. Barer (with T. R. Marmor and F. M. Morrison), *Social Science and Medicine*, Vol. 41, "Health Care Reform in the United States: On the Road to Nowhere Again?" pp. 453–460, copyright 1995, with kind permission from Elsevier Science Ltd., The Boulevard, Langford Lane, Kidlington oX5 1GB, UK.

1. The details of how the Wofford election affected the coverage of national health insurance are provided and analyzed in Hacker, J. (1996), Chapter 1.

2. For a summary of the debate over government health insurance from 1912 to 1920, see Burrows (1977). For an analysis of how organized medicine first embraced and then turned against compulsory health insurance, see Numbers (1978).

3. The most comprehensive history of this phase of the American debate over compulsory health insurance is Hirshfield (1970).

4. This is the story, told in considerable detail, in Marmor (1973).

5. These plans were the subject of enormous journalistic and scholarly scrutiny; see, Feder, Holohan, and Marmor (1980).

6. In this, they succumb to the so-called Rand Experiment fallacy. A major finding of the Rand health insurance experiment was that those *in the sample* faced with user fees used less care than those having to pay no user fees, and that the higher the user fee, the less care was sought. Despite the fact that the experiment precluded, by design, the extrapolation of such results to entire populations, generalizations have nevertheless become commonplace. The results of the experiment have been used to conclude that user fees can control costs, in spite of contrary *population-based* evidence from Canada, and the fundamental lack of logic in a conclusion that focuses exclusively on the demand side of this market. Analyses of the effects of extending coverage in the U.S. have fallen into the same analytical quicksand—differences in service use by sub-populations with different degrees of insurance coverage, have been extrapolated to estimate the global, population-based, implications of extending coverage to all.

7. For a specific critique of Ginzberg's reasoning about why national health insurance has failed to be enacted, see our chapter "American Health Politics: 1970–90" in Marmor (1994b).

References

Aaron, Henry J., & William B. Schwartz. (1993). Managed competition: Little cost containment without budget limits. *Health Affairs*, 12 [Supplement], 204–215.

Annas, George J. (1995). Reframing the debate on health care reform by replacing our metaphors. *New England Journal of Medicine*, 332 (March 16), 744.

Barer, Morris L. (1995). So near, and yet so far: A Canadian perspective on U.S. health reform. *Journal of Health Politics, Policy and Law*, 20 (Summer), 463–476.

Barer, Morris L., Robert G. Evans, Matthew Holt, and J. Ian Morrison. (1994). It ain't necessarily so: The cost implications of health care reform in the United States. *Health Affairs*, 13 (Fall), 88–99.

Barer, Morris L., Theodore R. Marmor, and Ellen M. Morrison. (1995). Health care reform in the United States: On the road to nowhere again? *Social Science and Medicine*, 41 (4), 453–460.

Brown, Lawrence D. (1983). *Politics and healthcare organization: HMO's as Federal policy*. Washington, DC: The Brookings Institution.

Burner, Sally T., Daniel R. Waldo, and David R. McKusick. (1992). National health expenditures projections through 2030. *Health Care Financing Review*, 14 (Fall), 1–30.

Burrows, James. (1977). *Organized medicine in the Progressive Era: The move toward monopoly*. Baltimore, MD: Johns Hopkins University Press.

Clymer, Adam. (1994). National health program, president's greatest goal, declared dead in Congress. *New York Times* (September 27), A1.

Consumer Reports. (1994). Health-care hucksters: What their ads say—and don't say (February), 116.

Employee Benefits Research Institute. (1993). *Source of health insurance and characteristics of the uninsured* (Issue Brief No. 133). Washington, DC: Employee Benefits Research Institute.

Fallows, J. (1995). A triumph at misinformation. *The Atlantic Monthly* (January 26).

Feder, Judith M. (1977). *Medicare: The politics of federal hospital insurance*. Lexington, MA: Lexington Books.

Feder, Judith, John Holahan, and Theodore R. Marmor. (Eds.). (1980). *National health insurance: Conflicting goals and policy choices*. Washington, DC: Urban Institute.

Feingold, Eugene. (1966). *Medicare: Policy and politics*. San Francisco, CA: Chandler.

Feingold, Eugene. (1993). *The health of nations: Public opinion and the making of American and British health policy*. Ithaca, NY: Cornell University Press.

Fox, Daniel M. (1979). From reform to relativism: A history of economics and health care. *Milbank Memorial Fund Quarterly/Health and Society*, 57 (3), 297–336.

Franklin, J. D. (1995). Tommy Boggs and the death of health care reform. *Washington Monthly* (April 31).

Friedman, Emily. (1991). Insurers under fire. *Health Management Quarterly*, 13 (3), 23–27.

Goldberg, Mark, Theodore R. Marmor, and Jerry Mashaw. (1994). The odd jargon of the 95% promise. *Los Angeles Times* (Washington edition) (August 4).

Hacker, Jacob. (1996). *The road to nowhere: The genesis of President's Clinton's plan for national health insurance*. Princeton, NJ: Princeton University Press.

Hamburger, Thomas, Theodore R. Marmor, and Jon Meacham. (1994). What the death of health reform teaches us about the press. *Washington Monthly* (November).

Henry J. Kaiser Family Foundation. (1994). News Release (November 15), 1.

Hirshfield, Daniel S. (1970). *The lost reform: The campaign for compulsory health insurance in the United States from 1932 to 1943*. Cambridge, MA: Harvard University Press.

Iglehart, John K. (1995). Republicans and the new politics of health care. *New England Journal of Medicine*, 332 (April 6), 972–975.

Jacobs, Lawrence. (1993). *The health of nations: Public opinion and the making of American and British health policy*. Ithaca, NY: Cornell University Press.

Kelley, Stanley. (1966). *Professional public relations and political power*. Baltimore, MD: Johns Hopkins University Press.

Lancet, The. (1993). Editorial: U.S. health reforms: Clichés, cost and Mrs. C., 341, 791–792.

Lefebvre, R. C. (1994). Health reform in the United States: A social marketing perspective. *Journal of Public Policy Marketing*, 13, 319.

Levit, Katherine R., Cathy A. Cowan, Helen C. Lazenby, Patricia A. McDonnell, Arthur L. Sensenig, Jean M. Stiller, and Darleen K. Won. (1994). National health spending trends, 1960–1993. *Health Affairs*, 3 (Winter), 14–31.

Light, Donald W. (1992). The practice and ethics of risk-related health insurance. *Journal of the American Medical Association*, 267 (May 13), 2503–2508.

Light, Donald W. (1994). Life, death and the insurance companies. *New England Journal of Medicine*, 330 (February 17), 498–499.

Marmor, Theodore R. (1973). *The politics of Medicare*. Chicago: Aldine.

Marmor, Theodore R. (1994a). The politics of universal health insurance: Lessons from past administrations? (Symposium on national health insurance). *PS* (June), 194–198.

Marmor, Theodore R. (1994b). *Understanding health care reform*. New Haven: Yale University Press.

Marmor, Theodore R. (1995). Murder, mayhem and medical care reform. *Journal of Health Politics, Policy and Law*, 20 (Summer), 817–819.

Mashaw, Jerry L., and Theodore R. Marmor. (1996). *Can the American state guarantee access to health care?* In Patricia Day, Daniel M. Fox, Robert Maxwell, and Ellie Scrivens (Eds.), *The state, politics and health: Essays for Rudolf Klein* (Chapter 5). Cambridge, MA: Blackwell.

Morone, James A. (1986). Seven laws of policy analysis. *Journal of Policy Analysis Management*, 5 (Summer), 817–819.

Morone, James A. (1990). *The democratic wish*. New York: Basic Books.

New York Times. (1994). Why health care fizzled: Too little time and too much politics (September 27).

Numbers, Ronald. (1978). *Almost persuaded: American physicians and compulsory health insurance, 1912–1920*. Baltimore: Johns Hopkins University Press.

Peterson, Mark A. (1931). Political influence in the 1990s: From iron triangles to policy that works. *Journal of Health Politics, Policy and Law*, 18 (Summer), 395–437.

Reinhardt, Uwe E. (1989). Health care spending and American competitiveness. *Health Affairs*, 8, (Fall), 5.

Rosenthal, Marilyn M. (1994). Whatever happened to the reform of American health policy? *British Medical Journal*, 309 (November 26), 1383.

Schieber, George J., Jean-Pierre Poullier, and Leslie M. Greenwald. (1993). Health spending, delivery, and outcomes in OECD countries. *Health Affairs*, 12 (Summer), 120–129.

Silver, George A. (1995). Topics for our times: Clausewitz vs. Sun Tzu—the art of health reform. *American Journal of Public Health*, 85 (March), 307–308.

Starr, Paul. (1994). Reform is dead. Long live reform. *New York Times* (September 4), E11.

Starr, Paul. (1995). What happened to health care reform? *American Prospect*, 20 (Winter), 20–31.

Steinmo, Sven, & Jon Watts. (1995). It's the institutions, stupid: Why comprehensive health reform always fails in America. *Journal of Health Politics, Policy and Law*, 20 (Summer), 329–372.

United States Congressional Budget Office (CBO). (1992). *Economic implications of rising health care costs*. Washington, D.C.: U.S. Congressional Budget Office.

White, Joseph. (1995). The horses and the jumps: Comments on the health care reform steeplechase. *Journal of Health Politics, Policy and Law*, 20 (Summer), 373–384.

Wolfe, Barbara L. (1993). Why changing the U.S. health care system is so difficult. *Social Science and Medicine*, 36 (3), iii–vi.

Yankelovich, Daniel. (1995). The debate that wasn't: The public and the Clinton health care plan. In Henry J. Aaron (Ed.), *The problem that won't go away: Reforming U.S. health care financing* (Chapter 4). Washington, D.C.: The Brookings Institution.

5

IDEAS

Movements and Influence

Ideas constitute one of our analytical trinity, and in this cluster of articles we treat very different notions of what health and health care policy ought to be and how it should be analyzed. Health policy—like policy in any important area—reflects normative and explanatory paradigms. In economic policy since the 1930s Keynesian formulations dominated. From the 1970s onward, monetarism became more powerful. By the first decade of the twenty-first century, balance between fiscal and monetary paradigms had changed yet again and will no doubt change further in the wake of the global financial debacle of 2007–9.

Health care policy has had its own sequence of competing paradigms. If we go back to the period just after World War II, the prominence of social democratic—and socialist—conceptions of how health care should be financed and organized is indisputable. From the NHS in 1948 to Sweden's universal health program of 1954, from the bitter disputes in Canada and the United States over national health insurance to the growth of publicly financed and regulated health insurance on the European continent, the dominant idea was that medical care was a merit good, one not to be financed by one's ability and willingness to pay. Allocation by medical need was the controlling idea, sharply contrasted with conventional market criteria for allocating scarce goods and services. The universalization of access to the wonders of modern medicine expresses the same ideas in different language.

Chronology—here as elsewhere in public life—makes a difference. By the 1970s, welfare state expansion met stagflation, and everywhere disputes raged over what to do about the relentless pressures on public and private budgets of medical inflation. This was true even in the United Kingdom, where NHS budgets were under tight control. Everywhere fiscal strain emboldened long-standing critics of the welfare states, and everywhere medical care's costs (and in some cases provision) were prominent topics of controversy. Critiques came from both the left and the right, from Marxists and libertarians, anti-capitalists and pro-capitalists, from those wanting to empower the state to reduce economic inequality to those seeking to limit the scope of the state to protecting legal contracts within market economies.

The selection of articles reflects both our own thinking about this range of ideas and the importance of changes in the relative influence of particular paradigms over time. So, for instance, we start with a review essay written in the 1970s that compares Marxist criticism of welfare state regimes under stress. The writers reviewed—Claus Offe from Germany, Ian Gough from the United Kingdom, and John O'Connor from the United States—were prominent figures in this period on the left and excited much comment. From the perspective of 2012 this writing appears an archeological relic. But that simply underlines how paradigms shift in appeal. And no one should state with certainty what will happen in the wake of the subprime financial scandals of the period 2007–9. The article on O'Goffe provides a reconstruction of ideas once central in European policy debates and regularly directed at health care. These ideas on the political left once provided a critical stance toward the national health insurance and national health services of the industrial democracies.

In the 1970s there was a resurgence of enthusiasm for using the market—and its instruments—in all sorts of realms. Under different names and labels, the virtues of market rather than bureaucratic allocation were extolled. One such version, which we have termed Manchesterian liberalism, launched full-scale attacks on efforts to deliver, finance, and regulate medical care under public programs. In the most libertarian version of this pro-market viewpoint, the role of government is reduced to enforcing contracts between consenting adults and letting the medical chips fall as they may. Selling kidneys would be legitimate, as would other unorthodox purchases and sales, but the controlling idea would be the consent of willing sellers and willing buyers.

Between these two divergent paradigms—represented here as social democratic and classic liberal conceptions of the proper role of government—are other views to be noted. Within the social democratic tradition, for example, there are disputes among defenders of the modern welfare state about using market instruments to promote accepted ends. The review essay illustrates the differences that set a postwar socialist like Richard Titmuss apart from a New Labor economist like Julian Le Grand. That turns out to be the extent to which welfare state programs can rely for their sensible operation on the goodwill of professional "knights" as opposed to self-seeking "knaves."

The article addressing the problem of medical inflation also explores how the tools of economics can be applied to public policy analysis. It describes the higher rates of inflation in medical care (in the 1970s) as a public "bad," using the collective terms that modern economists take for granted in distinguishing collective from individual benefits or burdens. That in turn gave rise to thinking of policies set in public markets, balanced or imbalanced, with material and nonmaterial stakes arrayed differently depending on the institutions where interests were in conflict. This article brings disciplinary modes of thought into comparison with what otherwise would be regarded as discussions of ideology. But what disciplinary and philosophical paradigms have in common is their impact on how we construct the questions asked and the answers given. It is worth noting too that the article was drafted in the 1970s, when economic strain was everywhere. In all of these instances, the impact of ideas on public policy is the topic at hand, whatever the decade and whatever the genre.

The other ideas discussed in this chapter are ones we labeled as fads and panaceas. By that the article calls attention to the speed and excitement with which many management notions and policy prescriptions are disseminated internationally. Some of those ideas are about dilemmas that are real, but for which there are no panaceas. Some are illusory efforts to mask real conflicts in managerial jargon and other linguistic sleights of hand. But there is no doubting that the movement of ideas across borders includes this category of international transfer.

Fads in Medical Care Policy and Politics

The Rhetoric and Reality of Managerialism

Theodore R. Marmor

INTRODUCTION

This article's topic is Fads in Medical Care Policy and Politics. I will introduce the broader topic of fads and then turn to how fashions in management commentary have shaped (and mis-shaped) understandings of medical care on both sides of the Atlantic Ocean.

By fads I simply mean outbursts of enthusiasm for particular ideas or practices. In clothing, we have no difficulty in identifying what is faddish. Either our adolescents or the press tell us what constitutes the current fad—or fashion. In the world of ideas, there are similar rushes of enthusiasm, though the character and pace of change of these fads differ greatly over time and space. There is a considerable sociological literature on the subject of fads in social practices.[1] There are fads in names for children, items of home consumption, television soap operas, and the like. But the fads that interest me in this lecture concern fashionable managerial ideas, particularly ideas that in their dissemination are presented as panaceas for longstanding policy and organizational problems.

THE PROBLEM OF MANAGERIAL FADS

My fundamental contention is that the managerial discussion of modern medicine's most prominent topics—cost, quality, access, and organization—is marked by linguistic muddle and conceptual confusion. Managerial jargon—and in the United States especially, marketing hyperbole—regularly threatens to drive out clear thought or reasoned argument.

One sees this most vividly as the managerial fads of one era give way to the enthusiasms of the next. As John Hunt of the London Business School has noted, there is what amounts to a "product cycle" in managerial fads.[2] New enthusiasms are promoted with high hopes, inflated rhetoric and competitive

Table 1: Managerial Fads "Strongly held but largely unfounded
beliefs and formulas about how to manage"

---

1.   Flatten the Structure—Eliminate Hierarchy
2.   Empowerment—Leaderless Teams
3.   TQ C/M?—V A/B M/?
4.   Vision, Mission, Values
5.   Customer Focused/Service Organization
6.   Trait Leadership
7.   Continuous Improvement—Learning Organization
8.   Process Re-engineering
9.   Cultural Transformation

Source: F. Hilmer and L. Donaldson. (1996). *Management Redeemed*. The Free Press.

zeal. These fads are soon abandoned without much regret, with promoters es-
caping chastisement for their prior hyperbole. Managerial gurus shed failed
models easily and embrace newer fashions promiscuously. Declarations of failure follow cycles of enthusiasm, as the scholarly literature documents.[3] Both
permit fame (and fortune) to be made out of distributing the managerial equivalent of snake oil. And, to complete the cycle, scholars then make academic
reputations by discovering the faddish patterns.[4] The first exhibit below sum-
marizes some of the well-known and widely used terms.

Many in the audience will be familiar with some of the shifting fads in
management—both for private and for public organizations. Let me briefly remind us of the shifts themselves. Twenty years ago or more, Management by
Objective (MBO) and Zero Based Budgeting (ZBO) were the rage in board-
rooms and bureaus. In recent years, the language of corporate seminars shifted
to such expressions as "re-engineering" and "core competencies." "Quality circles" were popular for a time, to be displaced by an emphasis on synergy, mergers and acquisitions. At one point, big was better. Politicians as well as managers
embraced larger scale operations, called conglomerates in the private sector
and "super-agencies" in the public sector. Within a few years, small became
beautiful. Divestiture, devolution, decentralization, and specialisation became
the watchwords of managerial correctness. One need not remind an audience
in the United Kingdom about the cycles and recycling of managerial models.
The list below illustrates the waves of ideas.

There is already a great deal of contemporary discomfort with managerial
fads, so I risk being accused of beating a dead horse. But perhaps the sort of
discomfort that has given rise to the popular "Bullshit Bingo" (see Figure 1)

Bullshit Bingo

**Do you keep falling asleep in meeting and seminars? What about those long and boring conference calls?
Here is a way to change all of that!**

How to play: Check off each block when you hear these words during a meeting, seminar or phone call. When you get five blocks horizontally, vertically or diagonally, stand up and shout **BULL****!!**

Synergy	Strategic Fit	Gap Analysis	Best Practice	Bottom Line
Revisit	Bandwidth	Hardball	Out of the Loop	Benchmark
Value-Added	Proactive	Win-Win	Think Outside the Box	Fast Track
Result-Driven	Empower [or] Empowerment	Knowledge Base	Total Quality [or] Quality Driven	Touch Base
Mindset	Client Focus[ed]	Ball Park	Game Plan	Leverage

Figure 1. Bullshit Bingo

circulating on the Internet indicates an audience receptive to more analytical discussion of why fads arise and what fads produce.

Realism about what management can and cannot do might guard against swallowing the more dangerous panaceas offered by managerial gurus. Dissecting the linguistic modes of managerial fads highlights fallacies that are more serious in their effects than simple exaggeration. Some disciplined review may help moderate disappointment that good management has not (and will not be able to) rid us of most of the world's evils. Here I want to elaborate the counter-argument that some have made about the effort this lecture represents.

Attention to the rhetoric of managerial thoughts is misplaced, I am told, because sophisticated audiences ignore the sloganeering and get on with the job. On this view, no one needs to worry about large numbers of misled and subsequently disappointed audiences. My topic, in short, could be thought of as an indulgence, a wasteful deflection of your time and mine.

My response to that is whether managerial gurus convince audiences or not, they take up time and energy, if only because their notions bewilder. I am reminded of a conversation I overheard in the waiting room at the Department of Health in Whitehall a few years ago. A group of four officials from a regional health authority were, to use its jargon, "debriefing." I listened as they tried to decipher the meaning of the bewildering terms used in the meeting from which they had just emerged. I could not help but hear their plaintive remarks and told them I was a student of managerial jargon and thought they would be better off if they proceeded with a more sceptical attitude. This appeared to give them some symptomatic relief. All too many audiences find themselves either fooled or furious about what turns out to be misleading, needlessly obscure, or downright fraudulent. At the very least, managerial obscurity directs discussion away from topics more worthy of the attention of those who provide medical care, receive care, pay for it, or manage those services.

WHY MANAGERIALISM (AND MARKET ENTHUSIASM) IN MEDICAL CARE?

I want now to turn to the context that proved to be such a fertile setting for the transfer of business models of allocation and management to medical care. My contention is that the decade of the 1970s—marked by stagflation and intense fiscal pressure in all the industrial democracies—provided such a context. In that decade medical care policy leapt to the forefront of public agendas for one or more of these reasons. First, the financing of medical care became a major burden on the budgets[5] of mature welfare states precisely when public revenues fell sharply from prior forecasts. When fiscal strain arises—especially from prolonged recession—policy scrutiny (not simply incremental budgeting) is the predictable result. Secondly, welfare states, as Rudolf Klein argued in the late 1980s,[6] under almost all circumstances came to have less capacity for bold fiscal expansion in new areas. This meant managing existing programs (in new ways perhaps, but in changing economic circumstances) necessarily assumed a larger share of the public agenda. Thirdly, there was what might be termed the wearing down of the post-war consensus about the welfare state.[7]

After the 1973–74 oil shock and consequent stagflation, bolstered by electoral victories (or advance) of parties opposed to welfare state expansion, critics assumed a bolder posture. Mass publics increasingly heard challenges to programs that had for decades seemed sacrosanct.[8] From Mulroney to Thatcher, from New Zealand to the Netherlands—the message was one of necessary change. The incentives to explore transformative but not fiscally burdensome options became relatively stronger. That, I would suggest, helps to explain the international pattern of welfare state review—including health policy—over the past two decades. It also helps to explain why the appeal to market mechanisms and business-like management became so much more compelling.

During the 1970s, there was a perceptible increase of proposals to improve the management of medicine by subjecting to market-like competition. Simultaneously, a dramatic shift took place in the language of medical commentary. This transformation can be presented as a case study of what George Orwell might have called "the politics of the medical language." To change thinking, one manipulates language. The traditional doctor-patient relationship becomes, in the language of competitive markets, provider-consumer, or buyer-seller, or supplier-demander. Medicine becomes just another business. The fallout from this refashioned language came to be a threat to the professional ethos of medicine, most obviously in America, but elsewhere as well.

Traditionally, much of the "income" doctors, nurses and other medical practitioners earned has been non-economic: self-esteem, respect from patients and the community and idealization as selfless professionals. In casting medical care as no different from other industries, medical professionals are reconceptualized. They no longer deserve (and increasingly no longer receive) the non-economic benefits of public esteem, patient idealization, and the gratitude of families. The stereotype of the medical professional as a self-interested (selfish) agent of business feeds on itself. And, over the quarter century we are surveying, the American public's esteem for medical practitioners indeed fell sharply.[9]

Part of the decreased satisfaction with American medicine undoubtedly arose from worries over very high and rapidly rising costs. Although it is impossible to establish a clear causal connection between the demystification of the medical profession and the increased incomes of doctors, the phenomena have gone hand in hand. Despite sharp increases in the number of new physicians, doctors' incomes grew by 30 per cent from 1984 to 1989. (This contrasted with an average 16.3 per cent increase for other full-time workers over the same period.)[10] It should not be surprising that to the extent professional medical work was increasingly regarded as ordinary commercial activity, higher physician fees (and incomes) were increasingly understood as the result of market power or greed rather than the professionals' just desserts.

External criticism and constraints on professional autonomy begat doctor dissatisfaction and the prestige of the American medical profession decreased over the 1970s and 1980s. Doctors complained that they no longer enjoyed the autonomy they once had. Rather, elaborate, intrusive and administratively expensive procedures proliferated, including utilization reviews, requirements for pre-admission certification and other forms of second-guessing. American Medical Association surveys in 1986, for example, found that 60 per cent of physicians strongly opposed third-party reviews of their hospitalization decisions.[11] In an often-quoted 1991 article in *The Atlantic*, Regina Herzlinger reported that despite increased incomes more than 30 per cent of current physicians said they would not have attended medical school had they known what their futures had in store.[12]

The language of industrial economics and competitive markets did not just affect doctors. Hospitals and hospital administrators recast themselves in new terms. The hospital administrator increasingly became the chief executive officer. Assistant administrators were refashioned as vice-presidents for their respective functions. These changes were not merely semantic. Rather, they represented a fateful change in the way Americans were encouraged to think of medical care. The vision of a hospital as primarily a business—and the concomitant shift in administrative power away from medical staff and toward professional managers—inevitably affected the way Americans regard medical care. It would be wrong to assume unanimity on this and equally wrong to presume that American physicians and nurses think of themselves as simply business figures. The point here is narrower. Over time, the attack on the professional standing of medicine helped to deflate public confidence and to increase the probability of proposals threatening professional autonomy.

As hospital administrators gave way to chief executive officers (CEOs), so too did their incomes change. By 1990, hospital CEOs earned an average base salary of over $103,000; those receiving incentive pay averaged $125,000. The salaries of these chief administrators increased by 8.5 per cent (on average) in

1989, while the Consumer Price Index grew by 4.6 per cent.[13] And this took place in the midst of a supposed "crisis" in health spending.

There are, of course, advantages to treating hospitals more like a typical business. Improved capital budgeting, financial and accounting systems are all vital in getting better value for health expenditures. Nor can one pretend medical practitioners are all selfless workers concerned only for the welfare of their patients. Clearly economic motives are important. Indeed, many of the concerns of those who subscribe to pro-competitive strategies are identical to my own. Asymmetries of information and bargaining strength between doctors and patients *do* require attention. Likewise, uncertainty about the efficacy of alternative treatments and the problems of moral hazard and adverse selection all need to be addressed whatever one's personal philosophy of entitlement to medical care.

But the rhetoric of the competitive market helped to disguise what sets medicine apart from other industries and it was that broader development that made it possible for a Democratic president like Bill Clinton to marry ideas of universal health insurance to "pro-market" ideology. No one can make sense Clinton's embrace of "managed competition" without appreciating just how much the celebrations of markets and management had depleted faith in ordinary public administration. It is worth noting that the very term managed competition is an example of an oxymoron or double talk, the holding of two contradictory ideas at once. A managed system is one whose parties control operations by various managerial techniques—for good or for ill. By contrast, the results of a competitive market are largely up for grabs. Under idealized competitive conditions, individual actors pursue their own interests without central direction. Whatever coordination occurs is not by managerial design, but as a consequence of individual adaptation to market conditions. The results are not planned and may not be desirable. We regulate competition, well or poorly. And we manage resources, well or poorly. What we do not do is manage competition.

In arguing against governmental provision (or government financing) of medical care, advocates of competition in health care regularly claim that governments are not competent as managers. The inevitable concessions of the political process, it is argued, deplete resolve and efficiency so that programs over time bear less and less resemblance to their initial design and purpose.

Ironically, from the 1970s to the present, advocates of competition in health care proposed a variety of detailed government programs, laws and regulations designed to address and eliminate the market failures that occur in unregulated medical markets. The dilemma, hardly addressed in public discussion of competition in medical care, arises precisely here. What happens to the logic of pro-competitive proposals when government incompetence contaminates the efforts to reform medical markets? How desirable can a plan for "managed competition" be when only half of its provisions get enacted and implemented, when insurance companies are not required to offer specific types of plans, when the government increases, rather than eliminates, the tax deductibility of medical insurance? What happens if experience rating is allowed (insurers can offer lower premiums to low risk groups) but the government sets up no provision for high risk groups who find it difficult to get insurance at all?

The answer is that most pro-competitive plans were not robust in precisely this crucial respect. They would not perform well unless conditions were just right. By the very detailing of the government actions required to eliminate market failures, backers of pro-competitive reform implicitly acknowledged that without these remedies, a competitive system does not work very well.

The characterization of medical care as just another business also had implications for the way in which the potential for improvement from government intervention came to be judged. The dichotomy drawn between private competition and public regulation invoked free choice and well-functioning markets on the one hand, and failed socialism on the other. But that dichotomy was, and is, artificial and misleading. The properties of the medical sector are such that regulation of some kind has always been regarded as inevitable by every serious writer on the subject. Ironically, the most popular pro-competitive schemes have all entailed a myriad of regulatory restrictions on practitioners and patients alike.

FROM IDEALIZED MARKETS TO MISLEADING MANAGERIALISM: THE CASE OF MANAGED CARE

I want now to return to the connection between market enthusiasm and managerial fads in health care. I have in mind the wide-spread and growing tendency to express ideas through misleadingly persuasive linguistic devices. Consider, for example, expressions like "managed care" or more general public management labels like "joined up" government. These are slogans, persuasive terms that imply success by their very use. In every case of such a slogan, however, the opposite or antonym has no appeal. So, for example, the appeal to integrated systems does not compete with defenders of "disintegrated" ones. Disease management is set against the non-management of disease, a null category. Even the familiar slogan in research circles—evidence-based medicine,

Table 2: Slogans/Antonyms

Managed Care	*NON-Managed Care*
Integrated Delivery System	DIS-Integrated Delivery System
Joined Up Government	DIS-Jointed Government
Empowerment of Employees	DIS-Empowerment of Employees
Evidence-Based Medicine	NON-Evidence-Based Medicine
Customer Focused	NON-Customer Focused
Learning Organization	NON-Learning Organization

policy, or whatever—has no credible antonym. The list below presents more examples of such terms.

Precisely because so much of the language used to describe medical care to-day is meant to convince rather than to describe or to explain, even thoughtful observers often end up endorsing claims whose validity they should be assessing. I cannot think of a better illustration of this process than the widespread appeal to "managed care" in medical reform circles.

The expression "managed care"—much like that ubiquitous reform phrase of the early 1990s, "managed competition"—is actually a product of market sloganeering, aspirational rhetoric, and managerial jargon. Insofar as it is an incoherent notion, most claims about managed care will suffer from incoherence as well. Although the exact provenance of "managed care" is uncertain, the term came into widespread usage only in the 1990s. The expression does not appear once, for example, in Paul Starr's exhaustive 1982 history *The Social Transformation of American Medicine*. The phrase first appeared in *The New York Times* in 1985 but surfaced in only a handful of articles during the decade. In the 1990s, however, the number of *Times* articles mentioning the phrase exploded, increasing from 27 in 1990 to 287 in 1994 to 587 in 1998. Because "managed care" has become something of a household term, it is difficult to recognize how recently it entered medical discourse.

What exactly managed care is, however, has never been entirely clear, even among its strongest proponents. To some, the crucial distinguishing feature is a shift in financing from indemnity-style fee-for-service, in which the insurer is little more than a bill-payer, to per capita payment methods. Yet there is nothing intrinsic to fee-for-service payment that requires that reimbursement be open-ended or insurers to remain passive. Many, if not most, American health insurance plans that are labeled "managed care" do not rely primarily on capitation. To others, the distinctive characteristic is the creation of administrative protocols for reviewing and sometimes denying care demanded by patients or medical professionals. But such micro-level managerial controls are not universal among so-called managed care health plans either. In fact, micro management may be obviated by payment methods like capitation or regulated fee-for-service reimbursement that create more diffuse constraints on medical practice. Finally, to some, what distinguishes managed care is the establishment of integrated networks of health professionals from which patients are required to obtain care. Yet some so-called managed care plans have no such networks. And what is called a network by many plans is little more than a list of providers willing to accept discounted fee-for-service payments—hardly a radical break with the past. In short, what constitutes the subject matter of managed care is utterly obscure.[14]

A more sensible interpretation of "managed care" is that it represents a fusion of two functions that had once been seen as separate: the financing of medical care and the delivery of medical services. This, at least, provides a reasonably accurate description of the most familiar organizational entity that marched under the managed care banner in the early 1980s: the health maintenance organization (HMO). When the majority of American health insurers used fee-for-service payments and placed few restrictions on patient or provider discretion, it was at least possible to identify a small subset of health plans that existed outside this insurance mainstream, however poorly the expression "managed care" described the organization of such plans or what they did. Today, however, that is decidedly no longer the case. Only two percent of private health plans in 1997 conformed to the traditional model of fee-for-service indemnity insurance. Another 16 percent use fee-for-service payment but employ some form of utilization review.[15] Thus between 80 and 98 percent of today's private health insurers appear to fall into the general category of managed care. The category does not, in other words, offer any guidance as to how to distinguish among the vast majority of contemporary American health insurance plans. From the patients' perspective, HMOs are more often focused on managing costs than on managing care.

Conflating organization, technique, and incentives within one term leads to unnecessary confusion. When contrasting health plans we often compare them across incommensurable dimensions (arguing, for example, that an HMO is somehow more "managed" than a fee-for-service plan with utilization review even when the latter may use much stricter controls on individual treatment decisions). It means, too, that we are tempted to presume necessary relationships between particular features of health plans (such as their payment method) and specific outcomes that are alleged to follow from these features (such as the degree of integration of medical finance and delivery)—even though such outcomes usually result from a complex of financial, organizational, and administrative factors. And finally, it encourages a wild goose chase of efforts to come up with black-and-white standards for identifying plan types. As health plans employ increasingly diverse payment methods and organizational forms, the search for the "essence" of a particular plan becomes all the more futile.

The "managed care revolution" was actually a set of related trends, few of which are accurately captured by the blanket term. When these trends are distinguished from one another, the evidence suggests that American health insurance has moved simultaneously in several different, perhaps even contradictory, directions in recent years and that many of the changes are longer standing than the rhetoric of managed-care celebrants implies.

The rapid changes taking place in American medical care place a special burden on analysts to be precise about the criteria and considerations that underlie their empirical evaluations and, ultimately, their judgments and assessments. Labels and categories are indispensable, but they should be designed to elucidate the techniques, organizational forms, and incentives that characterize alternative health plans, rather than to confirm or deny the claims of industry friends or foes. "Managed care" fails that test, and although I hardly expect my words to be heeded, I think that it—and other terms like it—should be banished from the medical care lexicon for good.

From this extended American example of linguistic muddle, let me turn to the use of managerial jargon in the UK context. First, let me contrast the policy contexts across the Atlantic. In the United States, the language of medical management—and managerial practices more generally—has produced a backlash, a sense of outrage in the late 1990s.[16] The disputes about the patient's bill of rights, for example, reveal this. Critics of the managers of health insurance plans portray them as greedy profiteers who extracted funds from the health insurance pools to line their pockets and obscured what they were doing under misleading labels like managed care, integrated delivery systems, and the like.

In the US, where no one is in charge of a national system of medical care financing, obscurantism more easily leads to dispersed rage and a search for scapegoats in the face of distress whose sources are not simple to identify. In the NHS context, the complaint is much more likely to express dismay at managerial changes recurrently imposed in the name of slogans, but with the force of budgetary authority. Here, sullen resentment—not diffused rage—appears the common response to managerial excess.

NHS MANAGEMENT: STYLES AND RESPONSES

Visitors from abroad should, in my view, be hesitant in commenting on the complexities of policy and management in another country with any certitude. For every Tocqueville, there are scores of others whose observations waste paper. So, what might this outsider say prudently about the reactions not only to the newly announced policy of dispersing managerial authority but also the style of policy making and management in the NHS more generally? Here the outsider has considerable help from a number of scholars who have written about the "New Public Management" in the United Kingdom. I have relied on that literature for both understanding the type of managerial rhetoric dominant and for making sense of why reactions to managerial fads are often so hostile.

My guides to the New Public Management in Britain are the writings of Michael Barzelay, Christopher Hood, and Michael Power.[17] Power has brilliantly summarized the central ideas, arguing that the new public management "consists of a cluster of ideas borrowed from the conceptual framework of private sector management."[18] Among the most commonly used ideas he found are:

> (i) cost control, financial transparency, decentralization of management authority, (ii) the creation of market and quasi-market mechanisms separating purchasing and providing functions and their linkage via contracts, and (iii) the enhancement of accountability to customers for the quality of service via the creation of performance indicators.

It does not take exhaustive research to see just how widely these ideas have spread in the world of the NHS. So, for example, consider this brief survey of faddish presentation of managerial ideas in recent years. In December of 1997, the white paper announcing the "New NHS" promised dramatic changes in the way Labour would manage things.[19] "Integrated care" would replace the internal market of the Thatcher reforms, building on "what has worked, but discard[ing] what has failed." This, we were told, would save huge amounts of red tape and put "money into frontline patient care." Here we have the familiar appeal to a persuasively defined action—"integration." Performance targets, quantitative measures, monitoring, and evaluating—these became watchwords of NHS reforms.

But the reality appears to contain more variability than these expressions suggest. The world of clinical audits promised wondrous improvement in patient care, but it was hardly embraced by those whose professional performance is the object of improvement. As Christopher Hood has argued, the new public management "is more a story of successive shifts in approach over the last twenty years than steady reinforcement of a single trend."[20]

Indeed, Hood observes a shift in emphasis over the 1980s "from efforts to . . . equip ministers to be effective managers of their departments . . . to the effort to take management away from ministers . . . by the creation of executive agencies at arm's length from the departments." The drumbeat of changing fads is evident in Hood's depiction of the themes of managerial innovation. He notes the "move from the stress on 'results' or 'outputs' that were the catchwords of public management reformers in the early 1980s to the stress on 'governance' (a euphemism for 'process') as the hot topic of the mid-1990s." Rather than a coherent doctrine, these persistent adjustments in doctrine might be regarded, Hood concludes, as "ceaseless activity to grapple with the unacknowledged consequences of yesterday's mistakes."

It is to the "ceaseless activity" that I want to call attention. It is striking to the visitor how unanimous NHS commentators are in both their criticism of and their cynicism about proposed NHS shifts in policy and management. Rudolf Klein, in discussing a "much advertised" speech about devolution by the Secretary of State for Health, Alan Milburn, predicted that "the first reaction to Mr Millburn's speech is . . . likely to be cynicism."[21] In published reactions to the Milburn policy during the summer of 2001, it seems, both analytical rage and policy skepticism was dominant.[22] This is true in the commentary from observers as different as Nicholas Bosanquet and Charles Webster, and across a wide spectrum of general political views. To this reader, it seems plain that Bosanquet and Webster are not ideological cousins, but they both find nothing to recommend in the NHS's mode of policy making. Bosanquet's claim that "there never has been a greater gap between the view of solutions at the center and the realities as they appear day to day at the local level" should, if true, worry the Blair government greatly. That critical stance is common from David Hunter (emphasizing the dismay of managers) and Charles Webster (emphasizing the secret and detached quality of the Blair government's policy making in healthcare) to Bob Sang's invocation of high managerial doctrine in lamenting what the NHS debate lacks. Only Jennifer Dixon saw a "chink of light," itself a qualifying metaphor for Dixon's effort to explain the "gripes" about what she describes as New Labor's "tendency towards hierarchy and centralism."[23] A sharpening of hierarchy and increase in centralism—that is the common theme of the criticism and the explanation of why these analysts were so cynical about the NHS plan to shift the balance of power.

What the outsider wonders about is whether there is any reason to think the 2001 plan of Milburn is any more than another centralist move in decentralist clothing. The NHS appears to have been on a centralizing mission for decades now, masking that for a time with one or another reorganization. And the reorganizations themselves have sapped morale and disturbed lives enough to make managers more likely candidates for psychotherapy than corporatist cooperators with central offices. None of these commentators found much to say about the announced aims of Shifting the Balance. Since paying more attention to "local level" actors—providers, patients, and payers—is what most of the commentators applaud, this inattention to the stated policy goals is striking testimony to the distrust of the NHS and its policy making modes.

There are good grounds for that distrust in the reviews of NHS history since the 1970s. First, as Webster notes, the rhetoric of local level decision making goes back to 1979, but the reality of both the Thatcher and Blair policies have not "been conducive to such decentralisation of power."[24] David Hunter emphasizes, as do others, what he calls "control freakery" and concludes that managers at the local level have been "unwilling to say what they think" about proposals like Mr. Milburn's on shifting the balance.[25] Most of the comments converge in disbelieving the commitment to devolution, whatever the rhetoric. The commentators believe that history, the Blair (and Thatcher) style of policymaking, and the structure of British government support their cynical reaction.

While appreciating these grounds, I want to offer two somewhat different perspectives on this evaluation. First, I want to call attention to the more general trends in national health decision-making that are not at all topic in this NHS debate. From Australia to New Zealand, from the US to Canada, from Holland to Germany, and from Sweden to Denmark, dismay about modern medical care financing, quality, and management is apparent. The attack on medical errors and the growing distrust of physician self-government are trends that are cross-national in the OECD world. What is more, the claim that good science, proper information, and appropriate monitoring can raise the quality of health care among industrial democracies is an article of faith among the devotees of the "New Public Management."

These views are neither new nor restricted to public management. They inform not only the development in the United States of new agencies of government devoted to the improvement of quality standards as well as the rise of private firms advertising their capacity to separate good from bad hospitals, competent from incompetent physicians, and worthy from worthless drugs. A UK audience will think of NICE, a Canadian audience of the Center for Health Information, and others will find their own acronyms. But, using Carolyn Tuohy's (1999) terms for alternative governance mechanisms, the common element is distrust of collegial authority combined with either a celebration of market mechanisms or government hierarchies as the right measure to address the lamentable state of "local self-government" of clinical matters.

What distinguishes the NHS is the degree of centralism in the day-to-day mode of policymaking. As David Hunter rightly notes, a non-political NHS is a fantasy, a goal that will not (and could not) be entertained in a democratic society.[26] But the extent of the political control in the UK has varied across time. There were decades when central budgetary control combined with considerable medical and managerial discretion about how to live within budgets. Not so for more than the last decade.

This brings us back to the question whether this new turn of policy is to be taken seriously. The only grounds for doing so is to see the connection, as Rudolf Klein did, between the "corset of control" that the Blair government has already established and a new freedom justified by the conviction that it will not be a "license for poor standards or inadequate performance."[27] This interpretation rests on the premise that no British government could ignore inappropriate variation in care standards. But, if the new Modernization Agency could count on prior constraints, then its posture could be one of promoting good practice and not hectoring.

This is the most generous interpretation of the logic of the Blair government's newest policy in 2001. It puts my sense of realism at the limit. But it also suggests a way of discussing such policy initiatives: namely, to add to justified criticism and cynicism a set of indicators of what would count as evidence that the new policy was actually carried out. Without that, commentary stays girdled by past disappointments and leaves little opportunity for those within government to show they mean what they say.

A RETURN TO REALISM: WHY SENSIBLE MANAGEMENT REQUIRES MODESTY, NOT ZEAL

The review of these cynical responses to recent shifts in NHS managerial directives does not mean I endorse all the criticism (or cynicism). But it does remind one of both the persistence of organisational changes and the weariness of those who are thereby affected. At the same time, the prominence of cynical commentary reminds one of the costs of massive gaps between what is claimed and what is true. It also leads me to comment on the incantation throughout contemporary management talk about the importance of having clear, measurable, and limited organisational objectives. An unfortunate consequence of the injection of managerial fads into medical care is the suggestion that there is

Table 3: What Is the Purpose of a Hospital?

---

1. A hospital is designed to contain the spread of contagious diseases.
2. A hospital is a place that provide hygienic surroundings for otherwise dangerous interventions.
3. A hospital is designed to economize on the cost of access to expensive technology.
4. A hospital provides respite from normal social roles that are producing physical or mental breakdown (strain) in patients.
5. Hospitals are intended to economize on the transmission of information and the process of learning among professionals who have clinical responsibilities and require multiple clinical encounters to validate their procedures.
6. Hospitals are designed to centralize medical activities sufficiently to achieve economies of scale in different healthcare tasks.
7. Hospitals provide symbolic reassurance that social effort is being devoted to the health of citizens in a culture with considerable faith in technological remedies.
8. Hospitals are institutions designed to improve the health of the population.

---

some one right way, some panacea, for a rational, decent, affordable delivery of medical care.

I want to challenge that contention directly and forcefully. The objectives of any institution are multiple, shifting, and often contradictory. It would be quite surprising if any single managerial approach could cope effectively with the entire range of such objectives, let alone with changes in priority among different objectives over time. To make this point clear, consider for a moment just how one might answer the following question: "What is a hospital's purpose?" The list above provides a selection of possible answers to that question.

Hospitals, in short, serve quite varied purposes, all of which cannot be pursued through the same internal authority structure, with the same information technology, or on the same scales. They give rise to starkly different images of what counts as a well-managed hospital. For example, emphasizing purposes 1 or 4 implies a relaxed approach to length of stay; stressing purposes 3 or 6 might mean treating longer hospital stays as evidence of managerial failure. Purpose 5 suggests a team approach to management, with authority centralized among the professionals; purpose 3 bolsters hierarchical forms of bureaucratic authority. Purposes 1 through 7 suggest allocations of authority within the hospital as a separate institution: purpose 8 suggests a much broader structure of authority, one including outside stakeholders with the power to define and redefine the institution's primary mission.

What should we make of this? The first lesson here is a simple one. Institutions such as hospitals have multiple tasks which imply different managerial approaches. Good management is not what slogan the administrator has emblazoned on the tee shirts of employees but how well the manager's particular approach balances the different demands of the multiple purposes of the institution. I would not belabor this simple point but for the overwhelming evidence that it is often, if not usually, forgotten. Indeed, when some clone of managerial guru Tom Peters next says to health care managers that to have multiple objectives, or even two objectives, is to have no objectives at all, he or she should be condemned to pursue one objective for the rest of their lives.

A second observation about managerial technique is the homily that every upside has a downside. For instance, when moving into a world of managerial cost containment, we should reflect on what can be lost as well as gained. Cost containment in practice seeks to reduce questionable doctor/patient encounters, duplicate diagnostic procedures, and dubious treatments. The bureaucratic routines required to implement these actions may or may not help to contain costs. But they may very seriously reduce the choices and negatively affect morale and satisfaction of both patients and health care professionals. Different managerial techniques and different organizational configurations will be required if old values are not to be unduly sacrificed to mindless cost control. Moreover, the managerial techniques imposed in the name of reducing costs do little to encourage innovation, patient control, or professional autonomy. Repeating the mantras of "total quality management" or "integrated systems management" every day will not eliminate the stress built into serving different purposes and clienteles with multiple objectives. Good management requires the balancing of the "goods" and "bads" of each approach. In other words, there are no managerial panaceas available—now or ever.

Finally, there is a deep ambivalence in managerial theorizing about the effectiveness of, very broadly speaking, *technological* as opposed to *cultural* solutions to managerial problems. Management theorists, ever since the so-called "scientific management" movement prompted hostility for treating people and machines interchangeably, have oscillated in their recommendations for change. On the one hand, there are recommendations based on improved structures, processes, and technologies and, on the other, those based on learning, motivation, and culture. One cannot decide which managerial strategy to believe in because both work some of the time, but neither works all of the time.

The same is true in the reorganization of health care systems. It is hard to believe that a cultural approach will be appealing from the standpoint of cost containment. Managing costs is mostly about information systems, the determination of what is cost-effective, and the delivery of incentives or coercion to act on those judgements. On the other hand, if there is cultural vision of the caring medical professional, there will be a need for internal structures that emphasize professional autonomy, team effort, group responsibility, and patient involvement in an overall culture of humane care. Under such circumstances, managerial arrangements will to some degree work at cross-purposes. The technology of cost containment confronts the professional culture of patient care. Good managers balance these perspectives in ways that cope with the conflicting purposes and competing and sometimes inconsistent desires (as illustrated by the following quotation):

> Something funny happened on the way to the future of business. It turned out to be hard work. Technology is not magical. There is no single catch phrase, whether "re-engineering" or "business-to-business software," that can automatically transform the nuts and bolts of how companies operate. And chief executives with "visions" cannot necessarily ride in on their white horses to save organizations single-handedly.
>
> If the latest offerings from management gurus are any indication, the whole focus of business is shifting from theory to practice, and it has nothing to do with terrorism or recession. It appears that the euphoric days of "revolutionary" and "radical" change in business are giving way to the painstaking and detailed work of reshaping companies, department by department and division by division.[28]

Management is not a solution to seemingly intractable stresses. Rather it is a means of coping with and sometimes improving only marginally tractable situations. This more modest vision of management has much to teach those in the reform business about the appropriate level of aspiration for anyone engaged in re-forming complex systems. But management thinkers cannot teach others that lesson until they give up the quasi-religious adoption of one management slogan after another as the solution to getting management right. There is no best management theory, technique, or slogan. In particular contexts, some are better than others. But that must be shown, not glibly claimed by persuasive definitions that presume that saying so makes something so.

Notes

The article is based on the Rock Carling Lecture given by Theodore R. Marmor, November 7, 2001.

1. To understand the "emergence, diffusion, and decline" of fads, see P. P. Carson, P. A. Lanier, K. D. Carson, and B. N. Guidry, "Clearing a Path through the Management Fashion Jungle: Some Preliminary Trailblazing," *American Academy of Management Journal*, 43.6 (2000): 1143–58.

   The diffusion or rejection of technologically inefficient fads is discussed in Eric Abrahamson, "Managerial Fads and Fashions: The Diffusion and Rejection of Innovations," *Academy of Management Review*, 35.3 (1991): 596–612.

   The stages in the life of a fad are discussed in Rolf Meyerson and Elihu Katz, "Notes on a Natural History of Fads," *American Journal of Sociology*, 62.6 (1957): 594–601.

   The psychology behind fads is examined in Herbert E. Krugman and Eugene L. Hartley, "The Learning of Tastes," *Public Opinion Quarterly*, 24.4 (1960): 621–31. For a more specific case study of what counts as a fad and why people participate, see B. E. Aguirre, E. L. Quarantelli, and Jorge L. Mendoza, "The Collective Behavior of Fads: The Characteristics, Effects, and Career of Streaking," *American Sociological Review*, 53.4 (1988): 569–84.

   For an examination of how language helped create and sustain the dot-com boom, see Neil Shister, "South Park: New-Economy Drivel Leaves a San Francisco Neighborhood High and Dry," *Boston Review* (February/March 2002).

2. John W. Hunt, "An Appetite for Ideas: US Research Shows That the Life Cycle of Management Fashions Are Getting Shorter," *The Financial Times* (16 May 2001). Hunt's analysis is very similar to my own. He reviews the research that identifies the "path" of managerial ideas "from invention through acceptance to disenchantment and decline." And he emphasizes the speeding up of the product cycle of fads, with chief executives "exploiting and rejecting fashions within three or four years."

3. As Richard Freeman has pointed out in Letters to the Editor in the *British Journal of Health-Care Management*, 8.2 (February 2002): 69–70, one of the intriguing aspects of fads is that they are not just rhetorically superficial, but also—by definition—short-lived. Still, the very process by which they are created helps ensure their danger later on. Fads arise, he postulates, through competition between management consultants and business schools, and then later, political competition (government officials looking to be viewed as "change makers"). Sadly enough, the very managerialism of medical care exacerbates this problem, since, as Freeman aptly puts it, managerialism serves as "an institutionalised cadre dedicated to the consumption and reproduction of the fad," thus allowing fads to feed off of and perpetuate themselves. See also P. P. Carson, P. A. Lanier, K. D. Carson, and B. N. Guidry, "Clearing a Path through the Management Fashion Jungle: Some Preliminary Trailblazing," *American Academy of Management Journal*, 43.6 (2000): 1143–58.

4. Two scholarly works were very helpful in identifying and documenting these developments. Staffan Furusten's *Popular Management Books* (London: Routledge, 1999) is a sociological study of the origins and dissemination of managerial ideas in the United States and Western Europe; Andrzej Huczynski's *Management Gurus* (London: Routledge, 1996) is more concerned with how particular marketers of management ideas promote the dissemination of their nostrums.

5. Technically, this is not strictly true of course, as is evident in the social insurance or sickness fund financing of care in Germany, the Netherlands, and elsewhere. But, since mandatory contributions are close cousins of "taxes," budget officials must obviously treat these outlays as constraints on direct tax increases.

6. R. Klein and M. O'Higgins, "Defusing the Crisis of the Welfare State: A New Interpretation," in T. R. Marmor and J. Mashaw, eds., *Social Security: Beyond the Rhetoric of Crisis*, (Princeton, N.J.: Princeton University Press, 1988), esp. pgs. 219–24.

7. The bulk of this ideological struggle took place, of course, within national borders, free from the spread of "foreign" ideas. To the extent similar arguments arose cross-nationally, as Kieke Okma

has noted, mostly that represented "parallel development." But, there are striking contemporary examples of the explicit international transfer and highlighting of welfare state commentary. Some of this takes place through think tank networks; some takes place through media
campaigns on behalf of particular figures; and, of course, some takes place through academic
exchanges and official meetings. Charles Murray—the controversial author of *Losing Ground*
(1984) and co-author of *The Bell Curve* (1994)—illustrates all three of these phenomena. The
medium of transfer seems to have changed in the post-war period. Where the Beveridge Report
would have been known to social policy elites very broadly, however much they used it, the
modern form seems to be the long newspaper or magazine article and the media interview.

8. This is the argument developed in T. R. Marmor, J. Mashaw, and L. Harvey, *America's Misunderstood Welfare State: Persistent Myths, Continuing Realities* (New York: Basic Books, 1992),
esp. ch. 3. The wider scholarly literature on the subject is the focus of a review essay, "Understanding the Welfare State: Crisis, Critics, and Counter-critics," *Critical Review*, 7.4 (1993):
461–77.

9. Public confidence in medicine and health institutions dropped from 73 to 33 per cent between
the mid-1960s and mid-1980s. While all major American institutions experienced a loss of public support, the medical profession lost support faster than any other professional group. Insofar
as high levels of public trust are associated with altruistic behavior and sense of social mission
of a profession, at least some of the lost support was no doubt due to the increasing commer-
cialization in the medical profession. In his analysis of a host of survey data. Blendon found
that while most (64 per cent of those polled) supported advertising by physicians, 58 per cent
did not expect it to be truthful. Robert Blendon, "The Public's View of the Future of Medical
Care," *Journal of the American Medical Association* 259 (1988): 3587–93. Physicians' fees for
procedures were approximately 234 per cent higher in the United States than in Canada, and
their take-home pay was more than 50 per cent higher than that received by Canadian doctors
(V. R. Fuchs and J. S. Hahn, "How Does Canada Do It?" *New England Journal of Medicine*,
323 [1990]: 888–90).

10. V. R. Fuchs, "The Health Sector's Share of the Gross National Product," *Science*, 247, no. 4942
[1990]: 534–38.

11. L. Harvey, *AMA Surveys of Physician and Public Opinion* (Chicago: American Medical Association, 1986).

12. Regina Herzlinger, "Healthy Competition," *The Atlantic*, no. 268 (1991): 71.

13. Regina Herzlinger, op. cit.

14. Even thoughtful critics of managed care reveal confusion. Donald Light's essay, "Managed
Care: False and Real Solutions," *The Lancet*, 344, 29 October, 1994, described managed care
as "the hot new export from the United States, promoted by major consultants as the most efficient way to integrate primary care, sub-specialization, and everything in between." He went
on to suggest that "these days [1994], the term managed care means any of several institutional
arrangements," but then employed the expression even though it is not clear which of the
"several" arrangements does constitute the relevant noun. It reminds one of the joke that if you
don't know where you are going, any road will get you there. If managed care has no settled
meaning, conversations about "it" are certain to be misleading.

15. HIAA, *Source Book of Health Insurance Data* 59 (1998).

16. See news reports from around the U.S., for example, Rob Hotakainen and Greg Gordon, "Patients' Testimony Helped Bill in Senate," *Minneapolis–St. Paul Star Tribune* (2 July 2001): A1;
or Howard Kurtz, "Some GOP Hopefuls Echo Democrats on Health Care," *The Washington
Post* (29 July 2000): A7.

17. Michael Power, *The Audit Society: Rituals of Verification* (Oxford: Oxford University Press,
1997). Michael Barzelay, *The New Public Management* (Berkeley: University of California
Press, 2001). Christopher Hood, *The Art of the State* (Oxford: Oxford University Press, 1998).

18. Power, op cit.

19. Department of Health, *The New NHS: Modern. Dependable: Beyond the Internal Market* (London: HM Stationery Office, 1997).

20. Hood, op. cit., 201.

21. Milburn, Alan, *Shifting the Balance of Power in the NHS*. Speech delivered on 25 April 2001. http://tap.ccta.gov.uk/doh/intpress.nsf/page/2001–0200. For a critique of the Milburn Plan, see Rudolf Klein, "Milburn's Version of a New NHS: Adopting the Missionary Position," editorial, *British Medical Journal*, 322 (5 May 2001): 1078–79.

22. Nick Bosanquet, Jennifer Dixon, Trevor Harvey, David Hunter, Allyson Pollock, Bob Sang, Andrew Wall, and Charles Webster, "Across the Great Divide: Discussing the Undiscussable," *British Journal of HealthCare Management*, 7.10 (2001): 395–400. David J. Hunter, "Policy-making in the NHS, Across the Great Divide: Discussing the Undiscussable," *British Journal of HealthCare Management*, 7.10 (2001): 397. Charles Webster, "Brave New NHS, Across the Great Divide: Discussing the Undiscussable," *British Journal of HealthCare Management*, 7.10 (2001): 399–400. Bob Sang, "Confronting Machiavelli's Dilemma: Are Managers Part of the Solution, or Part of the Problem, Across the Great Divide: Discussing the Undiscussable," *British Journal of HealthCare Management*, 7.10 (2001): 398–99. Jennifer Dixon, "Why the Gripes, Across the Great Divide: Discussing the Undiscussable," *British Journal of HealthCare Management*, 7.10 (2001): 396.

23. Dixon, *supra* note 22.

24. Webster, *supra* note 22.

25. Hunter, *supra* note 22.

26. Hunter, *supra* note 22.

27. Klein, *supra* note 21.

28. William J. Holstein, "Three Users' Manuals for Modern Management," *New York Times*, November 25, 2001.

The Politics of Medical Inflation

Theodore R. Marmor, Donald A. Wittman, and Thomas C. Heagy

THE PROBLEM OF INFLATION IN MEDICAL
CARE: INTRODUCTION

In the past twenty-four years the price of American medical services has risen 1.5 times as fast as the Consumer Price Index. The proportion of the gross national product devoted to health care has increased by 71 percent from 4.6 percent to 7.8 percent. Clearly, a continuation of these trends would have serious consequences. Moreover, many economists believe that the "continuing trend towards full or nearly full insurance coverage in the context of a nearly unregulated fee-for-service delivery system *is* likely to produce continued inflation in medical care."[1]

This article discusses the politics of anti-inflation policy in the medical care sector and the determinants of governmental responses to problems known jointly as medical care inflation. We attempt first to clarify the issue by distinguishing between four different concepts commonly used when discussing medical inflation. We then present some of the standard solutions to these problems suggested by economists.

Of necessity, a discussion of the political "market" and the political attributes of the solutions proposed go hand in hand with a discussion of inflation. The politics of medical inflation in our view produce persistent expressions of concern about inflation rates, but actions which at worst exacerbate the problem or at best are weak. The most decisive governmental reactions to medical inflation will continue to be reductions of medical care benefits in selected public programs rather than actions to reduce medical inflation generally, until or unless the budget for health is centralized at one governmental level. We find, in general, that a decentralized payment structure reduces the government's interest in effective implementation of anti-inflationary policies.

CLARIFICATION OF THE PROBLEM

Considerable confusion has arisen in the discussion of controlling medical inflation because commentators have discussed at least four different problems under the common rubric of "medical inflation."

Absolute price inflation. Absolute price inflation is measured by the Medical Services component of the CPI.[2] According to this index, the annual rate of medical inflation has averaged 4.4 percent over the past twenty-four years.[3] This measure seems clearly inappropriate. What we are concerned with is medical price inflation only to the extent that it exceeds general inflation. If the inflation rates are identical, the problem is one of general inflation, not medical inflation.

Relative price inflation. The difference between the annual rate of growth of the Medical Services component of the CPI and the total CPI measures relative price inflation. By this index, the rate of medical inflation has averaged 1.3 percent per year over the past twenty-four years.[4] This may appear small, but represents a total increase of 37 percent in the relative price of medical services over the twenty-four-year period.

Total real expenditures growth per capita. Measured by the percent growth in expenditures per capita on medical services deflated by the total CPI, the annual rate of expenditure growth over two decades has averaged 4.8 percent.[5] This measure is inappropriate for reasons similar to that cited in regard to absolute price inflation: the measure incorporates the general growth of real GNP per capita. Only if the real expenditures on medical services grow at a faster rate than total real income, is its growth noteworthy.

Relative expenditure growth. The increase of medical expenditures as a percent of GNP is an appropriate measure. The annual rate of growth has averaged 2.3 percent, from 4.6 percent of GNP to 7.8 percent of GNP, an increase of 71 percent. Relative expenditure growth can be divided into two components, relative price inflation (see 2 above), and relative quantity growth.[6] Over the past twenty-four years, both have been major contributors to relative expenditure growth.

Neither relative price inflation nor relative expenditure growth is a priori bad. People are concerned about relative price growth for at least two reasons. First, it redistributes income to health care providers from everyone else. Second, an increase in medical care's relative price has a disproportionate impact on the poor who spend a larger part of their income on medical care.[7] On the other hand, the assumption that relative prices are too high implies that prices can be too low. For example, a major part of the growth in the price of hospital services is explained by the increased wages of unskilled workers,[8] formerly among the worst paid workers in the economy. The relative increase in their wages may have been not only justified but insufficient.

People are also concerned about the reduced share of GNP available to other sectors. But as in the case of relative prices, growth in relative expenditures is undesirable only if relative expenditures are excessive on *Pareto optimal* or equity grounds. Critics of relative medical inflation argue that government subsidy, insurance, and other programs promote consumption of more and better quality medical services than are really needed; that expenditures on medical care bring rapidly diminishing marginal benefit; and that some of the money going to health care could be better used elsewhere in the economy.[9] It can also be argued, however, that the increase in relative expenditures has been the desirable result of increased access for the poor and better quality generally.

Despite disagreement concerning the optimal level of expenditures, it is clear that if relative expenditures increase at current rates without limit, they will soon become intolerable. For the remainder of this paper we will accept the argument that relative prices and expenditures in medical care are currently too high and that government action is justified to curtail further medical care inflation.

It is essential to note that limiting relative expenditures requires the simultaneous control of relative prices and relative quantity. However, some proposed policies would reduce relative price at the expense of increasing relative expenditures. If the goal is simply to control relative price, these are appropriate means. But, if the goal is to control relative expenditure, they are not. Ultimately, the choice of policy tools will depend on how the medical inflation problem is defined.

The appropriate response to the problem of medical inflation depends on its causes. Some observers have diagnosed six major causes of medical health inflation[10] (whether relative prices, relative expenditures, or high prices):[11] (1) wealthier societies tend to spend a larger fraction of their resources on medical care; (2) cost increasing technological developments in medical care in the post-war period, such as kidney machines and open heart surgery, have outweighed cost decreasing developments such as antibiotics; (3) doctors and hospitals have monopoly power; (4) the supply of doctors has been artificially limited and substitutes legally limited in scope; (5) greater use of medical insurance has reduced the marginal cost of medical care to the patients; and (6) the government supplies a substantial subsidy of health care. Only to the extent that health inflation is caused by numbers 3 to 6 is it a "problem" requiring or responsive to government action.

Cures. There are three broad types of responses to the problem so diagnosed. The first is to improve the market; that is, to make the market for medical care resemble efficient markets in other sectors where the interplay of people seeking private gain and paying out-of-pocket for their goods and services disciplines both the consumer and the provider. Such a strategy includes making patients more informed about the market and likewise giving them greater financial stakes in acting on that information. Typically such remedies include the suggestion of patient financial participation through substantial coinsurance and deductibles. This type of remedy is exemplified by Martin Feldstein's major risk insurance proposal where families would pay up to 10 percent of their income for medical care and anything above that would be paid for by the federal government in a catastrophic health insurance plan.[12] Other critics have argued for HMO expansion as part of the market improvement strategy.[13]

A second answer to this set of problems is to compensate for the poor market structure with public utility type regulation.[14] The standard site for such regulation is the states; electrical utilities are an example of such a regulated industry. The standard subjects of such regulation are health care facilities and the price they charge for their services. Many states are establishing commissions that deal with facility supply (Certificate of Need) and, in separate commissions, pricing (primarily for hospitals). Massachusetts, Maryland, Connecticut and other states have set up so-called rate commissions to regulate hospital prices.[15]

The third answer is to replace the economic market with a political market by effectively nationalizing the industry. In this case there is a constraining bilateral relationship between buyers and providers: the buyer is the government and the providers are the industry's constituent parts. The government bargains with the providers on price, supply, and quality, representing diffuse and decentralized consumers unorganized to influence health policy decisions. In effect, the government is dealing with the monopoly power of the providers by creating a monopsony for the consumers. The Kennedy-Corman bill (S.3, H.R. 21), for example, provides that the federal government pay for almost all medical care services and regulate the prices of those services by regional health boards in market areas throughout the country.

THE RESPONSE OF GOVERNMENT

For years economists have "supplied" solutions to medical care inflation, yet the government has largely ignored their advice. In some ways, as by granting tax subsidies for medical insurance, it has contributed to medical inflation.

Analysis of the political "market" suggests why there is little reason to expect bold government action against medical inflation (relative price or expenditure growth) in the future.

The theory of imbalanced political interests: concentrated versus diffuse benefits and costs. The political "market" refers to institutional arrangements—the relationships among organized pressure groups, voters, authoritative governmental agencies and affected citizens—which determine what governments do. As George Stigler says of governmental *regulation,* the theory of public policy ought to explain "who will receive the benefits and burdens of governmental [action.]"[16] Important is the emphasis on the natural imbalance between the interests of mass public and health care providers on issues like inflation.

An imbalanced political market is simply one where participants have unequal power. This stands in sharp contrast with the egalitarian theory of one man–one vote, implying equal power by all participants. Of the many theories of imbalanced political markets, one is especially applicable to medical care— that of concentrated versus diffuse interests. Those with concentrated interests feel the effects of a policy (whether subsidy or tax, compulsion or prohibition) significantly. Those with diffuse interests have no important stake, great as the aggregate costs or benefits may be. A $1 per capita tax would be a diffuse cost of large aggregate magnitude in the United States as a whole.

The incentives to press claims for concentrated interests are much greater than those for diffuse ones. The prospect of having one's well-being substantially affected creates powerful incentives to act to protect one's interest. An interest marginal to one's well-being—even though large when aggregated over the class of affected parties—provides insufficient incentives to act. This distribution of incentives results, then, in a systematic imbalance of the probabilities of interest representation. It is not the case that the theory of imbalance in the political market explains the outcomes of political struggles by itself. For the outcomes are a product not simply of the representation of interests, but also of other political resources—wealth, information, skill—that fuel the representation of those interests. But the structure of interests does largely determine which groups play a role in the channels of policy action and whose preferences are likely to count most in that process.[17] The theory of imbalanced interests holds that concentrated groups, other things being equal, will be more effective in the political process than diffuse ones.[18]

There are other concepts of imbalanced political markets. One stresses inequality of information among voters. Clearly, vote maximizing candidates for political office[19] will neglect the interests of the uninformed and cultivate those of the more informed voter. Obviously, groups differ in wealth as well. Other things being equal, the rich can exert greater influence per capita on election results and political decisions than the poor through donations. A group with extra-political purposes (e.g., a labor union) will have greater political capability than a solely political one. The first has already paid its overhead; the second must spend much of its resources on organizational maintenance. Since the results of most political activity constitute collective goods, the differential ability of various groups in overcoming the collective good problems of political activity creates an unbalanced power differential.[20]

These theories overlap; a cause in one may be an effect in another. For example, a group with concentrated benefits and costs has special incentives to be well informed. In addition, there is usually a substantial correlation among the characteristics that lead to greater political influence. For example, doctors are better informed (on health regulation issues), wealthier, better organized and have more concentrated interests than do patients. This obviously makes it difficult to pinpoint the specific effect of their concentrated interests on public policy as opposed to the effect of the other characteristics. This is why the care of welfare mothers is enlightening. On the basis of every criterion of political power except concentrated interest, one would expect them to have virtually no success in the policy arena. The extent to which they have been successful in increasing benefits in the post-war period might be explained by the theory of concentrated interests.[21]

IMBALANCED INTERESTS AND INFLATION

What is the connection between the theory of imbalanced political interests and the response to the problem of relative inflation generally?[22] The theory predicts that government will respond cautiously and ineffectively to relative inflation in any sector. In the past half decade, relative inflation, indeed, double digit inflation in the early 1970's has been a serious problem in both construction and medical care especially since these sectors together form a very large component of GNP. Substantial relative inflation in them preempts other national and individual spending.

Yet, any effective attack on this public "bad" mobilizes the resistance of concentrated interests in the affected industry.[23] Governmental action to control relative inflation in construction costs would save the average household far less than it would cost construction workers. Control of medical care inflation likewise would cost providers (hospitals, nursing homes, physicians, nurses, etc.) much more than it would benefit patients.

HOW DOES THIS APPLY TO MEDICAL CARE INFLATION?

Who will influence health care most? Doctors, hospital administrators, union officers and insurance underwriters will have power beyond their numbers; tax payers in general and patients in particular will be underrepresented. The reason is quite simple. The providers are very knowledgeable and concerned about health care policy since it is so important to their lives. On the other side, the expected benefits or costs of a health care policy are relatively unimportant to consumers in normal health. Their interests are diffuse including not only health, but also food, clothing, shelter, education, recreation, and employment. It does not pay the consumer to take strong action. Consumers do have a voice, but it is systematically underrepresented in the political process.

Political leaders, then, have little incentive to follow politically controversial economic advice on how to combat relative medical care inflation.[24] If it is everybody's problem — if the burdens are widely distributed among millions of health care purchasers — political rewards for improvement will be insufficient. A 10 percent decrease in health expenditures — an average of reduction from $400 per capita per year to $360 per year — would reduce the total health bill of the United States by a striking $10 billion. But, while "society" would "save" that much, the efforts to produce such a reduction would mobilize the powerful countervailing efforts of providers.[25] A 10 percent decrease in one's average health bill is of marginal concern to citizens in comparison to the preoccupation of providers with medical care pricing policy. As a result, governments have greater pressure upon them to resist anti-inflationary policy than to act on it.

The main exception is that governments in their buying capacity have a substantial interest in reducing their own program costs. Government departments, acting as if the total government expenditures are relatively inelastic, try to reduce expenditure increases by other departments. There is, therefore, an internal government market which partially serves to put a brake on programmatic expenditure increases. This means that the form of financing is very important. For example, non-health agencies will be less concerned about increased expenditures derived from payroll deductions than from those financed from general taxes. Not surprisingly, providers strongly prefer payroll deductions to financing from general revenues.

Theory suggests that the more any particular level of government pays for medical care, the more it will be concerned about price and expenditure increases. Again, there is some evidence to support the theory. Great Britain, with a centralized public finance payment structure, has a significantly lower inflation rate and level of expenditure than the U.S., Canada and Sweden, which vary in degree of public support (with Sweden being close to 100 percent government supported) but share decentralized financing.[26] Tables 1 and 2 present the changing proportion of resources spent on health care in several western industrial nations.

Table 1: Total Expenditures for Health Services as a Percentage of the Gross
National Product, Seven Countries, Selected Periods, 1961–1969

Country	WHO Estimates		SSA Estimates	
	Year	*Percentage of GNP*	*Year*	*Percentage of GNP*
Canada	1961	6	1969	7.3
United states	1961–62	5.8	1969	6.8
Sweden	1962	5.4	1969	6.7
Netherlands	1963	4.8	1969	5.9
Federal Republic of Germany	1961	4.5	1969	5.7
France	1963	4.4	1969	5.7
United Kingdom	1961–62	4.2	1969	4.8

Source: The Report of the Health Planning Task Force prepared under the auspices of the Research and Analysis Division of the Ontario Ministry of Health.
a. Brian Abel-Smith. An International Study of Health Expenditure, WHO Public Paper No. 32 (Geneva: 1967).
b. Joseph G. Simanis. "Medical Care Expenditures in Seven Countries," Social Security Bulletin (March 1973): 39

Medicare and Medicaid illustrate the complex interplay of the forces we have been discussing. During the period 1966–70 total government expenditures on both Medicare and Medicaid increased very rapidly; more beneficiaries were using more expensive services more often than planners had foreseen.[27] By the 1970's, the Nixon Administration was trying to hold down these program costs, first under brief price controls with no permanent effect, then merely by reducing Medicare and Medicaid benefits rather than cost inflation as such.[28] In constant dollars Medicare payments per beneficiary stopped growing. Medicaid payments per beneficiary actually declined. Because during the 1970's the number of beneficiaries continued to rise, total real expenditures also increased in both programs, though at a much slower rate.[29]

The theory of concentrated costs and benefits appears to predict past governmental responses to medical inflation and the impact on Medicare/Medicaid. It has more difficulty in predicting which of the two programs would be affected the most by concern over their program costs. Medicaid payment is more decentralized (federal, state, some cost-sharing by beneficiaries) but is financed by general revenues. Medicare payment is centralized but is financed by a payroll tax. The two factors tend to cancel out. Medicaid may have lost ground not because of its financing, but because the poor are less politically attractive than the old.[30]

Applied to the politics of inflation control in medical care, the theory of concentrated interests suggests that market improvement will be an unlikely strategy. It could work, and the diffuse public would pay lower insurance premiums and lower medical prices than otherwise. But precisely for that reason, the providers would probably mobilize their concentrated interests to defeat or sabotage it. The point about the market improvement proposals is not that they are all conceptually *ineffective*, but that the greater their likely effectiveness, if enacted, the greater the opposition of the concentrated interests and, therefore, the more *politically* unlikely their implementation.

The government—which would have to improve the market—would benefit from an anti-inflationary policy for medical care as fiscal agent for approximately one-quarter of total medical care expenditures.[31] But it would also incur all of the political costs of market improvement. So, the greater the share of costs a single level of government has in the medical care market, the greater its willingness to impose an anti-inflationary policy on medical providers.

Public utility type regulation, on the other hand, is politically feasible but questionably effective. The demand for state regulation is partly a gesture towards controlling relative medical care inflation and partly an expression of the belief that direct controls of supply and price can, through state commissions, actually moderate inflation.

Certificate of Need legislation and other supply restrictions will undoubtedly apply only to facility expansion and not to current hospital bed supply. This is protective legislation for present hospitals even if supply restraints will limit total expenditure growth, and supply constraints may even exacerbate relative price inflation.[32]

Rate review—medical care price setting—as proposed in the United States would be weak because independent of governmental payment in programs like Medicare and Medicaid. This separation of the payer from price regulator is likely in practice to lead to a weak price setting mechanism. The government agency with the greatest interest in relative prices is clearly the one which pays for medical care services. Again, state regulation of medical care inflation is possible; it just won't work and isn't working in states that are trying it because states pay a relatively small share of our medical expenditures.[33]

The third strategy—restraining inflation by fiscally centralized national health insurance—presents a mixed picture. On the one hand, the concentration of governmental responsibility of health expenditures is, on the basis of

Table 2: Increases in Relative Medical Expenditures. 1961–69

Average annual rate of increases of medical expenditure minus average annual increase for GNP

France	4.8
Sweden	4.2
Netherlands	4.2
Canada	3.3
Federal Republic of Germany	3.3
United States	2.8
United Kingdom	2.6

Source: Adapted from Table 7, page 31, of Michael H. Cooper. *Rationing Health Care* (New York. John Wiley and Sons. 1975).

our theory, likely to promote serious government interest in restraining inflation. On the other hand, the concentrated provider interests will be (and are) mobilized to resist precisely this feature of proposed national health insurance legislation. Again there is evidence to support our theory: most current providers resist the notion that health should be financed out of a single budget, whatever their views on the particular form of national health insurance. They point to Great Britain as a "starved" medical care system, where somewhere in excess of 5 percent of GNP is expended on health care despite the fact that it is all publicly funded.[34] Yet, as Rudolf Klein points out, this can be interpreted as an international achievement:[35] "The British National Health Service is remarkable for one achievement. In most other Western societies, expenditure on health care has been soaring over the past decade at a rate which has provoked an anxious search for ways of limiting the growth. In contrast, the NHS has been conspicuous for its success in containing the rate of increase in spending; in Britain the demand has been for an acceleration in the growth rate."

Health care expenditures in Sweden, Canada, and the U.S. are more than 8 percent of GNP, despite the range of financing sources from totally public (at various levels) to substantially private?[36] The Kennedy-Corman strategy makes concentrated or diffuse budgeting for health a significant issue:

To summarize, the greater the likely effectiveness of an anti-inflation policy, the less likely is its enactment. The market improvement strategy has some promise of effectiveness, but little likelihood of success. Public regulation at the state level has political appeal, but a much lower probability of effectiveness.

Controlling inflation through a single national health insurance program has some chance of effective constraint, but for that reason is likely to mobilize effective opposition.

The greatest chance of controlling relative medical inflation would appear to be through the back door of a national health insurance plan that is not necessarily passed for the purpose of controlling medical inflation and does not have a strong inflation control mechanism built into it, but which increases the effective pressure for controlling medical inflation in the future by increasing the portion of medical expenditures that flow through the federal budget.

For limiting relative expenditure growth (as opposed to price inflation) in the hospital sector, supply control is both effective and politically viable because its costs fall primarily on the prospective newcomers to the industry. Their opposition to supply control is outweighed by the support of established hospitals that want to curtail competition.

Nothing illustrates the futility of most conventional cost-control proposals better than the suggestions made by the September, 1974, HEW Summit Conference on medical inflation. Nearly all were in fact inflationary and beneficial mainly to health care providers, who contributed most of the prepared papers.

THE SUMMIT CONFERENCE ON INFLATION: ILLUSTRATIONS

The Conference made the following recommendations:

1. Increase the federal budget for health service programs. (This action will increase the relative expenditures on health and will increase the inflationary pressures in the health care industry. While there may be, depending on the program, some substitution from the private sector to the public thereby hurting some health care firms, increased federal activity will for the most part benefit health care providers.)
2. Keep operating costs as close to parity with increases in the Consumer Price Index as possible. (This is the goal of anti-inflationary policy, but no method of implementing it is contained in this section.)
3. Restructure reimbursement. For example, reimbursement should be on a total budget rather than a line item basis. This policy has been tried in some Canadian provinces with limited success.[37]
4. Shift emphasis to ambulatory and preventive care. (While there may be shift from the more expensive hospital care, the main effect is to bring more health care onto the "insurance gravy train." A good example of this problem is given by Lave for dental care.[38] The marginal costs of prevention are less than the benefits, inflation will be reduced; conversely, inflation will be increased if the reverse is true.

5. Initiate consumer education activities directed toward increasing consumer knowledge regarding what are realistic patient expectations from the health care system. (Inflationary and expenditure impact is insignificant one way or another, but it does create some jobs for health care researchers.)

6. Provide consumers with information on fees and prices. (It will probably result in a one-time reduction in prices of small magnitude. It should be noted that a footnote to the report mentioned that the providers showed considerable skepticism regarding this approach and suggested that it was, in fact, inflationary—no comment is necessary.)

7. Change the statutory definition of health maintenance organizations in order to allow for more flexibility in assembling benefit packages tailored to the needs and financial resources of particular population groups. (While this may be desirable, it is not clear what effect this will have on health care inflation. Essentially this law allows HMOs to use the optimal discrimination in pricing—a monopoly ploy to increase revenues and profits.)

8. Do not allow the quality of health care to become a casualty of zealous efforts to contain costs in the health sector. (Unfortunately, this is the crux of the matter, that increases in quality—more comfortable beds, better trained nurses, equipment which only brings very marginal increases in success rates—have been responsible for a substantial part of the increases in hospital care costs. *Not* to put a lid on quality improvement is *not* to put a lid on relative expenditure growth. On the assumption that hospital costs have risen because of increases in both quality and quantity demanded, then the desire to reduce relative expenditure increases without having any effects on quality improvement is a desire not to stop relative expenditure growth.)

9. Monitor the impact of the contribution to inflation in the health care sector. (This is a chance for the self-interested researcher to get in on the "anti-inflation gravy train." The main effect will be to increase trivially the relative amount of expenditures devoted to health care.)

10. Encourage comprehensive health planning coupled with regulatory power to reduce duplication of facilities via the innovative use of Certificate of Need and rate setting mechanisms. (This is essentially the hospital supply proposal we have already discussed.)

11. Increase supply of primary care providers and, in particular, third party reimbursement for the services of non-physician providers should be encouraged. (Economic theory predicts the first part of the suggestion would work but Canadian experience suggests the opposite.)[39]

12. Reconsider wage and price controls. (It was noted that a wide array of provider groups dissented from this view).[40]

CONCLUSION

Economic theory suggests that the economic market will systematically underproduce public goods. This conclusion is often used as a justification for governmental intervention. But the implication of this paper is that moving from the economic marketplace to the political marketplace does not necessarily solve problems. In the absence of some concentrated interest, the political market is unlikely to adopt a policy simply because it constitutes a public good.[41] The political market (like the economic one) will systematically underproduce public goods (and overproduce public "bads"). The political process is unlikely to right the distributive wrongs of the economic marketplace when a similar set of actors dominate both.[42]

The application of this theory to national health insurance suggests sober estimates about the government's ability to restrain national health care expenditures, which are increasing at the rate of more than $10 billion a year. The experiences of Canada and Sweden suggest that government financing on a large scale alone does not reverse the upward spiral in prices and expenditures. Certainly this has been the case when the government uses an insurance mechanism in which financing is diffusely shared among patients and different units of government. There is evidence that where financing is concentrated and service providers are directly budgeted (rather than reimbursed retrospectively by insurance) expenditures and the rate of medical inflation are lower. This has been the case in Great Britain, with its National Health Service. While one would not expect the United States to legislate a national health service, the experience of Great Britain has important implications for the degree of financing concentration desirable in a future national health insurance program.

Notes

This article was first published in *Journal of Health Politics, Policy and Law* 1, no. 1 (1976): 69–84. A version of this article also appears in *Health: A Victim or Cause of Inflation*, ed. M. Zubkoff (New York: Milbank Memorial Fund, 1975), as a chapter entitled *Politics, Public Policy, and Medical Inflation*.

1. Joseph Newhouse, *Inflation and Health Insurance*, in *Health: A Victim or Cause of Inflation*, ed. M. Zubkoff (New York: Milbank Memorial Fund, 1975).

2. Some analysts (including the authors of this paper) believe that the medical services component of the CPI overstates medical inflation because it does not fully take into account improvements in quality. However, since this assertion (if true) would not affect any of the conclusions of our paper, we will not consider it further.

3. Bureau of Labor Statistics, *Monthly Labor Review*, various issues.
4. Ibid.
5. U.S. Department of Health. Education, and Welfare, *The Health, Education and Welfare Income Security, Social Services Conference on Inflation Report* (Washington, D.C.: Government Printing Office, 1974).
6. Relative quantity growth is that growth in medical services as a percent of GNP that would have occurred in the absence of any change in the relative price level of medical services. It includes both quantity changes (in the strict sense) and quality changes.
7. Karen Davis, *The Impact of Inflation and Unemployment on Health Care of Low Income People*, in Zubkoff, *Health*.
8. Lester Lave, *The Effect of Inflation on Providers*, in Zubkoff, *Health*.
9. Joseph Newhouse, *Inflation and Health Insurance*, in Zubkoff, *Health*.
10. For example, U.S. Department of Health, Education, and Welfare, Social Security Administration, *Community Hospitals: Inflation in the Pre-Medicare Period*, by Karen Davis and Richard Foster, Research Report No. 41, Washington. D.C.: Government Printing Office. 1972; Martin Feldstein, "A New Approach to National Health Insurance," *The Public Interest* 23 (Spring 1971); Lave, *The Effect of Inflation*, and Newhouse, *Inflation and Health Insurance*.
11. Numbers 2 to 6 cause *high* relative prices (and/or expenditures), not *increasing* relative prices (and/or expenditures). For them to cause relative inflation they must increase in magnitude or effectiveness over time.
12. *A New Approach, op. cit.*
13. Newhouse, *Inflation*.
14. Fredric L. Sattler, *Hospital Prospective Rate Setting, Issues and Options*, working paper, SSA Interstudy Hospital Prospective Payment Workshop (Minneapolis: Inter-Study, 1975). For a survey of the extent of state rate review and certificate-of-need agencies see L. Lewin & Associates, *Nationwide Survey of Health Regulation*, NTIS Accession No. 236660-AS (September 1974), and *An Analysis of State and Regional Health Regulation* (February 1974). For analytical commentary on these developments see L. Lewin, Ann Somers and Herman Somers, *Issues in the Structure and Administration of State Health Cost Regulation*, Toledo Law Review Symposium (June 1975).
15. Sattler, *Hospital Prospective Rate Setting*.
16. George Stigler, "The Theory of Economic Regulation," *The Bell Journal of Economics and Management Science* 2 (Spring 1971).
17. These concepts are taken from the work of Graham Allison, *The Essence of Decision* (Boston: Little, Brown, 1971), especially the discussion of the organizational process model of politics. It further uses teaching materials prepared by Allison on *The Massachusetts Medical School Case*, Public Policy Program, Harvard University, 1973.
18. Compare the similar, but not identical views of George Stigler, "The Theory of Economic Regulation," and Richard Posner, "Theories of Economic Regulation," *The Bell Journal of Economics and Management Science* 5 (Autumn 1974): 335–58, for further discussion of economic approaches to the study of public policy policies.
19. Donald Wittman, "Political Decision-Making" in *Economics of Public Choice*, eds: Robert D. Leiter and Gerald Serkin (New York: Cyrco Press, 1975), pp. 29–48.
20. A government program to help farmers, to give a specific illustration helps a particular farmer whether or not he has contributed to lobbying for the passage of the bill. Since the farmer's individual efforts are costly and unlikely to change the outcome, he and all other farmers are likely to abstain from political activity. This is a variant of the "Prisoner's dilemma," a game theory problem where individually rational behavior results in collectively irrational behavior for the participants involved. Which groups will be most successful at overcoming the collective good behavior? Clearly, those groups which are best capable of internalizing the rewards and

externalizing the costs, i.e., making some of the good private instead of collective. For example, those who do not contribute are beaten up (a private bad to the person), while those who contribute receive a special citation or invitation to a dinner (a private good). The analysis takes on many subtle variations. Different kinds of groups are better at policing themselves for correct behavior (smaller groups versus larger and more physically concentrated groups than diffuse). See Mancur Olson, *The Logic of Collective Action* (Cambridge, Mass.: Harvard University Press, 1968). A monopolistic firm in an industry is thus capable of exerting great political pressure on behalf of the industry, because, first it is the industry and, therefore, the good is a private good and second, it does not have to organize a large number of firms for political action since it is already organized. For an excellent discussion, see William A. Brock and Stephen P. Magee, Mimeo, University of Chicago: Center for Mathematical Studies in Business and Economics, 1975, and for an insightful diagrammatic exposition, see John Chamberlynn, Mimeo, University of Michigan: Institute of Policy Studies, 1975.

21. There are of course other explanations for this particular phenomenon such as the one given by Frances Piven and Richard Cloward that welfare payments are a technique for "regulating the poor," or interdependent utility functions, i.e., other individuals have utility functions that are concerned with the welfare of mothers, *Regulating the Poor: The Functions of Public Welfare* (New York: Random House, 1971).

22. In order to use an essential static model to explain the response of the political system to a dynamic situation (inflation), we will assume that concentrated interests have not completely exhausted the benefits of concentration and still have marginal influence which is greater than that of the diffuse interests. There have been several papers written on the relationship of the political process to aggregate inflation and other macro-economics variables. For example, see Robert Gordon, *The Politics of Inflation*, National Bureau of Economic Research Conference on Economic Analysis of Political Behavior, 1975; Bruno Frey, "A Politico-Economic System: A Simulation Model," *Kyklos* 28 (1974): 227–254; and Gerald Kramer, "Short Run Fluctuation in U.S. Voting Behavior, 1896–1964," *American Political Science Review* 65 (March 1971): 131–143.

23. Sometimes there may be concentrated interests who will fight inflation (for example, the purchasers of intermediate goods). However, these are relatively weak in medical care and construction. Everyone would be for the public good (or against the public bad) if the gainers could bribe the losers; however, the high cost of bargaining across issues effectively prevents this theoretical possibility from taking place.

24. It may be in the interest of the politician to act as an entrepreneur in discovering public goods and offering policies that promote public goods. However, we doubt that it is complete—that all public goods are captured by politicians. For more information concerning entrepreneurialism, see Norman Froehlich, Joe Oppenheimer and Oran Young, *Political Leadership and Collective Good* (Princeton, N.J.: Princeton University Press, 1971).

25. Of course, some providers might benefit from a decrease in expenditures and clearly some customers would benefit from increased health expenditures; but we *believe* that intergroup conflict and variation is greater than the intragroup variation.

26. Odin Anderson, *Health Care: Can There Be Equity? The United States, Sweden and England* (New York: John Wiley and Sons, 1975); R. D. Fraser, *Overview: Canadian National Health Insurance*, paper presented at the Conference of Canadian Health Economists, Queens University. Ontario, September 1974; and Theodore Marmor et al., *Canadian National Health Insurance: Policy Implications for the United States, Policy Sciences* (December 1975). Also, in different form, see Spyros Andrepoulos, ed., *National Health Insurance* (New York: John Wiley and Sons, 1975).

27. U.S. Department of Health, Education, and Welfare, *Expenditures for Personal Health Services: National Trends and Variations—1953–1970*, by Ronald Andersen et al., U.S. Department HEW Publication No. (HRA) 74–3105, Washington, D.C.: Bureau of Health Services Research

and Evaluation, 1973; and U.S. Department of Health, Education, and Welfare, *Health Service Use: National Trends and Variations—1953–1971, by* Ronald Andersen et al., U.S. Department HEW Publication No. (HSM) 73–3004, Washington, D.C.: National Center for Health Services Research and Development, 1972.

28. Robert Stevens and Rosemary Stevens, *Welfare Medicine in America: A Case Study of Medicaid* (New York: The Free Press, 1974).

29. Karen Davis, "The Impact of Inflation and Unemployment on Health Care of Low Income People," in Zubkoff, *Health*.

30. Stevens and Stevens, *Welfare Medicine in America.*

31. Social Security Administration, *Background Information on Medical Expenditures, Prices and Costs*, Washington, D.C.: Office of Research and Statistics, September 1974.

32. Of course, there are models of hospital regulation which could have desirable effects on inflation. If unnecessary beds were excluded from cost reimbursement as one of our referees suggests is possible, both price and expenditure growth *could* be moderated.

33. L. Lewin, Ann Somers and Herman Somers. *Issues in the Structure and Administration of State Health Cost Regulation.*

34. Milton Friedman, "Leonard Woodcock's Free Lunch," *Newsweek*, 21 April 1975.

35. Rudolf Klein, ed., *Social Policy and Public Expenditure 1975: Inflation and Priorities* (London: Centre for Studies in Social Policy, 1975), p. 83.

36. U.S. Department of Health, Education, and Welfare, *Health Service Use: National Trends and Variations—1953–1971*; R. D. Fraser, *Overview: Canadian National Health Insurance*; and Marmor et al., *Canadian National Health Insurance.*

37. Andreopoulos, ed., *National Health Insurance* (especially chapters by R. G. Evans M. LeClair, and T. R. Marmor).

38. Lester Lave, *The Effect of Inflation on Providers*, in Zubkoff, *Health*.

39. Robert G. Evans, "Beyond the Medical Marketplace: Expenditure, Utilization and Pricing of Insured Health Care in Canada," in Andreopoulos, *National Health Insurance*.

40. For a discussion of how the controls worked, see Paul Ginsburg, "The Economic Stabilization Program," in Zubkoff, *Health*.

41. Robert R. Alford, *Health Care Politics: Ideological and Interest Group Barriers to Reform* (Chicago: University of Chicago Press, 1974).

42. The question of the precise comparative advantage of these respective markets has not been systematically studied.

The Great Transformation

Rudolf Klein

Over the past quarter century or so there has been, in Peter Hall's formulation (Hall, 1993), a paradigm shift in macro-economic policy making: a movement from a Keynesian mode of policy making towards one based on monetary theory. The latter was open to a variety of interpretations and has been modified in practice. However, there was clearly a transformation in the way we think about economic policy making. Is the same true of social policy? Has there been an equivalent paradigm shift in the way we think about social policy? The two books under review provide an opportunity for addressing this question.

The selection of Richard Titmuss's papers on the National Health Service illustrate what might be called the conventional wisdom—or operating paradigm—of the social policy community as forged in the post-war decades. Titmuss himself was, of course, largely responsible for articulating that paradigm: an enormously revered figure during his lifetime, his disciples at the London School of Economics dominated social policy studies after his death in 1973 and his views still have much resonance in the social policy community even today. Julian Le Grand, the Richard Titmuss Professor of Social Policy at LSE, has now produced a book that challenges many of the ideas of his predecessor and provides an alternative way of thinking not only about the NHS but also about social policy more generally. The contrast between the two books under review provides an opportunity to examine the transformation in the intellectual foundations of social policy that have taken place over the past decades.

Both Titmuss and Le Grand reflect the intellectual and policy environment of their time. Just as Titmuss provided an intellectual and moral justification for the post-war Welfare State, so Le Grand provides a rationale for the new social policy model that has emerged over the last 20 years or so. And just as LSE social policy staff of the Titmuss era was in an out of Whitehall during the Labour Governments of the 1960s and 1970s, so Le Grand served as policy adviser to Tony Blair. To state the obvious, intellectual development does not take place in a vacuum: ideas reflect the policy world—the success or otherwise of policy experiments (be it the creation of the NHS in 1948 or the invention of quasi-markets in the 1980s)—as well as influencing policy. Policy and ideas fertilise each other: there is no such thing as intellectual virginity when it comes to social policy discourse.

One important difference between Titmuss and Le Grand must be noted before addressing the specifics of their arguments. This is the difference in their styles of argument, reflecting partly their personal histories and partly changes in the academic environment in the 30 plus years that separate their writings. Titmuss was a self-made academic who had no university degree and eclectically drew on a variety of disciplines in the study of social policy. His publications ranged from rigorous statistical analysis to more general, speculative essays, the latter of which make up the bulk of the book under review. But I suspect that the quality that made him such an appealing figure was that he was a moralist, a sort of latter-day prophet. That, and the fact that he could write clearly and without technical jargon, appealing to his readers emotionally as well intellectually. Le Grand, in contrast, is a modern academic: a card-carrying economist with a Ph.D. to prove it. He is a more disciplined writer than Titmuss, building up his arguments step by step and acknowledging the strengths and weaknesses of any case that he is making. In contrast, as we shall see, Titmuss sometimes seems to avoid the logic of his own arguments and seldom acknowledges that there might be something to be said against them. If Titmuss is the master of persuasive rhetoric, very much in the mould of Tawney and others writing at the same time, Le Grand follows the rules of the academic game: he writes clearly but avoids arm waving gestures. Both are advocates—making a case for particular policies—but their ways of addressing the jury are very different.

Le Grand's book is an expanded and elaborated version of his influential article, "Knights, Knaves or Pawns? Human Behaviour and Social Policy" (Le Grand, 1997), based on his inaugural lecture. His starting point was the observation that in Britain—and elsewhere—there had been a significant shift in social policy: notably the introduction of competition in the delivery in social services—as epitomised by the invention of quasi markets—and the design of social security programmes. In turn, this implied a largely implicit shift "in the assumptions concerning motivation that underlay older models of welfare systems." The assumption of the founders of the post-1945 model Welfare State was that those providing the services or deciding on benefits—be they doctors, teachers or council house managers—were altruistic paternalists: they were considered to be, in Le Grand's terminology, knights. Contrariwise, the assumption of the quasi-market and other reforms of the 1980s and 1990s was that service providers pursued their own self-interest but would respond to incentives: they were considered to be (in Le Grand's phrase, borrowed from Hume) knaves. Finally, sticking to his chess analogy, Le Grand argued that recipients of services and benefits were seen as pawns—essentially passive—in the 1945 model, while later policy discourse challenged this assumption: a theme which he did not develop in his 1997 article but which he greatly amplifies in his book (see below). And these assumptions shaping policy needed to be made explicit, Le Grand argued, so that their validity and their implications could be tested.

Which is precisely what Le Grand's book does, as it develops "a theory of public service motivation." We start with a definition: "In our terminology, knaves can be defined as self-interested individuals who are motivated to help others only if by so doing they will serve their private interests; whereas knights are individuals who are motivated to help others for no private reward, and indeed who may undertake such activities to the detriment of their own private interests." In the former case it cannot be assumed that, for example, a doctor's decisions about treating his or her patients are not contaminated by self-interest. In the latter case, contrariwise, it is assumed that the doctor's decisions will be driven exclusively by what is best for the patient. Which assumption is empirically correct? Le Grand trawls the available evidence and concludes that the picture is mixed. The point is not that all doctors, teachers and other public service providers are knaves or knights, but that there is evidence of both knightly and knavish behaviour (often in the same person). So the policy trick is how to devise systems of rewards that provide incentives to knaves to behave in a more knightly fashion without turning knights into knaves by devaluing their dedication. The evidence for informing policy is, however, thin and mixed. On the one hand, there is evidence that incentives can change, or at least promote certain kinds of, behaviour: the experience of fundholding in the NHS is a case in point. On the other hand, it also suggests that there is a "threshold effect," that if knights are not going to be turned into knaves, incentives have to be set at a level which suggests public recognition for their dedication without being so high as to imply that they are being bribed to do worthy things. So policy designing incentives requires a fine balancing act.

The strength of Le Grand's analysis lies in its recognition that self-interest is a problematic concept and is defined by context (Wildavsky, 1994). Taking his arguments one step further, even altruistic, selfless behaviour can be seen as a form of self-interest if it is pursued in search of non-material rewards, whether in this world or the next (so the honours system can be seen as part of the public sector reward structure, shoring up the much-invoked public service ethos, a system which has the merit of being extremely cheap). But subtle and sophisticated as the exposition of his case is, it seems to me that he does not give sufficient weight to two considerations.

The first, which strengthens Le Grand's thesis, is the overwhelming evidence from the organisational literature that service deliverers make their own rules and policies (for example, Lipsky, 1980), which is why policies may subverted or even perverted in the process of implementation. Hence the proliferation of targets, indicators and so on as Governments try to control public services. The point is mentioned by Le Grand but not much elaborated, although the current interest in incentives largely reflects frustration with the shortcomings of a hierarchic, bureaucratic system of control.

The second, which complicates Le Grand's argument, is that knaves from the perspective of Governments (inasmuch as they subvert policy) may be knights from the perspective of patients and other clients (inasmuch as they bend rules in the latter's favour). Again, Le Grand touches on this, but does not explore the full implications, which is that both types of motivation may have undesirable consequences. From the perspective of public policy, I am inclined to argue, knightly behaviour may often be the problem rather than the solution. And from the perspective of users, knights may be authoritarian paternalists acting in the sure faith that they are altruists who know best. If the pursuit of self-interest at the expense of the public interest is the pathology of knavery, self-righteous rectitude is the pathology of knighthood.

From the theory of public service motivation, Le Grand moves on to addressing the problem of agency: the capacity of individuals for action and choice. Should power lie with the users of services or with the professionals and others providing them? Le Grand tends to argue the normative case for consumer power—though carefully qualifying the scope of that power—by building on the his analysis of public sector motivation. The case for paternalism (what Le Grand calls the welfarist case) rests on the assertion that professionals like doctors and teachers can, because of their expertise, do better than the users themselves. But this assumes, Le Grand argues, that professionals "face no conflict between their own interest and those of the users." They must be "something close to knights or perfect altruists." Failing that, "there is no guarantee that professionals will use their decision-making power in the interests of users." As indicated above, I tend to think that the same problem arises in the case of knights who may well see themselves as acting in the interests of consumers but who take it upon themselves to define what those interests are.

Le Grand's line of reasoning seems to flow from his desire to link the case for agency—the active participation of users in decisions affecting them—to his analysis of motivations. But, taking another tack, there is an even stronger normative case to be made by building on the principle of equal autonomy (Klein and Millar, 1995). As classically put by Weale (1983, 42): "This principle of autonomy asserts that all persons are entitled to respect as deliberative and purposive agents capable of formulating their own projects, and that as part of this respect there is a governmental obligation to bring into being or preserve the conditions in which this autonomy can be realized." This formulation has the merit of linking the case for individual decision-making to the general case for redistributive social policies: for what is the argument for redistributing income, if it is not to allow individuals to make the kind of autonomous decisions that the rest of society take for granted? And if lack of resources is one constraint on people's autonomy, paternalist public services are another.

So my main reservation about Le Grand's conclusion—that users should be queens rather than pawns—is that it could be strengthened by widening its conceptual base. But given this conclusion, what follows for policy? Here Le Grand is conspicuously—and rightly—cautious. There is no call for unlimited choice or unfettered competition. The existence of publicly funded services—like the NHS and the school system—is taken for granted. So in the case of the NHS he argues for something like the existing quasi-market, plus an incentive system combining a salary element and fee-for-service payments for consultants. In the case of schools, he argues for a positively discriminating voucher, where the value of the voucher would increase in areas with a high proportion of poor families. And he throws in proposals for demogrants and (most unconvincingly, to my mind) hypothecated taxes into the bargain. These are proposals that Le Grand has put forward at one time or another and there is inevitably a sense of pet ideas being recycled. In any case these policy specifics are of less interest for the purposes of this review—which is to ask whether there has been a paradigmatic change in the way we think about social policy—than the arguments leading up to them. To what extent does the new language of social policy, as articulated by Le Grand, challenge the traditional social policy paradigm as expounded by Titmuss?

Le Grand (like the present reviewer) would probably not quibble very much with Titmuss's vision of what social policy should seek to achieve—a more egalitarian, communitarian society, integrating all its citizens—though he might well demand tighter definitions of what these phrases actually mean and might even mutter something about utopian ambitions being an inadequate guide to policy-making. For the real difference lies in their assumptions of how to how to achieve these goals: the theories underlying the mechanics of policy (just as the monetarist challenge to Keynesian theories was about the mechanics of economic management). To exaggerate only a little, Titmuss saw economics as the enemy, rejecting the discipline's central assumption that the real world could be modelled on the basis of individuals pursuing their self-interest. Social policy started where economics left off: its role was to deal with the disbenefits of economic growth and to foster "those social institutions that foster integration and discourage alienation" (quoted in Reisman, 1977: 10).

The selection of Titmuss's writings in the book under review demonstrate the range, scope and depth of his work on the organisation and delivery of health care, and the humane spirit in which he writes. They range from his early work on rheumatic heart disease to an extract from his last, perhaps best-known book on the gift of blood, as well as essays on the origins and structure of the NHS. They show his ability to identify issues which still have much resonance and relevance today: notably inequalities in health. In what follows, however, I shall concentrate on those aspects of his writings challenged by Le Grand's revisionist analysis.

Titmuss never developed a theory of public sector motivation, and it would be anachronistic to expect him to have done so. And in trying to fillet out what his ideas were, there is a real problem: his failure to follow up the logic of his own insights. Despite his general thesis that the NHS owes its birth to the spirit of wartime solidarity, and should thus be seen and cherished as a symbol of social solidarity, he wrote (accurately), "The present structure of the Health Service owes more to the opinion of doctors than to political and public opinion." Despite his celebration of the fact that the NHS enlarged professional freedom, allowing doctors "to serve their patients according to their medical needs," he was far from uncritical about the way in which they actually treated patients. He wrote scathingly about hospital inertia and the survival of "primitive customs," citing a study which showed that "hardly any of the measures to prevent cross-infection recommended by the Medical Research Council were in operation in the 24 wards of the eight hospitals studied." "One of the new problems," he observed, "is the danger that hospitals may tend increasingly to be run in the interests of those working in and for them, rather than in the interests of the patients."

So would he have subscribed to the view that professionals might be knaves? The answer must be a firm "no." Having described some of the perverse (from a patient's point of view) hospital routines, Titmuss makes a crucial caveat: "I do not want to leave an impression that hospital staffs are deliberately callous to their patients. These things are done . . . unthinkingly by people who are devoted to their calling, working unselfishly and for long hours in the interests of the sick." So they should be seen as knights in Le Grand's terminology. The fact that this was not enough to ensure good care Titmuss attributes to a variety of factors: fragmentation of services, the absence of critical self-examination, administrative preoccupation with detail and so on. Behaviour, in short, depends on context. But how is that context to be changed in order to ensure that unselfish altruist can live up to the knightly ideal? Here Titmuss offered few clues. Some asides might suggest that he saw research as a tool for prompting reform—and this was indeed the route followed by his LSE social policy disciples—but he offered no coherent theory of the dynamics of organisational or policy change.

Was altruism the joker in the pack? Certainly Titmuss saw altruism as not only desirable in itself but as the cement of social policy. Hence his celebration of voluntary blood donation in *The Gift Relationship*, from which there is a short extract in the book. Here the problem is not so much doubt about whether voluntary giving is more efficient or effective than buying blood—although developments since the publication of his study suggest that the evidence is less clear cut than he suggested—but about how generalisable this particular example of altruism is. As Collard (1978: 148) has commented: "Generalising from the blood example, the relatively small band of Kantian altruists would find themselves bearing the whole cost of the welfare state," And given that voluntary contributions cannot be expected to generate sufficient funds for building hospitals or motorways, "The relevant gift relationship then becomes that implied in altruistic voting behaviour." Precisely, and one weakness of the Titmussian social policy tradition—whose effects are still observable today—has been the assumption that tax payers are indeed altruists and that Labour Governments are to be castigated for not committing political suicide by raising taxes more in order to redistribute income. There is an interesting study waiting to be done to investigate whether blood donors are readier to pay higher taxes than the rest of the population: whether altruism in one sphere breeds or reinforces altruism in another. Maybe if all taxpayers were blood donors. . . .

When it comes to the question of agency, the participation of users in decisions affecting them, there is once again some ambiguity about Titmuss's position. On the one hand, he saw the enlargement of freedom for patients as one of the achievements of the NHS, as indeed it was in the sense that it gave many the ability to opt for medical treatment when previously they had been unable to do so. So a commitment to positive freedom, the ability to make one's own decisions, was certainly one of his values: indeed it provides (as we have seen) the foundations of the case for income redistribution. On the other hand, he was emphatic in his rejection of consumer choice in health care, producing a list of 13 factors (citing Kenneth Arrow) which distinguish medical care from other goods. And most of the 13 factors implied that the doctor knew best. While Titmuss recognised that there was "a tendency for more people to adopt a questioning and critical attitude to medical care," and that this implied a somewhat different doctor-patient relationship than the submissive one of the past, he did not pursue the logic of his insight any further.

Titmuss's apparent rejection of choice in health care has to be put into context. It was made in the course of his battle with the Institute of Economic Affairs, which in the 1960s was the lonely flag-carrier for private markets in health care and other social services. For Titmuss this raised the spectre of American-style health care. And he devoted much energy to expounding the inadequacies of the US system. Similarly, the theme of money corrupting and contaminating other, higher motives in the provision of social services was illustrated in *The Gift Relationship* by counterpointing British and American experience. It was, in a sense, too easy: it encouraged a certain degree of chauvinistic complacency about Britain's NHS which might have been dispelled by comparing the UK with, say, Sweden or France. More important, perhaps, by using the United States case as a stick to beat the I.E.A. and others Titmuss left a legacy of suspicion in the social policy community towards anything which might be described (often wrongly) as the adoption of American-style ideas or policies. To use a vocabulary of competition, choice and markets was for long guaranteed to produce a knee-jerk reaction of indignation, as distinct from consideration of what these words might mean in a different context.

The knee-jerks are rarer these days, though there are still occasional twitches. And here the credit must, I think, go largely to the Conservative policies of the 1980s: an example, as argued at the beginning of this review, of the two way traffic between policies and ideas. In effect, the experiments with quasi-markets in publicly funded services — in education as well as health care — undermined the view that introducing competition and choice could be equated with privatisation and the path to the perdition of an unbridled capitalist economy (though some still confuse the two). Further, one of the weaknesses of the Titmuss social policy tradition, as I have argued, is that his prescriptions were not based on any analysis of politics and power, or of the relationship between social policy and economic performance. It is one of the strengths of the revisionism represented by Le Grand and others that they are attempting to fill this gap. Writing a decade ago my then colleague Jane Millar and I (Klein and Millar, 1995) entitled our review of the changing world of social policy "Searching for a New Paradigm?" I suspect that the question mark can now be removed.

References

Collard, David. 1978. *Altruism & Economy*. Oxford: Martin Robertson.

Hall, Peter A. 1993. "Policy Paradigms, Social Learning, and the State: The Case of Economic Policy-making in Britain." *Comparative Politics*, Vol. 25 (April), 275–296.

Klein, Rudolf, and Millar, Jane. 1995. "Do-It-Yourself Social Policy: Searching for a New Paradigm" *Social Policy & Administration*, Vol. 29, No. 4, 303–316.

Le Grand, Julian. 1997. "Knight, Knaves or Pawns ? Human Behaviour and Social Policy." *Journal of Social Policy*, Vol. 26, Part 2, 149–169.

Lipsky, Michael. 1980. *Street-Level Bureaucracy*. New York: Russell Sage Foundation.

Reisman, David. 1977. *Richard Titmuss*. London: Heinemann.

Weale, Albert. 1980. *Political Theory and Social Policy*. London: Macmillan.

Wildavsky, Aaron. 1994. "Why Self-Interest Means Less Outside of a Social Context." *Journal of Theoretical Politics*, Vol. 6, No. 2, 131–159.

O'Goffe's Tale

Or What Can We Learn from the Success of the Capitalist Welfare States?

Rudolf Klein

This paper starts with a puzzle. Looking back on the literature on the welfare state published in the 1970s and the early 1980s (Moran, 1988), there is a striking asymmetry. On the one hand, there are the grim prophecies of crisis—if not worse—threatening the welfare state in capitalist societies. On the other hand, there is the almost total silence about the likely fate of the welfare state in communist societies. Yet if we look around us now, there is a very simple observation to be made. On the one hand, the welfare state in capitalist societies has survived the crisis in remarkably good health. On the other hand, the welfare state in communist societies is going through precisely the same paroxysms of reconstruction as the regimes that created it. It is a contrast which, as I shall argue in this paper, has some important implications for both the practice and theory of comparative social policy studies.

The best starting point for exploring this puzzle is perhaps O'Goffe's tale.

In constructing O'Goffe's tale, I have taken the three leading exponents of the neo-Marxist thesis (O'Connor, 1973; Gough, 1979; Offe, 1984) and conflated the main features of their accounts. The result may not be fully fair to any individual member of the trio—and is not intended to be so—but it gives a sense of the logic of their argument. For what distinguished O'Goffe from the myriad of other scholars wringing their hands about the plight of the welfare state at a time of economic turmoil was that he sought to explain these troubles by invoking the nature of capitalist states. In O'Goffe's view this was not just a crisis. It was something much more serious: a contradiction. In other words, the difficulties of the welfare state did not just reflect contemporary or evanescent problems of capitalist societies but were inherent in their nature. They were inherent because of the in-built, inescapable conflict between the needs of legitimation, consumption and the demands of capital accumulation. To maintain political legitimacy, the capitalist state had to spend on welfare services and programmes; to maintain the machinery of capitalism, however, it had to promote capital accumulation and ensure profits. And all this was in addition to freeing enough resources for consumption. The development of the welfare state threatened the process of capital accumulation. While the Keynesian Welfare State had for 30 years created the illusion that both objectives of policy could be reconciled in an ever-more prosperous world, the loss of belief both in Keynesian theories of economic management and in the compound arithmetic of growth meant that conflict was inevitable. The conflict could be resolved and the welfare state saved, O'Goffe concluded, only in a new kind of socialist society.

There were important insights in this approach. It was a much-needed antidote to the kind of bland, historicist accounts of the welfare state typical of the hitherto dominant Marmuss School.[1] This tended to present the rise of the welfare state everywhere as an inevitable process: a milestone in the progress of mankind. O'Goffe rightly argued that welfare policies involved conflict about resources, and therefore raised questions about the distribution of power in society. Equally important, he pointed out that welfare policies could not be separated from economic policies, and that both are inevitably shaped by political institutions. In short, O'Goffe concluded, the welfare state could be understood only as the product of economic and political forces: as part of the total social environment.

The impact of O'Goffe's critique was all the greater because it echoed, and in many respects overlapped with, that of Hayman.[2] The New Right also argued that the welfare state would destroy capitalism. The growth of social spending, so the case ran, was undermining work incentives, sapping the ability to invest, creating self-serving welfare bureaucracies and fuelling inflation. Worse still, it was a threat to liberty: the political system was being corrupted (as well as being overloaded) by having to take decisions about the distribution of resources that should be left to the market. Not the least important common element between O'Goffe and Hayman was their shared distrust for the capacity of Western political systems. For very different reasons, they had little faith in politics—seen as a dialogue between groups with different interests but a common concern to solve societal problems—as a way of tackling the difficulties posed by rising social expenditures in times of economic stringency. Indeed, rising social expenditure was seen as a symptom of political failure: democratic politics, it was often argued (Brittan, 1977), generated extravagant public expectations which in turn led to excessive expenditure. O'Goffe had nothing to say, however, about the welfare state in communist states. Indeed, on his own premises, there was no need to say anything about this. For was not the whole point of his argument that the crisis—indeed contradictions—of the welfare state derived from the very nature of capitalist societies? There was no need to test the premises, even though some of us suggested at the time that it might be a good idea to do so (Klein, 1979): that communist societies might well have the same dilemmas—such as the conflict between meeting needs and maintaining work incentives and between the demands of capital accumulation and social spending—as capitalist ones. O'Goffe clearly took the premises to be self-evidently true. In fact, the events of the past few years suggest that they were self-evidently wrong: that the same conflicts, contradictions or crises afflicted the communist Welfare States (CWS) as the Keynesian Welfare States (KWS). The real difference lay in the fact that while the capitalist societies of the West were able to cope with the supposedly irreconcilable contradictions, the communist societies of the East collapsed under their weight. While the KWS has emerged virtually intact from the 1980s almost everywhere—a point to which we return below—the CWS is crumbling in the wake of the collapse of the regimes that created it.

A number of implications can be drawn out from O'Goffe's tale. The first is about the logic of political analysis. Before we can make a statement about cause-and-effect in a particular society—or class of societies—we surely have to be able to test it against a counter-factual. Otherwise, we are operating in a solipsistic universe. The point is as obvious as it is frequently neglected. The comparative method is not just a luxury add-on to the study of social policy but an essential component if we are to avoid repeating O'Goffe's blunder in over-predicting the crisis of the welfare state in the West while under-predicting its collapse in the East.

The point can be simply illustrated. Take O'Goffe's assertion about the conflict between the competing claims of political legitimation, capital accumulation and consumption. What evidence is there to support the assumption that this is somehow peculiar or unique to capitalism? None. But if O'Goffe had chosen to search for evidence that such conflict was also apparent in communist regimes, he might well have found it; certainly there are hints that communist regimes used welfare spending as a means of buying legitimacy and popularity (Ferge, 1986) when they failed to deliver the goods of economic prosperity or political acceptability. Indeed, it might quite plausibly be argued (using the O'Goffe line of reasoning) that, in doing so, they damaged their capacity for capital accumulation and further undermined their legitimacy, so creating what proved to be a fatal downward cycle.

But of course it may be argued in O'Goffe's defence that information about social policy in the communist bloc was remarkably scant at the time (as it still is). Therein, however, lies the second implication which can be drawn out from O'Goffe's tale. It suggests the need for self-examination in the social policy community. Why was there so little information in the 1970s and 1980s? And why, as anyone trying to teach comparative social policy soon found, were most of the available studies unsatisfactory in quality? Part of the answer lies, obviously, in the fact that communist regimes did not release accurate data or encourage research; even now it is extraordinarily difficult to establish with precision, for example, what percentage of the national income is spent on health care (or education and the social services) for purposes of comparison. But this is an incomplete answer. Even when there was evidence of the failure of the communist regimes in the welfare field—notably that provided by rising mortality (Wnuk-Lipinsky and Illsley, 1990)—it tended to be neglected in comparative social policy studies.

Similarly, the evidence of parallelisms between capitalist and communist welfare states tended to be overlooked: for example, Wilensky's conclusion (1975) that much the same (non-ideological) factors explained the growth of welfare state spending in capitalist and communist countries. It is therefore difficult to resist the conclusion that the under-prediction of crisis reflected both the linguistic incompetence and ideological predispositions of most of the scholars in the field. There has always been, and continues to be, a serious shortage of scholars in the field equipped with the languages required for the serious study of East European welfare systems. And there is a lingering tendency to use comparative studies as a search for ammunition in domestic political battles: to be able to cite examples of how much better things are done in other (preferably non-capitalist or left-wing) countries.

This is not to imply that O'Goffe was necessarily or invariably uncritical of the welfare state in communist societies. Indeed, some Marxists (Deacon, 1983) argued that the social policies of the Eastern bloc countries were, in themselves, evidence that these countries could not be considered to be fully communist or socialist societies. Despite the limitations of their analysis, dependent as they were on English-language sources, they were able to see the multiple inadequacies of the CWS. The analysis also conceded that, to establish a fully socialist welfare state, there would have to be a "class struggle" against the political leadership in Eastern Europe. But it crucially stopped short of considering whether a form of economic organisation that rested on the collective ownership of the means of production was compatible with a fully socialist welfare state. Might not the capture of the welfare state by the self-interest of the party bureaucracy represent an inherent, unavoidable contradiction in communist societies? Rather than conceding this point, the Marxist literature sought to argue that some communist regimes had demonstrated that truly socialist social policies were feasible. In Deacon's case, the examples cited were China, Cuba and (incredibly) Mozambique.

In short, the Marxist literature represents the search for a social policy Utopia, i.e. a society where there is no conflict between the self-interest of the welfare state producers and consumers or between competing claims on national resources. The quest for the "Eldorado banal de tour les vieux marxistes," to adapt Baudelaire, goes on—undiscouraged by the fact that infatuation inevitably leads to disillusion, as successive candidates for the "Eldorado" turn out to be flawed. While the failures or problems of capitalist societies are seen as being inherent in their very nature, the failures or problems of communist societies are seen only as evidence that they are not truly communist. In the first case, the system is showing its true face; in the second, it is a betrayal of what the system should be like—and therefore no conclusions can be drawn about the model's viability. It is a line of argument which, of course, can never be proved wrong by mere empirical evidence.

To summarise the argument so far, then, the paradox is that the neo-Marxist analysts of the welfare state developed an analytical tool-kit which might well have been quite useful in predicting the impending disintegration of the CWS—but chose not to use it. Instead, they applied their explanatory drill to the KWS, and it broke in their hands. And it broke in their hands precisely because of their assertion that the dilemma of choice was unique to capitalist societies. In doing so, they overlooked the possibility that these societies might have the political institutions and resources required to cope with the reconciliation of competing claims and the so-called "crisis of the welfare state": a rather overblown way of describing the problems of adaptation to new circumstances which faced Western societies in the wake of the global economic crisis of the mid-1970s. In contrast, the communist societies lacked these institutions and resources, which is, of course, why O'Goffe under-predicted the turmoil in the East and over-predicted the crisis in the West. In the next section, we therefore discuss in rather more detail what can be learnt from comparative studies of this success story for the capitalist societies of the West.

FROM CRISES TO SUCCESS

Although the 1970s spawned a formidable body of literature on the "crisis of the welfare state"—a phrase which also haunted the early 1980s—the actual story turned out to be one of successful adaptation (Jobert, 1991). The welfare state, on balance, turns out to have discomfited those who were writing its obituary (Ringen, 1987). The contradictions, it turned out, could be managed if not eliminated. If choice between competing claims on increasingly scarce resources could not be avoided—and where, except in Utopia, can it be avoided?—at least Western societies turned out to have the political capacity for dealing with the challenge.

Most important, perhaps, is what has not happened. There has been no crisis of legitimacy in the Western capitalist societies, in sharp contrast to the communist nations of the East. The existing political order has not been challenged. There is little evidence of massive disillusion with the political system. If one of the purposes of social spending is to legitimate the state, as O'Goffe would put it, then it appears to have been achieved. Bismarck's invention, "conceived of as an essay in practical politics" (King, 1983), has turned out to be a success. The welfare state has helped to maintain the political stability—and probably also the social cohesion—of the Western world.

The achievement is all the more remarkable if we consider that the period of the "crisis of the welfare state" was also the era of quite exceptional social change and dislocation in Britain and other countries of the West. The nature of the transformation is well known: the move from traditional industry to the service economy (Gershuny, 1978). So is the fact that it was accompanied everywhere by unemployment on a scale which, until the mid-1970s, would have been considered a threat to political stability: no government, so ran the conventional political wisdom of post-1945 Britain, could survive unemployment figures above 500,000—let alone 1 or 2 million. If the welfare state is conceived of as an instrument for insuring against the risks of change, or as a way of compensating those who bear the social costs (Baldwin, 1990), then again it seems to have earned its keep during these critical years. This is not to assert that the social costs of change were necessarily equitably or fully compensated everywhere; the level of unemployment benefits was one of the casualties of public expenditure retrenchment in many OECD countries (OECD, 1985). It is to argue, however, that—whatever its weaknesses or inequities—the welfare state did succeed in helping to smooth the social and political pains of a dramatic economic transformation.

Nor is there much evidence that social spending was at the expense—as both O'Goffe and the New Right argued—of capital accumulation (Cameron, 1985). The real conflict was between social spending and consumption; hence the famous tax back-lash of the late 1970s. It was this that seemed to vindicate

O'Goffe's prophecy. If the accelerating expansion of social spending characteristic of the 1960s and the early 1970s had been maintained, then clearly personal disposable income would have been severely squeezed: public consumption would effectively have replaced private consumption. Extrapolation could easily produce a doom scenario of government bankruptcy and falling personal incomes (Rose and Peters, 1978). In the event, governments did not go bankrupt and, on the whole, personal incomes continued to rise; one of the few countries in which the incomes of the "middle mass" have failed to rise substantially over the past decade is the United States, a notoriously low welfare spender. For what the predictions of crisis and collapse had overlooked was the institutional resilience of the welfare state and the effect over time of marginal, incremental changes. Nowhere was total welfare state expenditure reduced; everywhere, however, governments sought ways of reducing the inherited rate of increase.

On the one hand, the welfare state therefore emerged from the 1980s everywhere looking much as it had at the start of the decade. There were no dramatic changes in its institutions, policies and programmes. The welfare state, it turned out, had created a powerful political constituency for its own survival even in countries, like Britain (Hills, 1990) and the United States (Marmor, Mashaw and Harvey, 1990), which had governments ideologically committed to cutting it back. On the other hand, there turned out to be unexpected scope for decelerating the rate of growth in spending. In part, this was achieved by disguising retrenchment as technical change in the method of calculating benefits over time (for example, by decoupling them from movements in earnings); in part, it was done by concentrating economies on those groups with least political power (for example, welfare beneficiaries and the unemployed). On balance, the beneficiaries of the welfare state concentrated in strong, permanent constituencies—like the elderly and the service providers—seem to have emerged remarkably unscathed, while the shifting populations of those at the margins or outside the labour force appear to have done rather worse. The outcome, in fact, is what might be predicted if one sees the welfare state not as an instrument for "doing good"—let alone for achieving equality—but as both the product and the producer of coalitions of self-interest.

The welfare state also demonstrated, in the 1980s, its capacity for organisational adaptation. In response to economic stringency, it moved to meet some of the criticisms once again common to O'Goffe and the New Right: notably, the criticisms of a self-serving welfare bureaucracy imposing their own preferences on captive consumers. The current reforms of Britain's National Health Service (Day and Klein, 1991) are a case in point, as are the changes in the education system designed to tilt power towards parents, which in part at least inspired the health policies. The NHS changes are more likely to change the balance of power between managers and providers, rather than that between consumers and professionals. But, interestingly, Sweden is currently experimenting with a rather similar set of ideas (Saltman, 1990), if within a totally different ideological framework: there the intention appears to be to see how far it is possible to create choice for health care consumers by forcing public providers to compete for customers. There is, of course, a standard O'Goffe response to such changes. These are seen not as demonstrating a capacity for flexibility or innovation but as evidence that capitalism is trying to re-build the welfare state in its own image; that the welfare state has been saved only at the cost of distorting its real essence by introducing the values of the market place: by commodifying welfare. In short, the prediction of disaster has turned out to be correct, only the nature of the disaster was mis-specified.

The contradictions of capitalism have been resolved—if only temporarily—by invoking managerial efficiency. O'Goffe's capacity for salvaging predictions of impending doom from apparent success stories should not be underestimated.

But, of course, there are varieties of adaptive strategies and degrees of success. So far the discussion has been in terms of the "welfare state." It is useful shorthand, but a dangerous abstraction. The welfare state is a bundle of institutions, policies and programmes which varies in its composition from country to country (and some of its most important components, like labour market policies, may even be excluded under conventional definitions). As Figure 1 shows, countries reacted to the economic crisis of the 1970s in very different ways. Some, like the USA, "over-reacted" to the crisis, perhaps predictably: that is, the rate of increase in spending declined by much more than would be predicted from the fall in the rate of economic growth. Others, like Sweden, "under-reacted," again unsurprisingly: that is, the momentum of social spending continued relatively unaffected by economic problems. Similarly, there are significant variations in the pattern of retrenchment/continued expansion as between different programmes: pensions, health and education.

The pattern was much the same in the 1980s: common themes of concern about rising social spending, but many variations in the national solutions adopted. A recent analysis of developments—by a research group that included contributors to the original O'Goffe thesis (Pfaller, Gough and Therbom, 1991)—demonstrates considerable variations in both the nature of the policy debates and policy outcomes in a range of capitalist societies: Germany, France, the United States, Britain and Sweden. If there are conflicts between different societal goals and different interest groups in capitalist societies—as in all

	Pensions	Health	Education
Canada	△	▲	▲
France	○	▲	NA
Germay	▲	▲	▲
Italy	▲	▲	△
Japan	○	▲	△
UK	△	△	▲
USA	▲▲	▲▲	▲▲
Ireland	▲	▲	▲
Netherlands	▲	▲	▲
Norway	▲▲	▲▲	▲▲
Sweden	△	▲	△
Finland	▲	▲	△
Australia	▲	▲	▲
New Zealand	○	△	▲

△ 'Under-reactors': spending rate declines by less than the fall in GDP rate.
▲ 'Over-reactors': spending declines by more than the fall in GDP rate.
○ 'Non-reactors': spending rate increases even though GDP rate falls.
▲▲ 'Heavy over-reactors': spending declines by much more than the fall in GDP rate.

Figure 1. A Summary of Reaction Rations for Programme
Expenditure in 14 OECD Countries

societies—then, quite clearly, they are mediated by specific national factors: the nature of the political culture and the political system. The point is obvious enough, and needs stressing only because of past attempts to anchor all analysis and explanation in the nature of that mystical entity, capitalism.

Generalized theories—whether of the O'Goffe or Hayman variety—are not helpful in explaining such particular patterns, however ingenious the post hoc rationalisations offered when predictions fail. The history of the 1980s offers a special opportunity for comparative social policy studies precisely because it allows us to look at the way in which common economic problems were translated into policy change by very different political systems, and the relative weight given by these different political systems to equity and efficiency. It gives us an opportunity to explore different strategies of adaptation and to ask what kinds of social policies and welfare institutions provide most scope for flexibility. For not the least important reason why the crisis of the Western welfare state was over-predicted, while that of the communist welfare state was under-predicted, was that far too little attention was paid to the respective learning capacity of the two systems (Deutsch, 1966). And if it is indeed the case that an effective learning system, plus a well-developed capacity to adapt, is the necessary condition for the welfare state's survival, then perhaps we should be using the 1980s to draw some conclusions about the kind of conditions and institutions that best promote both learning and adaptation.

There is perhaps a further conclusion that we can draw from O'Goffe's tale, both for social policy discourse in general and for comparative analysis. We have noted throughout the surprising fact—given their ideological opposition to each other—that O'Goffe and Hayman agreed on so many issues. Why should that be? Fifteen or even ten years ago, one might have been tempted to answer the question by saying that they had intellectual insights denied to those of us in the soggy middle who rejected both approaches. Events since then suggest that this is not a plausible explanation. More recently Hirschman (1991) has provided a more persuasive explanation, which is that both O'Goffe and Hayman use the same type of rhetoric or style of argument. They tend to make apocalyptic prophecies based on the contention that, given the nature of mankind or of a particular class of society, change will inevitably be either futile or have perverse consequences. What this would suggest is that social policy needs a very different kind of theorising: one that is based not on large and often vacuous generalisations about the nature of capitalist or any other kind of society but on a rigorous analysis of the policy conflicts in particular societies and of the criteria used to justify specific choices (Weale, 1991). Diagnosing "contradictions," i.e. conflicts, in societies does not get us far. Investigating how different societies tackle those conflicts—their institutional capacity for so doing, the structure of power and the arguments used in the process—is likely to provide far more illumination.

Notes

I am grateful for the comments of all the participants at the conference which gave birth to this book, and for the specific suggestions from Bob Deacon, Nicholas Deakin and Richard Rose. This article was first published in Catherine Jones, ed., *New Perspectives on the Welfare State in Europe* (London: Routledge, 1993).

1. Otherwise known as T. H. Marshall and Richard M. Titmuss.
2. Otherwise known as Friedrich A. Hayek and Milton Friedman.

References

Baldwin, Peter (1990). *The Politics of Social Solidarity*. Cambridge: Cambridge University Press.

Britian, Samuel (1977). *The Economic Consequences of Democracy*. London: Temple Smith.

Cameron, David R. (1985). "Public expenditure and economic performance in international perspective," in Rudolf Klein and Michael O'Higgins (eds.), *The Future of Welfare*. Oxford: Basil Blackwell.

Day, Patricia, and Klein, Rudolf (1991). "The British health care experiment." *Health Affairs*.

Deacon, Bob (1983). *Social Policy and Socialism*. London: Pluto Press.

Deutsch, Karl W. (1966). *The Nerves of Government*. New York: The Free Press.

Ferge, Zsuzsa (1986). "The changing Hungarian social policy," in Else Oyen (ed.), *Comparing Welfare States and Their Future*. Aldershot: Gower.

Gershuny, Jonathan (1978). *After Industrial Society?* London: Macmillan.

Gough, Ian (1979). *The Political Economy of the Welfare State*. London: Macmillan.

Hills, John (ed.) (1990). *The State of Welfare*. Oxford: Clarendon Press.

Hirschman, Albert O. (1991). *The Rhetoric of Reaction*. Cambridge, Mass.: The Belknap Press.

Johert, Bruno (1991). "La Réstructuration des Stats Européens." Mimeo, University of Grenoble.

King, Anthony (1983). "The political consequences of the welfare state," in *Evaluating the Welfare State: Social and Political Perspectives*. London: Academic Press.

Klein, Rudolf (1979). "Welfare as power," a review of Gough op.cit., *New Society*, 20 September, 632–3.

Marmor, Theodore R., Mashaw, Terry L., and Harvey, Philip L. (1990). *America's Misunderstood Welfare State*. New York: Basic Books.

Moran, Michael (1988). "Crises of the welfare state." *British Journal of Political Science* 18(3): 397–414.

O'Connor, James (1973). *The Fiscal Crisis of the State*. New York: St. Martin's Press.

Offe, Claus (1984). *The Contradictions of the Welfare State*. London: Hutchinson.

Organisation for Economic Co-operation and Development (1985). *Social Expenditure, 1960–1990*. Paris: OECD.

Pfaller, Alfred, Gough, Ian, and Therborn, Goran (1991). *Can the Welfare State Compete?* London: Macmillan.

Ringen, Stein (1987). *The Possibility of Politics*. Oxford: Clarendon Press.

Rose, Richard, and Peters, Guy (1978). *Can Governments Go Bankrupt?* London: Macmillan.

Saltman, Richard B. (1990). "Competition and reform in the Swedish health system." *The Milbank Quarterly* 68(4): 597–618.

Weale, Albert (1991). "Principles, process and policy," in Thomas and Dorothy Wilson (eds.), *The State and Social Welfare*. London: Longman.

Wilensky, Harold L. (1975). *The Welfare State and Equality*. Berkeley: University of California Press.

Wnuk-Lipinsky, E., and Ilisley, Raymond (1990). "International comparative analysis: main findings and conclusions." *Social Science and Medicine* 31(8): 878–89.

6

VALUES, POLICIES, AND PROGRAMS

The role values play in politics has long been of interest. Appeals to basic values mark most democratic elections. Criticism of programs typically challenges the values expressed and offers more worthy aims. Liberty, equality, fraternity are not, for example, just historical notes from the French Revolution. They mattered—and continue to matter. In short, values—understood as fundamental doctrines about what is worthy and important—have inspired great reforms and guided the structure of institutions and the policies those institutions have created.

Interpreted in these terms, values play a foundational role in the politics of health and health care as well. But exactly what kind of role, one might well ask? That is the question the articles in this chapter pose and to which they provide somewhat complicated answers.

Values, the articles in common claim, are general views of what is worthy, enduring, and thus resistant to momentary shifts in sentiment. In health care, for example, the fundamental egalitarian appeal to access to care based on need is widespread. But, as is also noted, values compete with one another, which complicates the situation. Equal access clashes with freedom, whether to choose when to be treated, how to jump queues, or what treatment to apply. Equality and patient freedom conflict as well with the value of scientific professionalism, the claim that what is worth doing medically is for experts to decide, not patients or politicians claiming to act on behalf of citizens. One can easily enlarge the conflicts among values within an arena like health care. But, we note as well that values are general, broadly framed ideas, and that feature spawns ambiguity. There are at least eight different notions of equality in standard political philosophy. Scholars of liberty regularly distinguish its positive from its negative formulation. And, with this ambiguity comes ample grounds for disagreement about what an appeal to a health value entails in practice.

Finally, there is the question of to what degree the distribution of values—as opposed to the role of other ideas, interests, and institutions—determines what health care policies dominate a polity. The common conclusion reached in these articles is twofold. Fundamental values do rule out some practices and policies, but there remains a loose connection between a nation's health values and the practical policies and institutional arrangements of any one period or place. Understood as guides rather than straitjackets, values play an important role in understanding the world of health care.

Values, Institutions and Health Policies:
A Comparative Perspective

Theodore R. Marmor, Kieke G. H. Okma, and Stephen R. Latham

INTRODUCTION

Ideas, interests and institutions determine the shape and impact of social policies. All social policies are embedded in national institutional arrangements that reflect both cultural legacies and broadly supported values. For example, Canada's national health insurance program, it is often claimed, is special precisely because Medicare embodies distinctive, appealing Canadian social values. For some Canadians, it follows that any effort to alter Medicare substantially amounts to an attack on Canadian values and should therefore be rejected. At the same time, others claim that Canada's values have undergone substantial changes since the 1970s and that this shift in values may justify (or excuse) major amendments and alterations to Medicare.[1] Both assume a fairly tight connection between what are called "national values" and the particular structural features of the health care system. Other Western industrial democracies have engaged in analogous debates about the future of their fundamental medical care arrangements, with *anti-* and *pro-amendment* positions quite similar to those in Canada.

We have four main points to make about these debates: first, that core national values relating to the desirability of government providing (or safeguarding access to) medical care are quite similar across OECD nations; second, that in spite of the similarity in those underlying values, countries have developed a variety of medical care arrangements under the influence of different modes of policy-making and various contingencies of their institutional histories; third, that changes in medical care more often arise from shifts in political fashions and partisan power than from shifts in underlying values; and fourth, that the evidence we present shows that while there is no straight line from values to medical care policy, there are some policy measures that the core values rule out.

Section II first presents a methodological commentary on what is and can sensibly be meant by ideas and "national values." It also discusses other major forces that can shape public policy, most prominently the structure of interests and institutions.

Section III examines the broad array of institutional arrangements for medical care in most wealthy democracies. It starts with a brief overview of the historical developments of medical care arrangements in Western Europe. This shows how over time, different motives (including self-interest, compassion and moral obligation) prompted the development of a variety of solidaristic arrangements, ranging from mutual support schemes to voluntary and charitable activities and state-sponsored public schemes. This variety illustrates how loose the connections are between anything coherently termed "national values" and the concrete forms of social institutions. Many forces besides "values" are at work in shaping and re-shaping particular institutions of social policy, we argue. And, conversely, many quite differently shaped social institutions may reasonably be said to embody the same set of values.

Next, Section IV presents comparative evidence on how populations in industrialized countries understand the role of government in medical care. Here, we distinguish three sets of claims. First, we present polling data that directly measure beliefs about the proper role of government. These data show both high levels of public support for a governmental role in health care, and reveal a distribution of attitudes that provide indirect measures of values with which those beliefs are consistent. Second, we provide evidence of public opinion that varies according to specific welfare state programs. The contention here is that despite this variability, health care, as a core feature of the modern welfare state, continues to enjoy high levels of public support. Third, we discuss disputes about reform measures that are defended instrumentally, but raise problems for traditional welfare state values. So, for example, we address policy conflicts over efforts to exclude procedures from traditional health insurance coverage; we also discuss familiar conflicts over patient cost-sharing as an instrument of budgetary control.

Our conclusion is that there is a range of possible policy options in medical care that are perfectly consistent with the dominant social values we describe. Choosing among those options, however, requires prudence. That in turn requires attention to the political realities of conflicting interests and short-lived fads. That a social welfare institution expresses the right values, we contend, is a necessary, but not a sufficient, basis for its adoption—and its stable continuation.

WHAT ARE "NATIONAL VALUES?":
THE PRESUMPTIONS OF THE INQUIRY

Social scientists have long been suspicious of the notion of "national values" (Schumpeter 1908). After all, values are held by persons, not by corporate entities that have neither minds nor desires. It is true that we may speak loosely of the "values of the common law" or the "values of the Catholic church." By such usage we mean to locate fundamental doctrines that emerge from the writings, or from the beliefs of the elite, within a certain tradition. But in general, "values" refer to subjective views of individuals about what is worthy or important. In politics, these are views about the ends that collective institutions ought to advance and the virtues they ought to embody.

Values are general. They do not dictate preferences for particular institutional structures at any level of detail (Rawls 1971). That one values privacy in health care need not lead one, for example, to endorse a particular set of detailed privacy rules (those contained in the new United States *Health Insurance Portability and Accountability Act* of 1996 [HIPAA] regulations, say). It leads one only to prefer institutional arrangements that protect privacy over those that do not, and arrangements that protect privacy more over those that protect it less. One's values also *compete with one another* (Berlin 1998). Efficiency, for example, may need to be sacrificed to favor participatory governance or vice versa. A strong commitment to equality may limit someone's liberty to some extent. Multiple institutional arrangements may thus have equal claim to instantiating one's values, by giving prominence to them differentially. Precision in statements about "national values" is thus doubly imperiled: such statements are necessarily a summation across a broad population of varied individuals' general and potentially conflicting values.

These cautionary observations should not, however, blind us to the important role that values play in creating a political community and in guiding its actions. Statements of values may inspire, unite, or even "constitute" a people; think of the Declaration of Independence and the *Bill of Rights* in the United States, or the *Magna Carta* in Britain. And public statements of shared values—even if the values come to be shared only after they are publicly stated—may serve as important guides to action. The fact that values are general and may compete with one another does not render them meaningless. Values are no policy straitjacket, but there are certain choices they rule out.

The core values underlying the financing and delivery of medical care are, despite complicated debates, relatively simple. They include universal protection against being ruined financially by the costs of treatment, first of all. This one could call the common ground of income protection among nations that use sickness funds, those that have national health services, and those that combine nationwide insurance coverage for some but regulated private health insurance for others. Secondly, there is a core conception of allocation among competing claimants: medical need and ability to benefit rather than personal preference or willingness and ability to pay. No OECD nation makes it impossible for some to purchase preferential access through double coverage and other devices. But that such behaviour is open to sharp public debate illustrates the core presumption that medical care is mostly seen as a merit good, not to be allocated solely or largely by ability and willingness to pay in a market. These are the values we emphasize, but there are other policy preoccupations that regularly present themselves as fundamental. They include concerns about higher collective spending in this sector than would be socially desirable from investments in other sectors. Cost containment is a principle of prudence in all public spending; so is the aspiration for high quality of services. Some reformers highlight freedom of choice for patients and professional autonomy of health providers as well (OECD 1992). Others emphasize particular features of the Scandinavian welfare model, highlighting universality, solidarity and independence from the market (or, in fact, public funding) (Cox 2004).

In the context of the recent debate over Canada's Medicare debate, Michael Ignatieff expressed the core national values well: "We [Canadians] think that public taxation should provide for health care and that it is wrong for decent medical care to depend on the size of our bank balances" (Ignatieff 2000). Canadian provinces will only receive funding from the federal government if they adhere to the five criteria mentioned in the *Canada Health Act*—public administration, comprehensiveness, universality, portability and accessibility in the administration of the provincial health insurance schemes. Those criteria are themselves values, though perhaps narrower, more "instrumental" values. They give shape to the broad but fundamental public and egalitarian values expressed by Ignatieff. And, since their articulation in the Hall Commission Report of 1964 and the Canada Health Act (CHA) of 1984, these five criteria have gained widespread public support.

Both the core value of public finance and the "instrumental" values of CHA are, we believe, widely shared among OECD nations. Indeed, according to Johnson and Cullen (2000), "there is no lack of evidence [of solidarity] in 20th-century social policy and roots that go back both in theory and in practice to the original Elizabethan Poor Law." Because they are general and may have to be traded off against one another, however, these values have come to be advanced within a number of different institutional arrangements. Values, moreover, are relatively stable over time, changing only very gradually (Sabatier and Jenkins-Smith 1993).

Opinions are views — prudential or ethical — about states of affairs or courses of action. These are notoriously more subject to short-term change than either values or interests. Polling findings, of course, do not emerge in a vacuum (Altman and Brodie 2003). Rather, political leadership and real-world events shape poll results. Opinion polling can tell us where the public stands on an issue, but cannot tell us what is deeply felt or will be regarded as right. Polls tell part of the story of why policy takes the shape it does. Ordinary citizens may well rank issues quite differently from how experts or politicians would. But general opinions grounded in values ("as, for example, access to health care should be universal") appear to be more "sticky." Such opinion findings are less likely to change in the short term than opinions about particular states of affairs (e.g. "Canadian Medicare is working well") (Maioni and Martin 2001).

Before attempting to substantiate this claim, however, we pause to distinguish values from two other major forces that shape public policies: *interests* and *institutions*. Interests are states of affairs or courses of action that persons are motivated to pursue based on the powerful drive for self-aggrandizement (including self-aggrandizement's prerequisite, self-preservation) (Mansfield 1995; Hirschman 1992). Persons have multiple interests; these are calculable, predictable, objective, and — like values — can be traded off against one another (Mansfield 1995).

In addition to the ways in which different habits of governance affect the embodiment of values in public institutions, the play of interests among parties has considerable impact as well. In social policy, governments typically confront a large number of organized interests or *stakeholders* (Sabatier et al. 1993; Wilson 1990; Alford 1974). In many countries, provincial, regional and local governments and semi-autonomous governmental agencies share the responsibility for the administration of health care. In most industrial democracies, labor unions and private business associations, consumer advocacy groups, public interest groups, and many others lobby to influence health policy. The funding and provision of publicly financed or regulated services like housing, education and health care are not a governmental matter alone. Governments depend on others to make these systems work. The health policy arena is thus crowded with well-organized and competing interests, many of which have considerable power over their policy space.

Institutions are an obviously important factor in the shaping of social policy. Institutional arrangements created because they advanced shared values may of course survive partly because they further powerful interests. At the same time, institutions created from self-interested motives may well embody other values, and serve to entrench those values over time. A reciprocal relationship thus exists between institutions and interests: each shaping and influencing the other (Immergut 1992). Institutions are to some degree the products of the policymaking systems that create them, and those systems are, in terms of this contribution, value-informed. Thus centralist governments will more likely create centralized social welfare institutions; corporatist governments will more frequently create corporate entities whose bargaining will determine the particular means of implementing social values. Here then is another pathway by which societal values may shape public policy: namely, by influencing the modes and institutions of policymaking. So, for example, Douglas and Wildavsky (1989) distinguish what they term three distinct dominant value orientations: *competitive individualism, hierarchical collectivism* and *sectarianism*. The first emphasizes the rights and responsibilities of individuals and families that limit the role of governments. The second assumes that representative organizations in society act on behalf of their members in sharing certain responsibilities for social policy with the government. The third allows for a greater influence of sectarian movements in the framing of social policy.

The social democratic states of Northern Europe have, according to this line of argument, strong traditions of hierarchical collectivism, with moderate influence of individualistic norms and weaker embrace of sectarian modes of policy promotion (Okma 2002). The United States, by contrast, displays strong individualism, a weaker appeal to collectivism and an active streak of sectarian political mobilization. Indeed, market efficiency and individual liberty are, according to Douglas and Wildavsky, leading American values. Yet, as they acknowledge, it is a mistake to assume a very close fit between value-informed modes of policymaking and actual policy in specific areas. Even the United States, with its seemingly dominant competitive-individualist values, managed to enact Medicare, Medicaid, the Veterans Administration health program, the Indian Health service, law mandating emergency medical care regardless of patients' ability to pay, tax incentives to encourage the purchase of private insurance, tax incentives for the provision of private charity care, and publicly funded hospitals that give free or discounted care. No one could reason her way to this set of medical care institutions and programs from a premise of "competitive individualism" in policymaking. And this is so even if one concedes the relative accuracy of the characterization of American values. In short, the concrete details of policy are not tightly linked even to styles of policymaking that reflect dominant value orientations.

This warning also applies to efforts to categorize social policy models or welfare state models as a base for explaining variations in public support for social policy (Gelissen 2000). Esping-Andersen's widely noted typology of welfare states is a good illustration of this point. The typology distinguishes three groups: the social democratic model, the liberal regimes and the corporatist regimes (Esping-Andersen 1990). That categorization assumes a link between the type of regime and the legitimacy of particular welfare state policies. So, for example, the claim would be that universal social-democratic regimes offer benefits for the entire population and thus generate stable, strong popular support. By contrast, the typology presumes that more restricted residual (liberal) welfare states focus mainly on the working classes and the poor, and thus generate much lower levels of solidaristic support for welfare state programs. The conservative corporatist regimes, according to this formulation, are somewhere in the middle. There is, however, a sharp division of opinion about whether the empirical evidence about welfare states actually supports these claims. Some assert there is little or no evidence of such links, emphasizing that institutional structures never simply mirror individual preferences. Institutions are in any case at most a partial crystallization of individual preferences (Gelissen 2000; Marmor, Mashaw and Harvey 1990).

Finally, social and political institutions, once created, develop lives of their own (Tuohy 1999; Johnson and Cullen 2000; Cox 2004). For example, the historically contingent fact that Britain's National Health Service (NHS) emerged just after the Second World War made its centralized organization likely and shaped much of its subsequent development (Klein 1995). The long tradition of self-governing institutions in Western Europe has provided a solid footing to the neo-corporatist bargaining between the regional and national associations of the sick funds and health care providers. In the United States, the postwar development of private health insurance markets (driven, partly, by employers' tax benefits) has made it very difficult for government to assume as central a role in the delivery and financing of health care as in other developed countries. But the U.S. Veterans Administration and Medicare programs, once introduced, turned out to be such popular programs that politicians have not dared to propose major change for a long time. In Canada, the constitutional model for their national health insurance program, also called *Medicare*, required bargaining between provinces and the federal government. From the beginning, also, there was regular bargaining with medical associations. Those features have conditioned Canadian policymaking, and further developments of Medicare have emerged to a large extent out of these institutional processes and rules of the Canadian "game" (Tuohy 1999). And, the popularity of the Scandinavian welfare states remained high even though the intense fiscal and budgetary pressure of the 1980s required some retrenchment, as an example of what one scholar regards as programmatic "stickiness" (Cox 2004).

The next section turns to evidence of how different countries have, on the basis of similar values, established quite different national institutions of social welfare. Many of the core differences in national health care arrangements are not, we contend, the product of differences in fundamental social values. Rather, they reflect differences in political superstructure, differing accommodations of clashing interests, and of the historically contingent "accidental logics" (a term used by Carolyn Tuohy, 1999) of established social institutions. This section undergirds our core contention that national values, though surely important, do not constitute a policy straitjacket.

INSTITUTIONAL VARIATIONS IN MEDICAL CARE

This section starts with a brief summary of the historical development of the modern welfare states. Over time, an interesting mix of principles—mutual trust, moral obligation, compassion, self-interest as well as obligations imposed by voluntary organizations or state—laid the foundations for present day solidaristic arrangements. A wide variety of arrangements for the funding, providing and contracting of medical care in industrialized countries emerged. This reflected both strong popular support for universal access and solidaristic funding on the one hand and quite different periods of institutional reform.

The modern welfare states in Western Europe have their historical roots in the Middle Ages, with the craftsmen's guilds providing mutual support to their members, and churches and local communities creating hospitals as shelters for the poor, the homeless, the elderly and mentally deranged (De Swaan 1988). The 16th century Elizabethan Poor Law brought in the state by obliging local communities to take care of the poor. The 19th century mutual aid societies provided income protection and support for members. Germany was the first to introduce compulsory health insurance. It did so for low-income industrial workers in 1883 in part to protect the family incomes in case of illness, disability or death of the breadwinner, and to avert social unrest (Okma 2002). Over the course of decades, other countries followed the German example and developed mandatory social insurance schemes for the risks of disability, sickness, old age and death for the family income.

The so-called "Bismarckian" model of employment-related health insurance spread to Austria, France, Belgium, the Netherlands (as well as Japan and Korea). In this social health insurance model, legally independent and semi-autonomous bodies ("sick funds") administer the insurance and negotiate contracts with providers of care. Other nations expanded coverage beyond the working class and introduced population-wide schemes funded out of general taxation (the so-called "Beveridge model"). This, of course, is exemplified by the founding of the British National Health Service (NHS) in 1948. In a few countries—for example, the United States, Germany and (until January 2006) The Netherlands—access to social insurance is limited to specific population groups. In Germany, the insured whose incomes have surpassed a certain level, can opt out of the social scheme and take out private health insurance; about 10 percent of the population has actually done so. In The Netherlands, until 2006, two thirds of the population was registered with a sick fund, and one third (mostly self-employed and higher income groups) had to turn to the private market for health insurance. In January 2006, a population-wide compulsory social health insurance (administered by private insurance) replaced the former mixed model of public and private insurance. The United States has separate schemes for the older and disabled under social insurance principles of *Medicare*, categories of low-income Americans under *Medicaid*, programs for veterans and those on Native American reservations. In addition to the universal coverage of *Medicare*, Canada offers special arrangements to veterans and the armed forces, prison inmates, and First Nation populations.

By the end of the 20th century all industrialized nations had implemented state sponsored arrangements for financing and providing medical care. Over time, programmatic expansions and adjustments had led to widespread hybridization of the two basic models. And, in spite of the development of state-sponsored welfare, formal care has not fully replaced the provision of informal care to disabled family members, friends or neighbours. For example, a study shows that in The Netherlands the share of the adult population that is active in the care of dependent elderly of handicapped family members or neighbours rose from 8% in 1980 to 14% in 1995 (SCP, 1999).

The reports of the Organization for Economic Co-operation and Development, OECD, provide a useful way to portray the variety of arrangements for funding and contracting medical care (OECD 1992; OECD 1994). Funding sources include general taxation, earmarked taxation, public and private health insurance and out-of-pocket spending. In most OECD countries, general taxation and social health insurance are dominant compared to private health insurance or direct patient payments. As for contracting health care services, there are but three basic models. One is the integrated model in which (as in Britain until the 1990s) government handles both the funding and the provision of health care. The second is the contracting model (as in several health systems

Table 1: Funding, provision and contracting medical care in OECD countries, mid-1990s

Country	Main funding sources of health care	Provision of health care	Contracting model
Germany	Mix of public and private insurance; modest levels of out-of-pocket payment	Mix of public and private (independent, not-for-profit) providers	Public contracting and some reimbursement
The Netherlands	Mix of public and private insurance; modest levels of out-of-pocket spending. As of January 2006, one population-wide mandatory health insurance under private administration	Mostly private (independent, not-for-profit) providers	Mix of public and private contracting and reimbursement
Denmark, Finland, Greece, Iceland, Ireland, Norway, Portugal, Spain and Sweden	General taxation; modest levels of out-of-pocket spending	Mostly public providers	Integrated model, with some public contracting
Australia and New Zealand	Taxation and private health insurance (in Australia); higher levels of out-of-pocket spending	Mixed public and private providers	Public and some private contacting
Canada	General federal and provincial taxation (and supplemental voluntary private insurance); out-of-pocket spending	Mainly private providers	Mostly public contracting
Switzerland	Voluntary private insurance; higher levels of out-of-pocket spending	Mainly private providers	Public and private contracting
United States	Mix of private insurance and public schemes (Medicare, Medicaid, and Veterans Administration, Indian Health): high levels of out-of-pocket spending	Mainly private providers	Public contracting, reimbursement

Source: OECD (1992, 1994), Okma (2002a).

in continental Western Europe), in which third-party payers negotiate agreements with independent providers over the volume, quality (and sometimes, prices) of medical care. The third is the reimbursement model (as in private insurance for part of the population in Germany or the US), in which patients pay their health care providers and then seek financial indemnification from their public or private insurers. According to the OECD, the public contracting model has increased in recent decades, combining collective funding with independent providers of care.

The above table shows that, despite broad support for social solidarity in distributing and financing medical care in OECD countries (see the next section), the organizational features actually differ markedly. There is a wide variety of legal forms of ownership and management, ranging from private for-profit firms and religious and charitable not-for-profit institutions to local or regional government institutions providing community-based care. And some public financing arrangements cater to specific population groups, while others finance access for the entire population.

Policy and institutional variation across the OECD world, then, is indisputable. Similar baseline values have expressed themselves in very different social welfare institutions. The variation extends to the administrative models and style of policy-making as well. For example, the centralist policy processes of the United Kingdom and France sharply contrast with the *functionally* decentralized models of Germany, Belgium and The Netherlands or the *regionally* decentralized systems in Scandinavia (Klein 1995). In the latter three countries, in line with Douglas and Wildavsky's dominant cultural orientation of hierarchical collectivism, the label of *neo-corporatism* is broadly applicable, a decision-making model where governments and private actors (represented through their interest organizations) share responsibility for the shaping and outcome of social policies (Douglas and Wildavsky, 1989; Wilson 1990). This model implies that private actors are willing and able to take on public responsibilities in the form of active participation in the policy process as well as self-regulation. The main administrative bodies of social health insurance, the sick funds, are legally independent actors, and their organizations have collective bargaining power to contract health services on behalf of their insured. For example, the representative organizations or interest associations of the German hospitals and physicians represent their members in regional negotiations with the health insurance agencies over tariffs and volume of their services.

Germany's neighbor Holland has copied many of the features of this model. Until the 1980s, the Dutch social policy process provided "a striking model of corporatist arrangements," with private agencies empowered with public author-ity (Freddi 1989). These institutions were not only set up along functional lines, but also based on religious denominations (Lijphart, 1968). After mounting criticism of this model in the 1970s and 1980s, successive Dutch governments took steps to reduce or even dismantle this model of *"consociational corporat-ism"* (Baakman, Van der Made and Mur-Veeman 1989; Okma 1997). While Germany and Belgium kept most of their corporatist structures largely intact, The Netherlands eliminated the direct representation of organized stakehold-ers in government advisory bodies in an effort to streamline decision-making procedures. By the end of the 1990s, the main interest groups had lost much of their institutionalized veto power in social policies. Social insurance legislation in 1991 introduced selective contracting. Sick funds no longer had to contract with all providers, and under the rules of new competition law, the role of col-lective contracting reduced sharply. In Germany and Holland, medical associa-tions are empowered with public authority. They regulate access to the medical profession, set standards for medical education and for professional conduct, and police the professional conduct of all medical professionals (members and non-members alike) with rules and sanctions.

In contrast to such decentralized policy models, France and the United King-dom largely maintained their tradition of central state dominance. Under the French *étatisme*, interest groups have not developed a strong role as participants in social policymaking. The medical associations are fragmented and show lit-tle inclination to collaborate with each other or with government. In contrast, the British Medical Association has had a significant (if now diminished) role in health policies. It accepted the formation of the National Health Service (NHS) in 1948, a step that effectively nationalized most hospitals, but kept the self-employed status of general practitioners (Klein 1995). In the 1980s, policies aimed to reduce the direct role of government in the provision of health care included the return of independent hospital administration for Hospital Trusts. Further organizational change included the formation of group practices for general practitioners and, in a later stage, the creation of Primary Care Groups (PCGs) and next, Primary Care Trusts (PCTs). Yet, British physicians retained considerable professional autonomy and strong influence in the management of health care institutions (Klein 1995).

The Scandinavian countries have decentralized the administration of health care to the local and regional levels. Local and regional authorities bear the primary responsibility for funding and providing health care and related social services to their populations. They face the financial risk of acute medical and nursing care and have developed extensive social services, which include home care, adjusted housing for elderly or handicapped persons, and support for independent living.

As this brief historical sketch of social policy institutions suggests, mutual support, self-interest, solidarity, compassion and state sponsored obligation have been—and still are—major foundational bases of the modern welfare state. Organizational and institutional features, we have emphasized, differ substantially. Developed democracies have adopted very different models of administration and public institutions on the basis of quite similar national values. Why this is so is not a mystery. A tradition of statism promotes values through institutions governed by a central authority. A tradition of neo-corporatism promotes similar values as the outcome of a more-or-less structured bargaining game played among organized stakeholders, only one of whom is the government. On the other hand, decisions about whether values are to be advanced by central authorities or by a contest among individuals or sectors—or primarily by the public or by the private purse—are obviously not neutral. The shape of social institutions—even when promoting very similar values—can nonetheless affect the relevance and relative weight of those values.

The next section takes up the evidence about public ideas regarding the role of government in medical care across the industrialized countries. Values, after all, are hard to measure directly. Accordingly, we turn to indirect sources of value orientation in medical care from polling studies of public opinion. Second, we discuss policy disputes that reveal deeply held values indirectly, by which we mean instances where governments, facing strong opposition, felt obliged to soften or abandon measures altogether because of their expressed values.

GOVERNMENT'S ROLE IN HEALTH CARE:
VALUES, INTERESTS AND INSTITUTIONS

This section presents evidence from different sources that illustrate two generalizations: first, there is broad support for the view that medical care is a special responsibility of government. Second, there is substantial variation among nations over where this value is held in the strength of competing values. The section begins with an analysis of national surveys of popular support for welfare arrangements, concentrating on views of public (or publicly funded) health care. Next, it explores instances of policies where governments had to withdraw or to mitigate certain measures when facing opposition bolstered by accusations of violating widely shared values.

One of the core questions of this article is whether the changing context of the welfare state—from relative wealth and expansion to relative scarcity and retrenchment—has affected underlying popular support for health care. There are many, seemingly obvious, grounds to assume a decline in popular support for solidaristic arrangements. The aftermath of the oil crises of the 1970s, with stagnating economic growth and high levels of unemployment, provided ample reasons for extensive, fearful debate about the future of the welfare state. As one of the main categories of public spending, health care did not escape this critical reassessment. Indeed, in the 1980s and 1990s most industrial democracies had extended debates about health care reforms. (OECD 1992; OECD 1994; OECD 1995; Ranade 1998). Some scholars expected consensus about welfare policy to dissolve because of the rise of what they labelled "post-materialistic values" (Inglehart 1977). Others assumed that the middle class was no longer willing to extend its own security to the poor (Galbraith 1992). Still others argued that successful welfare states had reached their limits, with "diminishing returns." And there was considerable speculation that government's ability to provide policy solutions to economic insecurity had sharply declined (Beck 1986; Giddens 1994).

Despite such scepticism—plus extensive debate about the affordability of state welfare, criticism on the quality of public services, and in some countries, a general decline in trust in government—there is no evidence of a large scale popular backlash against the welfare state (Pierson 1999). Empirical studies of the welfare state legitimacy have not detected any substantial decline in popular support (Van Oorschot 2000). Comparative studies of the late 1980s and early 1990s all conclude that support for welfare has remained high from the 1970s (see e.g. Ringen 1987; Pierson 1991; Petterson 1995; Ferrera 1993; Ploug 1996; and Abrahamson 1997). In particular, the surveys show that in most industrialized countries—the United States included—citizens continue to expect the government to take responsibility for safeguarding access to health care services (Bergmark 2003:406).

Self-interest, social values and norms may go hand in hand, but the mix of motives differs across countries and social groups (Van Oorschot 2000). A national survey in 1995, for example, revealed that 82% of the Dutch population was willing to contribute to the welfare state. The strongest motive for doing so was self-interest, or the expectation to be a beneficiary at some stage of life. There was no sign of a middle class dropping out, with almost everyone a beneficiary, or expecting to benefit in the future. Two-thirds of the respondents mentioned moral grounds, in particular the moral obligation to help the needy, reflecting a strong sense of solidarity in the Dutch population. Forty-two percent of the respondents mentioned emotional grounds and compassion for the beneficiaries. The social groups did not differ much. Males were somewhat more motivated by self-interest than females. Both the elderly and the higher educated showed higher support levels for government-sponsored arrangements than did younger respondents. This turned out to depend especially on ideas of moral obligation and emotional resonance (and, interestingly, not so much because of self-interest). Income level was less important than might be expected, as self-interest played the same role for all income groups. All in all, the Dutch welfare state commands substantial legitimacy. The support differences between sexes or income levels are modest; but the elderly and highly education place greater emphasis on moral and compassionate justifications. Another study shows how across European countries, citizens reveal a strong and consistent pattern of ranking the deservedness of certain groups: first the elderly, closely followed by the ill and disabled, then at some distance, the unemployed and immigrants (Van Oorschot 2006).

Evidence from Sweden points in a similar direction (Bergmarck 2003). Public opinion on welfare provision is shaped by general ideas citizens have of what they want for themselves and others. The motivation is not just self-interest. The basic idea is that Swedish society has a responsibility to take care of its needy citizens, and that obligation cannot be handed over to the market (Bergmark 2003:400). After the economic recession in the 1990s, there was a fall in popular support for the Swedish welfare state, paralleling a general more negative attitude towards central authority. Following the upturn of the economy, that trend reversed (Bergmarck 2003:406). The core programs of education, health and pensions had continued to enjoy particularly strong support. There were lower levels of approval for social assistance or housing allowances. The overall popular reaction to social welfare cutbacks was mostly negative. Dismantling the Swedish welfare state was not on the agenda of any political party, with the solid majority of Sweden's population in favour of maintaining solidaristic welfare arrangements.

Similarly, British social attitude surveys indicate that public opinion on spending priorities have changed little. In 1996 health was the first or second priority for extra spending for 80% of the respondents (Judge et al. 1997, as cited in Johnson and Cullen 2000). The attitude surveys reveal substantial loyalty to the NHS among British citizens. Mau (1996) also found profound social and political support for the NHS over many decades, including more recently demands for sharp increases of the health budget. This loyalty may be closer to "enlightened self-interest" than altruism (Lipsey 1994 as cited by Johnson and Cullen 2000) since almost all British citizens use health services over their life-span

(Bergmark 2004). But whatever the actual mix of underlying motives, it reflects the ongoing commitment of the vast majority of the population to the core health component of welfare states. The findings, in short, do not support the fears of many commentators about a widening gap in British social attitudes.

In Western Germany, public support for governmental responsibility in health care is lower (Mau 1996). In health and old age pensions, about 50% of the population definitively wanted a role for government; 53% of the Western Germans supported increasing health care expenditures (versus 71% in East Germany). These data may well reflect a growing realism about what the welfare state can afford. As Mau notes these attitudes in Western Germany, seem "impregnated by a growing awareness that a further expansion of the welfare state is neither likely, nor affordable." The greater support in East Germany, according to Mau, reflects both a higher "egalitarian ethos" and a much higher expectation of receiving state support at some point. Ninety-one percent of the UK population, in contrast, supported increased government spending for health, with small differences between social classes.

The International Social Survey data confirm this picture for other countries as well. The levels of public support vary across countries, and across population groups within countries. Nonetheless, in all countries studied, a solid majority has continued to believe that government should (definitively or probably) be responsible for making sure that sick people have access to medical care when needed. The table below presents relevant data from those Surveys in 1985, 1990 and 1996.

Public attitudes towards "government provision" (or financing) of medical care throughout Western Europe show, according to other research, "surprisingly constant patterns of popularity" (Ardigo 1995 and Coughlin 1980, *cited in* Gevers et al. 2000). Data from seven European countries (and the United States) portray "citizens [considering] good medical care 'very important' and its provision an: 'essential responsibility' of the government" (Ardigo 1995). Coughlin's earlier research had come to the same conclusion. There are grounds then for believing that the "Western European welfare state [can] be regarded as an organized system of solidarity" in the sense of redistribution from the healthy to the sick, from the young to the old, and from the employed to the unemployed and those not in the labor force (Gevers et al. 2000, 302).

Gevers et al. presented more detailed data on contemporary sentiments in Western Europe that reflect broad support for the role for government in safeguarding universal access to health care (see Table 3 below).

The next table below presents evidence about the degree of agreement concerning the role of government in *assuring access* to medical care. Here, while

Table 2: Popular support for government provision of health care,
selected countries, 1985–1996

	definitely should	probably should	probably should not	definitely should not
Australia				
1985	60.3	33.0	5.4	1.3
1990	37.6	56.2	5.6	.6
1996	42.4	51.7	5.4	.4
(West) Germany				
1985	53.7	43.9	2.1	.3
1990	56.8	38.6	3.7	.8
1996	50.6	46.0	2.9	.5
Great Britain				
1985	85.4	13.7	.6	.3
1990	85.0	14.5	.4	.1
1996	81.7	16.9	1.1	.3
United States				
1985	35.9	47.0	12.8	4.3
1990	40.3	48.8	8.0	2.9
1996	38.5	46.1	11.7	3.7
Italy				
1985	86.6	13.0	.1	.3
1990	87.9	11.4	.3	.3
1996	81.0	17.7	1.0	.4

Note: The support for government provision of health care is captured by the question: "On the whole, do you think that it should be or should not be the government's responsibility to provide health care to the sick?"
Source: ISSP 1985/1990, 1996 Role of government, V49; www.geis.de

there is a wider variation in views, the majority of populations still rejects a limited role of government in this policy arena.

The proportion which "disagree[s] completely" varies among the samples, which provides some basis for the study's emphasis on a dispersion of values and beliefs among the nations of the European Union. Yet, in spite of retrenchment efforts, and varying levels of support for the welfare state arrangements across these countries, health care and old age pensions are invariably popular (Gevers et al. 2000:301). General secular trends like individualization and changes in so-

Table 3: Government responsibility to safeguard
universal access to medical care

Country	*Percent choosing alternative 1*	*Mean*
Sweden	94.80	2.84
Spain	90.10	2.68
Greece	87.20	2.86
Denmark	86.50	2.75
United Kingdom	85.90	2.94
Finland	79.60	2.88
Netherlands	77.70	2.83
France	76.20	2.70
Portugal	72.00	2.67
West Germany	71.80	2.55
Italy	71.70	2.79
Austria	65.00	2.84
Ireland	58.90	2.59

Note: The Government's responsibility is captured by the statement: "Here are three opinions. Please tell me which one comes closest to your own? (1) government has to ensure that health care is provided to all people residing legally here, irrespective of their income; (2) government has to ensure that health care is provided only to those people residing legally here, with low income; (3) government does not have to ensure that health care is provided to people residing legally here, not even those with low income"
Source: Gevers (2000), based on Eurobarometer 44.3/1996.

cial relations seem not to have affected this position much. Yet, while solidarity is the bedrock of Western European welfare state values, there remain bases for making distinctions among both programs and nations as well.

Indeed, the variations in respondents' answers suggest clear differences between the less extensive welfare states of southern Europe and the more extensive social policy regimes of other European countries. This picture reflects, of course, the long-standing typologies of welfare states (Esping-Andersen 1990). The degree of egalitarian sentiment seems to differ between the south and the north of Europe. This is especially so between Sweden and Denmark on the one hand, and the more conservative Austria and Germany, and southern states like Portugal and Italy on the other.

The problem with this interpretation is, however, that there are as many exceptions as confirmations to this pattern. Spain and Greece, two of the southern states in Europe, belong to the staunchest supporters, whereas Austria and West

Table 4: Restricted role of government in providing medical care

Country	Percent disagree completely	Mean
United Kingdom	44.90	3.98
Italy	41.90	3.44
Denmark	41.90	3.71
Netherlands	39.00	3.54
Sweden	36.80	3.98
Spain	35.20	3.82
Greece	29.20	3.60
France	26.60	3.44
West Germany	25.60	3.50
Ireland	25.00	3.40
Finland	23.30	3.28
Portugal	21.30	3.48
Austria	18.60	3.10

Note: The level of disagreement is captured by the statement: "The government should provide everyone with only essential services such as care for serious diseases and encourage people to provide for themselves in other respects" (1 = agree strongly, to 5 = disagree strongly).
Source: Gevers (2000), based on Eurobarometer 44.3/1996.

Germany belong to the least supportive group (and not to the middle group as the Esping-Andersen ranking would predict). In addition, Gelissen (2000) does not find any convincing systematic variation between the levels of popular support for the welfare state and its institutional design. Rather, support levels are more closely linked to the individual's demographic characteristics, moral view and position in the social stratification (Gelissen 2000).

This pattern is not limited to Europe. In the United States, levels of popular support for collective health care arrangements, while lower than in Europe, remain substantial. Between 1975 and 1991, for example, Schlesinger finds that between 44% and 58% of the American population favoured government responsibility for health care, and between 28% and 36% supported a split public and private responsibility. (This was in answer to the question: "Is it the responsibility of the government in Washington to see to it that people have help in paying for doctors and hospital bills?"). By contrast, 16 to 21% favoured individual responsibility only (Schlesinger 2004). Gallup polls over the period 2000 to 2005 found that 58 to 64% of the Americans polled agreed with the idea

Table 5: Support for federal role in providing health care coverage,
2000–2005, in percent

	Jan. *2000*	*Sept.* *2000*	*Nov.* *2001*	*Nov.* *2002*	*Nov.* *2003*	*Nov.* *2004*	*Nov.* *2005*
Yes, government responsibility	59	64	62	62	59	64	58
No, not government responsibility	38	31	34	35	39	34	38

Note: The question is: "Do you think it is the responsibility of the federal government to make sure all American have health care coverage, or is it not the responsibility of the federal government?" Source: Gallup (2005) (www.poll.gallup.com, Jan. 2006).

that the federal government should make sure that all citizens have health care coverage (Gallup 2005).

The average numbers, to be sure, disguise variations across the American population. Political background, gender and health status all shape these views (Gallup Polls 2005). In 2005, for example, 39% of the Republicans, 68% of the Independents and 83% of the Democrats supported an expansive role of government in health care. The percentage was 61 for men between 18 and 49 years of age, 57 percent of men older than 50, 71 percent of women between 18 and 49, and 55 percent of women over 50. Of those who reported fair or poor health status, 75 percent agreed, and of those in good or excellent health, 59 percent.

It is important to note that little or no direct relation exists between high levels of popular support for a strong or even expanding role of government in safeguarding access to medical care with satisfaction with the health care system. The following tables present findings about overall public satisfaction with American health care and satisfaction with the care actually received. One recent Gallup poll, comparing surveys in the US, Canada and the UK, found that while only small majorities in all three countries think their health care system is excellent or good, the rating for the care people have actually received is much higher.

Eurobarometer surveys of citizens' views on health care confirm this general picture (Mossialos 1997). There is wide variety in levels of satisfaction with the health care across European countries. The share of the population very (or fairly) satisfied ranges from a low of 16.3 in Italy, 17.4 in Greece, to a middle

Table 6: Satisfaction with health care system, and
with own experience in health care

	2003	2004	2005
US	60	59	53
Canada	54	54	52
UK	49	54	55
Rating personal care actually received			
US	82	80	78
Canada	76	72	75
UK	74	67	76

Note: Percentage of population who thinks that the quality of
health care in their country is excellent or good.
Source: Gallup (2005) (www.poll.gallup.com, Jan. 2006).

level of 48.1 in the UK, 65.6 in France, 66.0 in Germany, to higher levels in
Belgium (70.1), Denmark (90.0), Netherlands (72.8) and Sweden (67.3). In particular, 59.4 % of the Italians, 53.9 % of the Greeks and 40.9 of the UK population are fairly or very dissatisfied with their health care.

We should note that populations in countries with high and low levels of satisfaction still support substantial public spending on health care. Indeed, support for more (or the same level of) government spending on health care ranges
from 95.9 percent in the UK, 94.4 in Greece, 94.0 in Sweden, 93.4 in Denmark,
90.2 in The Netherlands, 85.0 in Belgium, 82.1 in Spain, 81.9 in France, 79.2 in
Germany and 76.3% in Italy.

The overall picture is one of broad approval of more or the same level of
spending—both in countries where the population is less satisfied with the current system and where public spending levels are already fairly high. Again,
these findings confirm that values of solidarity are longer lasting than shorter-
term opinions about the actual state of health care. There are clear differences
in the popular assessment of the quality of the health care system, people's own
experience with care, and their support for government involvement in health
care (Blendon et al. 2001). The views on quality can change rapidly on the
short term (under the influence of direct experience, media reports or political
rhetoric). The attitudes toward government involvement appears more reliant
on underlying values that do not change easily. Over all, the data we found

support the view of wide and lasting popular approval of the European welfare state, with little evidence of a popular backlash.

Another source of evidence that indirectly confirms that popular values played a major role is resisting efforts to reduce the scope and funding of the welfare states since the 1970s. There is little question that in the late 1970s, the modern welfare state was under attack. A confluence of economic, demographic and ideological factors reshaped the policy environment of the welfare state and emboldened its critics. The oil crisis of 1973–1974 brought economic stagnation. Demographers projected a rapid ageing of society, which critics took as proof of the unaffordability of the welfare state. For some commentators, the welfare state was no longer seen as the *solution* for economic problems, but as one of its *causes* (Timmins 1995). Markets, not governments, were for neoliberal critics the best agents to represent the interests of individual citizens. In this period, after decades of expansion, traditional social welfare arrangements came under mounting attack and in some instances started to contract. The golden era of expansion turned into the era of accountability, control and attempted retrenchment (Marmor, Mashaw and Harvey 1992).

The rise of a pro-market, anti-government ideology in the 1970s, with Ronald Reagan as its iconic American leader and Margaret Thatcher as his European counterpart, provided the base for widespread if not very successful retrenchment efforts (Pierson 1999). Those anti-welfare state ideas were exported to other countries, too. At first, the retrenchment efforts seemed to exclude health care, focusing on other social sectors instead. But over time, the attention also turned to health care as a major category of public spending (Okma 2002). Several countries, including New Zealand, Sweden, Australia, Germany and The Netherlands joined the search for ways to reduce the role of government in health care and increase the role of the private sector (Ranade 1998; Maarse 2004).

On the funding side, there were efforts to encourage private insurance (e.g. in the UK), to eliminate certain services from social insurance coverage (in almost all OECD countries), to introduce or increase co-payments for certain services (in almost all OECD countries), and to introduce administration by competing agencies (e.g. in Germany and The Netherlands). On the contracting side, new models were tested that separate the function of funding from the provision of medical care (the "purchaser-provider split") and strengthen the role of third payers by allowing them to selectively contract with health care providers (Sweden, UK and The Netherlands).

On the provision side, the 1990s and early 2000s saw a bewildering succession of organizational models. In the UK, after the separation of the purchasing and provision functions, independent Health Care Trusts and groups of general practitioners had to enter the "managed market" and negotiate with governments and each other. Other countries offered insured citizens the option to change health insurance organizations (Germany and The Netherlands) but the increased consumer choice was offset by the creation of regional monopolies and thus fewer providers from whom to choose. In many instances, increased competition and increased state control went hand in hand. Mergers and other forms of vertical and horizontal integration of health services generated new institutions and much organizational change. Hospitals and other health facilities faced increased external pressure to improve the quality and patient-friendliness of their services, to reduce medical errors and to increase the transparency of their operations.

The organizational upheaval in the world of medical care has been described elsewhere more extensively (see e.g. Okma and De Roo 2009). For our argument, the main point is that efforts of governments to reduce public health care funding have been far less successful than efforts to change organizational and administrative features of health services (Ranade 1998).

That result itself is crucial to our argument. Governments, when trying to reduce the share of public funding, faced strong popular opposition and had to change when their policies seemed to depart too much from generally accepted beliefs and values. The pro-market health reformers seemed to have underestimated the deep popularity (or even iconic status) of certain programs, especially in medical care. In many cases, governments reversed the de-listing of entitlements from social health insurance or exempted certain population groups from co-payments for prescription drugs (Jacobzone 2000). In spite of government efforts to reduce the public share of health care spending in four European countries, that share did not decline (Maarse and Paulus 2003). Both the expansion of entitlements and expansion of populations covered more than offset the effect of delisting. In fact, the Dutch experience in this area can be labelled a "catalogue of failures" (Maarse and Okma 2004).

In general, cost containment efforts have not led to radical rollback of the welfare state (Pierson 1999). In Sweden, facing some backlash against its retrenchment efforts, the government reversed its policy. "People did not like what they saw" was the way one scholar described this situation (Bergmark 2003:406). The strong support for the Swedish welfare state clearly limited the range of policy options. What is called the "stickiness" of the Scandinavian model arises from widely and strongly felt core values of universality, solidarity and market independence—and those values continue to dominate the expectations of the Swedes of what should happen. They have created a *"logic of appropriateness"* for the consideration of policy options (Cox 2004:207). Because of the strong attachment to core values, some policy options will be viewed more favourably than others. How core values work out in policies and programs is of course a matter of interpretation and political dispute. For example, there can be a broad or a narrow interpretation of the notion of universalism that will lead to a wider or narrower range of entitlements offered to all. And reversely, a broader interpretation of solidarity that translates into a wide pooling of the risks of illness can create strong political coalitions across classes.

For our purposes, this interpretation buttresses a point central to our article. Both survey data and actual policy outcomes indicate a broad similarity in the central, solidaristic conception of the role of medical care in the Western European and North American welfare states. This general value orientation exists side by side with substantial differences in the detailed administration, policies and rules of medical care arrangements.

All OECD countries, we have suggested, publicly express basic commitments to universal access to care and relatively equal treatment of similarly ill citizens. Their citizens, as we have noted, embrace such attitudes at a very general level. There is expressed concern that any care given be of high quality, even though there is little basis for believing that paying for care can ensure that care is appropriate. Leaders of these countries also voice concern about patient satisfaction; they call for some degree of choice of provider (in some cases, also choice of health insurance) and typically acknowledge the importance of preserving physician autonomy in professional decisions (OECD 1992, 1994). (The operational definition of what would count as appropriate autonomy, satisfaction or quality is far from settled, one must add, but the appeals to these values are real.) With public funds the largest single source of funding, cost control is a generally acknowledged goal as well. And, finally, there is implicit or explicit sponsorship in most of the OECD for health promotion and consumer safety. These are presented as worthy—or at least appealing—national policy goals. But, as we showed in *Section III*, these strikingly similar sets of expressed values have not resulted in similar social institutions for the delivery of health care.

CONCLUSION

Our contribution's major claim is that national values and medical care policy are only loosely associated. The experience of OECD countries reveals a substantial variety of institutional forms and policy practices, all of which developed alongside with broadly shared social values. Values may serve as the foundation for social programs, we have argued in reviewing the experience of

Western European democracies, but they do not supply programmatic architecture or detailed recipes for policy adjustment.

Differences in social institutions reflect not only fundamentally different ideologies, but also historical (and contingent) differences in the initial construction of programs, and in the subsequent play of political and social interests.

It is not surprising that calls for reform arose in the last three decades in the aftermath of the turbulent 1970s. It is to the political advantage of every interest group to attempt to secure a larger share of public financial resources by stressing the sacrifices it has made and the fiscal challenges it faces. "Crisis talk"—allegations to the effect that times are extraordinary, and extraordinarily dangerous—is in fact a quite ordinary tool of interest-group politics. By every indication we reviewed, OECD medical programs stand firm on their foundations of still-shared national values.

The question for health-policy reformers, we suggest, is not whether to abandon or re-think their values. It is, instead, how best to embody those values in 21st century institutions. That question requires, for its answer, a prudent attention to the ground-level political and economic realities of each nation. It also calls for a prudent review of the managerial and financing arrangements that have been tried, for better or for worse, by others. That is not to claim, as we have emphasized throughout, that national values are consistent with just any prudential or managerial adjustment. There is little doubt that some of the reform suggestions for national health programs are actually threats to their continuation and express values inconsistent with those that national systems currently embody. Most citizens of OECD nations, the data show, do not believe that access to medical care should depend on the size of their bank accounts. That, we say in conclusion, is a fundamental value.

Notes

This article was first published in *Sociology of Health and Illness* (*Kölner Zeitschrift für Soziologie und Sozialpsychologie*), May 9, 2006. The authors express their gratitude for the comments and suggestions of Heinz Rothgang and Claud Wendt and anonymous reviewers. We also acknowledge the editorial contributions of Nicholas Gerry-Bullard, our research assistant at Yale University.

1. This is precisely the debate that took place in Canada in the wake of the Chaoulli decision, a Supreme Court ruling of 2005 holding that overturned the Quebec government's ban on double-coverage of publicly financed medical care. See Flood et al. (2005).

References

Alford, R. 1974. *Health Care Politics. Ideological and Group Barriers to Reform.* Chicago: University of Chicago Press.

Altman, D., and M. Brodie. 2003. Opinion on public opinion polling. *Health Affairs*, p. W276.

Ardigo, A. 1995. "Public attitudes and changes in health care systems: a confrontation and a puzzle," in *The Scope of Government*, edited by O. Borre and E. Scarborough. Oxford: Oxford University Press. Pp. 388–409.

Baakman, N., J. Van Der Made and I. Mur-Veeman. 1989. "Controlling Dutch health care," in *Controlling Medical Professionals: The Comparative Politics of Health Governance*, edited by G. Freddi and J. W. Björkman. London: Sage Publications.

Bergmark, A. 2000. Solidarity in Swedish welfare—Standing the test of time? *Health Care Analysis* 8:395–411.

Berlin, I. 1998. My intellectual path. *New York Review of Books*, May 14.

Blendon, R. J., M. Kim and J. M. Benson. 2001. The public versus the World Health Organization on health system performance. *Health Affairs* 20, no. 3: 10–20.

CIHI. 2001. *Health Care in Canada 2001: Annual report.* Ottawa: Canadian Institute for Health Information.

Clair Commission. 2001. *Les solutions émergentes.* Commission d'étude sur les services de santé et les services sociaux. Available at http://www.cessss.gouv.qc.ca/pdf/fr/oo–109.pdf.

Conference Board of Canada. 2001. Universality, Quality and Efficiency—Top Values for Health Care. News release.

Coughlin, R. 1980. *Ideology, Public Opinion, and Welfare Policy: Attitudes Toward Taxes and Spending in Industrialized Societies.* Berkeley: University of California, Institute of International Studies.

Cox, R. 2004. The path-dependency of an idea: Why Scandinavian welfare states remain distinct. *Social Policy & Administration*, 38, no. 2: 204–219.

Douglas, M., and A. Wildavsky. 1989. Chapter 10 in *Controlling Medical Professionals: The Comparative Politics of Health Governance*, edited by G. Freddi and J. W. Björkman. London: Sage Publications.

de Swaan, A. 1998. *In Care of the State: Health Care, Education and Welfare in Europe and the USA in the Modern Era.* New York: Oxford University Press.

Esping-Andersen, G. 1990. *The Three Worlds of Welfare Capitalism.* Cambridge: Polity Press.

Flood, C., K. Roach and L. Sossen (eds.). 2005. *Access to Care, Access to Justice: The Legal Battle over Private Health Insurance in Canada.* Toronto: University of Toronto University Press.

Freddi, G. 1989. "Problems of organisational rationality in health systems: Policy controls and policy options," in *Controlling Medical Professionals: The Comparative Politics of Health Governance*, edited by G. Freddi and J. W. Björkman. London: Sage Publications.

Freddi, G., and J. W. Björkman (eds.). 1989. *Controlling Medical Professionals: The Comparative Politics of Health Governance.* London: Sage Publications.

Gailbraith, J. K. 1992. *The Culture of Contentment.* Houghton Mifflin.

The Gallup Poll Healthcare System. 2005, November. www.poll.gallup.com

Gelissen, J. 2000. Popular support for institutionalised solidarity: A comparison between European welfare states. *Int J Soc Welfare* 9:285–300.

Gevers, J., J. Gelissen, W. Arts and R. Muffels. 2000. Public health care in the balance: exploring popular support for health care systems in the European Union. *Int J Social Welfare* 9:301–321.

Giddens, A. 1994. *Beyond Left and Right.* Cambridge: Polity.

Graves, F. 1988. *Canadians and Their Public Institutions.* Ottawa: Ekos Research Associates and Paul Reed, Canadian Centre for Management Development.

Halman, L. 2004. *Attitudes Towards Welfare in the European Values Study.* Paper prepared for the ESPAnet Expert Seminar, Tilburg University, October.

Hinrichs, K. 2003. *Bounded Solidarity: The Demand for and the Presence of Solidaristic Motivations in the Welfare State.* Paper prepared for the Conference New Challenges for Welfare State Research, Toronto, August.

Hirschman, A. O. 1992. "The concept of interest: From euphemism to tautology," in *Rival Views of Market Society.* Cambridge: Harvard University Press.

Hospital Quarterly. 2000. Canadians and the Canada Health Act: Renewed commitment to national principles. *Quarterly Index* (Fall): 80.

Houtepen, R., and R. Ter Meulen. 2000. The expectations of solidarity: Matters of justice, responsibility and identity in the reconstruction of the health care system. *Health Care Analysis* 8:355–376.

Ignatieff, M. 2000. "Does history matter?" in *Great Questions of Canada*, edited by R. Griffiths. Toronto: Stoddart.

Inglehart, R. 2000. Globalization and Postmodern Values. *The Washington Quarterly*, 23(1):215–228.

Immergut, E. M. 1992. *Health Politics. Interests and Institutions in Western Europe.* Cambridge Studies in Comparative Politics. New York: Cambridge University Press.

ISSP 1985; ISSP 1990; ISSP 1996. Role of Government. www.gesis.org

Jacobzone, S. 2000. Pharmaceutical Policies in OECD Countries. Social and Industrial Goals. Labour Market and Social Policy Occasional Paper, no. 40. Paris: Organisation for Economic Cooperation and Development.

Johnson, M., and L. Cullen. 2000. Solidarity put to the test: Health and social care in the UK. *Int J Soc Welfare* 9:228–237.

Klein, R. 1995. *The New Politics of the National Health Service* (3rd ed.). Harlow, Essex: Longman.

Lijphart, A. 1968. *Verzuiling, pacificatie en kentering in de Nederlandse politiek.* Amsterdam: J. H. De Bussy.

Maarse, H. (ed.). *Privatisation in European Health Care. A Comparative Analysis in Eight Countries.* Elsevier gezondheidszorg, Maarssen, The Netherlands, 2004.

Maarse, H., and K. G. H. Okma. 2004. "The privatization paradox in Dutch health care," Chapter 6 in H. Maarse (ed.), *Privatisation in European Health Care. A Comparative Analysis in Eight Countries.* Maarssen, The Netherlands: Elsevier. Pp. 97–116.

Maarse, H., and A. Paulus. 2003. Has solidarity survived? A comparative analysis of the effect of social health reform in four European countries. *Journal of Health Politics, Policy and Law* 28 (4):585–614.

Maioni, A., and P. Martin. 2001. *Is the Canadian Health Care Model Politically Viable? Some Evidence from Public Opinion.* Ottawa: Canadian Political Science Association.

Mansfield, H. C. 1995. Self-interest rightly understood. *Political Theory* 23(1):48–66.

Marmor, T. R. 2002. Medicare: Suspect messages. *The Globe and Mail* and *La Presse.* February 12.

Marmor, T. R., R. Freeman, and K. G. H. Okma, eds. 2009. *Comparative Studies and the Politics of Modern Medical Care.* New Haven: Yale University Press.

Marmor, T. R., J. L. Mashaw and P. L. Harvey, eds. 1990. *America's Misunderstood Welfare State: Persisting Myths, Enduring Realities.* New York: Basic Books.

Mau, S. n.d. Attitudinal cleavages and the welfare state: A comparison between the United Kingdom and Germany (unpublished paper). mau@datacomm.iue.it

Mazankowski Commission. 2001. *A Framework for Reform.* Report of the Premier's Advisory Council on Health. Edmonton.

Mossialos, E. 1997. Citizen's views on the health care systems in the 15 member countries of the European Union. *Health Economics* 6:109–116.

OECD. 1994. *The Reform of Health Care. A Comparative Analysis of Seven OECD Countries.* Health Reform Studies no. 5. Paris: Organisation for Economic Cooperation and Development.

———. 1992. *The Reform of Health Care: A Comparative Analysis of Seven OECD Countries.* Health Reform Studies no. 2. Paris: Organisation for Economic Cooperation and Development.

Okma, K. G. H. 2002a. *What Is the Best Public-Private Model for Canadian Health Care?* Montreal: Institute for Research of Public Policy.

———. 2002b. Health care and the welfare state: Two worlds of welfare drifting apart? In J. Berghman et al. (eds)., *Social Security in Transition.* Leiden: Kluwer Law International. Pp. 229–238.

———. 1997. *Studies on Dutch Health Politics, Policies and Law.* Ph.D. thesis, Utrecht University.

Pierson, P. 2001. Coping with permanent austerity: Welfare states restructuring in affluent societies. In Paul Pierson, ed., *The New Politics of the Welfare State.* New York: Oxford University Press.

Ranade, W., ed. 1998. *Markets and Health Care: A Comparative Analysis.* New York: Longman.

Rawls, J. 1971. *A Theory of Justice.* Cambridge: Harvard University Press.

Romanow Commission. 2002. *Shape the Future of Health Care.* Interim Report. Saskatoon: Commission on the Future of Health Care in Canada.

Sabatier, R., P. A. Jenkins-Smith and H. C. Jenkins-Smith, eds. 1993. *Policy Change and Learning.* Boulder: Westview Press.

Schlesinger, M. 2004. Reprivatizing the public household? Medical care in the context of American public values. *Journal of Health Politics, Policy and Law* 29(4–5):961–1004.

Schumpeter, J. 1908. On the concept of social value. *Quarterly Journal of Economics* 23:213–32.

Taylor, M. G. 1987. *Health Insurance and Canadian Public Policy: The Seven Decisions That Created the Canadian Health Insurance System and Their Outcomes.* Montreal: McGill-Queen's University Press.

Timmins, N. 1995. *The Five Giants: A Biography of the Welfare State.* London: HarperCollins.

Tuohy, C. H. 1999. *Accidental Logics: The Dynamics of Change in the Health Care Arena in the United States, Britain and Canada.* New York: Oxford University Press.

———. 1993. "Social policy: Two worlds of welfare," in *Governing Canada. Institutions and Public Policy*, edited by M. A. Atkinson. Toronto: Harcourt Brace Canada.

Van Oorschot, W. 2000. Why pay for welfare? A sociological analysis of the reasons for welfare solidarity. *The Netherlands' Journal of Social Sciences* 36(1):15–36.

Van Oorschot, W. 2006. Making the difference in Social Europe: Deservedness perceptions among citizens of European welfare states. *Journal of European Social Policy* 16(1):23–42.

Wilson, G. K. 1990. *Interest Groups.* Oxford: Basil Blackwell.

Values Talk in the (English) NHS

Rudolf Klein

We start with our values—the values of a health service funded by all of
us, available to each of us, equally, free at the point of treatment, with
care based on our need and not our ability to pay. Those values are non-
negotiable. They make the NHS unique—the institution that makes people proud to be British. They are a beacon of compassion and an ethic
of care, of fairness and of social solidarity, mutual responsibility for one
another, in times that so often feel harshly individualistic.

In everything we do, in every change we make, we will not compromise those values. Indeed I go further, because I believe that the changes
we are making are not simply consistent with our traditional values: they
are the best way of securing our values in a rapidly changing world.

—*Patricia Hewitt, Secretary of State for Health*

So there we have it. Whatever is driving the changes that are currently transforming the English National Health Service (ENHS)—and no lesser word
than transformation will do—it is seemingly not a change in the *values* inspir-
ing policy makers. So we have a puzzle, prompting a series of questions. What
is the relationship between policy making and values, if a dramatic shift can
take place in the former without any change in the latter? How useful is the notion of values as an analytic tool when it comes to explaining policy variations
either over time or between different jurisdictions? While values may only be
a rubber tin opener when it comes to *explaining* change, are they nevertheless
significant as the language of *justification* for policy makers? If so, does their
invocation represents a kind of moral path dependency—note the use of the
word "traditional" in Patricia Hewitt's speech—and thus help us to understand
continuities across time, as distinct from disruptions, in policy? "Values are no

policy straitjacket but there are certain choices they rule out," as Marmor et al. have argued.[1]

THE CHANGING NHS

While policy rhetoric stresses traditional values, the institutional changes in the English NHS represent a break with the past. A Trinitarian mimic market model is emerging, based on consumer choice, a plurality of providers competing for custom and money following the patient). Having created a command and control system in their first five years in office, successive Labour Secretaries of State spent the next five years chipping away at the structure. Power is to be devolved to the periphery; independent regulators will increasingly take over the supervisory role previously played by the central bureaucracy; the target-ridden, top-down-directed ENHS is to become "self-inventing."

So much for the theory. How the model works out in practice remains to be seen, of course, and its drawing-board elegance will no doubt be greatly modified in practice. But for the purposes of this analysis it is not so much the institutional characteristics of the new NHS that matter as their intellectual underpinning: the changes in the way the policy community in the widest sense (academics included) has come to think about health care over the past 20 years or so. I have tried to encapsulate what I see as the main elements in this intellectual shift by counterpointing what I see the traditional way of thinking about the NHS as a church.[2] The former include trust, planning, and need; those characterising the latter include choice, demand, contract.

None of these words or concepts appear in Patricia Hewitt's list of values, nor in other analyses of ENHS values (see below). But they do capture what I see

Model 1

Model 1: NHS as church	Model 2: NHS as garage
Paternalism	Consumerism
Planning	Responsiveness
Need	Demand
Priorities	Choice
Trust	Contract
Monolithic	Pluralistic
Stability	Adaptability

as a decisive shift in our collective "appreciative system"[3] when thinking about health care, and not just health care. Here it is crucial to distinguish between policy goals and policy means. The move from the church to the garage model certainly represents disillusion with traditional policy tools but does not necessarily imply abandoning the traditional values shaping policy goals.

To elaborate. Introducing his legislation for the creation of the health service in 1946, Nye Bevan did not use the language of values. Neither, for that matter, did the 1979 Royal Commission on the NHS—a reminder that the proliferation of values talk is a relatively recent phenomenon. The master rhetorician contented himself with enunciating the principle that no one ought to be deterred from seeking medical help by "financial anxiety" and pointing out that the NHS would "keep very many people alive who would otherwise be dead."[4] The implicit ethical imperative was subsequently spelled out by Barbara Castle, one of Bevan's disciples, when Secretary of State for Health in the 1970s: "Intrinsically the National Health Service is a church. It is the nearest thing to the embodiment of the Good Samaritan that we have in respect of our public policy."[5]

To achieve this "embodiment of the Good Samaritan" vision, the NHS as conceived in 1946 relied on a mixture of technocratic paternalism, faith in rational planning and trust in medical professionals to determine who needed what. It was these intellectual pillars that crumbled over the decades, as the ration-book society gave way to the credit-card society. Enter the garage model with its emphasis on consumerism, choice, responsiveness and so on. Does this represent a change in the ENHS values as set out by Ms. Hewitt and others? Or does it represent a rise in public expectations, on the one hand, and a perceived failure of the church model to meet those expectations, on the other hand, so leading to a search for new ways to meet traditional goals? Ms. Hewitt would certainly take the latter view, and I am inclined to agree with her. Moreover, in stressing the radical nature of the institutional changes, it is all too easy to ignore the very strong element of continuity: the fact that the ENHS remains a tax-financed service, free at the point of delivery.

On this interpretation, the real change in our "appreciative system" has been in the way we think about the mechanics of public service delivery as distinct from the goals. Hence the emphasis on introducing the dynamics of the market into the public sector, as well as using the private sector to supply public services. Whether this undermines or corrupts public sector values is another question, where the answer may depend largely on how we define those values and whether we think that they shape behaviour, and how, as distinct from rhetoric: knights have their pathologies as well as knaves.[6]

In all these respects, it is important to emphasise, change in the ENHS (as in other countries) is the by-product of wider changes in the way we think about public policy, which have affected all public services. In turn the way we think about public policy—the successive waves of reform starting with the New Public Management—reflect wider changes in society: notably the shift from production to consumption as the centre of political gravity, as symbolised in the decline of organised labour. So one question to consider is whether this is as true of Scotland and Wales as it is of England: if the transformation of the ENHS reflects a transformation in the political culture of its environment, do divergent directions taken by Scotland and Wales reflect distinctive local political cultures—i.e. assumptions about appropriate mechanisms and tools of policy—rather than different sets of values?[7] Maybe the neo-Hegelian formula of the Third Way—reconciling what had appeared to be opposites and creating a new synthesis as between State purposes and market dynamics—has not caught on there.

The reason for stressing the role of political culture, political institutions and political process is simple. This is that the language of values does not translate directly into the language of policy making, as distinct from policy justification. As Deborah Stone has put it: "Behind every policy issue lurks a contest over conflicting, though equally plausible conceptions of the same abstract goal. The enduring values are aspirations for a community, into which people read contradictory interpretations."[8] In short, to introduce the theme of the next section, values do not drive policy but are revealed in the process of making policy.

WHAT DO WE KNOW ABOUT VALUES?

Values are a plasticine concept. There is little agreement about how to define a "value," as distinct from a principle or a goal. Following Bill New's analysis,[9] a sensible working definition appears to be: "values are conceptions of the morally desirable." And his list of specifically ENHS values, filleted out by him from official documents, runs as follows:

- Health
- Universalism (compulsory cover etc.)
- Equity (social justice, fairness etc.)
- Democracy (accountability, answerability etc.)
- Choice (autonomy, freedom etc)
- Respect for human dignity (honesty, consideration, fair dealing etc.)

- "Public service" (public service ethos, altruism, non-commercial motives etc.)
- Efficiency (cost-effectiveness, waste avoidance etc.)

It is, conceptually, a very mixed bag (even not counting the etceteras). Some of the values appear to be about promoting desirable outcomes, like health and equity. Others appear to be primarily about processes, like accountability. Some are about ways of doing things that are desirable in themselves, like respecting human dignity. Others are about the means for achieving desirable ends: so, for example, efficiency would simply seem to be necessary conditions for achieving other goals, given resource constraints.[10] Some of the values cited by Patricia Hewitt, and not included in this list, appear to me to fall into the same category: so, for example, I would argue that "free at the point of delivery" falls into the class of values, if indeed they can be called such, which are not intrinsically morally desirable but may or may not be a necessary condition for achieving others that are, such as equity.

End-state values tend to command universal support inasmuch as they have become the rhetorical platitudes of health care policy-making across countries. So, for example, the 25 Health Ministers of the European Union have agreed on the "overarching values"—universality, access to good quality care, equity and solidarity—which, they claim, are shared across the EU, as well as a set of operating principles.[11] Everyone can subscribe to them because they are essentially vacuous in the abstract. As the EU Ministers acknowledged, "the practical ways in which these values and principles become a reality vary significantly . . . and will continue to do so." Further, they conceded that "decisions about the basket of healthcare to which citizens are entitled and the mechanisms used to finance and deliver that healthcare, such as the extent to which it is appropriate to rely on market mechanisms and competitive pressures to manage health systems must be taken in the national context." In short, value convergence is consistent with a large degree of policy divergence: policies cannot, for sure, be "read off" values.

Inevitably so, for values become contentious and fuzzy when it comes to giving them meaning in the process of interpreting and implementing them. What does equity mean in practice and how should it be measured? What is the role and responsibility of a healthcare system in promoting health? If such questions could yield a once and for all answer, commanding general assent, there would be mass unemployment in the academic health care industry. However, there is no prospect of that. The instrumental values are contentious for somewhat different reasons. This is that their claim to be *morally* desirable often appears to rest on an (undeclared) assertion about causal relationships, and as such is vulnerable to empirical challenge. Do we know, for example, that abjuring profit motivation necessarily and inevitably contributes to respect for dignity or any of the other end-state, intrinsically desirable values?

Not only are values ambiguous. Not only do they yield many different, competing interpretations. But there is another reason yet for arguing that we discover our values—and the weight we attach to them—in the process of policy making and implementation. This is that our values are often in conflict. There are trade-offs between them. For example, the existence of privately-financed health care indisputably offends against the equity principle—that need should be the only criterion for allocating health care resources. However, abolishing privately financed health care would undoubtedly offend against the choice/ autonomy principle as well as being politically dangerous (as Barbara Castle found out when she attempted to phase out pay beds from the NHS in the 1970s, a never-to-be-repeated policy experiment). Similarly, promoting health may come into collision with autonomy, raising questions about the extent to which the State should control individual behaviour and what relative weight should be given to the two conflicting values.[12]

A PROLIXITY OF VALUES

So far I have been discussing what might be called big-picture, systems values. However, within systems there are nests of professional and other values. And again there is no reason to expect harmonious congruence. Most obviously, there is tension between managerial and professional values.[13] The clash of competing and conflicting values is apparent in the on-going debate about rationing. On the one hand, there are the values of the medical profession: these tend to rest on an ethical individualism, which stresses the doctor's responsibility to do the utmost for the individual patient—for example, the rule of rescue. On the other hand, there are the managerial values (shared by many policy makers and academics) derived from a utilitarian calculus, which stress the cost-effectiveness of interventions not in terms of individuals but in their effect on the community of patients, actual and potential. Interestingly, the one point of near convergence appears to be agreement on process values: i.e. that decisions about rationing should be transparent, reasonable and publicly defensible.[14] This may suggest a more general conclusion: that process values are more robust—in terms of clarity and precision—than many other members of the value family.

Overall, the ENHS is remarkable for the explosion of value statements produced by its component organisations, in particular provider trusts. Box 1 presents two such statements (chosen because they are short, in contrast to the prolixity that marks most others) plus some individual examples. What these suggest is that the concept of "values" is in danger of losing any precise meaning it might ever have had, and is becoming synonymous with any declaration of organisational ambitions, aspirations and goals, however general or platitudinous: who could object to striving for excellence, for example? Clearly those responsible for producing such litanies believe that they are useful in terms of defining an organisational culture and perhaps even shaping individual behaviour. Maybe they are. But it is difficult to resist the conclusion that they also reflect managerial fads or fashions[15]—like organisational visions and mission statements—and one which is not exclusive to the ENHS.

The ENHS—like the health care arena internationally—may be a particularly highly developed example of values introspection and proclamation. But it has no monopoly of values talk. The Civil Service, among others, has proclaimed its core values: integrity, honesty, objectivity and impartiality. Nor is values-talk limited to the public sector. When the retiring chairman of the John Lewis Partnership gave a farewell speech, he entitled it "Combining established

---

Box 1. English NHS Trust Value Statements

Guy's and St. Thomas'

1. Put patients first
2. Take pride in what we do
3. Respect others
4. Strive to be the best
5. Act with integrity

St. George's

*   Treat all people with respect and dignity
*   Deliver care in partnership with others
*   Continually strive for clinical excellence
*   Ensure probity and transparency in spending public money
*   Be an exemplary employer
*   Be committed to excellence in education, training and research
*   Be open and honest with each other and those outside the organisation

"Balance technical excellence with consideration and compassion for those we serve" *Cambridge University Hospitals*
"We will recognise and celebrate the achievements of individuals, teams, departments and directorates across the Trust" *Salisbury NHS Trust*

---

values with modern retailing."[16] Google gives more than 1,000,000 references to values. Yet this appears to be a relatively new phenomenon in the case of the ENHS, as noted earlier and perhaps more generally. Speculatively this might suggest that values that used to be taken for granted are made explicit when institutions have to cope with change: they represent an attempt to define the parameters of the acceptable and desirable in times of turmoil, moral life-boats in rough seas.

CONCLUDING COMMENT

Scepticism about values talk should not be taken for nihilism. To sum up the main theme of this chapter, my argument is not that values don't matter but that the starting point of any comparison of the four UK systems should be *revealed* values, not officially promulgated ones (which, I suspect, would not show up many differences). To repeat: values may constrain but do not drive policy. It is policy that reveals the meaning and weight attached to often ambiguous and conflicting values. For example, if equity is one of the professed values, policy makers are constrained inasmuch as they would incur politically damaging charges of dishonesty and betrayal if they introduced measures that patently made access to health care more difficult for the worst-off. More than that, a commitment to equity as a value is likely (at a minimum) to mean that other things being equal policy makers will lean towards measures likely to promote this goal: it establishes a presumption that policy will move in a particular direction. But it will tell us little (if anything) about the degree of enthusiasm that policy makers will show , the resources they will be prepared to invest or the instruments they will choose for achieving their goal.

In exploring why countries adopt different policies even while proclaiming the same values, one starting point is history. Even when countries share the same broad institutional framework (as in the case of the United Kingdom), policy-making styles may differ. For example, while in the ENHS relations between policy makers and professionals have become more antagonistic over the decades, the same does not appear to apply in the smaller UK countries. And if policy communities differ,[17] then so may policy priorities or directions. Again, it cannot be assumed that the health services of the UK countries face exactly the same challenge. On the contrary: there is a relatively higher concentration of deprivation and ill-health in the peripheral countries, so it would not be surprising if different weights were attached to competing values. Similarly, the public in the four countries may have different expectations: the exit strategy of opting for private health care is very much an English phenomenon whereas loyalty appears to be the norm elsewhere. Institutions matter, too: proportional representation leading to coalition government is less likely to produce the kind of dramatic policy switches in the organisation of health care characteristic of the Westminster winner-takes-all system.

In exploring differences in policy outcomes the emphasis should surely, therefore, be on analysing the politics of values: the way in which institutions, coalitions of interests, established networks and ways of handling conflict shape the interpretation and implementation of shared values in the four countries. Above all, I would suggest, attention should be paid not to the values of the health care systems but to the ideas in good currency about the management of public services in the different countries of the UK. To the extent that many, perhaps most, so-called health care values are instrumental—means of achieving end-state goals—so the key variable may be notions about what are effective policy instruments (notions which may, in turn, depend on the context: small, homogenous countries may have different options than large, heterogeneous ones). So different paths to achieving the same end-state values—whether in health care or in education—will be taken depending on whether it is assumed that they can best be achieved by a strategy of co-operation and consensus or by competition and diversity: A judgment not so much about what should count as a good society as about what is best calculated to achieve shared ends.

Notes

The article was a chapter in Scott L. Greer and David Rowland, eds., *Devolving Policy, Diverging Values? The Values of the United Kingdom's National Health Services*, London, The Nuffield Trust, 2008, pp. 19–28. Epigraph from Patricia Hewitt, *Annual Health and Social Care Lecture—Investment and Reform: Transforming Health and Healthcare*, London School of Economics, 13 December 2005, Mimeo.

1. Theodore Marmor, Kieke Okma and Stephen Latham, *National Values, Institutions and Health Policies*, Discussion Paper No. 5, Ottawa: Commission on the Future of Health Care in Canada, July 2002.

2. Rudolf Klein, "The goals of health policy: Church or garage?" in A. Harrison, ed., *Health Care UK 1992/1993*, King's Fund 1993. Since then the model has been revised, and the most recent version appears in the *New Politics of the NHS*, 5th ed., Radcliffe, 2006.

3. The phrase and concept is derived from Geoffrey Vickers, *The Art of Judgment*, Chapman & Hall, 1965. As he argues (p. 4), an appreciative system will include reality judgments and value judgments: "The relationship between judgments of fact and of value is close and mutual; for facts are relevant only in relation to some judgment of value and judgments of value are operative only in relation to some configuration of fact."

4. Hansard, *Official Report*, 5th Series, Vol. 422 National Health Service Bill debate, 30 April 1946, cols. 43–63.

5. Quoted in Klein (2006), p. 86.

6. Julian Le Grand, *Motivation, Agency, and Public Policy*, 2nd ed., Oxford, 2006. See also Rudolf Klein, "The Great Transformation," reprinted in this edition.

7. This would be consistent with the findings of Scott L. Greer, *Territorial Politics and Health Policy*, Manchester University Press, 2004.

8. Deborah A. Stone, *Policy, Paradox and Political Reason*, Scott, Foresman/Little Brown 1988.

9. Bill New, "Thinking about values," in Bill New and Julia Neuberger, *Hidden Assets: Values and Decision-Making in the NHS*, King's Fund, 2002.
   See also, his earlier *A Good Enough Service: Values, Trade-offs and the NHS*, King's Fund/IPPR 1999.

10. Rudolf Klein, "A Babel of voices: values, policy-making and the NHS," in New and Neuberger *op.cit.*

11. Council of the European Union "Council Conclusion: common values and principles in EU Health Systems," 2733rd Employment, Social Policy, Health and Consumer Affairs Council Meeting, Luxembourg, 1–2 June 2006.

12. For example, the recent case of an actor playing Churchill being banned from smoking a cigar on stage at the Edinburgh Festival suggests to me that in Scotland greater weight is given to the health promotion value than to autonomy, and I would be surprised (and disappointed) if there had been a similar decision had the performance taken place in London.

13. David. J. Hunter, "A tale of two tribes: the tension between managerial and professional values," in New and Neuberger, *op. cit.* See also Rudolf Klein, "The conflict between professionals, consumers and bureaucrats," *Journal of the Irish Colleges of Physicians and Surgeons* ,Vol. 6, No. 3, 1977, 88–91.

14. Norman Daniels, "Accountability for reasonableness," *British Medical Journal*, Vol. 321, 25 November 2000, 1300–1301.

15. Theodore Marmor, *Fads in Medical Care Management and Policy*, London: The Stationery Office, 2004.

16. Sir Stuart Hampson, "Combining established values with modern retailing," Lecture, 28 February 2007, The John Lewis Partnership website.

17. Greer, *op.cit.*

THE STATE AND THE
MEDICAL PROFESSION

The relation between physicians and the governments that fund some or all of their citizens' medical care depends critically on how one construes the fundamental starting point. Does one begin with doctors as members of a learned profession, self-governing, largely trusted to serve their patients' interests, and immensely respected as pillars of their local community? Do we therefore stress the autonomy of this corporate guild, no longer financed by client payment, but still guided by peer consensus rather than managerial review and public accountability for their performance? Were the title of this chapter reversed, we would have a defensible starting point in the period just after World War II. Medicine had proven itself effective during war to save lives and limbs, and all over the industrial democracies there were determined efforts to expand access to the doctors whose scientific qualifications and trusted status were so impressive.

Writing in the early twenty-first century justifies beginning with the state, the prime regulator and financier of modern medical systems costing rich countries between 8 and 15 percent of their national incomes. Everywhere there is commentary about getting more value for money and doing so by holding physicians to account for their performance according to targets and audits set by public authorities. While physicians remain more trusted than any other profession, their autonomy has everywhere been challenged and the reliance on peer control weakened. There has been a shift from status to contract. So understood, such change has been breathtakingly substantial from the perspective of physicians familiar with the earlier order. From the standpoint of business management and economists skeptical of the claims of professions, it is a change long overdue.

The changes noted varied, of course, in timing and intensity across the globe. How to understand the general shift requires asking what is common across the democracies over these decades. Dealing with particular episodes requires by contrast more detailed analysis, not only of changing ideas, but of the differing priorities and organization of states and doctors.

For the general shift in the standing and influence of physicians on whether and how they are to be governed, the clash of basic ideas has been very important. The more individualistic notions from classic liberalism held sway (see Chapter 5), the more threatened medical autonomy was. The fiscal crisis welfare states faced in the wake of the stagflation of the mid- and later 1970s bolstered pro-market enthusiasts critical of expensive social welfare regimes and persistent demands from physicians for both greater budgets and continued autonomy. Within the profession itself there were critics of peer review without scientific backing, especially from randomized clinical trials. And there were continuing attacks on professional self-government, with ever more common belittling in the United States of the "cottage industry" they controlled. These developments bolstered those outside the medical profession in their efforts—varying in success, of course—to control what was done, paid for, and proscribed.

The variation across countries in how medical autonomy has been restricted is a substantial subject, and we have not covered much of that variation in this chapter or others. We know that American doctors face more micro-regulation than their Canadian counterparts and that, by contrast, traditional autonomy is more a feature of German and Austrian medicine than would be imaginable to counterparts in anglophone countries. There are also variations across time. While Britain initially lagged behind the United States in circumscribing clinical freedom, the pace of change has picked up since the British article in this chapter was written in the 1990s. Thus the General Medical Council—the profession's regulatory body and the citadel of medical autonomy—has been forced by government pressure to change the composition of its governing body, the method of selecting it, and its methods of ensuring the competence of doctors and disciplining those who offend against the professional code. But while this transformation of the regime of professional self-regulation reflects a more general shift in the balance between managers and doctors in the NHS, the medical profession has been spectacularly successful in distributional conflicts: medical earnings have soared.

But whatever the differences between countries and across time, there is one common element. This is the imbalance, as between physicians and funders, in the centrality of some issues. One is explored in the first essay in this chapter, which distinguishes between the politics of constitutional and distributional conflicts. Another illustrative example, addressed in the article on doctors' pay, is the methods by which physicians are rewarded. The reality is that doctors are paid by different methods across the board—whether by fee-for-service, capitation, salary, or some mix of these methods. But which methods are used at any one time are of greater symbolic interest to the profession than they are to their financiers. The legacy of meaning attached to methods of payment is something the sociologists of professions understand but governments regard as less important than how much is paid and how much credit comes from that.

This issue—the determinants of how (as distinct from how much) doctors are paid—turns out to be a good test, as well, of the comparative approach to explanation. Whereas the particular mix of methods varies, as noted, the fact that doctors have almost always got their way on such issues means that national accounts of pay disputes may give a misleading picture. The profession may on occasion allow itself to be bribed into accepting modifications to the rewards system—no one has ever accused doctors of lacking interest in money—but only if this does not threaten its influence over that system.

Doctors, Politics and Pay Disputes

"Pressure Group Politics" Revisited

Theodore R. Marmor and David Thomas

This article reports on an inquiry into the outcomes of conflicts over the methods by which doctors are paid in western industrial countries. England, Sweden and the United States provide the primary comparative data. And the theoretical starting point is Harry Eckstein's widely known study of the British Medical Association, from which he derives some broader generalizations about the determinants of pressure group effectiveness. Eckstein's contention is that the effectiveness of the BMA in dealing with the Ministry of Health is largely dependent on the extent to which negotiations are private conversations between the two parties. To the extent that the arena of conflict opens up, so the BMA's influences diminishes. In short, it is a pressure group theory which puts the emphasis on the style of negotiation and the relationship between the two principal actors. In what follows, we challenge this emphasis on the intimacy of negotiations as a key differentiating explanatory factor.

THE DOCTORS' PAY CRISIS IN BRITAIN 1965–6

This section of the paper presents a research report on the doctors' pay crisis in Britain (1965–6) as well as a commentary on both when and why the BMA is successful in getting its way on the methods and amount of its remuneration. We want to know—through the use of remuneration disputes in England—why it is that Eckstein's local, national explanation of BMA influence is faulty (the "closest imaginable relationship" between the BMA and the Ministry). And we want to suggest, through the use of comparative data in the next section, a more promising account of the unquestionable success doctors in Western Europe and America have in controlling the form and amount of their remuneration by the state.

Neither internal nor external evidence supports Eckstein's view that bargaining structures determine much of the British Medical Association's effectiveness. The internal evidence—remuneration disputes over time within England—already has suggested that intimacy of negotiations is not a crucial factor in accounting for BMA success on pay. External evidence is another check on this causal scheme. We have taken three countries for study—Great Britain, Sweden, and the US—and analyzed three policy decisions about how doctors are to be paid by the state: (a) the changes in methods of remuneration following the general practitioner crisis (1965–6) in Great Britain, (b) the fee-for-service policy of the National Health Insurance Act in Sweden (1955), and (c) the Medicare "reasonable charge policy" in the US. Two features of this type of comparative study should be made clear at the outset. First, the countries differ markedly in the setting and atmosphere of negotiations about medical remuneration.[1] Second, the policy decisions in each case are strikingly similar, when measured by the intentions of the medical organizations. That is to say, methods known to be preferred by the respective medical organizations were, broadly speaking, what the government policy became in each of the three episodes. Here we have a common burden on a political system—the requirement of settling methods of remunerating physicians in public programs—and three different decision-making structures which cope with this burden. The existence of a common outcome suggests that the causal factor lies in the first of Eckstein's three categories—the nature of the pressure group and the resources which doctors, as opposed to other producer groups in the society, share. The question of why it is that doctors in different national settings prefer different methods is a separate issue in the history and sociology of professions, which some sociologists have explored, particularly Mark Field and Talcott Parsons. For present purposes, it is enough to know that knowledge of their preferences is the single best predictor of policy decisions in this area.

The politics of medical remuneration methods involves three separate areas of argument, not all of which are equally at issue in remuneration disputes in the three countries. Method may refer to the *unit* of payment: whether by person, by item of service, by time, etc. The *source* of payment may be the method feature at issue, either in the sense of whether the patient should transfer funds to the doctor and be reimbursed by the public program, or whether the doctor should be paid by the state directly or by agencies mediating between the profession and the government. Finally, the *bases of differentiating doctors* for payment may be the issue; the dispute may involve whether age, training, setting of work, etc. should count in the amounts paid physicians. The political influence of medical organizations in remuneration policy may be understood as the ability of physician groups to raise issues, suppress issues, delimit alternatives, and produce desirable policy outcomes in these three types of conflict.

What does the British case of 1965–6 tell one about the influence of the BMA, when influence is understood in the terms suggested above? The very creation of a dispute was the work of the BMA, its answer to the Review Body's decision in 1965 to give doctors a net 10 per cent increase and to leave the methods of remuneration substantially unchanged.[2] No changes in unit, source, or bases of differentiation were made in the fifth report of the Review Body on Doctors' and Dentists' Remuneration. Interviews with government actors suggest the conclusion that hesitancy about changing the methods of remuneration grew out of the unwillingness to pay the doctors in ways they themselves had not suggested. The response to the Fifth Review Body Report was unexpectedly heated; the BMA asked for signed but undated letters of resignation from the National Health Service, and demanded that a complete review of methods and amount of remuneration take place. Approximately 16,500 of Britain's 22,000 general practitioners sent in these letters by 17 March 1965,[3] and the stage was set for raising a wide variety of issues about method and amount of state payment to general practitioners.

How did the BMA fare in delimiting the range of issues considered and getting its way on those which were at issue? On the question of the unit of payment, the BMA was able to get consideration of all three of the typical possibilities: capitation, item-of-service, and salary. The outcome was, first, the continuation of capitation and, second, the expression of the Ministry's willingness to pay doctors in health centres by salary (subject to later negotiation). Finally, the government rejected the BMA demand that item-of-service payment be permitted. The latter result superficially suggests a BMA defeat. But it should be added that no widespread enthusiasm for item-of-service payment was evident in the profession, except among the numerically insignificant Fellowship for Freedom in Medicine. In the course of BMA-Ministry negotiations on units of payment during the summer of 1965 it became clear that item-of-service recommended itself to the BMA only insofar as it involved lifting any ceiling on the income of doctors who used it. When the Ministry cited the case of dentists to suggest it would be unwilling to let amounts of remuneration expand without control, the BMA leadership quickly gave up. BMA leaders then asked the Ministry to write up its argument so that they could explain how unappealing the necessary control would be, and how irrelevant this means was to their general aim to reduce workloads, an aim unlikely to be satisfied if doctors' pay varied largely with respect to the incidence of their consultations. In this case, the issue of payment amount was dominant, both in the sense of the global increases attributable to this unit of payment, and in the sense of the uneven distribution of income which item-of-service payment would entail if it were not limited by an income ceiling.[4]

The source of payment was not raised as an issue during the course of negotiations, except for occasional laments that patients had no financial incentives to avoid excessive medical consultations. The profession was not interested in patients actually paying physicians. In England, payment by the patient was not so much an issue of remunerating doctors as controlling the distribution of medical services. The decisive argument raised against patient payment was that such pecuniary arrangements always present a dilemma. If costly enough to dissuade hypochondriacs, payment would also dissuade those who really needed medical attention. If inexpensive enough to avoid that latter problem, direct payment would not prevent nasty or casual consumers from pestering doctors. From a comparative standpoint, the striking fact is that source of payment was not a controversial matter. Doctors raise this issue in both the US and the Swedish context; in both cases the patient is involved in the actual transfer of money to doctors, a practice at the insistence of the medical organizations, and done against the original intentions of the government health reformers. In Great Britain, the source of payment is not a political issue in that there is no conflict over what source ought to be used.

But, if there is consensus on the source of payment, there is disagreement between the BMA and the Ministry on what sorts of doctors ought to be differentially regarded. This disagreement arises on all three of the most common ways of discriminating one general practitioner from another: the nature of his output (health measure, quality), the nature of his practice setting (shoddy, under-doctored group), and the characteristics of the doctor himself (age, training, etc.). Since the Royal Commission (1957–60) there have been persistent attempts to reward something called superior general practitioners. Both the Ministry and the Review Body have encouraged this form of differentiation, using tactics from persuasion to ear-marked funds, as in 1966. The recent outcome, a rejection of ear-marked merit awards to general practitioners (by a BMA vote of 16,000 to 4,000), illustrates the capacity of the BMA and its membership to shape public policy. But note that merit awards represent a small expected expenditure, and as such fall under the conditions whereby the government is not constrained financially from conceding medical wishes on the methods of their payment.[5]

The use of merit awards is but one of the controversial ways by which physicians may be differentiated for payment purposes. Another attribute of the physician that the BMA has made relevant to general practitioner remuneration is age. Seniority payments have never been a Ministry of Health preference, and because such payments would have financial implications for a very large proportion of the participating physicians, they are worrisome from a budgetary standpoint. The fate of seniority payments during 1965–6 is an excellent illustration of the limited ability of the government to resist medical preferences on methods when the profession is acknowledged to be angry, militant, and prepared to create difficulties for the continuation of normal health services. The precise timing of the demand for seniority payments is difficult to establish, but it is absolutely clear that the BMA took the initiative in pressing for this type of differentiation during negotiations with Minister of Health, Robinson, in the summer of 1965. The Ministry, on the other hand, was anxious that differentiation by type of doctor should reflect differences in quality. Either subjective judgments of physicians or objective measures of training (to become better doctors presumably) were the preferred methods. In the end, the subjective judgment approach (merit awards) was rejected by a vote of the profession, and the training criterion was incorporated into seniority payments. After a short delay, seniority payments would only be paid to physicians who took a prescribed number of refresher courses. Here was a case in which the Ministry was able to add a quality consideration to a method of remuneration which only very indirectly measured ability (through experience) and was unable to get more direct measures of quality practice.

The same pattern is evident in the other methods of payment which the Ministry and the BMA agreed upon during the summer and fall of 1965.[6] Either the BMA was able to satisfy its charter demands fully, or the government, while agreeing in principle, placed constraints on the amount or scope of special payments. The BMA demanded full reimbursement for practice expenses, but the Ministry was unable to recommend this to the Review Body, arguing for some proportion below 100 per cent to avoid the necessity of direct supervision of the expenditures and reimbursement. The BMA insistence on special payment for work outside the hours of a normal working day met with substantial but not unlimited success. The government reluctantly agreed to pay physicians both for being responsible for patient cases between 8:00 p.m. and 8:00 a.m. and for actually going out on home visits between midnight and 7:00 a.m. The BMA had requested actual payment for any night call during the whole period outside the normal working day.

The evident pattern is that of the government intermittently qualifying or slightly adjusting the requests that the BMA makes on method. These requests may well be those which the government at an earlier date has suggested. But the timing of their serious consideration is determined by the BMA. In short, the BMA exercises both positive and negative influence, determining what is done through suggestion and veto. Typically, the government manages to get its way only when a preferred method of payment is known to be favored by only a small proportion of the physicians, as was the case in item-for-service remuneration. Only a small proportion favored salary, but the Ministry itself approved of this unit, and the lack of sharp disagreement produced the expected outcome. Until the profession had given up its crusade against salary, the Ministry avoided serious suggestion of it.

As with the old issue of salary, the use of a pool in establishing a desirable average physician income was sacrosanct until the profession itself recommended its abolition. As early as 1960, discussions took place within the Treasury and the Ministry of Health on the anomalies of the pool. But the government refrained from suggesting to the Royal Commission that the pool be either done away with or substantially changed. Instead, discussion took place with BMA leaders on whether the pool would be changed so that practice expenses could be reimbursed more directly. These discussions proceeded in the early 1960s, and there was substantial agreement by 1965 that this change should take place. When the profession took the view, after the crisis over the Fifth Report, that the pool should be abolished, the government acceded to their wishes. Here was another illustration of the veto and initiating power of the professional organization. Since 1948 they had been able to foreclose the suggestion of doing away with the pool. In 1965, they were able to go beyond the limited Ministry suggestion of extracting practice expenses from the pool payments.

It is idle to provide further illustrations of BMA influence during the 1965–6 period. What should be clear is the basis for their successes. None of the variables mentioned by Eckstein changed between 1964 and 1966, except the constituency resources of the BMA. The style of negotiations leading up to the 1965 crisis was the same, regular consultations at the top floor of the Ministry of Health that took place in the summer of 1965. The Review Body was the authoritative decision-maker on the amount of payment both in 1965 and 1966. What had changed was the mobilization of professional opinion. The threat to strike had intervened. The Ministry at no time was worried about the resignation of 17,000 doctors, and the BMA was never confident that more than a third of that number would actually go out of the NHS.[7] But the fear was that substantial sections of the country would be faced with a crisis of medical supply, that a government with only a bare majority would face a crisis of confidence. Even after the election of 1966 the government was not willing to face such a NHS catastrophe, although it is clear that some members of the Cabinet were willing to consider a rejection of the Review Body recommendations on amount, and hence the negotiated methods that had preceded the determination of amount. But these pressures were, it appears, rejected almost as soon as they were brought forward.

The 1965–6 crisis represents an almost unbroken string of BMA victories. These victories support the hypothesis that doctors get their way on methods of payment when two conditions are satisfied: when intense and widespread doctors' preferences are known by the actors in the decision-making process, and when large additional public funding is not entailed. We would offer this hypothesis as one covering all medical-political systems in the democratic and developed world except Israel, where the relative oversupply of physicians reduces the threat of a breakdown in the public provision of medical care. In fact, large Exchequer contributions were also conceded in the 1965–6 crisis, but the victory on amount is *analytically and temporally distinct* from the policy changes on method. The granting of a 35 per cent payment increase in a time of general wage squeeze can only be interpreted as an extraordinary concession to medical demands. This is doubly evident when one considers that the profession was given a 10 per cent increase just a year earlier, and no criteria used to establish the 10 per cent figure had changed to promote an upward revision; rather, pressure had arisen for lower payments to all government employees.

The comparative study of the US and Swedish cases offers support for both the positive hypothesis and the rejection of the Eckstein emphasis on the "style" of bargaining in explaining medical policy decisions. In the United States, any method other than item-of-service payment was foreclosed by what might be termed *tacit* bargaining. The medical profession did not in fact take part in the detailed drafting of the Medicare law, and only consultation took place at the administrative stage in 1966–7. But the outcome was precisely what the AMA would have demanded had they been asked, and these implicit preferences were recognized by all the legislative and administrative actors concerned: a clear case of anticipated reaction. Interviews show that, although many of the executive officials would have preferred other methods (a limited fee schedule), they were unwilling to precipitate an open dispute with the profession. And they recognized that members of the profession were not simply income maximizers (at least in the short run) when they insisted that patients be permitted to be the source of payment under the Medicare program. A reimbursement plan (direct billing option) involved the possibility that some patients would not pay their doctors, while billing the insurance companies (assignment option) would have insured 100 per cent payment, but up to the reasonable charge standard. The AMA contended that patient payment would keep the doctor further removed from the state. It also meant that some of the aged would be faced with either borrowing the money to pay the physician directly or signing promissory notes to the physician. In either case, the doctor was trading off income certainty for a preferred source of payment and risking money losses for the gain of distance from the federal government program. However odd such insistence may appear by international comparison, this demand illustrates the goals of status and independence which doctors seek to maximize in payment method disputes. What they prefer for these ends varies with the cultural definition of status and independence. But that they seek non-income ends and are successful in securing them against the insistence of the state holds for all three of the countries studied.[8]

The Swedish case testifies as well to the influence of medical organizations on payment policy. Without going into detail, it is apparent that the Swedish experience parallels that of England and the United States. The Swedish medical profession, a small and disciplined group, has obligingly accepted both a national health insurance scheme and expansion of its numbers, but has retained most of what it values in high status and remuneration. Swedish doctors have been successful in its attempts to retain a mixed system of employment and compensation methods. Options are kept open by retaining a sector of private practice not rigidly bound to a fee schedule. Thus, doctors, in both the private and public sector, are able to retain an important bargaining lever, a lever that has been used by the SL to resist government-sponsored schemes to increase ambulatory medical care in the hospital polyclinics.[9]

The very fact of similar successes by medical organizations in very dissimilar political settings is evidence against the local explanation of Eckstein and support for the hypothesis we have put forward. Decisive support would come from a comparison of effectiveness of those pressure groups which can withhold vital services (through limited substitutability or supply) and those, like teachers, who share national styles and methods of bargaining, but do not have the resources of a producer group like physicians.

It should be clear that the most promising tests of pressure group theory are not single-country studies, but those which use the comparative data that, at a theoretical level, are the only type of data that could confirm hypotheses like those Eckstein has put forward. When one reviewer commented that the Eckstein book is an "excellent example of how to conduct a case study if it is to have analytic value,"[10] he was surely unclear about the logical requirements of a study of pressure group effectiveness. What Eckstein provides is a conceptual introduction which is little more than the substitution of words like "all" and "every" for singular adjectives referring to the British case. He provides a case illustration of the use of a would-be universalistic theory which proceeds to individual cases without the intervention of comparative data and determinate hypotheses. As such, it is a book with a crippling methodological flaw. And, since it is widely read as a description of medical politics, its assumptions and conclusion are legitimate objects of analysis for those interested in explaining public health policy decisions in Western Europe and America.

THE DETERMINANTS OF GOVERNMENT PAYMENT METHODS FOR PHYSICIANS: BRITAIN, SWEDEN AND USA

This section sets forth more formally our findings about medical remuneration disputes in the above three countries and assesses the implications of these findings for scholarly analyses of health politics and of future policy decisions about how doctors ought to and will be paid.

The method of paying physicians in government programs is an important political issue in every society in which there are substantial public programs of personal medical care services. The issue of method is important, first, because there are substantial conflicts over the appropriate ways of paying physicians, conflicts both between the state and medical organizations and within the medical organizations. Second, it is important because the preferences for particular payment methods are intensely held, particularly by physicians. Hence disagreement over how to pay doctors usually becomes not only a public issue, but a strikingly bitter type of issue. Finally, decisions about payment methods are important because they have significant financial implications for both the governments and physicians involved. Western industrial nations typically spend more than 5 per cent of the gross national product on medical care services.[11] Health is thus a substantial industry within these nations; it is an industry with expensive component services, and the costs of those services are almost certainly going to continue to rise rapidly in the foreseeable future. As a result controversies over medical payment methods are likely to continue to be deeply divisive and important. Increasing prices and their fiscal impact on public programs ensure that much.

THE PROBLEM

This discussion focuses upon controversies concerning methods of pay and does not concentrate on disputes over the amount of income doctors should receive from the state. Both issues are important, and the decision to exclude the question of total payments in no way reflects the judgment that the latter topic is unimportant. The chief reason for excluding the amounts of payment as the object of investigation is that public decisions on methods of pay, while obviously affecting total expenditures, are not always about the amounts of pay that doctors receive. That is to say, governments make explicit decisions about the total income of physicians in some societies, or the total income physicians can expect to receive from the state. But this is not the case in all western industrial societies with substantial medical care programs. In some societies, notably the United States, decisions are in fact made about methods of pay (e.g., Medicare, 1965) and no explicit recognition is given to the likely implications of such methods for the total income physicians will enjoy. The latter issue becomes important if use of payment methods generates unexpectedly high program costs, as for example took place in the United States after 1966.[12] Hence, if one is interested in illustrating the workings of various political systems by taking into account the way they cope with a common burden, the common burden most easily discussed in the medical remuneration area is the public methods of paying doctors, not the amounts paid.

All governments must make decisions about how doctors are to be paid, whether those decisions are negative ones to exclude alternatives or positive ones to select among logical possibilities one method rather than another. By method of payment we mean the unit of payment (by person, by item-of-service, by salary units), the source of payment (patient, intermediary, government), and the bases of differentiating doctors for payment purposes (by type of practice, type of doctor, or type of result).[13]

Public medical care programs must answer, even through tacit acceptance, the question of which unit, which source, and which basis of differentiation are to be used in state payment of doctors. One way of framing the issue for comparative politics is to say: there are a finite number of logically possible units, sources, and bases of differentiation to be chosen among by governments; among these options governments must and do choose; hence the outcome of the decision process can be seen as the way by which a given political system copes with a burden common to a large class of political systems. Such studies offer the bases for estimating both the determinants of payment method decisions and, through comparative analysis, the constraints on what is not possible for western industrial countries to do in this controversial area of public policy.

CENTRAL ISSUES

The central research interest was in the following hypothesis: "Whatever the political and medical structure of a western industrial country, physician preferences determine the governmental methods of payment." This outcome takes place except when the preferences stated express views known by both doctors and government bargainers to represent only a minority of physicians within the relevant physician group. A striking example was the demand for item-of-service payments made in the course of the general practitioners' crisis in England in 1965.[14] The British government knew that this demand did not represent a widely held physician preference; so did the BMA. In the end, the BMA, to deal with its militant members, asked the government privately to set forth in writing the reasons why such a unit of payment could not be granted.[15]

As producers of a crucial service in industrial countries, and a service for which governments can seldom provide short-run substitutes, physicians have the overwhelming political resources to influence decisions regarding payment methods quite apart from the form of bargaining their organizations employ. The hypothesis thus links directly the economic and political attributes of physicians to public policy outcomes, and asserts that intervening bargaining variables are not central to explaining public policy decisions in this area. This hypothesis challenges the assumption that bargaining conditions are key factors in medical policy outcomes, an assumption set forth explicitly in Eckstein's *Pressure Group Politics.*[16]

The evidence gathered in the testing of this hypothesis is of two sorts. First, we have investigated the pattern of payment method decisions since World War II in three western industrial countries—Sweden, Great Britain, and the United States. Data from these countries include broad patterns of medical payment methods over time in the postwar period, reported in the secondary literature, and our own analysis of three extraordinarily controversial instances of payment method decisions in each of the three societies: the Medicare payment method decisions in the United States in 1965, the payment policy changes following the general practitioner strike crisis in Great Britain in 1965–6, and the payment methods introduced at the outset of the Swedish national health insurance program in 1955. The second major type of data collected was secondary analysis of payment methods used in other industrial countries, notably the Netherlands, West Germany, France, Switzerland, Spain, Italy, Canada, Greece, Poland, the Soviet Union and Israel.[17] We have considered our hypothesis in the light of both the secondary evidence and our fuller data on Swedish, English, and American decision patterns. We have analyzed the decisions on the basis of a model of payment method decisions, and tried to estimate the conditions under which the premises of the model are true—and hence the conclusion (our hypothesis) entailed. The model may be described as follows.

THE MODEL OF EXPLANATION

Premise 1. Doctors in western industrial countries prefer payment methods in public programs with which they were familiar before the onset of the public program in question.

Premise 2. Doctors are presumed[18] to be willing to strike over government efforts to change these familiar payment methods or to prevent changes which the overwhelming majority of the profession is thought to want and has expressed the desire for programs outside the public sector.

Premise 3. Western industrial states will never risk a medical strike because of the high political costs associated with the interruption of personal health services, irrespective of government views on the merits of physician demands concerning payment methods.

Premise 4. Such governments, while often disagreeing with physicians and their organizations about desirable methods of payment, prefer gaining medical concessions on the amount of expenditures in exchange for concessions on methods of payment.

Premise 5. The failure to satisfy widely understood medical preferences on payment methods is presumed in western industrial countries to be a sufficient condition for a physicians' strike.

Premise 6. In general, government medical officials prefer a salary method of payment.

Conclusions. Hence, whatever the political and medical structure of the western industrial country, medical preferences determine the methods of payment used in public medical care programs (subject to the constraint cited above). Worldwide, the methods for paying physicians are extraordinarily diverse. What they share, however, is a remarkably close resemblance to what physicians were used to before the programs began.[19]

The application of this model to the three national settings we have investigated highlights our disagreement with two prominent types of political science analysis:

a. Individual country studies cannot logically test the explanatory power of hypotheses which emphasize distinctive features of the individual political systems. On the basis of our model, the relevant structural attributes are the central elements in an explanation of payment method decisions by western industrial governments. If factors common to these countries account for common patterns of decision making, it is impossible to find this out by studying decisions of individual nations. In addition, there is no way of testing the superfluity or centrality of one or another attribute of a political system in explaining the pattern of decisions within a nation in the absence of comparison.

b. Studies which focus on political culture as a causal variable are called into question by our model, or more precisely, by the data used in testing our model. Political culture may well be an important variable in the explanation of some public policies, but our findings suggest that the economic power of physicians is an overriding political resource which washes away the effects of both the bargaining styles employed by physician organizations and the attributes of the political culture such as mass and elite conceptions of the nature and legitimacy of physician demands.

THE EXPLICATION OF THE MODEL

We now turn to an explication of both the premises and the conclusions of the model. First, in the most general terms, the argument is simply that doctors get their way on the methods of their pay. This generalization has very wide scope: the Western European industrial countries, North America, and the countries of the British Commonwealth at comparable levels of industrialization. The reason for this can be deduced from an analysis of the economic producer position of physicians (what it is they can produce, withhold, and whether or not their services are substitutable in the short run) and the ranking of goals on the part of bargaining antagonists, represented abstractly in the model as doctors and governments (see Figure below). Generally put, we argue that the political resources of physicians in western industrial countries are so overwhelming that institutional differences among the countries are rendered unimportant in accounting for public policies regulating the payment of physicians.

These comments on the geographic and economic limits of the application of the model should be extended to discussions of the limits of the model related to timing. The conditions under which the hypothesis is most likely to be true are twofold: (1) the initiation of a public medical care program in which the political costs of noncompliance by doctors are at their highest, given the expectations aroused by the statutory enactment of such a program and the increased likelihood that opposing doctors could be mobilized in preventing the initiation of such a program; and (2) circumstances in which mass physician protest is expressed, thus making salient again the possibility of a medical strike, a possibility that always exists on payment disputes, but neither is nor is perceived to be equally probable under all circumstances. A premise of the model is that a strike threat is a credible possibility. We argue that such a strike threat is always credible when traditional medical demands are violated or initiatives blocked, but that this constraint on government behavior is most evident at the time of mass protest or the initiation of a new public program.

Under what conditions are the other premises of the model true? Since the conclusion of the model follows logically from the premises, the description of the conditions under which the premises are true permits predicting the outcome we have described. Our factual premises concerning the preferences of

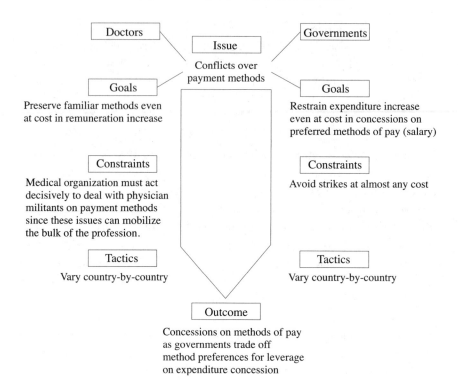

physicians and governments do not arise from either polling data concerning mass publics or structured interviews with a random sample of involved bureaucrats in the countries studied. Rather this distribution of preferences is inferred from secondary country studies[20] and interviews with key officials in England, Sweden, and the United States. We take confidence in these findings because only preferences widely understood are relevant to the model we have used. Typically, medical organizations and their government counterparts articulate the issues that shape medical care disputes. Our presumption about preferences is not restricted to these subgroups, but extends to widely held presumptions concerning the preferences of governments and doctors. Secondly, the description of preferences concerning methods of pay applies not to all features of the transmission of income from states to doctors, but rather to the three above-mentioned types of method issues. That is to say, preferences are relevant if and only if they deal with the unit, source, or basis of differentiation in the payment of doctors. Disputes about which unit to use, whether in England, for example, to pay general practitioners by salary or by capitation in the 1940s, exemplify the type of payment issue for which the model is relevant. Disputes about whether or not physicians paid by salary ought to be compensated every week or every two weeks are not relevant to the model. In short, mechanisms used in the administration of the type of unit, source, and basis of differentiation are not subject to the constraints to which the selection of the unit, source, or differentiation basis themselves are subject. We should add that why it is that doctors prefer the method they are used to is an issue in the sociology of the profession separable from the question of whether or not their preferences predict public policy results. It is worth adding, perhaps, that fee-for-service preferences have a logical relationship to market ideologies and may well be more extensive in societies where the social distance between physicians and patients is less marked, and where the imposition of market relationships is part of the subordination of patient by doctor, and doctor by patient. Likewise, the source of payment may well be more at issue in market-oriented societies because of the obligations generally entailed by the transfer of cash from consumers to producers (patients to doctors). Finally, differentiation of doctors for payment purposes may well reflect the degree to which there is wide acceptance of formal training accomplishment as an accurate indicator of medical ability, beliefs more typical in societies with marked class differences and aristocratic legacies.

The proposition that doctors prefer concessions on methods over concessions on amounts when they are forced to choose and are thought willing to strike over method disputes is true for all the cases investigated. But the political costs of an interruption of medical care services are reduced in societies like the USSR, where the supply of physicians has been expanded enormously through the revolutionary takeover of the medical profession. Israel is another exception. There the *per capita* supply of doctors is comparatively high, and hence the bargaining position of governments is comparatively stronger. By stronger, we mean that the government has a larger pool of physicians to call upon for emergency purposes. The ability of medical organizations to cripple health programs is thus diminished; the political costs of strike efforts are, as a result, lower for the state.

The third type of limit on the political costs of medical strikes is the degree to which politically relevant consumer groups take medical care to be a vital public service, one whose interruption counts as an extraordinary failure of the government in power. Non-modern societies, with major population groups outside the market economy, are what we have in mind. Public medical programs in such societies usually focus on environmental health problems (sanitation, epidemic control, and so forth) and the relevant elite groups are usually not dependent upon the public health service for their personal health care. This means that the interruption of public medical care programs is a burden for those sectors of the population least powerful politically and less likely than urban, middle class groups to consider the restriction of public health services decisive grounds for militant political protest.

Finally, we ought to make clear that in describing bargaining agents as governments and physicians we are well aware of the lack of descriptive realism. We have made use of simplifying abstractions for purposes of clarifying the main line of argument. We have specified the model in such terms while recognizing that qualifications could be made throughout. We are saying, however, that the bargaining process can be represented as if the relevant agents were in a dyadic relationship (doctors and government), and the test of the model is not the realism of the premises, but whether the model accurately predicts public policies governing medical pay methods.

RESEARCH PROCEDURES

Our research design specified the analysis of instances of medical payment conflict in three dissimilar institutional settings. Our purpose was to vary the political setting so as to test for the impact of what we took to be the comparable economic power of physicians in the three societies studied. Our second strategy was to use secondary information on the patterns of medical payment policy for a wider range of countries. Here our aim was to provide secondary confirmation (or disconfirmation) of the scope of the hypothesis we applied to the British, Swedish, and American experiences. Finally, our concern was to give case analyses of the initiation of issues, the limitation of what became at issue, and the policy outcomes in the three settings. Our design involved detailed analysis for three national arenas of medical payment policy and more summary evidence from the rest of the western industrial countries.

RESEARCH FINDINGS

The most important research finding was that the conclusion of the model accurately described public policy outcomes in the three countries studied. This was the case not only for the three instances studied in depth, but also for medical care payment conflicts over time in these countries. Moreover, the secondary evidence supported the extension of the hypothesis to the larger class of western industrial nations.

The major implications of these findings, first, is that national explanations of public policy in this controversial area are invalid, that explanations must use structural and economic variables rather than political and cultural ones in accounting for why it is that doctors get their way on how they ought to be paid. Second, there are methodological implications, the primary one being that

Table 1: Present payment methods

	Type of public medical System	Specialists		General practitioners	
		Unit of payment*	Source†	Unit of payment	Source
France	Insurance	Fee	Reimbursement	Fee	Reimbursement
Germany (Fed. Rep.)	Insurance	Fee	Direct	Fee	Direct
Great Britain	Health Service	Salary‡	Direct	Capitation	Direct
Israel	Insurance	Salary‡	Direct	Salary‡	Direct
Netherlands	Insurance	Salary, Fee, Case	Direct	Capitation	Direct
Sweden	Insurance	Salary, Fee	Reimbursement	Fee	Reimbursement
Switzerland	Insurance	Fee	Direct, Reimbursement	Fee	Direct, Reimbursement
USSR	Health Service	Salary‡	Direct	Salary‡	Direct
USA	Insurance	Fee	Direct, Reimbursement	Fee	Direct, Reimbursement
Canada	Insurance	Fee	Reimbursement	Fee	Direct Reimbursement

* Method of payment: salary, capitation, fee for service, case payments.
† Source of physician remuneration: direct government payment or patient payment and government reimbursement.
‡ In these cases changes have been made in public programs to introduce salaries instead of fees.
Source: adapted from Glaser, *Paying the Doctor*, p. 24.

cross-national research is essential for the adequate explanation of public policy outcomes. Finally, the policy implications are extraordinarily important.

POLICY IMPLICATIONS

First, the most important thing for governments to understand is both the nature of medical power and the limits on that medical power. We conclude that certain features of payment method controversies are, in fact, not negotiable however much these disputes are raised in the course of medical–government confrontations. That is the negative case we want to claim, the limits on what governments are able to do. Why governments are not able to control medical payment methods is accounted for in terms of the different priorities and economic power of the bargaining antagonists.

Knowing what governments cannot do, and what outcomes will take place, is of obvious importance to government officials involved in controversial negotiations. In health policy, such knowledge may permit concentrating on alternative means to the goals which traditional government payment preferences express. There are two alternatives to continually disputing the choice of payment methods. One is to concede the choice of method to physicians and concentrate on administrative technique to make undesirable methods less so. The other is to seek alternative ways to accomplish the goals which payment methods were to serve: reward of quality education, limits on excessive services, and so on. The application of this perspective in individual cases is best left out of this article. We want to suggest here only the direction such applications should take, based on our findings.

Notes

An earlier version of this article was published in the *British Journal of Political Science*, 2:421–442, 1972. An earlier version of the concluding section, "The Politics of Paying Physicians: US, UK, Sweden," was published in the *International Journal of Health Services*, 1 (1971):71–78. This version is from Theodore R. Marmor, *Political Analysis and American Medical Care* (Cambridge: Cambridge University Press, 1983).

1. Highly structured and regular in Great Britain and Sweden; diffuse and irregular in the United States, where consultation may take place in congressional hearings or through ad hoc meetings with executive officials responsible for public medical care programs.
2. Interview with Sir Donald Fraser, formerly Permanent Secretary of the Ministry of Health (April 1967).
3. David Mechanic and Ronald Faich, "Doctors in Revolt: The Crisis in the British Nationalized Health Service," *Medical Care*, VIII (1970), p. 444. Ralph M. Goldman, "Review of *Harry Eckstein, Pressure Group Politics*," *American Political Science Review*, LX (1961), 141.
4. Interviews with both BMA and governmental officials in 1967 provided the basis for this account. These officials understandably prefer to remain anonymous. See Mechanic and Faich, "Doctors in Revolt," for a similar interpretation.
5. For information on this episode, see Mechanic and Faich, "Doctors in Revolt."
6. For documentation of these decisions, see Mechanic and Faich, "Doctors in Revolt."
7. Interviews with BMA Secretary and National Health Service officials, Spring 1967.
8. See Glaser, *Paying the Doctor*, and "The Problem" section in this article.
9. David J. Thomas, *Postwar Swedish Medical Politics*, unpublished research report for US Public Health Service, 1968.
10. Ralph M. Goldman, Review of *Harry Eckstein, Pressure Group Politics*, 141.
11. B. Abel-Smith, "Health Expenditure in Seven Countries," *The Times Review of Industry and Technology*, March 1963, p. vi.
12. Department of Health, Education and Welfare, *A Report to the President on Medical Care Prices* (Government Printing Office, February 1967), and a report published by the Ways and Means Committee, July 1971, for evidence of interest in physician incomes and the impact of public programs on those incomes. See also L. H. Horowitz, "Medical Care Price Changes

During the First Year of Medicare," Research and Statistics Note No. 18, pp. 3–4 (Social Security Administration, 31 October 1967); E. T. Chase, "The Doctors' Bonanza," *The New Republic*, XV (1967), 15–16.

13. Theodore R. Marmor, "Why Medicare Helped Raise Doctors' Fees," *Transaction*, September 1968.

14. British Medical Association, *A Charter for the Family Doctor Service* (London: British Medical Association, 1965), p. 1.

15. Confidential interviews with British Medical Association officers and Ministry of Health officials, Spring 1967.

16. Eckstein asserts that negotiations with the British Medical Association are typically "intimate," that the issues are "treated as a matter between the Ministry and the profession . . . the powers of the profession [are] at their maximum, those of the Ministry at their minimum" (8, p. 125). The two case studies Eckstein presents to illustrate this generalization provide ambiguous support. More important, varying the bargaining tactics and atmosphere across the three countries does not coincide with differences in medical influence on the salient question of payment methods.

17. B. Abel-Smith, "Paying the Family Doctor," *Medical Care*, I (1963), 27–35; B. Abel-Smith, "The Major Pattern of Financing and Organization of Medical Services That Have Emerged in Other Countries," *Medicare Care*, III (1965), 33–40; Glaser, *Paying the Doctor*; J. A. Schnur and R. D. Hollenberg, "The Saskatchewan Medical Care Crisis in Retrospect," *Medical Care*, IV (1966), 111–19; Badgley and Wolfe, *Doctors' Strike*.

18. The actors whose views are referred to here are government officials responsible for payment decisions concerning doctors. References to the government are broader, meaning the whole range of actors involved in the fiscal decisions of a modern industrial state.

19. Marmor, "Why Medicare Helped Raise Doctors' Fees," p. 25; Abel-Smith, "Paying the Family Doctor," p. 27.

20. Abel-Smith, "Paying the Family Doctor," p. 27; "The Major Pattern of Financing and Organization," p. 36; Glaser, *Paying the Doctor*, p. 26.

Constitutional and Distributional Conflict in British Medical Politics

The Case of General Practice, 1911–1991

Patricia Day and Rudolf Klein

In the twentieth century there have been three major confrontations between the state and the medical profession in Britain: in 1911, 1945 and 1989. These have been major in two quite different senses. First, they involved disputes about the structure of the health care system itself: the way in which it should be organized and run. Secondly, they involved disputes about the structure of the decision-making process: the rights of various actors to participate in the health care policy arena. On both counts, they can be said to be fundamental in the sense of being concerned with the constitution of the health care system. There have, of course, been other disagreements, some of them extremely sharp. Wrangles over pay have punctuated the history of the National Health Service (NHS). In the 1960s there was much hullabaloo over the Family Doctors' Charter, the manifesto of disaffected general practitioners; in the 1970s the Wilson government and the medical profession came into collision over private practice. Indeed one of the characteristics of the NHS is precisely that it tends to politicize issues: denied the option of exit, since there are few alternative sources of employment, its providers use voice. However, the conflicts of the 1960s and 1970s were contained by consensus about the structure, organization and financing of the NHS.[1] They were distributional rather than constitutional, so distinguishing them from the events of 1911, 1945 and 1989 even though money featured in all three.

We concentrate on these three episodes because, by so doing, it may be possible to resolve a central puzzle in the history of political theory as applied to health care policies: the failure of political theory (here used in the sense of conceptual tools designed to explain or account for policy) to make any sort of consistent sense of events. In part, this may simply reflect the neglect of this policy area over the decades in the mainstream political science literature; a neglect which would have been total until the 1970s but for the activities of American scholars. But it may also reflect the susceptibility of political science to fashion. Going through the literature on health policy is rather like leafing through the back issues of magazines and noting when hemlines moved or male models stopped wearing ties. In the 1950s and 1960s, it was all about pressure groups—a kind of protocorporatism. In the early to mid-1970s, it was all about incrementalism, with just a dash of Marxism. In the later 1970s and 1980s, it was all about corporatism. In the 1990s, we seem to have moved into an era of post-modern eclecticism, marked by the use of the prefix "neo": so we get neo-elitism, neo-pluralism, neo-Marxism, and so on.[2] It is therefore tempting to resurrect the conclusion, drawn by one of the authors 17 years ago, that all the theoretical tools "explain something but that none explains everything."[3] Perhaps we should just reconcile ourselves to theoretical polytheism, and abandon hope of explanatory parsimony. Furthermore, it may be argued that the various theories are not necessarily in conflict but may even complement each other.

It may just be that explanatory promiscuity or prodigality reflects confusion about what is being explained. In other words, the finding that divergent theories all have some plausibility may mean that there is no such thing as health politics; that this is simply a loose (and in some ways deceptive) label for a great many diverse types of activity. The fact that issues crop up within the health policy arena does not, after all, mean that they are the same conceptually. Indeed even to talk about a "health care arena" may be misleading; it would be more accurate to conceptualize it as a complex of different if related arenas, with different if overlapping sets of actors. So the medical arena is a subset of the health policy arena and the general practice arena is a subset of the medical arena. In Marmor's formulation, "there are political struggles in the arena termed health, but not a politics of health."[4] Moreover, these "political struggles" will inevitably vary as the political, economic and social environment changes. In other words, the reason why different theories may all appear to work, but only inconsistently or partially, is that they are temporally contingent, as well as specific to particular types of situations or particular kinds of issues. If so, the way out of postmodernist confusion may be not to try to glue different pieces of theory together but to state more precisely the conditions under which specific explanatory tools may be expected to be useful. By taking the events of 1911, 1945 and 1989—and by comparing them with what happened in the years between these dramatic, confrontational crises—we intend to identify two different types of situations and policy outcomes, calling for different explanatory tools.

In doing so, we distinguish between the politics of structural innovation and the politics of adaptation, between abnormal and routine politics.[5] Our contention is that what happened in 1911, 1945 and 1989 cannot be explained in terms of the norms, routines and power relationships of the health policy arena (obviously so in the 1911 case since it was precisely the Liberal government's national insurance legislation that created the health policy arena). In each of these three cases, the explanation has to be sought in the wider political, economic and social environment; in each case, too, there was the kind of political landslide that transformed the contours of the policy scene and made it necessary to draw new maps, and not just in the health policy arenas. However, the periods of policy implementation and adaptation between and after these epochal years call for a very different kind of interpretation. They can best be understood, in our view, in terms of the politics of the double bed.[6] By this, we mean the corporatist style of policy-making[7] that became one of the hallmarks of the NHS but was already evident in the circumstances of its creation; a partnership of mutual dependence between the state and the medical profession which conceded a large degree of veto power to the latter.

THE BIRTH OF NATIONAL HEALTH INSURANCE

The introduction of national health insurance is a classic case study of pressure group politics. Lloyd George first introduced his scheme in 1908 and the legislation came into effect in 1911, but as Gilbert's account demonstrates, the final product bore little resemblance to the original plan. "The total reconstruction of the Liberal Government's first plan for health care for workers was . . . the result of the powerful and conflicting political pressures exerted by the three great social institutions most affected by health insurance—the friendly societies, the commercial insurance industry and the British medical profession."[8]

The events, Gilbert concluded, illustrated the thesis put forward by the Webbs that "the real government of Great Britain is nowadays carried on, not in the House of Commons at all, not even in Cabinet but in private conferences between Ministers with their principal officials and representatives of the persons specifically affected by any proposed legislation or by any action on the part of the administration."[9]

The details of the negotiations between 1908 and 1911—and the subsequent conflicts with the British Medical Association (BMA) over scales of pay which staggered on until 1913—are of no concern here. We shall only bring out those characteristics of this episode relevant for our general theme. First, the outcome marked the successful assertion by the BMA of the right to be involved in negotiations affecting its members. While formulating the Bill, Lloyd George "consulted the doctors as little as possible."[10] Indeed they were seen as less important than the Approved Societies and the insurance industry. It was the militant reaction of the medical profession that forced Lloyd George to change tack. The BMA mobilized its members in 1911, collecting the signatures of 26,000 practitioners ready to boycott Lloyd George's scheme. It successfully edged its way into the "private conferences" with ministers and their officials and in so doing asserted its right to be involved in the policy-making process. The structured relationship that emerged from the conflict was already well established by the 1920s. Interestingly, James Smith Whitaker, the BMA's Medical Secretary during the years of conflict, became a Senior Medical Officer at the Ministry of Health in 1919. It is not surprising that the official history of the BMA, published in 1932, sums up the outcome of the conflict as follows:

> In retrospect the achievement of the Association must be regarded as of the first importance. It was able to secure the acquiescence of the great majority of the medical profession of the country to its acting as the voice of the profession, no serious attempts being made during the fight to dispute its authority. Its action radically altered the original nature of a system which provides medical attendance for a third of the population, and the alterations were all of a nature which brought the system more into line with the wishes of the profession. The position thus secured by the Association has never been lost—on the contrary, each successive Government has acknowledged the Association as the representative organisation of the whole profession, a gain which in itself would justify all the energy and money expended during the struggle.[11]

Secondly, quite apart from establishing its place as a leading actor in the policy arena, the BMA won a number of victories on points of substance. Specifically, it won the battle against lay dominance in the administration of the insurance scheme and successfully asserted the right of doctors to be involved in the implementation of health policy. Lloyd George's original plan had been based on the assumption that the administration of the new system would be carried out by the Approved Societies, since these would have a direct interest in limiting medical discretion in treatment and prescribing in order to protect their own funds (Lloyd George was greatly obsessed with the problem of malingering). And it was precisely because the medical profession did not want its discretion limited by the Approved Societies—old antagonists, in any case—that they fought Lloyd George's proposals so strenuously. In the outcome, the BMA was successful. Control of the system was given to the newly created Insurance Committees, on which the medical profession was strongly represented; a system of administration which was to persist with remarkably little alteration, albeit under various names, until the changes of the 1990s. As Lloyd George noted: "This is the first occasion I think in the history of this country in which a body of persons engaged in any calling have been secured, by statute, the opportunity of being represented and consulted by the local authority as to the lines on which local administration of public work should be conducted."[12]

In addition, the BMA secured one of its other main objectives, designed to protect the autonomy of the doctor against lay interference. This was the principle that patients should be free to choose their own doctors and vice versa. It is not surprising that this has been the aim of medical professions cross-nationally, since it protects the doctor's freedom to decide whom to treat and how.

Following the introduction of national health insurance, the period between the wars was one of much discussion but little substantive change in the organization of health care or the place of the general practitioner in it.[13] The right of representation in the policy process, established by the pre-1914 struggle, was in no way weakened. The BMA played an active part—demonstrating its ability to use veto power—in the events leading up to the creation of the NHS.

THE CREATION OF THE NHS AND OF CONSENSUS

The 1911 legislation introduced a system of health insurance that gave the employed working-class population access to general practice. By the outbreak of war in 1939 there was general agreement that this system would have to be extended to the rest of the population and to the hospital sector. The years of the wartime coalition government were a period of continuous planning that saw the production of a series of draft proposals and white papers.[14] In strong contrast to the events leading up to the unveiling of Lloyd George's plans, the medical profession was soon involved. In effect, their right to be represented in the policy-making process was conceded. Moreover, of all the interest groups whose meetings with officials and ministers are recorded in the massive departmental files, the BMA was clearly the most powerful. The Approved Societies and the insurance industry, key actors 30 years earlier, were fading fast from the scene; the voluntary hospital and local authority lobbies were surprisingly ineffective. The key to reform, it was accepted, was to win the consent of the BMA and with it the cooperation of the medical profession in the implementation of post-war policy.

Despite these intensive private negotiations, there was also public confrontation, but by the time the 1945 Labour government arrived in office and its Minister of Health Aneurin Bevan prepared his plans for the NHS, the

BMA had achieved victory in the main issue concerning general practice that emerged during the negotiations. It successfully defended the 1911 settlement and defeated the attempt to turn general practice into a public service. Sir John Maude, the Ministry of Health's Permanent Secretary, had pushed hard for a salaried general practitioner service working out of local authority health centers.[15] This was a vision of bureaucratic rationality calculated to enrage the BMA—and so it did. For the effect of the Maude proposals would have been to rob general practitioners of their independent contractor status as enshrined in the 1911 settlement, guaranteed by the fact that they were paid not salaries but capitation fees for the patients on their list. Moreover, it would have replaced Insurance Committees—on which doctors were strongly represented, as previously noted—by local authorities as the administrative agencies responsible for the delivery of health care. The proposals thus raised the twin spectres of lay control and diminished medical autonomy. No other issue was so central to the medical profession. There were other issues on which the BMA fought, such as the abolition of the right to buy and sell general practices, but on most of these it was prepared to compromise or even to accept defeat. The independent status of the general practitioner, guaranteed by capitation payments and by a separate administrative machinery, was a very different matter. The BMA fought and won.

By the time Bevan took office, the Maude proposals were dead and he did not attempt to resurrect them.[16] The paradox of the confrontation between the Labour government and the medical profession—which was to lead to an extremely vicious public debate (on both sides) and a series of strike threats by the BMA—is that it largely hinged on the least radical part of Bevan's plan. It was his proposals for nationalizing the whole hospital system that represented a break with the past. Endless ingenuity had previously gone into attempts to maintain both voluntary and local authority hospitals while unifying planning, but these aroused surprisingly little opposition, perhaps because of Bevan's willingness to square the Royal Colleges and to buy off the specialists with financial and other concessions. Instead, there was a two-year battle with the BMA largely over general practice issues, despite the fact that Bevan's proposals accepted the contractor status of general practitioners and the survival of the Insurance Committee machinery. The battle did not end until 1948, when Bevan introduced amending legislation—abjuring all intention of introducing a salaried service—and the BMA's troops started to desert its leadership, so forcing it to abandon its aggressively combative stance (much of the same pattern as in the years after 1911 and, as we shall see, 1989).

It is difficult to explain the anger and bitterness of the confrontation between Bevan and the BMA in terms of the substantive issues involved. True, his

scheme did include provision for a salary element in general practitioner remuneration, in addition to the capitation payments—a method of remuneration
happily embraced by the medical profession in the 1960s. True, it also included
proposals for experimenting with local authority health centres. True, too, there
was much conflict about how to calculate capitation payments and compensation for the abolition of the right to buy and sell practices. But all this would
seem fairly small change in a settled system of corporatist-style negotiation; precisely the kind of shocks that such a system is designed to absorb. The main
explanation for the confrontation therefore seems to be that Bevan's approach
challenged the system: in effect, he announced his decisions without first going through the ritual of consultation and negotiation. More important still, it
challenged the right of the medical profession to participate in policy-making.
To the BMA, Bevan appeared to be redefining the relationship between the
state and the medical profession. Again, the BMA's official history is instructive
on this point. Writing more than 30 years after the events, the history concedes
that the "pretexts of the dispute were technical," but argues that "so long as
the Minister of Health exhibited a high-handed, truculent attitude towards the
medical profession the doctors were united against him."[17] The 1948 amending
legislation was thus important not for what it said but for what it symbolized:
an act of ministerial penitence, acknowledging the special status of the medical
profession, a status which, as the profession was subsequently to argue successfully, had to be reflected in its rewards.

Created amidst controversy, the NHS was soon cocooned in consensus. Over
the following decades, the NHS not only established itself as Britain's most
popular institution next to the monarchy—invariably receiving top ratings in
all public opinion surveys—but increasingly came to be strongly supported by
those who had fought its creation: the medical profession. (This is a recurring
pattern: in 1945 general practitioners went into battle in order to preserve the
1911 settlement which they had fought so strenuously at the time of its introduction.) There were, of course, frequent conflicts between successive governments and the doctors, but these were, for the most part, about money, not
about the structure of either the NHS itself or of the relationship between the
medical profession and the state. In effect, the medical profession had achieved
the ability to veto policy change by defining the limits of the acceptable and
by determining the policy agenda. Whether this reflects the structure of the
relationship between the state and the profession (as corporatist theory might
demand), or simply the dependence of the state on doctors to implement policy
and to keep the NHS running, is perhaps an open question. But it may not be a
particularly important or interesting question. If indeed the state is dependent

on the medical profession (and other providers), then the precise institutional forms or patterns of interaction that emerge may not be all that critical.[18]

Certainly the pattern of policy into the 1980s can best be described as corporatist in style, defined as conflict contained by consensus: an awareness by both sides that they could not risk pushing their differences to the point where they might threaten the survival of the NHS itself. The result, almost always, was compromise. So the Family Doctor Charter battle of the 1960s[19] both gave the profession much of what they wanted (more money, higher status, seniority payments for long-serving GPs) and allowed the Ministry of Health to start changing the organization of general practice (by introducing incentives for group practice, for training and for postgraduate education). There were, in short, no conflicts which could not be solved through the normal machinery of negotiation and by an injection of extra funds.[20] Perhaps the best definition of a constitutional or fundamental conflict—of the kind identified in 1911, 1945 and 1989—might therefore be that it is one which cannot be resolved by giving the medical profession more money (although this is always a useful prescription for dealing with subsequent bruises). The reasons why the 1989 Review of the NHS falls into the category of constitutional confrontations are now explored.

BREAKING THE MOULD—AND STICKING IT TOGETHER AGAIN

In April 1990 the government, for the first time in the history of the NHS, imposed a new general practitioner contract on the medical profession. The defeat for the medical profession, as represented by the BMA, was all the more humiliating given that it followed a campaign against the government unprecedented in its relentless ferocity, as well as in the scale of expenditure on mobilizing public opinion. But the BMA had taken to the advertising hoardings only to advertise its own impotence in the face of a government determined to impose its own programme of change. Moreover, it was a double defeat. On the one hand, the government's policies involved changes in the structure of the NHS that threatened the autonomy of doctors as traditionally defined by the medical profession itself. On the other hand, the government had demonstrated its willingness, and ability, to push these changes through without involving the medical profession in the policy-making process. In both respects, Kenneth Clarke—then Secretary of State for Health—established his claim to be considered alongside Lloyd George and Aneurin Bevan in the history of health policy in Britain, as someone responsible not just for incremental change but for pushing policy in a new direction.

The main features of this drama can be presented as a play in three acts. In the first, the government sets about reforming general practice in the traditional corporatist style by involving the medical profession and seeking to build consensus. It is a cosy family play. In the second, this limited exercise is caught up in the more comprehensive and radical Review of the NHS, with the result that the curtain falls on a scene spattered with blood and littered with corpses. It is the end of Hamlet. In the third, the corpses have got up and are beginning to talk to each other. We seem to be back to the beginning of the first act, but both actors and audience know that things will never be quite the same again. While there may be a return to traditional process, there has been a decisive shift in the terms of the debate.

ACT 1. OVERTURE TO CHANGE

The government's green paper, setting out its first thoughts for change in the organization of general practice, was published in April 1986.[21] The proposals there set out were intended to achieve three main policy aims. First, they were designed to improve the quality of general practice, by means of a "good practice allowance" paid to those doctors who met certain criteria. This represented a resurrection of an idea that had been killed by the medical profession during the Family Doctor Charter negotiations in the 1960s but which now had the support of the Royal College of General Practitioners. Secondly, they were designed (in line with the government's general stance, as evident in its policies towards schools) to make professional providers more sensitive to consumer preferences. This was to be done by making it easier to change doctors and to make complaints, as well as by increasing the proportion of general practitioners' incomes drawn from capitation payments (which had slumped to 45 per cent as a result of changes made in the 1960s and subsequently). Thirdly, they were designed to bring greater managerial control over the activities of general practitioners, in particular over their prescribing. Most of the primary health care budget is not covered by cash limits, and throughout the 1980s this open-ended commitment grew at a much faster rate than spending on the hospital and community services. There was therefore widespread concern, not least in the Treasury, about whether this investment was bringing value for money, for example, by relieving pressure on hospitals.

After the publication of this green paper, there followed an elaborate round of consultations. Norman Fowler, the Secretary of State, and his Ministers went on a tour of Britain to elicit reactions at a series of local meetings. When the government published its white paper in November 1987,[22] it was clear that it was determined to stick to its main policy aims, while making concessions to the medical profession. The main themes of the green paper were, if any-thing, spelled out more emphatically: for example, the increased managerial responsibilities of Family Practitioner Committees (lineal descendants of Lloyd George's Insurance Committees). But some of the most contentious means for achieving them were either dropped—notably the proposal for a good prac-tice allowance, which the BMA resolutely opposed as divisive—or modified. The scene appeared to be set for a prolonged round of negotiations between the Department of Health and the General Medical Services Committee of the BMA: the kind of gritty wrangling about the details of the general practitioner contract—and, in particular, over the small print of financial provision—that had become institutionalized over the decades. It was the kind of negotiating process that severely tested the stamina and temper of the participating civil servants and doctors, since it could be expected to go on for years. But in this case the process was brutally cut short by the NHS Review.

ACT 2. ENTER PRIME MINISTER, PURSUING DOCTORS

In January 1988 the Prime Minister, Margaret Thatcher, announced a Review of the NHS.[23] This had nothing to do with general practice initially, although pri-mary health care policy subsequently became involved. It was largely a response to the mounting political pressure on the government—orchestrated as much by the medical profession as by the opposition parties—about the "underfund-ing" of the NHS's hospital services. The NHS, it was argued, was on the point of collapse because of the government's financial parsimony. More specifically, the Prime Minister's announcement of the Review—which surprised both her own Cabinet colleagues and the Department of Health's civil servants—was precipi-tated by a public denunciation of the government's policies by the Presidents of the Royal Colleges. This represented, in Mrs. Thatcher's view, a repudiation of the implicit concordat[24] between the state and the medical profession forged by the creation of the NHS whereby the state accepted the right of the medical pro-fession to use the available resources without question, while the medical profes-sion in exchange accepted the right of the state to set the budgetary constraints within which it worked. In short, the medical profession was assured almost total autonomy—with virtually no accountability—while the state could delegate to doctors the job of rationing. Decisions about resource allocation were, in effect, disguised as clinical decisions. By challenging the government's budgetary con-straints, the profession—in Mrs. Thatcher's view—was in effect reneging on the deal. The review itself reflected, in both form and substance, the impulse that had given birth to it, as well as the Prime Minister's more general suspicion of professional power. The medical profession was excluded from it and its claims of autonomy came under challenge. There were no representatives of the BMA or of the Royal Colleges in the working group that Mrs. Thatcher assembled around her. There was no call for evidence from any of these bodies, either. Even the Department of Health, with its institutionalized links to the profession, was peripheral to the exercise: it submitted papers, and responded to proposals that came up but did not play a leading role in the development of policy ideas. When the Review was finally published in January 1989[25] many of its proposals affronted the medical profession. It was suspicious of the notion of an internal market; it was hostile to the creation of trusts, which would be free to set their own salary levels and terms of service (so threatening the role of the national negotiating bodies like the BMA). Above all, it was threatened by the increasing emphasis on the accountability of doctors, as evident in the proposals for medical audit, a new and much more specific consultant contract and a revised system for making distinction awards which would actually involve managers, as well as doctors, in the process.

We shall later explore these specific proposals, in so far as they concerned general practitioners, but it is difficult to escape the impression that the medical profession's violent reaction to them was largely coloured by the style in which they had been produced; by the fact that the Review, as such, represented a challenge to its position as a leading player in the health policy arena. It is a point well made by Kenneth Clarke:

> The BMA, the Royal Colleges, never recovered from the feeling that they had not been consulted. They were deeply shocked that we weren't going down the traditional path. They were easily persuaded during this secret period that this was some group of ideologues, producing a market-based solution to health, which they were going to fight and they prepared to fight it even before they even knew what it was. . . . We would have found the whole thing easier had we consulted. On the other hand, experience I think would show, had we consulted we'd have taken two, three years over the process, and the input from the interest groups, as well as from the rest of the political world, would largely have been in favour of the status quo, slightly amended with more money, and we would never have come up with any reforms at all.[26]

Indeed the medical profession's reaction to the Review only makes sense if it is seen as a response to an affront to its collective sense of self-esteem. The Review signaled, in effect, that doctors had lost their right of veto over policy. Many of their charges against the government's specific proposals were extravagant nonsense. Perhaps the most remarkable (and neglected) aspect of the Review was that, despite having been set up to consider new ways of funding health care in Britain, it concluded by endorsing the universal, tax-financed system created in 1948. But behind the hysteria there was a totally realistic recognition that the profession had been beaten; in future, it could not rely merely on its status but would increasingly be tethered by contract.[27]

The case of general practice illustrates these points well. The Review's proposals for general practice were, in the main, variations on themes already developed in the previous policy documents. There is remarkable consistency over time in these, reflecting the fact that they were mostly the product of evolutionary departmental thinking rather than of Conservative ideological impulses. If there is any ideology shaping the general practice proposals it is, indeed, the ideology of the public health profession, with its emphasis on encouraging preventative medicine and the development of better quality practice, particularly in inner cities. So, for example, the original good practice allowance—killed by the medical profession, as already noted—became transmuted into a system of performance-related pay, which made some payments contingent on the achievement of fixed targets for immunization and vaccination and cervical cytology.

However, there were a number of specific innovations in the Review that were to cause a great deal of suspicion and aggravation, souring subsequent negotiations about the new contract. First, there was the introduction of general practice budgets: practices above a certain size (originally 1 1,000 patients, subsequently lowered to 9,000) could opt to become fundholders, allocated a budget out of which they would then buy the services required by their patients. This was very much Kenneth Clarke's personal idea, which he had long been pushing.[28] It was bitterly attacked by the medical profession on the grounds that it would introduce financial considerations into what should be purely clinical decisions (as well as raising the danger of adverse selection). Never mind that consultants had always to balance competing needs within constrained budgets; never mind that general practitioners had in the past put other trade-unionists in the shade with their unrelenting preoccupation with the financial small print of their contract. The BMA managed to convince itself that fundholding would introduce the canker of profit-seeking into the medical Eden.

Secondly, there was the introduction of indicative prescribing budgets for all general practitioners. The proposal was that all practitioners should be allocated budgets to cover their prescribing costs. Here the objective was "to place downward pressure on expenditure on drugs, particularly in those practices with highest expenditure, but without in any way preventing people getting the medicines they need."[29] It was a proposal that revived all the BMA's fears that the hidden agenda of the government's whole exercise was to put a cap on primary health care spending and to bring it under the same tight control that was already being exercised over the hospital and community services. The spectre of Treasury control certainly roamed the corridors of BMA House and helped to shape the subsequent campaign against the government's proposals; a campaign that caused much alarm among the elderly population of Britain threatened (according to the BMA) by the possibility that doctors would not be able to prescribe the drugs they needed or that they would turn away expensive patients.

Thirdly, there was the reshaping of the administrative machinery. Family Practitioner Committees (FPCs) were to be replaced by Family Health Service Authorities (FHSAs). These, in line with developments in the rest of the NHS, were to be managerial rather than representative bodies. FPCs were the product of the 1974 reorganization of the NHS, a reorganization that was planned in concert with the provider interests, in true corporatist fashion, and that gave those provider interests strong representation at all levels in the NHS.[30] Not surprisingly, therefore, FPCs—like the Insurance Committees before them— had a very strong element of professional representation. FPCs consisted of 30 members, of which eight were appointed by the Local Medical Committee (the body representing local general practitioners), while a further seven were nominated by the other primary health care professions like the dentists and the opticians. In sharp contrast, the Review promulgated that FHSAs would be small, managerial bodies, with a total membership of 11. Only one member would be a general practitioner and even that solitary figure would be appointed not by the Local Medical Committee but by the Regional Health Authority and would serve "in a personal, not a representative, capacity."[31] The great victory of 1911—the assertion that general practitioners would have a strong voice in the implementation of policy at the local level—had seemingly been largely undone. The corporatist machinery of local administration, first devised in 1911, was being dismantled. It was all the more disturbing for the medical profession, given that the responsibilities of FHSAs were to be greatly enlarged, in line with policy pronouncements from the time of the green paper onward, with more power to plan the pattern of primary health care provision and to call individual practitioners to account for their use of public funds.

The last point can be simply illustrated. In the regulations laid before Parliament in the autumn of 1989—and which came into effect at the same time as the new contract in April 1990—the responsibilities of general practitioners were spelled out as never before.[32] FPCs simply had the duty to ensure that GPs provided "all necessary and appropriate personal medical services of the type usually provided by general medical practitioners": the responsibilities of general practitioners were defined in terms of their own customs. But their successor bodies, the FHSAs, had the duty of policing a contract which laid down in great detail what general practitioners should do. So, for example, the contract required not only that general practitioners should invite all patients over 75 to participate in an annual assessment but also spelled out how that assessment should be carried out. In other words, FHSAs could call individual practitioners to account and indeed had a statutory duty to do so.

Not surprisingly the BMA's General Medical Service Committee (GMSC) rejected the new contract package, although the Secretary of State offered to make concessions provided that the medical leadership was prepared to recommend any agreement reached to the profession.[33] Perhaps the leadership knew that any recommendations it made were likely to be ignored. Instead the BMA polled its members in May 1989. Over 82 per cent took part in a ballot organized by the Electoral Reform Society. The result was an overwhelming vote—by 76 per cent to 24 per cent—against the government's package. There followed months of further negotiations. The Department offered a series of concessions to the profession on points of detail. So, for instance, it abandoned its original intention of abolishing seniority payments—originally introduced, on the insistence of the BMA, during the Family Doctor Charter negotiations of the 1960s—and payments for night visits. Similarly, it showed flexibility about the way in which the performance targets for immunization and vaccination were to be calculated. The GMSC leaders who had taken part in the negotiations recommended acceptance of the new terms, albeit with little enthusiasm, as the best obtainable. However, the conference of Local Medical Committees—called in March 1990 to consider the revised terms—rejected them "without a dissenting vote . . . as being ill considered and harmful to patients."[34] However, the Conference also rejected—if only by 153 to 148 votes—a call for sanctions against the imposition of the new contract. The government's calculation that the medical profession's opposition would be rhetorical rather than effective turned out to be correct. The new contract duly came into effect in April 1990.

ACT 3. BUSINESS AS USUAL

After the drama of confrontation came anti-climax—a return to the traditional politics of mutual accommodation. Having marched its troops into battle, the BMA found that its troops had no stomach for a prolonged campaign—a repeat of the pattern in the two previous confrontations. Indeed many deserted. Although the BMA had denounced fundholding as subversive of the principles of the NHS, there was no shortage of practices willing—often eager—to take part in this experiment. Even after winnowing out applications not considered suitable, almost 300 practices were on the starting line when the fundholding experiment started in April 1991. Moreover, general practitioners discovered that the contract was highly rewarding. The winners were in a majority. Indeed, in the first six months of the new contract, the average earnings of GPs were £3,000 higher than had been expected.[35] Conversely, the Department of Health—with a new Secretary of State at the helm, William Waldegrave— emphasized its concern to restore mutual confidence.[36] While insisting that the principles of the new contract were not negotiable, the new Secretary of State emphasized his flexibility in discussing the details with the profession. It was back to business as usual: a continuous process of niggling away about the small print of the contract, very much the same situation as that described by Eckstein in the 1950s[37] following the turmoil of the 1940s.

Again, the point can be simply illustrated. The Bible of every FHSA manager (and of every general practitioner) is what is known, from the colour of its covers, as the Red Book, which sets out the details of how payments should be made.[38] It is produced in a loose-leaf format to allow amendments to be slotted in as they are made. By the autumn of 1991, there were over 250 pages of such amendments. Most of these were relatively trivial or minor in character but overwhelmingly about money. So, for example, changes were made in the calculation of payments for minor surgery and health promotion clinics. The mass of amendments is testimony to the sheer complexity of running general practitioner services, as well as to the pertinacity of the BMA in getting the best possible financial deal for its members. It helps to explain, furthermore, why both the Department and BMA were prepared to resume their normal relationship: their bickering and differences constrained by the need to keep the show on the road and to sort out the problems of administering a uniquely complex organization dependent on the cooperation of the providers. We are back, in effect, to the theme enunciated at the start of this paper: that the NHS compels mutual dependence which brings about a particular style of corporatist incremental policy adjustment. Following the confrontational crisis, it was in the self-interest of government to be conciliatory and to revert to administering policy through the medical profession.

IMPLICATIONS FOR THEORY

Our analysis suggests that the initial distinction made between the politics of constitutional crisis and the politics of distributional conflicts in the NHS is sustained by the evidence of the past 80 years. The politics of constitutional crisis are, indeed, marked by disputes which call into question not just the structure of the health care system but the place of the medical profession within it. In all three cases—1911, 1945 and 1989—the confrontation between the state and the medical profession involved the latter's right of representation, both in the policy-making process itself and in its subsequent implementation. In all three cases, too, the medical profession's view of its own position—independent, autonomous and accountable only to itself—was at issue. In a sense, the medical profession, certainly as represented by the general practitioners and the BMA, were fighting, in these constitutional confrontations, to establish or maintain a corporatist-style, routine relationship with the state, which acknowledged their special position and their role in both making and implementing policy. It is therefore not surprising that a corporatist style is indeed the usual pattern in the health policy arena, as well as the preferred pattern as far as the medical profession is concerned. Leaving aside the crisis periods, corporatist theory appears to be vindicated.

Yet our analysis also underlines the limits of this type of theory. Corporatist theory is essentially descriptive, not explanatory—far less predictive. It tells us that change in the NHS is usually likely to be adaptive because the product of institutionalized compromise. Issues that can be resolved by an injection of extra money will be tackled. Issues that involve the distribution of power are likely to be side-stepped. But corporatist theory (in all its 57 varieties) does not help us to say very much about the likely direction of change or about the specific issues that are likely to appear on the policy agenda. If we are to explain change, we have to adopt a very different strategy of inquiry. We might, for example, have to analyse the economic and demographic pressures on health care systems internationally and to consider why there appears to be a cross-national drift to greater emphasis on managerialism and market competition.[39] We might, further, want to invoke the role of information technology in transforming all kinds of organizations; in particular by transforming the capacity, in terms of both speed and quantity, to monitor the performance of producers, doctors among them.

There are other problems about applying corporatist theory. They stem from analytical ambiguity about why corporatist-style arrangements come into being in the first place. Is it (as we have tended to argue) simply a functional response to the problems of creating and running institutions like the NHS? Such institutions, it might be argued, are characterized by their complexity and their dependence on groups of providers with monopolies of particular kinds of skill, a monopoly which, in the case of the medical profession, is based not just on statute but also its successful assertion of its special place in society. Like most functionalist-type explanations, this may be just a touch too bland. As we have seen, the emergence of corporatist-style arrangements has not just happened automatically or without pain. It is the result, rather, of active campaigning by the medical profession in pursuit of its own interests. However, once in place, corporatist-style arrangements appear to offer benefits to both sides. They are highly functional, in that they provide a machinery for routinizing the solution of the kind of problems that are inevitably and continuously thrown up in an organization as complex and large as the NHS. They are a recognition, as previously argued, of mutual dependence: the doctors dependent on the state for their legal professional monopoly and for resources; the state dependent on the doctors for the delivery of services and the acceptance of responsibility for rationing. This would certainly explain the rapid reversion to the invariable pattern of the politics of the double bed after periods of crisis.

However, puzzles remain. There are other areas of mutual dependence between state and providers (the universities might be one example) where corporatist-style arrangements have either never developed or have broken down. Even within the NHS, it would be difficult to argue that other providers have achieved the same position as the medical profession. So what is so special about doctors? Is the medical profession's place in the policy arena the result of its functional or of its social position? Does mutual dependence lead to corporatist-style arrangements only in the case of those monopolists of skill with a special place in the country's elite and in the hierarchy of power? Here the case of general practice, examined in this paper, is especially instructive. General practitioners in 1911 were the proletariat of the medical profession[40] and their subsequent rise in status and income is the product of their participation in the health policy arena, not its cause. It is therefore much more difficult to invoke elite theory to account for the bringing into being of corporatist-style arrangements in their case, in contrast to high prestige consultants. Even in the case of consultants, the evidence seems to be at best inconclusive.[41]

Above all, the theories which seem reasonably successful in explaining routine policy processes and outcomes offer very little help when explaining why corporatist-style arrangements broke down in 1945 and 1989. Nor is this problem limited to Britain. It does not reflect, as might plausibly be argued, the fragility of corporatist-style institutions in Britain. Our Black Swan is that paradigm of corporatism, Sweden. There the 1968 Seven Crowns Reform of the Swedish health care systems[42] was introduced without any of the customary exercises in consensus-building and discussion which are the normal pattern of policy-making, not just in the health arena. The result was a collision with the medical profession—not surprisingly, since the reform meant a move towards salaried doctors. In sharp contrast to Britain in 1989 (and offering a warning against looking for explanations exclusively in the New Right ideology of the Thatcher administration), the changes were introduced by a Social Democrat government committed to a corporatist style of policy-making, not by a radical Conservative government committed to a crusade against corporatism of all kinds.

It is beyond the scope of this paper to investigate how, and in what respects, the governments of 1911, 1945 and 1989 differed from their predecessors and successors. Even more so, it is beyond the scope of this inquiry to analyse the economic, social and political factors which produced these radical, reforming administrations whose policies changed the political landscape so that policy debate in all spheres, and not just the NHS, started from a new base.[43] But it is clear that the kind of political theories normally invoked to explain steady-state policy-making in the health care arena do not hold for these times. Such political theories are revealed as being contingent on specific circumstances: in particular, continuity and stability in the economic, political and social environment. No wonder, for example, that most studies of health policy in the 1960s and 1970s leant heavily on theories of incrementalism, since this was the period of Butskellism and attempts to create tripartite institutions of national policy-making. No wonder, either, that subsequent fashions in theory-building rapidly changed in an attempt to keep up with changes in the environment of policy-making.

The contingent nature of so much theory, ad hoc explanations stitched together to meet unexpected developments, would suggest a number of conclusions for the methodology of political theory as applied to policy practice, not just in the health policy arena. First, comparative policy studies are essential if we are to avoid the dangers of ethnocentric over-explanation, anchored in the circumstances of individual countries. Secondly, historical studies are essential if we are to avoid the dangers of temporal over-explanation, anchored in the circumstances of a particular political, economic and social epoch. Thirdly, we have to distinguish sharply between the characteristics of different policy arenas (even within such an umbrella concept as the health policy arena) and of the actors that inhabit them. Fourthly, we have to develop a taxonomy of issues cutting across arenas, so that we can analyse the relative contribution of arena characteristics. Our distinction between constitutional and distributional issue is one such attempt but there have been many others.[44] Unless we move in this direction, theoretical prolixity and incoherence will remain the norm, since we will not know precisely what it is we are trying to explain.

Notes

The article was first published in *Political Studies* 40(1992):462–478. We are grateful for the comments of Stephen Harrison, the journal's anonymous referees and the participants in the Politics of Health Care panel at the 1991 Political Science Association Conference, where this paper was first given. The research was funded by ESRC grant No. 600232419.

1. Rudolf Klein, *The Politics of the National Health Service*, London, Longman, 2nd edn, 1989, Chs. 3 and 4.

2. The first study to bring health policy into the mainstream of political science was Harry Eckstein, *Pressure Group Politics* (London, George Allen & Unwin, 1960), who argued that the power of the medical profession rested on the structured relationship between the Ministry of Health and the British Medical Association. Its thesis was subsequently challenged by Theodore R. Marmor and David Thomas, *Doctors, politics and pay disputes*, British Journal of Political Science, 2:4 (1972), 421–42, on the grounds that the medical profession appeared to enjoy similar power to veto change in pay arrangements in countries where there was no such structured relationship. An attempt to compare the explanatory power of different theories, reflecting the contemporary bias towards trying to explain micro-decisions rather than political turning-points, was made by Rudolf Klein, *Policy making in the National Health Service*, Political Studies, XXII:1 (1974), 1–14. A similar bias towards explaining the micro-implementation of policy is evident in David J. Hunter, *Coping with Uncertainty*, Chichester, Research Studies Press, 1980. Rather more ambiguous, and Marxisant, are Lesley Doyal, *The Political Economy of Health*, London, Pluto Press, 1979, and Chris Ham, *Health Policy in Britain*, London, Macmillan, 1982. The corporatist theme creeps in with Rudolf Klein, *The corporate state, the health service and the professions*, New Universities Quarterly, 31:2 (Spring 1977), and is subsequently developed in Alan Cawson, *Corporatism and Welfare*, London, Heinemann Educational Books, 1982. The most recent study of health policy-making is that of Stephen Harrison, David Hunter and Christopher Pollitt, *The Dynamics of British Health Policy*, London, Unwin Hyman, 1990. This explores the explanatory power of different theoretical approaches, concluding that no one theory can explain everything—though with a tentative bias towards neo-Marxist theory.

3. Rudolf Klein, *Policy problems and policy perceptions in the National Health Service*, Policy and Politics, 2:3 (1974), 219–36, especially p. 219.

4. Theodore R. Marmor, *Politics Analysis and American Medical Care*, Cambridge, Cambridge University Press, 1983, p. 54.

5. For a similar approach, which has influenced our thinking, see Ellen M. Immergut, *The Political Construction of Interests. National Health Insurance Politics in Sweden. France and Switzerland, 1930–1970*, Unpublished manuscript, Department of Political Science, Massachusetts Institute of Technology, 1990.

6. Rudolf Klein, *The state and the profession: the politics of the double bed*, British Medical Journal, 301 (3 Oct. 1990), 700–2.

7. The phrase "corporatist-style" has been used very deliberately in order to avoid becoming a casualty in the definitional battle about what "corporatism" means. For this, see Andrew Cox, *The Old and New Testaments of corporatism*, Political Studies, XXXVI: 2 (1988), 294–308, and Alan Cawson, *In defence of the New Testament: a reply to Andrew Cox*, Political Studies, XXXVI: 2 (1988), 309–15. We would accept Cawson's definition of corporate representation, as distinct from pressure group involvement in policy-making, as meaning that "corporations are involved in negotiation with the state not simply to press their demands but to act as agents through which state policy is implemented"; see Cawson, *Corporatism and Welfare*, p. 38. In short, there is a structured relationship of mutual dependency. Although we tend to identify the medical profession with the British Medical Association, in practice the picture is more complex: the BMA is certainly the main political voice of the profession but it has not got a complete

monopoly of representation since other bodies, like the Royal Colleges, may also be involved at times. Moreover, whereas the strong definition of corporatism would require the BMA to be able to deliver its troops, in practice the history of health care politics is notable for its failure to do so. At critical points, the BMA has often been at cross-purposes with its membership and the troops have refused to follow their leaders into battle.

8. Bentley B. Gilbert, *The Evolution of National Insurance in Great Britain*, London, Michael Joseph, 1966, p. 290.

9. Sidney and Beatrice Webb, *A Constitution for the Socialist Commonwealth of Great Britain*, London, Longman, 1920, p. 69, quoted in Gilbert, *The Evolution of National Insurance*, p. 291.

10. Gilbert, *The Evolution of National Insurance*, p. 363.

11. Ernest Muirhead Little, *History of the British Medical Association, 1832–1932*, London, British Medical Association, 1932, pp. 329–30. Quoted in Rudolf Klein, *Complaints against Doctors*, London, Charles Knight, 1973, p. 68. For this period, see Bentley B. Gilbert, *British Social Policy, 1914–1939*, London, B. T. Batsford, 1970, and Frank Honigsbaum, *The Division in British Medicine*, London, Kogan Page, 1979.

12. Honigsbaum, *The Division in British Medicine*.

13. Ibid.

14. John E. Pater, *The Making of the National Health Service*, London, King's Fund, 1981.

15. Frank Honigsbaum, *Health, Happiness and Security: the Creation of the National Health Service*, London, Routledge, 1989.

16. Charles Webster, *The Health Services Since the War*, Vol. 1, London, HMSO, 1988. See also the same author's *Conflict and consensus: explaining the British Health Service*, Twentieth Century British History, I:2 (1990), 115–5 1. This argues, although offering little evidence, that the labour movement had a larger role in creating the NHS than is conventionally assumed.

17. Elston Grey-Turner and F. M. Sutherland, *History of the British Medical Association*, Vol. 11, London, British Medical Association, 1982, p. 65.

18. Marmor and Thomas, *Doctors, politics and pay disputes*, p. 428.

19. Gordon Forsyth, *Doctors and Slate Medicine*, London, Pitman Medical, 1973, Ch.3.

20. It might be argued that the conflict over private practice between the Wilson government and the consultants was in a different category: that is, that the government's policies were challenging the existing consensus. But even this dispute ended in compromise: see Rudolf Klein, *Ideology, class and the National Health Service*, Journal of Health Politics, Policy and Law, 4: 3 (Fall 1979), 464–90.

21. Secretary of State for Social Services, *Primary Health Care: an Agenda for Discussion*, London, HMSO, 1986, Cm. 9771.

22. Secretary of State for Social Services, *Promoting Better Health*, London, HMSO, 1987, Cm. 249.

23. For an analysis of the background to this, and its outcome, see Patricia Day and Rudolf Klein, *The politics of modernisation: Britain's National Health Service in the 1980s*, The Milbank Quarterly, 67: 1 (1989), 1–34.

24. The concordat is implicit; see Klein, *The Politics of the NHS*. However, it is said that the Prime Minister—in her anger at the statement by the Presidents of the Royal Colleges—sent her civil servants scurrying in search of it.

25. Secretary of State for Health, *Working for Patients*, London, HMSO, 1989, Cm. 555.

26. Kenneth Clarke, *Talking Politics*, Radio Four, 12 Jan. 1991, BBC transcript.

27. Rudolf Klein, *From status to contract: the transformation of the British medical profession*, in Hugh L'Etang (ed.), *Health Care Provision Under Financial Constraint*, London, Royal Society of Medicine Services, 1990, pp. 127–34.

28. Although the notion of fundholding was very much Kenneth Clarke's personal obsession, the idea did not originate with him. It was very much part of the general soup of ideas cooked up in the years before the Review. If anyone can claim credit for first putting it forward, it is probably Alan Maynard. See, for example, his "Performance incentives in general practice," in George Teeling Smith (ed.), *Health, Education and General Practice*, London, Office of Health Economics, 1986.

29 Secretary of State for Health, Working for Patients, Para. 7.15, p. 58.

30. Klein, *The Politics of the NHS*, pp. 90–9.

31. Secretary of State for Health, *Working for Patients*, Para. 7.24, pp. 60–1.

32. General Medical Services Committee, *NHS Regulations*, London, British Medical Association, 1989.

33. General Medical Services Committee, Report to a Special Conference of Representatives of Local Medical Committees on 21 March 1990, London, British Medical Association, March 1990.

34. *Meeting just fails to back ballot on sanctions*, British Medical Journal, 300 (31 March 1991), p. 880.

35. Trevor Holdsworth (chairman), *Review Body on Doctors' and Dentists' Remuneration:* Twenty First Report 1991, London, HMSO, 1991, Cm. 1412.

36. *Taking the bureaucracy out of the GP contract*, British Medical Journal, 302, 16 Feb. 1991, p. 367.

37. Eckstein, *Pressure Group Politics*.

38. Department of Health, National Health Service General Medical Services, *Statement of Fees and Allowances payable to General Medical Practitioners in England and Wales*, London, Department of Health, 1989 onward.

39. Chris Ham, Ray Robinson and Michaela Benzeval, *Health Check: Health Care Reform in an International Context*, London, King's Fund Institute, 1990.

40. Bernard Shaw, *The Doctors Dilemma*, London, Constable & Co., 1911, "Preface," pp. xxv–xxvi: "Better to be a railway porter than an ordinary English general practitioner. A railway porter has from eighteen to twenty-three shillings a week from the Company merely as a retainer; and his additional fees from the public . . . are equivalent to doctor's fees in the case of second-class passengers, and double doctor's fees in the case of the first." For more scholarly evidence that a substantial proportion of doctors had very low incomes, see Guy Routh, *Occupation and Pay in Great Britain*, 1906–1960, Cambridge, Cambridge University Press, 1965, pp. 62–3.

41. Klein, *Ideology, class and the National Health Services*. See also Harrison et al., *The Dynamics of British Health Policy*.

42. Mack Carder and Bendix Klingeberg, *Towards a salaried medical profession*, in Arnold J. Heidenheimer and Nils Elvander (eds.), *The Shaping of the Swedish Health System*, London, Croom Helm, 1980, Ch. 60. Note, however, that this stresses that the Swedish medical profession at the time was divided and that the exclusion of the Swedish Medical Association may therefore, at least in part, have been self-inflicted.

43. Previous attempts, based on historical case studies, to develop a theory of "crisis politics" have not been encouraging. See, for example, Gabriel A. Almond, Scott C. Flanagan and Robert J. Mundt, *Crisis, Choice and Change*, Boston, Little, Brown and Company, 1973. Nor does "neo-Marxism," as invoked by Harrison et al. in *The Dynamics of British Health Policy* help very much in our view. This approach stressed the importance of change in the social and economic environment—and who could disagree?—but stops well short of providing a coherent theory of the linkages between environment and policy.

44. Constructing policy typologies is, of course, an old game. See, especially Theodore J. Lowi, *American business public policy case studies and political theory*, World Politics, 16 (1964), 677–715. The game has often proved frustrating, but may be due for a revival.

8

NO ANALYSIS WITHOUT COMPARISON

The articles in this chapter make explicit and amplify the logic of analysis that has informed previous chapters and which provides the rationale for the selection of articles in subsequent ones. This is the logical impossibility of making a causal statement about policy in any one country without testing it against the experience of another. If there are different policy outcomes in countries with similar institutions, then clearly an institution-based explanation will not wash. The same conclusion follows if similar policy outcomes are found in countries with different institutions. And what goes for institution-based explanations also goes for other explanatory variables. The point is as simple as it is obvious and would not be worth making but for the fact that it is so often ignored when country-specific claims are made. Explanatory ethnocentrism will usually lead to misleading interpretations.

So far the chapters have mostly concentrated on two country comparisons, playing off the United States' experience against that of Britain. In the remaining chapters, we continue with the Anglo-American theme, but the arc of comparison widens, and we examine (among other issues) the politics of contaminated blood and rationing a new drug across a wider span of countries. The two articles in this chapter, however, take a different tack. They address directly the promise and perils of comparison — outlining an anthropology, as it were, of the use and misuse of comparisons by both policy makers and academics.

In doing so, the articles also analyze the many and mixed reasons for the explosion of interest in the experience of other countries in recent decades. Negatively, there is the polemical use of foreign experience (real or, as often, imagined) as a warning exemplar in domestic political battles. Positively, there is the drive to learn from the experience of others: to see the health care arena of other countries as a laboratory from which useful lessons (both about what to do and about what not to do) can be drawn. Diagnostically, shared cross-country trends can help to identify problems common to all health care systems, though, as the articles warn, this cannot be taken to mean that there are necessarily common solutions.

Indeed if there is any general conclusion to be drawn from this chapter's two articles—and others in this volume—it is that they underline the complexity and subtlety of the interplay between the shared characteristics and shared problems of health care systems, on the one hand, and the way those characteristics and problems are perceived and addressed in specific institutional and cultural settings, on the other. The free flow of information and ideas across frontiers deceptively and seductively suggests that health policy makers and academics everywhere are all using the same language. In fact, words often change meaning at the frontier. And one of the functions of the academic analyst is to act as a border guard, making sure that those who cross borders are not smuggling misleading or counterfeit pictures of the world.

Comparative Perspectives and Policy Learning in the World of Health Care

Theodore R. Marmor, Richard Freeman, and Kieke G. H. Okma

None of us can escape the "bombardment of information about what is happening in other countries" (Klein 1997). Yet, in the field of health policy that is the subject here, there is an extraordinary imbalance between the magnitude and speed of the information flows and the capacity to learn useful lessons from them.[1] There is, moreover, a considerable gap between promise and performance in the field of comparative policy studies. Misdescription and superficiality are all too common.

Unwarranted inferences, rhetorical distortion, and caricatures—all show up too regularly in comparative health policy scholarship and debates. Why might that be so and what does that suggest about more promising forms of cross-national intellectual exchange? The main point of this article is to explore the methodological questions raised by concerns about the above weaknesses in international comparison in health policy. The core question is how competent learning from one nation to another can take place in health care policy.

To address that question, this article first describes the political context of health and welfare state reform debates during the past three decades. Section I argues that in almost all industrial democracies rising medical expenditures exacerbated fiscal concerns about the affordability of mature welfare states. Those concerns turned into increased pressure for policy change in health care and, with that, the inclination to look abroad for promising solutions of domestic problems. Section II takes up the topic of cross-national policy learning more directly, addressing some of the promises and methodological pitfalls of such work. The third section focuses on recent debates about health reform, skeptically reviews the claims of convergence among OECD health care systems, and explains the growth of scholarship on comparative health policy. The fourth section addresses the purposes, promises and pitfalls of comparative study in health policy. Section V groups these studies in categories that highlight the character, possibilities and limits of the comparative health policy literature. The concluding section returns to the article's basic theme: the real promise of comparative policy scholarship and the quite mixed portrait of the performance to date.

THE POLITICAL CONTEXT: WELFARE STATE DEBATES AND HEALTH REFORMS, 1970–2000

There is little doubt about the prominence of health policy[2] on the public agenda of most if not all of the industrial democracies. Canada's universal health insurance is a model of achievement for many observers, the subject of considerable intellectual scrutiny and the destination of many policy travelers in search of illumination. Yet both the national government and a majority of its provinces in recent years have felt sufficiently concerned about the condition of Canadian Medicare to set up advisory commissions to chart adjustments. The United States has been even more obvious about its medical care worries, with crisis commentary a fixture for decades on the national agenda. Fretting about medical care costs, quality, and access is not limited to North America. Disputes about reforming Dutch medical care have been ongoing for decades. Any review of the European experience would discover persistent policy controversies in Germany (burdened by the fiscal pressures of unification), in Great Britain (with recurrent debates about the NHS), and in Italy and Sweden (with great fiscal and unemployment pressures).[3]

The puzzle is not whether or why there is such widespread interest in health policy, but why now. And why has international evidence (arguments, claims, caricatures) seemed more prominent at the turn of the twenty-first century than, say, during the fiscal strains of the mid-1970s or early 1980s? What can be usefully said not only about the substance of the experience of different nations, but about the political processes of introducing and acting upon policy change in a national context?

There is a simple answer to these questions that, one hopes, is not simple minded. Medical care policy came to the forefront of public agendas for one or more of the following reasons. First, the financing of personal medical care everywhere became a major financial component of the budgets[4] of mature welfare states. When fiscal strain arises, policy scrutiny (not simply incremental budgeting) is the predictable result. Secondly, mature welfare states, as Rudolf Klein (1988: esp. 219–224) argued in the late 1980s, face restricted capacity for bold fiscal expansion in new areas. This means that managing existing pro-

grams in changing economic circumstances necessarily assumes a more prominent place on the public agenda. Thirdly, there is what might be termed the
wearing out (perhaps wearing down) of the postwar consensus about the welfare
state. We see the effects of more than two decades of fretfulness about the affordability, desirability, and governability of the welfare state.[5]

Begun in earnest during the 1973–74 oil shock, with high levels of unemployment and persistent stagflation, bolstered by electoral victories (or advance) of
parties opposed to welfare state expansion, critics assumed a bolder posture.
Mass publics increasingly heard challenges to programs that had for decades
seemed sacrosanct.[6] From Mulroney to Thatcher, from New Zealand to the
Netherlands—the message of serious problems requiring major change gained
support. Accordingly, when economic strain reappears, the inner rim of programmatic protection—not just interest group commitment, but social faith—
weakens, and the incentives to explore transformative but not fiscally burdensome options become relatively stronger. Those factors help to explain the
pattern of welfare state review—including health policy—over the past three
decades across the industrialized world. But, even accepting this contention,
there still remains the question of why these pressures gave rise to increased
attention to other national experiences.[7]

Recent experience illustrates how times of policy change increase the demand
for new ideas—or at least new means to old ends. Rudolf Klein once argued "no
one wants to be caught wearing yesterday's ideas" (Klein 1996). Everywhere,
policy makers and analysts looked increasingly across the border to search for
the latest policy fashion. Just as some American reformers turned to Canada's
example, so a number of Canadian, German, Dutch, and other intellectual entrepreneurs reviewed American, Swiss, and Swedish experience in recent years.
In the 1990s, many conferences followed this pattern. Conferees were interested
in getting better policy answers to the problems they faced at home. For example, participants in one such conference held in the Netherlands in the mid-
1990s were explicit about their aspirations for cross-border learning: how to find
a balance between "solidarity and subsidiary," how to maintain a "high quality
health system in times of economic stress," even an optimistic query about "what
are the optimum relations between patients, insurers, providers, and the government?" (Report Four Country Conference 1995). Understood as simply wanting
to stretch one's mind—to explore what is possible conceptually, or what others
have managed to achieve—this is unexceptionable. Understood as the pursuit of
the best model, absent further exploration of the political, social, and economic
context required for implementation, this is wishful thinking.

Others saw the opportunity for an informational version of this intellectual stretching: quests for "exchange of policy information" of various sorts without commitment to policy importation, "exchanging views with kindred spirits," and explicit calls for stimulation. All of this is the learning anthropologists have long extolled—understanding the range of possible options and seeing one's own circumstances more clearly by contrast.

But what about drawing policy lessons from such exercises? What are the rules of defensible conduct here and are they followed? The truth is that, whatever the appearances, most policy debates in most countries are (and will remain) parochial affairs. They address national problems, they emphasize national developments in the particular domain (pensions, medical finance, transportation), and embody conflicting visions of what policies the particular country should adopt. Only occasionally are the experiences of other nations—and the lessons they embody—seriously examined.[8] When cross-national experiences are employed in such parochial struggles, their use is typically that of policy warfare, not policy understanding and careful lesson-drawing. And, one must add, there are few knowledgeable critics at home of ideas about "solutions" abroad. In the world of American medical debate, the misuse of British and Canadian experience surely illustrates this point. The National Health Service was from the late 1940s the specter of what "government medicine" or "socialized medicine" and "rationing" could mean. In recent years, mythmaking about Canada has dominated the distortion league tables in North America.[9]

The reasons are almost too obvious to cite. Policy makers are busy with day-to-day pressures. Practical concerns incline them, if they take the time for comparative inquiry, to pay more attention to what appears to work, not academic reasons for what is and is not transferable and why. Policy debaters—whether politicians, policy analysts or interest group figures—are in struggles, not seminars. Like lawyers, they seek victory, not illumination. For that purpose, compelling stories, whether well substantiated or not, are more useful than careful conclusions. Interest groups, as their label suggests, have material and symbolic stakes in policy outcomes, not reputations for intellectual precision to protect.[10] Once generated and communicated, however, health policy ideas are adopted more readily in some contexts than in others. These patterns of adoption and adaptation have to do with the machinery of government, as well as with local cultural understandings. The autonomy and authority of government in parliament in the UK, for example, as well as its position at the apex of a nationalized health service, means that "ideas can make a difference more quickly in Britain than in America" (Marmor and Plowden 1991: 810). It may be, too, that policy ideas transfer more easily between similar types of health systems. Institutional similarity—however notional—seems to have facilitated the spread of managed competition ideas among the national health services of northern and southern Europe (Freeman 1998).

This argument must be qualified, however. Lessons from abroad often meet strong local cultural resistance. Giaimo and Manow (1997: 197), for example, observe that "while the market has won in international terms, the national answers to the economic pressures resulting from economic globalization demonstrate that national 'markets for ideas' have yet to be fully liberalized." Morone (1990: 141) similarly remarks of Canada's experience with universal health insurance:

> It is difficult to imagine a lesson that is more foreign to the American experience. Instead of hard conscious choices, we have sought painless automatic solutions.
>
> Rather than explicit programmatic decisions Americans prefer hidden, implicit policies. Rather than centralize control in governmental hands, we would scatter it across many players. In short the Canadian lessons . . . are not just different—they challenge the central features of American political culture, at least as they have manifested themselves in health care policy.

It is not clear, then, whether what matters is administrative infrastructure as such or the values and assumptions it appears to embody. For it matters a lot not only how systems are configured in organizational terms but also how they are construed mentally (Freeman 1999). This probably amounts to something more than ideas and values as such, pointing to the significance of ways of thinking or "framing." Different national policy communities—however well networked internationally—simply see problems differently.

For all this, the field of health policy is notable for the absence of studies which set out to investigate the process of transfer or learning in any specific instance. Bennett refers to the "paucity of systematic research that can convincingly make the case that cross-national policy learning has had a determined influence on policy choice in a particular jurisdiction at a particular time" (Bennett 1997). But, paucity of studies on policy learning does not apply to cross-national studies of policy origins, implementation, and change. Indeed, for that broader field of work, there are large and growing clusters of quite different sorts of scholarship and advocacy that address medical care cross-nationally.

None of these considerations are new—or surprising. But the increased flow of cross-national claims in health policy—both in the world of academia and politics—generates new reasons to consider the meaning of cross-national policy learning.

THE PROMISE AND PERILS OF CROSS-NATIONAL
COMPARATIVE POLICY RESEARCH

The presumptions of such cross-national efforts are important to explore, even if briefly. One is that the outside observer can more easily highlight features of debates that are missed or underplayed by national participants. The other is that comparative commentary may bring some policy wisdom as well as illuminating asides about national debates. The common assumption is that cross-cultural observation, if accurate and alert, has some advantages. It brings a different, "foreign" and arguably illuminating perspective to the debate.

A similar rationale lies behind much of the enthusiasm for contemporary comparative policy studies. Welfare state disputes—over pensions and medical care most prominently—are undoubtedly salient on the public agendas of all industrial democracies. There is in fact a brisk trade in panaceas for the various (real and imagined) ills of welfare states. As will be obvious in later comments on the comparative literature, however, many cross-national investigations are not factually accurate enough to offer useful illumination, let alone policy wisdom. But, properly done, studies that compare what appear to be similar topics have two potential benefits not available to the policy analyst in a single nation inquiry.

First, how others see a problem, how options for action are set out and evaluated, how implementation is understood and undertaken—all offer learning opportunities even if the policy experiences of different polities are not easily transplantable as "lessons." Secondly, where the context is reasonably similar, comparative work has features of a quasi-natural experiment. So, for instance the adaptation of reference prices for pharmaceuticals in Germany and in the Netherlands—two countries with very similar institutional arrangements in health care—provides an interesting example of policy learning. The policy of reference pricing constrains drug outlays in the short term. But those gains are somewhat dissipated as the actors strategically adapt to the new policy reality (Report Four Country Conference 2000).

Cross-national sources of information have proliferated to the extent that it has become almost impossible for a policy maker in any given country not to know something about what is going on elsewhere. But know what, exactly? What part can and should comparative policy analysis play in these debates? Ruud Lubbers, the former Dutch prime minister, provides a striking example of trying to draw lessons from American experience, apparently without much understanding of its policy realities (Lubbers 1997). In a 1997 article for the *International Herald Tribune*, Lubbers contrasted what he called the "lean welfare state . . . with rapid job growth" of the United States with "costly social welfare system[s] with persistently high unemployment in most of Europe." He went on in the rest of the article to laud Holland's "third way," one that "tackled" the unemployment problem while "remaining within the European tradition that emphasizes quality of life rather than growth at any cost." This rather self-congratulatory theme seems odd in comparison with contemporary Dutch complaints. But the point here is that the United States functions as a poorly analyzed symbol of a type of welfare state to avoid. Citing President Clinton as his source, Lubbers went on to write most of the article about the so-called Dutch miracle: a more flexible workforce, less unemployment, and a somewhat more restrained welfare state, all the result of the famous corporatist Wassenaar Agreement of 1982.

The American example is in fact hardly discussed, treated mostly as a negative symbol of what the Dutch have avoided.[11] Nowhere is there any recognition that the American welfare state is in fact quite extensive fiscally, concentrated on its older citizens, and with spending levels that—when properly accounted for in tax expenditures, direct program outlays, and the like—are hardly lean. Indeed, the point of recent books like Hacker's *The Divided Welfare State* (2002) is precisely to set aside this common but mistaken impression of American social policy as concentrated on the poor; miserly in its levels of benefits; and, depending on one's ideology, splendid or horrible in its social and economic results.[12]

The paradox is that the post-1970 decades witnessed the rapid expansion of public policy research, of which a significant proportion claimed to provide comparisons across countries as a base for drawing lessons. But most of those studies, in fact, consisted of mere statistical and descriptive portraitures of health systems, ignoring the methodological issues of comparison. So the argument here underlines the truism that policy making and policy research are often—if not always—pursued with little reference to each other. Nevertheless, the question remains as why that truism should apply so fully in this particular, costly area of public policy: health care. Why are claims about system convergence so widespread in the face of persistent patterns of continuity in national models of health care?

CONVERGENCE IN THE HEALTH REFORM DEBATE: CLAIMS AND REALITIES

The bulk of the ideological and fiscal debates about health reform took place within national borders, largely free from the spread of "foreign" ideas. To the extent that similar arguments arose cross-nationally, these mostly represented what might be described as "parallel thinking." That is to say, the common questioning of health policy reflects similarities in circumstances and problem definition. This was obvious in the common preoccupation with rising medical care costs. Figure 1 portrays the upward pressure of medical care expenditures in four OECD nations since the early 1970s. Even while the four countries' health expenditure rose steadily, they also varied in the growth rates over time. Obviously, some countries, in some periods, were more successful than others in reigning in health costs. This raises the question whether—and if so, to what extent—common pressure will cause system convergence.

One can think of convergence as "a kind of soft technological determinism," the logic of which is that, across systems, "the common features will increase at the expense of the differences" (Field 1989: 13). This sense of convergence has intensified by the emergence in the late 1980s and 1990s of active international and supranational actors in both general welfare state disputes and, in particular, health policy. These actors include the European Union (EU), the World Health Organization (WHO), the Organisation for Economic Co-operation and Development (OECD), and the World Bank. But, however powerful these institutions are in some areas, their role in domestic policy making within the OECD world remains indirect and limited. The European Commission has established a policy competence in public health and has become a sponsor of biomedical research. Yet recent rulings of the European Court of Justice have had important spillover effects on national healthcare policies. EU legislation designed originally to ensure the freedom of goods, people, capital and services across borders no longer exempts the domain of health care (Report of Workshop on EU Law and National Health Policy 2004).

The WHO struggles to lead health policy discussions, but remains a minor actor in the funding of medical care. And the World Bank, particularly powerful in the transformation of health care in eastern Europe, expresses some of the reform ideas found in the western industrial democracies, but does not wield its influence there. Finally, OECD reports certainly affect the discussion of welfare state issues, but at one step removed from policy decision making. But in spite of their limited direct role in health policy, the international agencies have become platforms for debate and carriers of policy ideas across borders.

Almost everywhere, health care became relatively more expensive as public budgets were more constrained—but how much more expensive and how much more constrained has varied substantially between countries. These pressures, in turn, are mediated by different sets of actors and institutions. It is important to note that debates over controlling health care expenditures took place every-

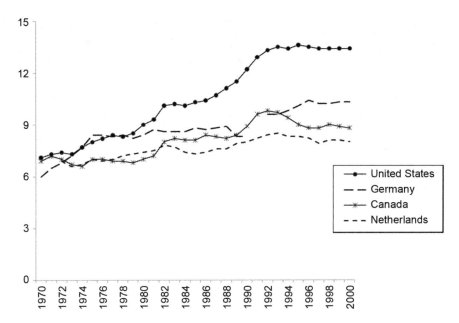

Figure 1. Health Expenditure in The Netherlands, Germany, Canada, US, 1970–2000 (percentage of GDP). Source: OECD Health Data 2003.

where, regardless of actual levels or growth rates of health spending. In short, the apparently common pressures on health systems are themselves uneven and indirect. And this is the essential difficulty in taking convergence as a framework for studying—or advocating—reforms in health policy. Quite simply, there is as much evidence of continued difference (or divergence) in national arrangements for the finance, delivery and regulation of health care as there is of increasing similarity. As a former official of the OECD's health policy unit claimed, "[T]he delivery and finance of healthcare vary between nations more than any other public policy" (Poullier 1989). One does not have to agree with Poullier's conclusion to see that reducing variation has been neither the purpose nor the effect of health reform in the past decades. In health care no more than in other areas of public administration are there good arguments or evidence that "one size fits all."

To be fair, this variation is one of degree rather than of kind. At the most general level, it seems perfectly clear that some countries with roughly similar constellations of political interests, economic and political institutions and resources develop broadly comparable arrangements for health care. And so, in turn, when social structures, patterns of economic organization, and expressions of political interest begin to change, health care arrangements will face pressures to change also. But what matters is what that formulation leaves unsaid. While there is value in pointing to the structural and technological context of health policy, policy makers faced not only with multiple pressures but also with myriad proposals for change tend to choose options that are politically feasible in the short term. To them, an appeal to convergence seems anodyne, reductionist or superficial. Conditions are not determining. They explain only why there should be pressure for reform, but not whether or not change will indeed occur, let alone what shape or direction it will—or should—take.

Nonetheless, these conditions do help to explain why—if not when or where or how—cross-national trade in policy ideas should be going on and why it is increasing. For the more similar countries become in general, the more they may believe they can learn from each other. Getting it right in health policy—ensuring universal access to high quality health care without breaking the bank—makes for significant competitive advantage in the domestic political arena as well as in the international economy. Convergence in circumstances creates opportunities for learning, as well as an increased interest in applying lessons from abroad. Convergence theory, then, offers useful clues about why adaptive change might take place. It says much less, however, about the form it takes, about why one solution to a problem should be preferred over others. And for that topic, the next section addresses the purposes, promises and pitfalls of comparative studies in health policy.

PURPOSE, PROMISE AND PERILS OF COMPARATIVE INQUIRY IN HEALTH POLICY

The emphasis in this part of the discussion is on the following, perhaps obvious, distinctions among the purposes comparative analysis in health policy can serve: learning about national health arrangements and how they operate, learning why they take the forms they do, and learning policy lessons from those analyses. While these distinctions should be obvious to scholars of the subject, much of the comparative commentary on health care neither clarifies the different modes of comparison nor addresses the difficulties of drawing policy lessons from the experience of other countries.

First, there is the goal of learning about health policy abroad. Comparative work of this sort can illuminate and clarify national arrangements without addressing causal explanation or seeking policy transplantation as aims. Its comparative element remains for the most part implicit: in reading (or writing) about them, we make sense of other systems by contrasting them with our own and with others we know about. The process of learning entails, which is obvious once noted: appreciation of what something is by reference to what it is like or unlike. This is the gift of perspective, which may or may not bring explanatory insight or lesson drawing.

The second fundamental purpose served by comparison is to generate causal explanations without necessarily seeking policy transplantation: that is, learning why policies develop as they do. Many of the historical and developmental studies of healthcare fall into this category. This approach uses cross-national inquiry to check on the adequacy of nation-specific accounts. Let us call that a defense against explanatory provincialism. What precedes policy making in country A includes many things, from legacies of past policy to institutional and temporal features, that "seem" decisive. How is one to know if a feature is decisive as opposed to simply present? One answer is to look for similar outcomes elsewhere where some of those factors are missing or configured differently. Another is to look for a similar configuration of precedents without a comparable outcome.

A third and still different approach is to treat cross-national experience as quasi-experimental. Here one hopes to draw lessons about why some policies seem promising and doable, promising but impossible, or doable but not promising. All of these approaches appear in the comparative literature. And, with the growth of such writing, there was widespread optimism about the promise of lesson drawing from comparative policy analyses. But is that optimism justified?

One useful starting point to address this question is a cross-national generalization that at first sight seems misleading but, upon reflection, helps to clarify differences in the framing of policy problems. A 1995 article on European health reform, for example, claims that "countries everywhere are reforming their health systems" (Hunter 1995). It asserts that "what is remarkable about this global movement is that both the diagnosis of the problems and the prescription for them are virtually the same in all health care systems." These globalist claims, it turns out, were mistaken (Jacobs 1998, Marmor 1999). But the process of specifying more precisely exactly what counts as national healthcare problems—whether cost control, poor quality of care, or fragmented organization of services—turns out to be quite clarifying. In this instance, the comparative approach first refutes the generalization, but then helps to discipline the process of describing national health "problems." So, to illustrate further, the European researcher coming to investigate Oregon's experiment in health care rationing would soon discover that it was neither restrictive in practice nor a major cost control remedy in the 1990s (Jacobs, Marmor and Oberlander 1999). To do so is to see the issue of rationing more clearly.

Offering new perspectives on problems and making factual adjustments in national portraits are not to be treated as trivial tasks. They are what policy craftsmen and -women might well spend a good deal of time perfecting. All too many comparative studies are in fact caricatures rather than characterizations of policies. A striking illustration is the 2000 WHO report mentioned above on the ranking of the performance of health systems across the globe. Not only was the ambition itself grandiose, but its execution evoked sharp criticism from serious scholars[13] (Williams 2001). That criticism in itself should not serve as a deterrent to serious scholars who seek to compare experiences. But it is a warning against superficiality.

An often cited advantage of comparative studies is that they serve as an antidote to explanatory provincialism. An example from North American health policy provides a good illustration of how and how not to proceed. Some policy makers and academics in North America regard universal health insurance as incompatible with American values. They rest their case in part on the belief that Canada enacted health insurance and the US has not because North American values are sharply different. In short, they attribute a different outcome to a different political culture in the US. In fact, the values of Canada and the United States, while not identical, are actually quite similar (Lipset 1990). Like siblings, differences are there, sure, but Canada's distribution of values is closer to that of the United States than any other modern, rich democracy. In fact, the value similarities between British Columbia and Washington State are greater than those between either of those jurisdictions and, say, New Brunswick or New Hampshire along the North American east coast. Similar values are compatible with different outcomes, which in turn draw one's attention to other institutional and strategic factors that distinguish Canadian from American experience with financing health care (White 1995, Maioni 1998). One can imagine many other examples of such cautionary lessons, but the important point is simply that the explanatory checks are unavailable from national histories alone.

The third category of work is directly relevant to our inquiry. Drawing lessons from the policy experience of other nations is what has financially supported a good deal of the comparative analysis available. The international organizations have this as part of their rationale. The WHO, as noted, is firmly in the business of selling "best practices." The OECD regularly produces extensive, expensive, hard to gather, statistical portraits of programs as diverse as disability and pensions, trade flows and the movement of professionals, education and health care. No one can avoid using these studies, if only because the task of collecting data and discovering "the facts" in a number of countries is so daunting. But the portraiture that emerges requires its own craft review. Does what Germany spends on spas count as public health expenditure elsewhere or does it fall, as in the United States, under another category? Often the same words do not mean the same things. And different words may denote similar phenomena.

For now, it is enough to restate that learning about the experience of other nations is a precondition for understanding why change takes place, or for learning from that experience. Looking at the large and growing volume of comparative studies in health policy, we found that the vast majority of studies do not deliver on their claim to provide a sound base for drawing lessons from the experience of other countries. The section below categorizes the studies in four groups, each with its distinct purpose and applications. This grouping shows that the majority of reports and studies available (the first and second categories) provide, at best, a sound base for further analysis but hardly any ground for learning from experience abroad. The few studies that are based on more solid analysis (the third and fourth group) are less frequent, less wide in their geographical application and more modest in their claims about policy lessons.

COMPARATIVE HEALTH POLICY ANALYSIS: CLUSTERS OF WRITING

Health policy in the OECD world is, at the same time, a matter of insistent national debate, a frequent topic of descriptive, statistical portraiture for international organizations, a sometime subject of publication in the comparative journals, and only very infrequently in its cross-national comparative form the object of book length treatment. For many years, readers had to turn to Anderson's (1972) treatment of Swedish, British and American medical care developments in the post–World War II period for acute, well-informed judgments.[14] There were many other individual country studies, but few if any that employed a systematic, comparative method of policy analysis. In contemporary debates about Dutch health care, for instance, there appears little evidence of detailed understanding about German—or American—policy experience with health care reform in the 1990s. What is true for medical care applies just as well to other fiscally important areas of the welfare state. So, for example, American discussions of disability policy in the early 1980s drew very little from Dutch experience, though there were knowledgeable scholars in both countries who sought to have influence (Wilensky 2002).[15]

By the end of the 1980s, political scientists—particularly North American ones—had become interested in comparing relations between the medical profession, as a particular kind of interest group, and the state (Tuohy 1974, Stone 1984, Freddi and Bjorkman 1989, Wilsford 1991, Immergut 1992, Pierson 1994). Their theoretical focus was by and large on the institutions of government and the different ways in which they shape health care politics. Slowly, the field began to produce genuinely comparative political analyses of substantial industry and competence.

The ten years and more since then have witnessed a rapid expansion of cross-national health policy literature. The quality of these works varies enormously — whether measured by the standard of intellectual rigor, theoretical perspective, descriptive accuracy, or concern for systematic policy learning across borders. There are, roughly speaking, four separable but not mutually exclusive categories of such writing (Marmor and Okma 2003).

The first includes the well-known statistical, largely descriptive documents that provide data on a number of countries assumed to constitute a coherent class. It also includes more specialized surveys that deal with public opinion, health care and health policy (Blendon and Brodie 1997). In that way they supply much of the basic information that policy commentators explore. The OECD Health Data series has become a staple of both academic and more applied analyses alike. These studies typically neither provide behavioral hypotheses nor test explanations for why certain patterns exist. Nor do they, generally speaking, explicitly deal with the promise and pitfalls of cross-border learning. In a wider sense, the recent efforts to rank systems, countries or institutions by means of benchmarking techniques belong to this group, too. In the report we noted above, the WHO used its comparative data to rank the performance of national health care systems (WHO 2000).

The second category of comparative studies — by far the largest number — includes collections of international material, that we label as "parallel" or "stapled" national case studies. Examples of this kind of cross-national study are the volumes by Ham et al. (1990), OECD (1992, 1994), Wall (1996), Altenstetter and Bjorkman (1997), Ham (1997), Raffell (1997) and Powell and Wessen (1999) as well as the national portraits of the WHO European Observatory. These are usually country reports bound together, accompanied by an editorial introduction and summary conclusion. For the most part, the authors are intent on setting out "how things work" in whichever country they are writing about. They are mostly descriptive, but with some assessment of performance and the flagging of issues prompting political concern. As such, they represent a qualitative correlation of the quantitative statistical studies described above. Done carefully, they are an invaluable resource for cross-national understanding. In many cases, they leave readers to find what is relevant and, as far as policy learning is concerned, leave them to do the work.

Thirdly, there are books about a number of individual countries that employ a common framework of analysis, usually addressing a particular theme in health policy, for example competition or privatization. That means, in principle, that comparative generalizations are possible, though not all such works actually draw them.[16]

Fourthly, there are cross-national studies with a fundamental theoretical orientation that take up a specific medical care theme or question as the focus of analysis.[17] One of the interesting features of this fourth category of comparative studies is that there appears a necessary trade-off between theoretical depth and the number of nations studied. The disciplined treatment of broad topics by a single author almost inevitably addresses a more limited set of countries.[18]

In this latter category, Tuohy's (1999) *Accidental Logics* offers both a theoretical and empirical analysis of policy change and continuity in three English-speaking nations. The book addresses a limited range of countries but combines theoretical sophistication with command of the relevant factual data, and causal analysis in addressing the quite different patterns of policy change during the post–World War II years in Britain, Canada and the United States. The likelihood of major policy changes, for Tuohy, differs according to each nation's particular "institutional mix." By that, she means the degree of governmental hierarchy, market forces and professional collegiality in medical decision making and the "structural balance" between the state, medical providers and private financial interests. Directed at understanding, Tuohy's work is of clear relevance to policy makers concerned with questions of timing for reform initiatives.

Works in this fourth category of scholarship typically use comparative methods to explore and to explain policy developments. Their practical limitations for policy makers include the relatively restricted range of countries studied and, to some degree, their reliance on the theoretical perspective known as historical institutionalism. There is some irony in the fact that the most careful cross-national analyses tend to have reinforced a sense of the contingency and specificity of the way things work out at different times in different places. This kind of comparison seems to ignore (if not implicitly deny) the cross-national exchange of information and ideas in health policy that is so much part of the very intellectual environment in which it has been produced. The most powerful studies are at the same time the most academic; the practical learning which might result from comparison is largely left implicit. Often, those books do not reach the desks of policy makers. There is much less here which speaks directly to the policy maker seeking to use evidence and experience from elsewhere in any straightforward way. Nonetheless, in the course of little more than a decade, the comparative analysis of health policy became a specialized field of academic inquiry, highly developed and successful in its own terms, but limited so far in its policy impact. So, we turn back to the question: how should we evaluate the purposes and performance of comparative policy research?

Perhaps the most important lesson we can draw from the overview in the current literature is that the development of a serious body of comparative work takes more time and effort than health policy makers are willing to spend. They feel pressures to take action and feel they cannot wait. At the same time, policy errors based on misconceptions of the experience abroad can be costly. The eagerness of some health ministers to embrace and import policy models from the US like the managed care models, the benchmark methodology or the medical savings idea without a proper assessment of how those ideas and models worked out in practice may lead to policies that will require repair action soon, can force politicians to reverse policies and can erode the popular support for health policy altogether. The unwillingness of some politicians to delay action in order to study experience with similar policy elsewhere contrasts sharply with the practice of some Asian countries that have spent much time and attention before adjusting certain measures to their own national policy environments. The good news is that the last two decades have brought a large body of comparative research that can serve as the base for the next generation of studies that take the above warnings into account. The statistical data are there, the materials are there, the experience in drawing portraits of individual countries is there and all of these are necessary conditions for the next phases of learning about policy causation and the crossnational transfer of policy experience.

SUMMARY AND CONCLUSIONS

The last decades have seen a growing body of comparative study in health policy, but this growth was not matched by a growing understanding of the processes of policy learning from the experience of other countries. There is, in fact, little attention to methodological questions about this learning process.

The confluence of economic, demographic and ideological factors that led to extensive debate about the future of the welfare state also created pressure to reform health care systems. Fiscal strains and declining political support for an active role of the state undermined support for welfare state expansion and that strain also affected health policy. There was, indeed, growing pressure to seek out new policy solutions abroad. That pressure also gave rise to a new body of research within national communities as well as international agencies like the World Bank, OECD, WHO and European Union. However, to date most of that research consists of merely descriptive studies of health care systems and policy measures within national boundaries. The studies pay little attention to the question of what experience can be applied in another country under what circumstances. Institutional and cultural factors are important elements in the policy context as determinants of successful reception and implementation of ideas.

In practice, there is much mislearning and misrepresentation by omission. Policy makers and politicians feel pressured to change, but have little or no time (or willingness) to critically assess claims about policy experience across the border. Potentially, comparison can bring learning opportunities as other countries can serve as natural experiments, in particular when the policy contexts are similar. Some lessons apply across many different countries. Similar pressure can create opportunities for learning, and international organizations serve as platforms for debate and potential sources for comparative studies. Existing research largely ignores the important difference between the process of learning about other countries' experience, learning why certain change takes place, and drawing lessons from that experience. But the basic ingredients for improved policy learning are there: the statistical database, the first generation of descriptive country studies and the experience of academics and international organizations.

Notes

This article was first published in *Journal of Comparative Policy Analysis* 7, no. 4 (2005):331–448. The authors want to thank Avi Feller, our research assistant and Yale undergraduate, for his helpful assistance with this article.

1. This skeptical argument is advanced, with Anglo-American examples from medical care and welfare, by Marmor and Plowden (1991: 807–812). On the other hand, there is very rapid communication of scientific findings and claims, with journals and meetings regarded as the proper sites for evaluation. As yet, there is no journal in the political economy of medical care that has enough authority, audience, or acuteness to play the evaluative role assumed in the medical world by *The New England Journal of Medicine, Lancet, BMJ,* or *JAMA.*

2. Readers may be puzzled by our reluctance in this note to treat "reform" as the object of commentary. This paragraph's parade of substitutes—health policy concerns, worries and so on—reflects discomfort with the marketing connotations of the "reform" expression. That there are pressures for change are obvious and understanding them is part of our gathering's point, but reforming can obviously be a benefit, a burden, or beside the point.

3. In the 1990s work in English on health policy learning was for the most part concerned with a single topic, managed competition. This topic dominated reform discussion across countries between the mid-1980s and the mid-1990s. However, the focus was largely on the transatlantic relationship between the US and the UK (Klein 1991 and 1997; Marmor and Plowden 1991;

Mechanic 1995; Marmor 1997; Marmor and Okma 1998; O'Neill 2000). There were complementary treatments of western Europe (Freeman 1999), southern Europe (Cabiedes and Guillen 2001) and New Zealand (Jacobs and Barnett 2000).

4. Technically, this is not strictly true of course, as is evident in the sickness fund financing of care
in Germany, the Netherlands, and elsewhere. But, since mandatory contributions are close
cousins of "taxes," budget officials must obviously treat these outlays as constraints on direct tax
increases. Moreover, the precise level of acceptable cost increases is a regulatory issue of great
controversiality.

5. The bulk of this ideological struggle took place, of course, within national borders, free from the
spread of "foreign" ideas. To the extent similar arguments arose cross-nationally, as Kieke Okma
has noted, most represent "parallel development" (Report Four Country Conference 1995). But
there are striking contemporary examples of the explicit international transfer and highlighting
of welfare state commentary. Some of this takes place through think-tank networks; some takes
place through media campaigns on behalf of particular figures; and, of course, some takes
place through academic exchanges and official meetings. Charles Murray—the controversial
author of *Losing Ground* (1984) and co-author of *The Bell Curve* (1994)—illustrates all three of
these phenomena, as our British conferees can attest. The medium of transfer seems to have
changed in the postwar period. Where the Beveridge Report would have been known to social
policy elites very broadly, however much they used it, the modern form seems to be the long
newspaper or magazine article and the media interview.

6. This is the argument developed in Marmor, Mashaw and Harvey (1990: esp. ch. 3). The wider
scholarly literature on the subject is the focus of a review essay (Marmor 1993).

7. The turning to US health policy experience for lessons about cost control or insurance coverage seems particularly puzzling to American scholars preoccupied with health care problems
at home.

8. Some readers have suggested this article is too pessimistic about the field of cross-national policy
learning. And it is certainly true that some cross-national investigations have been enormously
illuminating and helpful. For example, the 1964 Royal Commission on Health Services was an
exemplary investigator of the experience of other countries. In the 1990s comparative policy
investigations by Japanese and German analysts were important in nursing home reforms in
both countries.

9. For an elaboration of this point, see Marmor (1994: ch. 12). A particularly careful and extensive
treatment of the North American experience is the review article by Evans, Barer, and Hertzman (1991).

10. The political fight over the Clinton health plan vividly illustrates these generalizations. The
number of interest groups with a stake in the Clinton plan's fate—given the nearly $1 trillion
medical economy—was enormous; there were more than 8,000 registered lobbyists alone in
Washington and thousands more trying to influence the outcome under some other label.
The estimates of expenditures on the battle are in the hundreds of millions; one trade association, The Pharmaceutical Manufacturer's Association, spent $7 million on "public relations"
by 1993. The most noted effort was that of the Health Insurance Association of America, which
produced the infamous Harry and Louise advertisements. Washington was awash in interest
group activities during the health care reform battle of 1993–94, but the character, impact and
meaning of those activities are far from clear.

11. One of the Dutch policy commentators in a chapter dealing with cross-national perspectives on
the Dutch welfare state and its health system strikingly illustrates how one can oddly justify not
learning much from comparative policy studies. "Comparative studies," he writes, "are generally backward looking, so don't always provide us with the right answers for the future" (personal
interview 2004). The restrictive definition of the purpose of comparative inquiry—getting the
"right answers"—limits greatly what this Dutch public servant would consider useful.

12. As Hacker (2002: 7) rightly points out, the "share of the US economy devoted to social welfare spending is not all that different from the corresponding proportion in even the most generous of European welfare states." The "sources" of the spending—tax expenditures and employment-benefits especially—are what distinguishes the American case. The same myth of the "lean" American welfare state was the object of criticism in a book published a decade earlier (Marmor, Mashaw and Harvey 1990).

13. The 2000 WHO report seeks to rank health systems across the globe. The WHO posed good questions about how health systems work: are they fair, responsive to patient needs, efficient, and do they provide good quality health care. But it answered those questions without much attention to the difficulties of describing responsiveness or fairness or efficiency in some universalistic and reliable manner. What is more, the report used as partial evidence the opinions of WHO personnel to "verify" what takes place in Australia, Oman, Turkmenistan or Canada. Moreover, while the report claims to provide data in order to improve health systems across the globe, it is hard to see how a health minister of a country ranked, say, at place 125, has any stake to climb the ladder. Predictably, most of the uproar about the report was the battle between the countries that ranked high but not highest. Many journalists and members of parliament quoted the report as a critical comment on the failures of the national health system whereas, unsurprisingly, the French minister saw the number one ranking of his country (that in the end turned out to be based on a calculating error) as proof of the effectiveness of his policy. With comparisons like that, one can easily understand why some funders of research regard comparative policy studies as excuses for boondoggles. But that should not drive out the impulse for serious cross-national scholarship and learning.

14. For a retrospective appreciation of Anderson, see Freeman and Marmor (2003).

15. There is a rich scholarly disability literature, with a good deal of knowledgeable commentary on comparative policy developments. See especially Aarts and De Jong (2003).

16. Good examples are Freddi and Bjorkman's *Controlling Medical Professionals* (1989) and Ranade's *Markets and Health Care* (1998); another is White's *Competing Solutions* (1995), written at the Brookings Institution to draw lessons from OECD experience for the universal health insurance debate in the United States. Sometimes journals present work of this kind: see the case studies of priority setting in *Health Policy* (1999), for example, and the *Journal of Health Politics, Policy and Law* (2001) for international commentary.

17. A good example of this genre is the book edited by Bayer and Feldman (1999) on the politics of contaminated blood in Germany, France, Japan, Canada, Denmark, and the United States: *Blood Feuds*. The theme is taken up in Bovens, 't Hart and Peters's (2002) *Success and Failure in Governance*, which also looks at medical professions and health care reform.

18. For instance, Pierson (1994) compares retrenchment politics in Reagan's America and Thatcher's England; Immergut (1992) compares the disputes over national health insurance in France, Switzerland and Sweden in the early part of the twentieth century; and Maioni (1998) the different paths to national health insurance taken in Canada and the United States. Moran (1999) assesses the political economy of health care in Britain, Germany and the United States, Freeman (2000) the politics of health care in five European countries.

References

Aarts, L., and De Jong, P., 2003, *Able to Work? How Policies Help Disabled People in 20 OECD Countries* (Paris: OECD).

Altenstetter, C., and Bjorkman, J. W. (Eds), 1997, *Health Policy Reform, National Variations and Globalization* (Basingstoke: Macmillan).

Anderson, O., 1972, *Health Care: Can There Be Equity? The United States, Sweden and England* (New York: John Wiley).

Bayer, R., and Feldman, E., 1999, *Blood Feuds: Aids, Blood and the Politics of the Medical Disaster* (Oxford: Oxford University Press).

Bennett, C. J., 1997, Understanding ripple effects: the cross-national adoption of policy instruments for bureaucratic accountability, *Governance*, 10(3), 213–233.

Blendon, R. J., and Brodie, M., 1997, Public opinion and health policy, in: T. J. Litman and L. S. Robins (Eds.), *Health Politics and Policy* (Albany, NY: Delmar).

Bovens, M., t' Hart, P., and Peters, B. G. (Eds.), 2002, *Success and Failure in Governance: A Comparative Analysis of European States* (Cheltenham: Edward Elgar).

Cabiedes, L. and Guillen, A. M., 2001, Adopting and adapting managed competition: health care reform in southern Europe, *Social Science and Medicine*, 52(8), 1205–1217.

Evans, R., Barer, M., and Hertzman, C., 1991, The 20-year experiment: accounting for, explaining, and evaluating health care cost containment in Canada and the United States, *American Review of Public Health*, 12, 481–518.

Field, M. (Ed.), 1989, *Success and Crisis in National Health Systems: A Comparative Approach* (New York: Routledge).

Freddi, G., and Bjorkman, J. W. (Eds.), 1989, *Controlling Medical Professionals. The Comparative Politics of Health Governance* (London: Sage).

Freeman, R., 1998, Competition in context: the politics of health care reform in Europe, *International Journal for Quality in Health Care*, 10(5), 395–401.

Freeman, R., 1999, Policy transfer in the health sector. European Forum conference paper WS/35, Florence: European University Institute.

Freeman, R., 2000, *The Politics of Health in Europe* (Manchester: Manchester University Press).

Freeman, R., and Marmor, T., 2003, Making sense of health services politics through cross-national comparison, *Journal of Health Services Research and Policy*, 8(3), 180–182.

Giaimo, S. and Manow, P., 1997, Institutions and ideas into politics: health care reform in Britain and Germany, in: C. Altenstetter and J. W. Bjorkman (Eds.), *Health Policy Reform, National Variations and Globalization* (Basingstoke: Macmillan).

Hacker, J., 2002, *The Divided Welfare State: The Battle over Public and Private Benefits in the United States* (New York: Cambridge University Press).

Ham, C. (Ed.), 1997, *Health Care Reform: Learning from International Experience* (Buckingham: Open University Press).

Ham, C., Robinson, R., and Benzeval, M. (Eds.), 1990, *Health Check: Healthcare Reforms in an International Context* (London: King's Fund Institute).

Health Policy, 1999, 50 (1–2).

Herrnstein, R. J. and Murray, C., 1994, *The Bell Curve: Intelligence and Class Structure in American Life* (New York: Free Press).

Hunter, D., 1995, A new focus for dialogue, *European Health Reform: The Bulletin of the European Network and Database*, No. 1, March.

Immergut, E. M., 1992, *Health Politics Interests and Institutions in Western Europe, Cambridge Studies in Comparative Studies* (Cambridge: Cambridge University Press).

Jacobs, A., 1998, Seeing difference: market health reform in Europe, *Journal of Health Politics, Policy and Law*, 23(1), 1–33.

Jacobs, K., and Barnett, P., 2000, Policy transfer and policy learning: a study of the 1991 New Zealand Health Services Taskforce, *Governance*, 13(2), 229–257.

Jacobs, L., Marmor, T. M. and Oberlander, J., 1999, The Oregon Health Plan and the political paradox of rationing: what advocates and critics have claimed and what Oregon did, *Journal of Health Politics, Policy and Law*, 24(1), 161–180.

Journal of Health Politics, Policy and Law, 2001, 26(4).

Klein, R., 1991, Risks and benefits of comparative studies: notes from another shore, *Milbank Quarterly*, 69(2), 275–291.

Klein, R., 1996, Commentary at Second Annual Meeting of the Four Country Conference on Health Policy, Montebello, Canada.

Klein, R., 1997, Learning from others: shall the last be the first? *Journal of Health Politics, Policy and Law*, 22(5), 1267–1278.

Klein, R., and O'Higgins, M., 1988, Defusing the crisis of the welfare state: a new interpretation, in: T. R. Marmor and J. Mashaw (Eds.), *Social Security: Beyond the Rhetoric of Crisis* (Princeton, NJ: Princeton University Press).

Lipset, S. M., 1990, *Continental Divide: The Values and Institutions of the United States and Canada* (New York: Routledge).

Lubbers, R., 1997, In seeking a third way, the Dutch model is worth a look, *International Herald Tribune*, September 9.

Maioni, A., 1998, *Parting at the Crossroads: The Emergence of Health Insurance in the United States and Canada* (Princeton, NJ: Princeton University Press).

Marmor, T. R., 1993, Understanding the welfare states: crisis, critics, and countercritics, *Critical Review*, 7(4), 461–477.

Marmor, T. R., 1994, Patterns of fact and fiction in the use of the Canadian experience; and Implementation: making reform work, in: *Understanding Health Care Reform* (New Haven, CT: Yale University Press), pp. 179–194.

Marmor, T. R., 1997, Global health policy reform: misleading mythology or learning opportunity, in: C. Altenstetter and J. W. Bjorkman (Eds.), *Health Policy Reform, National Variations, and Globalization* (Basingstoke: Macmillan).

Marmor, T. R., 1999, The rage for reform: sense and nonsense in health policy, in: D. Drache and T. Sullivan (Eds.), *Health Reform: Public Success, Private Failure* (London: Routledge), 260–272.

Marmor, T. R., and Okma, K. G. H., 1998, Cautionary lessons from the west: what (not) to learn from other countries' experiences in the financing and delivery of health care, in: P. Flora, P. R. De Jong, J. Le Grand and J. Y. Kim (Eds.), *The State of Social Welfare. International Studies on Social Insurance and Retirement, Employment, Family Policy and Health Care* (Aldershot: Ashgate).

Marmor, T. R., and Okma, K. G. H., 2003, Review essay: health care systems in transition, *Journal of Health Politics, Policy and Law*, 28(4), 747–755.

Marmor, T. R., and Plowden, W., 1991, Rhetoric and reality in the international jet stream: the export to Britain from America of questionable ideas, *Journal of Health Politics, Policy and Law*, 16(4), 807–812.

Marmor, T. R., Mashaw, J., and Harvey, P., 1990, Crisis and the welfare state, in: *America's Misunderstood Welfare State: Persistent Myths, Enduring Realities* (New York: Basic Books), pp. 53–81.

Mechanic, D., 1995, The Americanization of the British national health service, *Health Affairs*, Summer, 51–67.

Moran, M., 1999, *Governing the Health Care State* (Manchester: Manchester University Press).

Morone, J. A., 1990, American political culture and the search for lessons from abroad, *Journal of Health Politics, Policy and Law*, 15(1), 129–143.

Murray, C., 1984, *Losing Ground: American Social Policy 1950–1980* (New York: Basic Books).

OECD, 1992, *The Reform of Health Care. A Comparative Analysis of Seven OECD Countries*, Health Policy Studies (Paris: OECD).

OECD, 1994, *The Reform of Health Care. A Review of Seventeen OECD Countries* (Paris: OECD).

OECD, 2003, *OECD Health Data 2003* (Paris: OECD).

O'Neill, F., 2000, Health: the "internal market" and reform of the national health service, in: D. Dolowitz (Ed.), *Policy Transfer and British Social Policy* (Buckingham: Open University Press).

Pierson, P., 1994, *Dismantling the Welfare State? Reagan, Thatcher and the Politics of Retrenchment* (Cambridge: Cambridge University Press).

Poullier, J. P., 1989, Managing health in the 1990s: a European overview, *Health Service Journal*, 27 April, 6.

Powell, F., and Wessen, A., 1999, *Health Care Systems in Transition* (Thousand Oaks, CA: Sage).

Raffell, M. W. (Ed.), 1997, *Health Care and Reform in Industrialized Countries* (University Park, PA: Pennsylvania State University Press).

Ranade, W. (Ed.), 1998, *Markets and Health Care. A Comparative Analysis* (Harlow: Longman).

Report Four Country Conference, 1995, Health care reforms and health care policies in the United States, Canada, Germany and the Netherlands, Amsterdam, February 23–25, The Hague: Ministry of Health, Welfare and Sports.

Report Four Country Conference, 2000, Pharmaceutical policies in the US, Canada, Germany and the Netherlands, Amsterdam: Four Country Conference.

Report Workshop EU Law and National Health Policy, 2004, The Hague: Ministry of Health, Welfare and Sports.

Stone, D., 1984, *The Disabled State* (Philadelphia, PA: Temple University Press).

Tuohy, C., 1974, The political attitudes of Ontario physicians: a skill group perspective. PhD thesis, New Haven, CT: Yale University Department of Political Science.

Tuohy, C., 1999, *Accidental Logics* (Oxford: Oxford University Press).

Wall, A. (Ed.), 1996, *Health Care Systems in Liberal Democracies* (London: Routledge).

White, J., 1995, *Competing Solutions: American Health Care Proposals and International Experiences* (Washington, DC: Brookings Institution).

Wilensky, H. L., 2002, *Rich Democracies: Political Economy, Public Policy, and Performance* (Berkeley, CA: University of California Press).

Williams, A., 2001, Science or marketing at WHO? A commentary on "World Health 2000," *Health Economics*, 10(2), 93–100.

Wilsford, D., 1991, *Doctors and the State: The Politics of Health Care in France and the United States* (Durham, NC: Duke University Press).

World Health Organization, 2000, *The World Health Report 2000, Health Systems: Improving Performance* (Geneva: World Health Organization).

Learning from Others

Shall the Last Be the First?

Rudolf Klein

Learning about other countries is rather like breathing: only the brain dead are likely to avoid the experience. None of us can escape the bombardment of information about what is happening in other countries. The process of learning takes many forms. There is the systematic diffusion of information by international bodies like the Organization for Economic Cooperation and Development (OECD 1992, 1994). There is the annual pilgrimage of academics from conference to conference. There are the formal contacts between politicians and civil servants within the framework of European Union and other international organizations, as well as informal contacts in other settings. In effect, there is a series of overlapping health care policy networks. No one belongs to all of them but almost everyone in the health care policy business belongs to at least some of them. There is even a common language: English. Learning *about* other countries must, of course, be sharply distinguished from learning *from* their experience. The former activity is about collecting information; the latter is about reflecting on that information. Still, even allowing for this distinction, lesson-drawing is an expanding industry.

And yet interest in comparative studies—as reflected both in the academic literature (e.g., Marmor 1994; White 1995) and in the conference trade—continues to proliferate. Despite the availability of so much information about what other countries are doing and the accelerating speed of its diffusion, we worry about our capacity to learn from the experience of others and search for ways of improving our ability to do so. Rather like health care itself, supply creates its own demand: the appetite for learning seems to grow as the menu of information expands. In what follows, this article will reflect on this paradox. It is not intended to be, in any way, a systematic analysis of policy learning—let alone the comparative—literature but instead seeks to explore some of the is-

sues and problems encountered in the process of seeking to use the experience
of other countries to inform or shape national decision making.

WHY DO WE WANT TO LEARN?

There is something extremely seductive about the notion of policy learning
(Rose 1993). Given the limited scope for policy experiment in any one country
(and the considerable costs, political as well as economic, often involved) what
could be more sensible than to draw on the experience of other nations? From
this perspective, other countries are to policy makers what laboratories are to
scientists: places where policy theories or techniques are tested. Depending on
the success or failure of the experiment, the theories or techniques can then
be tried out in one's own country. So, at least, runs the naive version of policy
learning. But, of course, the metaphor of scientific experiments is misleading.
In the health care policy field, no two laboratories are the same. No two experiments can therefore be replicated with anything even remotely approaching exactitude. The simplistic utopian model of policy learning therefore leads
to a nihilistic conclusion: if health care policy making is indeed contingent
on its institutional, political, and social context—in other words, the national
laboratory—then learning, seen as the transfer of ideas and techniques, would
seem to be a recipe for disaster. If a particular technique of cost control is contingent on the cooperation of the medical profession in a corporatist system (as in
Germany), there is no point in exporting it to a country (like the United States)
which totally lacks such a system. If the opportunities for radical changes in
health policy are constrained by constitutional arrangements (Immergut 1992),
then again the scope for transferring experience would seem to be very limited.

As these examples suggest, policy learning—if it is to be successful—is at
least as much about the analysis of the *circumstances* in which particular innovations succeed (or fail) as about the innovations themselves: in Peterson's
terminology (Peterson 1997), substantive learning seems to be contingent on
situational learning. To argue that health care policy is shaped by the national
context is therefore not to conclude that the transfer of experience is impossible, but that an understanding of that context is a necessary condition for
drawing any transnational conclusions about the exportability (or otherwise)
of any lessons learned. Before transplanting any policies, we have to make sure
that there is institutional compatibility between donor and recipient. So, for
instance, the ability to implement policy changes depends on political institutions such as electoral systems: it will be much higher in countries like Britain
where the executive commands an automatic majority in the legislature than in

countries like the Netherlands, where coalition politics greatly complicate the task of implementation. Again, policy notions deeply embedded in a century-old culture of social solidarity (as in Germany) will not be easily transferable to countries (like the United States) lacking such a tradition.

All this would suggest that an analysis of the environment of health policy—by which I mean taking account not just of political institutions but civic traditions, tax systems, and administrative resources—must have priority over the analysis of specific health care policy issues in any learning process. The test of any model of health care is its appropriateness to a particular setting; consequently, the challenge to improving our capacity to learn from the experience of other countries is to deepen our understanding of the respects in which they differ or are similar. The point would seem obvious enough, but for the fact that there are a variety of institutions such as the World Bank (1993), which tend to advocate all-purpose models (usually designed by economists) supposedly applicable to all countries. Real learning, I would argue, is about *distinguishing*, about knowing when a particular model is relevant or irrelevant to the specific circumstances of a country.

Policy learning, I would further suggest, is as much a process of self examination—of reflecting on the characteristics of one's own country and health care system—as of looking at the experience of others. Indeed, the experience of other countries is largely valuable insofar as it prompts such a process of critical introspection by enlarging our sense of what is possible and adding to our repertoire of possible policy tools. For policy learning in practice is not about the *transfer* of ideas or techniques (in this respect the transplantation metaphor is misleading), but about their *adaptation* to local circumstances. The experience of other countries stimulates the policy imagination and nudges policy makers in particular directions. But the process of naturalizing foreign experience tends also to transform it into forms that are suitable for the national environment. The case of competition in health care—that new master idea seemingly sweeping the globe—illustrates the point well. The meaning given to this notion (inherently many-layered) has been very different in the various countries that have seemingly embraced it: if the vocabulary is international, the way in which it is translated into policy remains national. So, for example, the health care system that has emerged in the United Kingdom, under the flag of the internal market, is very different from that emerging in the Netherlands: it is all too easy, as Jacobs points out (1998), to lose sight of national differences in the search for global trends. Similarly, many European countries have flirted with the idea of importing Diagnosis Related Groups (DRGs) as a policy tool from the United States, but they have done so in very different ways and with different purposes in mind, depending on local circumstances (Kimberley and Pouvourville 1993). Translation often means transformation.

Above all, cross-national learning is not pursued for its own sake. First, it presupposes a coincidence of concerns in the exporting and importing countries. Interest in the experience of other countries is a function of discontent or anxiety about conditions in one's own country. Second, cross-national curiosity is not a neutral intellectual exercise. Receptivity to foreign ideas is a function of the extent to which they reinforce or fit in with existing policy predilections and prejudices. The experience of other countries may be used in domestic policy debate to inspire either emulation or repudiation. As Marmor and Plowden have argued, "Ideas are elements in policy warfare whose take-up is determined not by their intrinsic validity but by the local setting—its present moods and circumstances, and structures" (1991: 812). Thus, in Britain, the experience of the United States is often invoked in political debate to elicit a kneejerk repudiation of anything which looks remotely like a market, while conversely, in the United States, the experience of Britain's National Health Service (NHS) is invoked to provoke horror at the very idea of "socialized medicine" (Klein 1991).

For learning from other countries is not just about adopting or adapting new ideas. Negative learning—avoiding the mistakes of others—may be just as important as positive learning. But in either instance, as the above quote from Marmor and Plowden suggests, the experience of other countries serves to provide ammunition for domestic conflicts. They are battles to impose a particular view of the world in a universe of multiple versions of the truth. Some policies or techniques are unambiguous failures or successes. But in most cases there are complex balance sheets, and success or failure may be contingent on particular local conditions. Not surprisingly, therefore, selective perception and disputes about the interpretation of evidence characterize the use (and misuse) of cross-national comparisons in the world of policy debate. Even if we are driven by shared problems and anxieties to examine the experience of other countries, what we find will be viewed through the prism of national values and presented in the rhetoric of politics.

THE CHALLENGE TO ACADEMIC ANALYSTS

This analysis helps to explain the challenge to, and frustrations of, academic comparative analysts concerned to influence policy debate. Two recent, distinguished examples make the point. Consider, first, Marmor's attempt to use the Canadian experience of combining comprehensive coverage with successful cost containment (at least when compared to the United States) to draw policy lessons for the United States as part of a wide-ranging review of health care reform options (Marmor 1994). As he points out, the United States shares with Canada "a common language and political roots, a comparably diverse population with a similar distribution of living standards, increasingly integrated economies and a tradition of fractious but constitutional federalism that makes political disputes similar though obviously not identical." Canada's experience with national health insurance, Marmor therefore argues, "provides American policy makers with a perfect opportunity for cross-national learning" (ibid.: 185).

Marmor is far too sophisticated to advocate that the United States should adopt the Canadian single-payer model lock, stock, and barrel. Instead, his strategy is to draw out the principles underlying the Canadian health care system and to explore ways in which these could be applied in the context of the United States. These, he argues, are three-fold: universal access, a responsible financing agency, and accountable political leaders. However, these principles could be translated—and adapted—to the American environment in a variety of ways. In effect, he argues, the United States could move toward something like the Canadian universal system by aggregating existing schemes like Medicare and Medicaid and by introducing a new insurance plan for those not covered by these schemes. The case for accepting second or even third best choices has seldom been put more persuasively. In other words, he uses the Canadian experience not as a template but as a way of stimulating thought about how to move toward achieving certain policy objectives in full awareness of American exceptionalism in health care.

A somewhat similar strategy is pursued by White (1995) in his study of health care systems in Australia, France, Japan, and the United Kingdom. Again, the aim is not to construct a model for the United States, but to distill some general principles from international experience. These are what White calls "international standards": universal coverage, contributions to a national system of insurance related to income, and the central regulation of budgets. These "standards" are, in practice, translated into very different institutional arrangements in the countries concerned, reflecting their history and culture. Again, therefore, they do not provide an off-the-peg solution for adoption in the United States. But they do provide criteria for assessing proposals for reform, such as managed competition—a task which White carries out with relish.

The list of distinguished contributions to the American lessons-from-abroad literature could be greatly extended: Glaser's recent (1994) article is only the latest in the long list of his contributions to the topic. The aim here, however, is not to review the literature but to make the simple point that all this activity appears to have made little impact on policy making in the United States. Despite all the intellectual rigor deployed, despite the acknowledgment that foreign experience cannot be directly translated into policy recipes for the United States, the debate (and proposals like the Clinton plan) have been shaped by other considerations. There are some fairly obvious explanations for this. If only the United States had not declared independence in 1776 and if, like Canada, it had been endowed with a Westminster-type constitution—assuring the government of the day of an automatic majority in the legislature—the story might be very different. Absent that, there is an inverse relationship between the capacity of the American academic industry to produce outstanding studies of foreign experience and the ability of the American political system to make use of the resulting products.

Some consolation may perhaps be drawn from the argument that policy makers only make use of ideas when they have forgotten their source: when they have persuaded themselves that they are the product of their own ratiocinations, untainted by foreign influences. If so, the lesson drawing literature may have a long-term sedimentary effect. But it is a thin consolation.

LEARNING ABOUT WHAT FROM WHOM?

So far this article has used the notion of cross-national learning in an undifferentiated and rather promiscuous way. Now the time has come to unpackage it and to define more precisely the specific characteristics of what is being learned. For, as I will argue in this section, the various dimensions of cross-national learning may differ in important respects. In particular, the learning circuits—the networks of people involved in the process of acquiring and interpreting information about what is happening in other countries—will differ, as will the audiences involved. Deciding *whom* to learn from may also decide *what* we learn.

The most comprehensive form of cross-national learning is when we compare *systems* of health care provision—that is, the way in which they are financed and organized—in the search for that elusive formula which will allow us to reconcile cost containment, efficiency, equity, and effectiveness. And this is what I have concentrated on so far. However, much of policy learning is more limited in its ambition and more narrowly focused on specific problems or programs. So, for example, the onset of AIDS in Britain sent politicians and civil servants scurrying to the United States to discover what could be learned from American experience. Similarly, the Oregon approach to limiting the menu of health care attracted a long procession of international tourists. Again, there may be much interest in comparing experience about the impact of introducing charges for services on patterns of use. In all these instances, the focus of attention is on policy issues. But much of cross-national learning may be about organizational processes or managerial techniques: the introduction and international marketing of DRGs provide the most obvious example. Lastly, there is the continual frenzy of cross-national learning that characterizes the delivery of medical care itself: the rapid transfer of new technology (in its widest sense) from country to country.

Finally, it must be stressed that policy learning is as much about the past as about the present. That is, although it is easy to get excited about policy innovation, and to focus on what is new, some of the most policy-relevant questions can only be answered by looking at the experience of different countries over decades. There are, therefore, different worlds of cross-national learning within the health care arena. And one of the explanations for the paradox noted at the start of this article—that the appetite for the exchange of information grows as the supply increases—may well be that there is too little contact between these worlds. The introduction of new management tools has obvious implications for public policy: Should DRGs, for example, be used simply in order to prompt critical self-examination by managers and clinicians, or as a reimbursement mechanism? The transfer of medical technology, similarly, has very obvious implications for health care budgets—but the policy makers who will pick up the bill (or seek ways of restraining its growth) are not involved in the process of cross-national learning.

So it may well be that *controlling* cross-national learning—constraining the adoption of imported ideas—is at least as important as promoting free trade in information. Perhaps we should be putting more emphasis on studying the way in which different countries test and make use of imported ideas and techniques to see what we can learn from their successes (or failures) in preventing the adoption of half-baked or untried notions or technologies—a point discussed further in the next, and final, section of this article.

If we accept that cross-national learning is rather like a multi-ring circus, with different actors performing in each ring—then some other implications may follow as well. In particular, it may be that the problems of such learning (the evaluation of what is happening in another country) are compounded by the fact that different actors use different languages and have different perspectives. Practical policy makers—by which I mean both civil servants and politicians—do not, for example, have the same agenda as academics. Neither do they necessarily draw on the same kind of knowledge (Lindblom and Cohen 1979). They may both operate in the field of health policy, but their concerns

and questions will be rather different. Civil servants may perhaps be more concerned with questions of feasibility and implementability than academics (just
as among academics, political scientists pay more attention to this dimension of
policy making than economists do). There may well also be differences in their
views about who counts as an authoritative interpreter of reality. Just as academics will naturally look to their peers, so will civil servants. And, of course, both
policy makers and academics will differ, in turn, from medical practitioners and
managers.

The testing of ideas may therefore depend precisely on having a confrontation of perspectives, occupational and disciplinary as well as national. Explicitly
acknowledging and identifying the differences between the various groups may
be a better way forward than attempting to reduce the language of discourse to
a bland international Esperanto.

Precisely because learning from other countries is such a value-laden exercise, precisely because there are so many different reasons for wanting to look
at the experience of other countries, it is important to know who wants to know
what and why, rather than assuming that a common interest in comparisons
necessarily involves a commonality of purpose or a shared assumptive world.

HOW DO WE KNOW WHEN TO LEARN?

There is another factor in cross-national learning that has so far not been
considered: the time dimension. During what stage in the policy cycle, and at
what point in the life history of a program or technical innovation, should we
start getting interested and seeking out any lessons? The obvious temptation is
to rush in as quickly as possible. Policy making (and even more so the academic
study of policy making) has a lot in common with the fashion industry. No
one likes to be caught wearing yesterday's ideas. The adoption of new policy
models, new programs, or new techniques commands attention and generates
intellectual excitement. The searchlight of academic inquiry—and the consequent flow of information to the policy community—therefore tends to focus
disproportionately on what is new. And, to an extent, this is only right. If one of
the most important roles of policy learning is (as argued earlier) to stir up our
own ideas and to stretch our imagination, then the shock of the new provides
an appropriate stimulus.

But there is also a case for arguing that policy learning should only take place
when the new models, programs, and techniques have been tested and evaluated over time in their country of origin (White 1995). What is the point of rushing in to study a new experiment, much less to adopt a new model, before there

is any evidence about its outcome? If no policy is better than its implementability, then why not wait to see how it works out in practice? After all, the durability
of an institutional innovation or program may be one of the most important
tests of its desirability; there seems little point in rushing in to adopt something
which may ultimately be abandoned by the originating country. And if we accept this line of argument, the real beneficiaries of cross-national learning will
be those countries who come last in the queue of would-be adaptors.

There is a further twist to this argument. A cautious approach to the import of
foreign models might even suggest waiting until several countries have tried out
a particular policy or program model in order to test its robustness and its sensitivity to different institutional environments. A careful analysis of the life cycles
of policy experiments in a variety of countries might help to identify the common elements that characterize the most successful models. In other words,
the most valuable form of cross-national policy learning may be the study of
the patterns of success and failure over time, not in any single country but in a
whole population of countries: the intellectual model being not the laboratory
experiment, but historical epidemiology.

It is an argument which, on balance, I find convincing. It cannot be swallowed whole, however. It applies much more strongly to policy learning about
health care systems as a whole than to policy learning about the design of programs to handle crises. If policy makers are in a situation where they must take
immediate action, as in the case of AIDS, then it is futile to argue that learning should be delayed until there has been an opportunity to study evaluation
reports on what has been done in a range of other countries. There is, in any
case, a problem about the notion that cross-national learning should be filtered
through evaluation studies. One of the characteristics of many programs is that
they change over their life cycles: in other words, there is a constant process
of adjustment in the light of experience. The same is even more true of the
introduction of new models for the organization or financing of health care
systems. So, for example, Britain's new model National Health Service is an
institution that is constantly reinventing itself: it is a car that is being reengi-
neered even while it is roaring around the test track (Klein 1995). Evaluating
what happened in the past might thus be a poor guide to the model's likely
future performance.

But the example of Britain's new model of NHS suggests that there may
be another dimension to cross-national learning. So far in this essay the emphasis has been on learning about the substance of new models, programs,
or techniques and on asking the question, Are they successful (whatever that
may mean) or not? But there is another question, which is about the *process* of

introducing change. There may be much to be learned from the experiences of different countries about the balance of advantages and disadvantages of trying to introduce carefully crafted new models, with every detail fully worked out, as against designing framework institutions which evolve over time. A comparison of the experiences of the United States and the United Kingdom might suggest that the advantage lies on the side of designing flexible framework institutions which allow for adaptation over time. Or it might simply demonstrate that different models of change are contingent on the political institutions in which the health care systems are embedded. But whatever the conclusion reached, this is a case where learning need perhaps not wait on history.

Note

This essay is an expanded version of a paper given at the Four Country Conference on Health Care Reforms, the Netherlands, February 1995. In revising the article, I have gratefully drawn on the comments of the participants at the conference. It was first published in *Journal of Health Politics, Policy and Law* 22, no. 5 (October 1997).

References

Glaser, William. 1994. Universal Health Insurance That Really Works: Foreign Lessons for the United States. In *The Politics of Health Care Reform: Lessons from the Past, Prospects for the Future*, ed. James A. Morone and Gary S. Belkin. Durham: Duke University Press.

Immergut, Ellen M. 1992. *Health Politics: Interests and Institutions in Western Europe.* Cambridge: Cambridge University Press.

Jacobs, Alan. 1998. Seeing Difference: Market Health Reform in Europe. *Journal of Health Politics, Policy and Law* 23(1):1–33.

Kimberley, John R., and Gerard Pouvourville, eds. 1993. *The Migration of Managerial Innovation: Diagnosis Related Groups and Health Care Administration in Western Europe.* San Francisco: Jossey-Bass.

Klein, Rudolf. 1991. Risks and Benefits of Comparative Studies: Notes from Another Shore. *Milbank Quarterly* 69:275–291. 1995.

———. 2010. *The New Politics of the NHS,* 6th ed. London: Longman.

Lindblom, Charles E., and David K. Cohen. 1979. *Usable Knowledge.* New Haven: Yale University Press.

Marmor, Theodore R. 1994. *Understanding Health Care Reform.* New Haven: Yale University Press.

Marmor, Theodore R., and William Plowden. 1991. Rhetoric and Reality in the Intellectual Jet Stream: The Export to Britain from America of Questionable Ideas. *Journal of Health Politics, Policy and Law* 16:807–812.

Organization for Economic Cooperation and Development (OECD). 1992. *The Reform of Health Care: A Comparative Analysis of Seven OECD Countries.* Paris: OECD.

———. 1994. *The Reform of Health Care Systems: A Review of Seventeen OECD Countries.* Paris: OECD.

Peterson, Mark A. 1997. The Limits of Social Learning: Translating Analysis into Action. *Journal of Health Politics, Policy and Law* 22:1077–1114.

Rose, Richard. 1993. *Lesson-Drawing in Public Policy: A Guide to Learning across Time and Space.* Chatham, NJ: Chatham House.

White, Joseph. 1995. *Competing Solutions: American Health Care Proposals and International Experience.* Washington, DC: Brookings Institution.

World Bank. 1993. *World Development Report 1993.* Oxford: Oxford University Press.

9

RESOURCES AND RATIONING

If we were to try to organize the politics of health care around one theme, it would most likely be that of how to raise, contain, and distribute resources. In some countries, like the United States, the policy concern is about inexorably rising costs; in others, like Britain, it is about inexorably rising demands. In all countries, the concern is how to make the better use of existing resources. Driving policy cross-nationally is the hope that if only health care systems could deliver scientifically validated treatments efficiently—while eliminating those where there is no evidence of efficacy—costs could be contained and the political dilemmas of allocating limited resources among competing demands resolved.

The hope represents the triumph of naive optimism over hard facts. Squeezing out waste is not the simple remedy that political rhetoric suggests. Rather, as the first article in this chapter demonstrates, it diverts attention from the complex reality. The politics of making hard choices about resource distribution are here to stay and may even become more fraught as demography, technology, and the pharmaceutical industry combine to generate new pressures on resources.

The politics of hard choice have one characteristic common to both the United States and Britain: blame avoidance for rationing (by which we mean the denial of potentially beneficial treatment; refusing to prescribe snake oil is not rationing in our vocabulary). The United States is in a state of denial about rationing; there is a reluctance even to acknowledge its existence. In Britain, the existence of rationing is openly acknowledged, though its scale is not. In both, it is the reality, even while the strategies pursued to make rationing as politically invisible as possible reflect the very different organizational characteristics of health care in the two countries.

In the United States, the traditional freedom of physicians to decide whom to treat and how has become increasingly constrained over time. "Managed care" in effect means managed rationing. Physician decisions about the treatment to be offered are subject to both ex ante and ex post review. Insurance policies have long lists of exclusions, while at the same time lack of insurance coverage limits access to medical care for many. If the United States is in a state of denial about the existence and scale of rationing, as it largely is, it is because of the diffuse nature of this process. Institutionally, there is no political focus for directing blame for the extent and form of rationing.

The situation in Britain is very different, though in the process of change. The freedom of physicians in the NHS has always been circumscribed by having to work within fixed budgets. But within their budgets, they have been less subject to external constraints and checks than their American counterparts. In effect, they maintained medical autonomy by internalizing resource constraints—and presenting denial or dilution of treatment as the exercise of clinical discretion. Rationing in Britain carried low political costs for the government because— long, highly visible waiting lists apart—it was largely invisible: central political decisions about the level of resources to be allocated to the NHS were transmuted into clinical decisions at the point of delivery.

This traditional rationing strategy is, as of the turn of the millennium, under challenge. Implicit decisions about what to provide for whom have become explicit as the NHS has adopted an internal market, with budgets delegated to Primary Care Trusts. The PCTs are responsible for buying health care on behalf of their populations and therefore have to make decisions about which drugs or treatments will or will not be funded; in turn, doctors are constrained by these decisions. The resulting visibility of geographical variations in what is or is not provided leads to public outcries and demands for government action to end "postcode rationing." Enter therefore another strategy for avoiding blame falling on central government and minimizing the political costs of hard choices: the creation of the National Institute for Health and Clinical Excellence (NICE), whose remit is to recommend the use or non-use of drugs and medical interventions in the NHS on criteria of cost effectiveness. In effect, this is an attempt to transmute political decisions about the use of resources into expert decisions.

This is not the first attempt to depoliticize rationing decisions, and will certainly not be the last. The search for a formula to define health care entitlements, invoking science and economics in the name of rationality, is global. Today it is NICE, which is attracting international policy tourists; in the 1990s it was Oregon. The Oregon experiment, as discussed in the article in this chapter, was an attempt to define a package of health care for those covered by the state's Medicaid scheme. It sought to marry cost-effectiveness analysis and popular participation in ranking different procedures. It achieved almost mythical status, attracting widespread international attention. In the outcome, however, the model never worked as advertised. Its final ranking of eligible Medicaid procedures turned out to be the product not of cost-effectiveness analysis or even popular values, but rather an opaque juggling act designed to achieve a politically acceptable package.

Paradoxically, the reason for analyzing the Oregon experience in detail is precisely the fact that it provided a warning rather than an example, but this warning was largely ignored. The myth of Oregon achieved much greater prominence than the reality: it was an example of the overenthusiastic, undercritical circulation of ideas as described in Chapter 5 and a reminder of the need for careful scrutiny of innovative models before rushing to import them, as argued in Chapter 10.

Neither the history of the Oregon model nor the experience of NICE is, however, likely to halt the search for ways to depoliticize rationing. What might be described as an intellectual interest group—an alliance of the evidence-based medicine movement with economists—has continued to lobby for rationing to be based on so-called rational criteria of effectiveness and cost: a good example of a campaign to change the assumptive world of policy making. It remains to be seen whether this succeeds. There are, as the articles in this chapter argue, formidable difficulties. Ethical arguments cut across cost-effectiveness considerations; applying any criteria involves taking into account the specific circumstances of individual patients, such as differing capacities to benefit from treatment.

Perhaps the most important single conclusion to be drawn from the articles in this chapter is that all health care systems will remain dependent on the exercise of the medical profession's discretion in the use of resources. The case of Viagra, analyzed in one of this chapter's essays, reinforces this conclusion. It shows that the process of policy making differed considerably in different health care systems—institutions matter—and that the resulting criteria for funding (or mostly refusing to fund) Viagra varied somewhat. But what seems to have made even the most severe decisions politically acceptable—the special character of this drug apart—was an escape clause allowing doctors to exercise their clinical judgment.

Cutting Waste by Making Rules

Promises, Pitfalls, and Realistic Prospects

Jan Blustein and Theodore R. Marmor

American medical costs, one hardly needs to say, continue to rise relentlessly. In 1990, health expenditures consumed approximately 12.2% of America's GNP.[1] A decade earlier, the share was 9.1%.[2] In 1970, we spent approximately 7.4%.[3] There has developed an apparent consensus—among government, labor, and profession leaders—that costs must be contained. At the same time, there is widespread agreement that access must be universalized. As a result, many believe that excruciatingly hard choices are unavoidable.

This perceived dilemma has led to a great deal of talk about rationing.[4] The tenor of the commentary indicates that it is a fearsome solution to our present troubles—painful and divisive, entailing choices that no one wants to make but which must be faced due to inescapable scarcity.[5] Both contemporary rhetoric and current health policy, however, hold out the hope of a far more agreeable alternative. Galvanized by the realization that much medical care is of uncertain value, and bolstered by findings that show significant variation in medical practice patterns, a coalition of policymakers, politicians, and researchers is now actively engaged in seeking to contain costs by eliminating wasteful care. This appears an attractive course. Waste-cutting, unlike rationing, does not connote the cruel denial of necessary care. On the contrary, it suggests saving people from medical interventions that would not have done them any good. If "rationing" is the fearsome alternative, "cutting waste" is the benign one.

While consensus grows that wasteful practice is a problem, there is considerable disagreement about the solution. Such disagreement is hardly surprising, since cutting waste is merely a goal, not a program. Cutting waste can mean any of a number of things. It can mean regionalizing services, instituting yearly expenditure targets, implementing managed care systems, or developing elaborate review mechanisms to constrain the diffusion of new technologies. Indeed, the idea of "cutting waste" is so broad in its potential scope that it can subsume many hotly debated reforms in the field of health policy. Like Health Maintenance Organizations, competition, and Diagnostic Related Groups before it, it is another vaunted panacea, the new great answer to arrive on the American health policy agenda.[6]

This essay critically assesses the widely advertised plan to cut waste by making microallocational rules for the provision of medical care. Such rules, variously denominated "practice parameters,"[7] "clinical guidelines,"[8] and "standards of care,"[9] are aimed at ensuring that no patient is subjected to "wasteful" care by specifying what treatments particular patients should receive. For example, the rule that "healthy patients under 40 years of age without a family history of heart disease should not be given an electrocardiogram" is a practice parameter. It could be used by physicians to guide day-to-day treatment decisions. It could also be used by payers to control reimbursement, and by policymakers to appraise aggregate data about medical care utilization.[10]

Our analysis raises the fundamental but too-little discussed question of what constitutes waste. Our central claim is that so called "wasteful" practice is a conceptual hodgepodge, which encompasses treatments that are (1) ineffective; (2) of uncertain effectiveness; (3) ethically troubling; or (4) not allocationally efficient.[11] From this starting point, we address issues of rule making and resource allocation and ask the following questions: Can all four of these types of wasteful care be identified in ways that are scientifically defensible and administratively practicable? What obstacles must be faced to make cutting waste by making rules into a policy in each case? Are there American institutions and attitudes that would make such rule making more costly, and therefore less attractive, than it seems? And can any (or all) of these four types of waste be cut without confronting the dilemma of difficult choices? But before approaching these questions, we begin by briefly reviewing the ways in which the problem of wasteful care has been framed by health care analysts, providers, and policymakers.

LOOSE TALK ABOUT "WASTE"

Terms like "wasteful," "ineffective," "inappropriate," "of unproven effectiveness," "unnecessary," and even "irrational" are used loosely and often interchangeably in the literature that is critical of current medical practice. Commentators have lamented the prevalence of unnecessary elective surgery,[12] gratuitous "little ticket" diagnostic tests,[13] and expensive treatments for AIDS patients.[14] It is tempting to assume that these practices share some fundamental characteristic that places them within a unified category of wasteful medical treatments.

Although the temptation is evident, assimilating various "inappropriate" types of care within the rhetoric of waste cutting is at best confusing. Take the example of the rules that determine when physician office visits are "medically necessary."[15] As one physician explained it:

> Medicare has set guidelines that for a given condition, you're only allowed to see patients so many times. That doesn't mean that you can't see them more often—you certainly can—but they won't pay for it. . . .
>
> It takes a great deal of time . . . because I have to explain to them why Medicare may not pay for their visit to me. You're legally obliged to explain to the patient that this is considered medically unnecessary. Well, that choice of words implies to most patients that you're giving poor medical care. You're making them come back too often. And I think it's terrible.
>
> It wastes 20 minutes of my time explaining to them that no, its not really medically unnecessary, that that's just how Medicare has chosen to word the new form. . . .[16]

Making "expensive" synonymous with "medically unnecessary" seems a particularly troubling example of bureaucratically sanctioned linguistic drift. But it is not just linguistic territory that has been invaded by the waste cutters. Utilization review companies have moved beyond the realm of previewing surgical procedures and into the field of making allocational choices in the cases of very sick and dying patients. They employ "case managers" to direct the costly care of their sickest enrollees. This strategy can pay off handsomely. "[M]any cost-management companies are strengthening their 'case management' of patients who are seriously ill, with advanced cancer or AIDS, for example, or recovering from a stroke. 'The savings can average $10,000 to $15,000 per case and be as high as $400,000.'"[17] While some case managers may be truly well intentioned, intervening to help patients and save them from painful overtreatment, they also represent economic interests that will inevitably conflict at times with the interests of the patient. In the future, we are likely to hear more from case managers about "inappropriate," "ineffective," and "medically unnecessary" care. When we do, it will be hard to know exactly what this means. Is the proposed treatment harmful or worthless? Is it futile or just too costly?

These ambiguities must be faced in formulating a sensible strategy for controlling the cost of medical care in America. It would be enormously agreeable if cost containment could be achieved by cutting out a homogeneous wedge of present practices (Figure 1). But our analysis suggests that waste is heterogeneous (Figure 2), a claim worth exploring at some length. We need to know more about the four different types of waste. How prevalent are they? How do

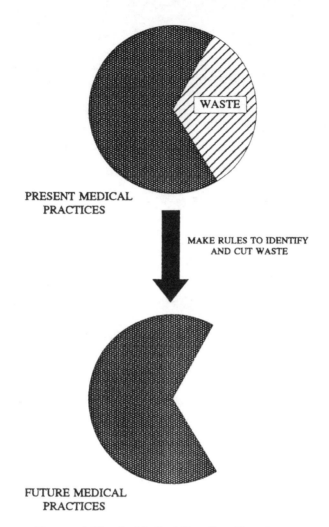

PRESENT MEDICAL
PRACTICES

WASTE

MAKE RULES TO IDENTIFY
AND CUT WASTE

FUTURE MEDICAL
PRACTICES

Figure 1. A Plan for Medical Care Cost Containment

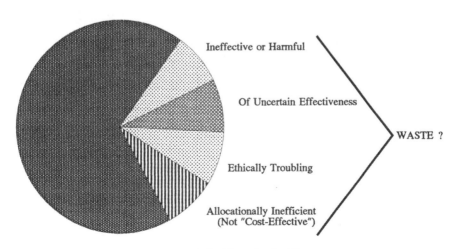

Ineffective or Harmful

Of Uncertain Effectiveness

WASTE ?

Ethically Troubling

Allocationally Inefficient
(Not "Cost-Effective")

Figure 2. A Problem for the Plan

Table 1: A Taxonomy of Wasteful Care

Type of Waste	Amount of Waste	Issues in Identifying Waste	Costs of Cutting Waste by Making Rules	Does Cutting Waste Mean Denying Benefit?
Ineffective or harmful	Unknown, since the effectiveness of most intervention is uncertain.	Requires an extensive scientific database. "Clinical judgment" introduces uncertainty.	Relatively few. Public probably will accept physicians have accepted the strategy (RAND/AMA cooperation).	No.
Of uncertain effectiveness	Abundant, since the effectiveness of most intervention is uncertain.	See above.	Many. Physicians likely to resent intrusion on clinical judgment. Public unlikely to accept denial of care perceived to be beneficial.	Not known (hard choices).
Ethically troubling	Growing.	Requires an ethical consensus.	Many (need to distinguish between guidelines and rules to cut waste). Public discussion of rules to cut waste is controversial.	Perhaps (depends on values; hard choices).
Allocationally inefficient ("not cost-effective")	Unknown, since cost-benefit analysis and cost-effectiveness analysis work better in theory than in practice.	Requires the acquisition of scientific and economic data, as well as development of a consensus about values and an agreement about budgetary constraints.	Many. Rulemaking can be bitterly divisive. Public expects to get beneficial care regardless of costs. There may be legal obstacles to rulemaking. Physicians feel that consideration of costs taints of professionalism.	Yes (hard choices).

we determine that particular treatments fall into one of the four categories? What political, social, and professional obstacles will arise when standards are introduced forbidding wasteful practices? Will waste-cutting erect barriers to beneficial care, or can waste-cutting bypass such choices in medical care allocation? These four questions are at the core of the following section. Our main findings are summarized in Table 1.

A TAXONOMY OF "WASTE"

INEFFECTIVE (OR HARMFUL) TREATMENT

Some Americans, expert and lay, believe that much of medical care is ineffective or positively harmful. In part a generalized rebellion against authority of the 1960s, and nurtured by the consumer health movement of the 1970s, this view found a passionate voice in Ivan Illich's 1976 book, *Medical Nemesis.*[18] His scathing critique of the medical profession's "poisons"[19] and "black magic"[20] never found widespread public acceptance. But the 1980s brought a wider condemnation of the medical profession. Today's conventional wisdom is that doctors have little idea of what they are doing.

Consider what doctors, to say nothing of patients, don't know about the value of just one procedure. Every year about 80,000 Americans get a carotid endarterectomy, a kind of Roto-Rooter job on clogged neck arteries. Typically costing $9,000, counting the bill for a hospital stay, the operation is designed to prevent strokes. Another triumph of modern medicine? Or an overly risky, overdone alternative to cheaper drug therapy? Incredibly, no one knows for sure, and no one is tracking the patients on a systematic basis to find out.

The same holds true for scores of other medical ministrations. Food companies know the impact of a redesigned ketchup bottle on sales. But the virtuosos performing hysterectomies, installing pacemakers, and bypassing diseased coronary arteries have only patchy information about the real payoffs. "Half of what the medical profession does is of unverified effectiveness," asserts Dr. Paul M. Ellwood, Jr. of Minneapolis, one in a phalanx of physicians who want to cut down on the guesswork.[21]

Academic medicine is trying to answer this criticism. Researchers in a relatively new branch of investigation, clinical epidemiology, are trying to sort out which medical maneuvers are effective.

Ideally, the research involves systematic and painstaking testing of therapies through randomized controlled clinical trials. But these experiments, the "gold standard" for determining clinical effectiveness, are events of epic proportion, lasting for years, costing millions of dollars, involving thousands of patients, facing monumental bureaucratic barriers, and raising serious ethical issues.[22] Often, by the time clinical trials are completed, the technology they studied is outmoded.[23] Although other methodologies have been developed and can yield useful information,[24] physicians must regularly weigh the preponderance of imperfect evidence in order to estimate whether a particular patient might benefit from a particular intervention.[25] It is often possible to entertain some reasonable doubt (or to hold out some reasonable hope) that a treatment will be effective. While there is currently a great deal of enthusiasm about improving the scientific basis of medicine, and while there is surely room for improvement, a vast project to make medicine scientific can never keep up with innovations in medical practice. Nor is it likely to provide firm ground for determining correct choices in most clinical situations. Medical decision-making is simply too complex.[26]

Given these limitations, how can ineffective treatments be identified? One approach is to augment imperfect information with the judgments of experts. Distinguished physicians, well-versed in the scientific literature, can use their clinical judgment and their beliefs about what works, based on their own past practices—to produce estimates of effectiveness. And groups of physicians can combine their expert judgments to arrive at consensus. A group of researchers at the RAND Corporation has developed a method for generating this kind of professional consensus about what works (and what doesn't work) in medicine.[27] Because their innovative method has been so widely acclaimed and so often held up as a model for cutting waste by making rules, it warrants a brief review.

The RAND group's goal was to develop practice parameters for several widely used operations. They assembled a panel of distinguished physicians for each of the operations, and each panel member reviewed the available scientific literature about the procedure.[28] With a list of all of the possible clinical scenarios in which each procedure might be performed, each panelist made an assessment of the appropriateness of the intervention for each of the scenarios, based on the literature review and clinical judgment. After making independent assessments, the panel members met to discuss the cases and compare their ratings. They found there was substantial disagreement among them about the appropriateness of performing the operations in many clinical settings.[29] And so, after reviewing the cases together, the individual physicians rated each scenario again, and the revised ratings were combined into a group consensus rating of the appropriateness of treatment in each situation. For each clinical scenario, the surgery was rated as "appropriate," "inappropriate," or "equivocal." "Inappropriate" care was treatment in which "the expected health benefit[s] (i.e., increased life expectancy, relief of pain, reduction in anxiety, [and] improved functional capacity) [were] exceeded [by] the expected negative consequences (i.e., mortality, morbidity, anxiety of anticipating the procedure, pain produced by the procedure, and time lost from work)."[30] Roughly speaking, then, "inappropriate" was defined to mean ineffective or harmful.

The ratings have been used successfully in pilot programs to identify "inappropriate" care: Two prominent RAND researchers recently left the Santa Monica think tank to found Value Health Sciences, Inc., bringing along the RAND methodology. They then developed some innovative software that uses the expert consensus on appropriateness to deliver second opinions about physicians' treatment choices. Value's clients employ utilization review nurses to quiz physicians about referrals for the selected procedures. Using Value's computer-driven questionnaire while talking over the telephone, the nurses gather information about prospective patients and then match each prospective patient to a previously rated clinical scenario. If the prior consensus suggested the operation was "appropriate" for that patient, the patient's insurance company pays for the hospital admission. If the rules identified the operation as "inappropriate," the procedure is not covered. The referring physician may then appeal the decision regarding coverage with a doctor representing the utilization review company. In a trial run by the Aetna insurance company, 15% of 1,000 referrals for procedures were judged "inappropriate"; physician appeals brought the number of actual refusals down to 9%.[31]

The successful implementation of the RAND/Value method is one of the first achievements of what has been called the "outcomes movement."[32] This informal coalition of academic researchers, government officials, physician professional organizations, and members of the health insurance industry has come together over the past three years in an effort to study what works in medicine, to define "appropriate" care, and to use that definition of appropriateness to eliminate allegedly wasteful care through the use of practice guidelines. While each participant has a slightly different sense of the movement's mission,[33] most share Paul Ellwood's ambitious vision:

Outcomes management is a technology of patient experience designed to help patients, payers, and providers make rational medical care–related choices based on better insight into the effect of these choices on the patient's life. Outcomes management consists of a . . . language of health outcomes; a national data base containing information and analysis on clinical, financial and health outcomes that estimates as best we can the relation between medical interventions and health outcomes, as well as the relation between health outcomes and money; and an opportunity for each decision-maker to have access to the analyses that are relevant to the choices they must make.[34]

Federal officials have been enthusiastic supporters of what has been hailed— perhaps somewhat grandiosely—as "the third revolution in health care."[35] Former Health Care Financing Administration ("HCFA") director William L. Roper, under pressure to contain Medicare's explosive growth, announced a major initiative to "evaluate and improve medical practice" by using HCFA's mammoth databases to study the outcomes of care given under that program.[36] In a related later development, the Department of Health and Human Services' National Center for Health Services Research ("NCHSR") was renamed the Agency for Health Care Policy and Research ("AHCPR") and charged with "promoting the quality, appropriateness, and effectiveness of health care" and directing studies that would lead to the development of clinical guidelines for "treatments or conditions that account for a significant portion of Medicare expenditures."[37] With the new name came an increase in federal funding. In 1991, the agency received over sixty million dollars to investigate the outcomes of medical care and develop parameters to guide clinical practice.[38] Three years earlier, as the NCHSR, the agency had been given less than two million dollars to support such efforts.[39] Many leaders of private industry and health insurance firms are enthusiastic about these developments, and foresee using the results to cut costs.[40]

The American Medical Association ("AMA") is perhaps the least likely of the coalition's members. Historically a staunch advocate of physician auton-omy, the AMA has teamed up with the RAND Corporation and the Academic Medical Center Consortium, a group of major teaching hospitals,[41] to develop practice guidelines for use by "payers and utilization and medical reviewers to define a range of practice options physicians could use without incurring finan-cial or other sanctions. . . ."[42] The AMA's embrace of the parameters initiative is somewhat puzzling—few physicians wish to do their patients harm, but none seem to want to be told what to do—organized medicine's position probably reflects the recognition that "if you can't beat 'em, join 'em." As AMA Executive Vice President James Todd explained, physicians must lead the effort to de-velop practice standards because they "can't afford to abdicate this responsibil-ity to [the] bureaucratic computer screens of HCFA or commercial insurance companies."[43] Although support for the initiative must be viewed primarily as a kind of preemptive strike, practice parameters do offer some attractive features from the physicians' perspective.[44] First, they have a substantial educational potential. In a bewilderingly complex and rapidly changing technical environment, parameters can provide physicians with a simple, easily accessible reference guide. Second, in a hostile legal environment, adherence to "appropriate" practices may protect practitioners from malpractice liability.[45]

In summary, parameters do hold some promise in curbing ineffective or harmful care, and there is clearly energetic activity in support of their development. But the amount of time and money required to develop and implement the RAND/Value approach on a large scale, though unknown, is surely substantial. According to AHCPR officials, it has taken three years to move from the process of identifying conditions for guideline development to early pilot testing of those guidelines; the agency released two guidelines in March 1992, intending to make several more available this summer.[46] If such guidelines were to be widely used to audit physician choices, the degree of bureaucratization in medical care would increase substantially. The requirement that physicians "clear" a large proportion of their decisions could impose significant additional costs in a system where, experts estimate, as much as 20% of expenditures already go to administrative matters,[47] and where provider frustration with the micromanagement of care is already intense.[48] Still, the movement has generated tremendous enthusiasm and significant funding. It is worth exploring the probable consequences of extending its approach to other types of "wasteful" care.

TREATMENT OF UNCERTAIN EFFECTIVENESS

Dr. Ellwood's estimate that "half of what the medical profession does is of unverified effectiveness"[49] is undeniably provocative. If that were the case, policymakers might well be advised to discontinue such practices pending scientific demonstration of their worth. Although this could mean waiting decades for research results, the successful implementation of this policy might cut medical costs dramatically.[50]

There is ample room for doubt about the effectiveness of many medical treatments. For some treatments, there is very little data on effectiveness. For most treatments, there is disagreement as to how to interpret the available data. In the face of this uncertainty, how feasible is it to talk about cutting waste with rules prohibiting payment for treatments of undetermined effectiveness?

Most physicians would almost certainly oppose this approach. Because of the lack of scientific knowledge about disease, the practice of medicine is not a "cookbook" endeavor. Clinicians extrapolate beyond scientific data in "the large portion of cases . . . [that] are clinically gray and require clinical judgment."[51] Judging how to proceed in questionable cases is part of what constitutes the art of medicine. Physician Donald Berwick of the Harvard Community Health

Plan has rightly warned that in choosing to cut waste by overriding clinical judgment, "we [may] gain control of care patterns only to find that care is being given by doctors who have lost pride and heart."[52] And while the specter of disheartened physicians might not forestall officials intent upon cutting costs, public opinion would likely inhibit this approach to "cutting waste." Some patients would surely be outraged at being denied treatment simply because scientific data is lacking. The relatively minor turbulence that has attended the denial of "questionable" drugs to AIDS patients, along with the success that AIDS advocates have had in modifying and bypassing bureaucratic obstacles, foreshadows the uproar that would attend widespread denial of "questionable" care. For example, the constituency of patients with heart disease is unquestionably broader and more powerful than those with AIDS; many of the well established technologies in this area are of uncertain benefit for many types of patients. It is implausible to expect that heart-disease victims would quietly forego potentially lifesaving treatment in the name of scientific purity. In short, if "wasteful" means "of uncertain effectiveness," cutting waste by making rules faces substantial popular and professional opposition.

TREATMENT THAT IS ETHICALLY TROUBLING

The explosive growth of the bioethics field, an area that was virtually nonexistent a generation ago, testifies to the proliferation of ethically troubling medical treatment.[53] The use of aggressive medical therapies in treating the very old, the very young, and the very sick has engendered some of the most vehement charges of "waste," "inappropriateness," and "irrationality" in American medicine.

Rulemaking in this area requires an ethical consensus concerning an appropriate level of care. For people who are intimately acquainted with instances of gross overtreatment, this often seems a trivial problem. Waste is apparent and outrageous. Something like Justice Stewart's standard for obscenity—"I know it when I see it"—seems to hold. But experience shows that even the seemingly clearest cases can evoke controversy (if not litigation), bringing into conflict those most intimately familiar with the patient's situation. These controversies often reflect fundamental disagreements about the goals and obligations of providers, payers, and patients, or even disputes about the significance of human life, including a "right to life." We will not recapitulate the bioethical debates surrounding these issues.[54] It is enough to note that the term "wasteful" is used here in an entirely different sense than in the previous two sections. No literature search or scientific experiment satisfactorily speaks to this issue of "waste."

No consensus panel can settle the ethical question of what is futile, desirable, or even cruel.

What then are the possibilities for policy in this area? What kinds of rules can be made to cut waste in ethically problematic cases? Significant progress has been made in defining when it is *permissible* to terminate care. Guidelines developed in the bioethics community have informed court decisions and state statutes.[55] Such policies undoubtedly can help in guiding individual decisions, but their impact on the overall allocation of medical resources is unknown. Such guidelines, however, are not analogous to the RAND/Value procedures to "cut waste." Little progress has been made in developing analogous rules in this area, rules that would say when wastefulness makes it *obligatory* to deny or terminate care. (It should be emphasized, moreover, that no one connected with the landmark RAND studies has proposed that any such rules be made.)

Their very suggestion is enormously controversial, as illustrated by the reception that greeted Daniel Callahan's proposal that age be a criterion in the allocation of public funds for medical care.[56] Highlighted on the op-ed pages of the *New York Times*,[57] the proposal drew vociferous attacks from gerontologists, senior-citizen advocates, and the elderly themselves. Social critic Nat Hentoff branded the scheme "morally depraved," a comment that was duly noted in the American Association of Retired People's *News Bulletin*.[58] Further discussion was effectively ended. If "wasteful" means "ethically troubling," cutting wasteful care means facing hard and bitter choices. In matters of life and death, when values clash, proposing allocational rules can place those rules beyond reasonable public discussion. It is difficult to imagine how such a process could lead to public consensus.

TREATMENT THAT IS NOT ALLOCATIONALLY EFFICIENT

Notwithstanding the above difficulties, bread-and-butter medicine is not about complex ethical issues. Rather, increasingly it is about expensive medical care options. Today's physicians must choose daily from among various costly treatments and tests, many of which are unquestionably beneficial. Consider these lifesaving treatments:

(1) *Early Cancer Detection* (e.g., annual mammography for women aged 40–50). Since women in this age group have a low incidence of breast cancer, annual mammography offers a modest improvement in life expectancy at a significant financial and social cost. Screening 25% of all American women in this age group on an annual basis would save 373 lives each year. Costs (in

1984 dollars) would be $408 million for mammography, surgical workups, and continuing care. Savings from early detection of cancer would be $6 million annually, resulting in a net annual cost of $402 million to save 373 lives.[59]

(2) *Safer Diagnostic Tests* (e.g., nonionic contrast medium). Contrast medium is a liquid which, when injected into the bloodstream, circulates throughout the body making blood vessels and certain organs more visible on x-ray. Injection with the dye carries a certain risk of a fatal allergic reaction. Recently, a nonionic contrast dye was introduced that is safer for patients. The risk of death from injection with the new dye is 1 in 250,000 (an improvement over the risk of 1 in 30,000 with the older dye). The newer dye costs 10 times as much as the older one, and widespread adoption could cost as much as one billion dollars annually nationwide.[60]

(3) *Organ Transplantation* (e.g., heart transplantation). Heart replacement is surprisingly effective in the treatment of end-stage heart disease. Recipients enjoy a 75–80% one-year survival rate. Although only 346 cardiac transplants were performed in 1984, an estimated 50,000 people could benefit from the procedure each year. Heart transplantation costs between $70,000 and $200,000 per patient.[61]

When do expensive maneuvers become "wasteful?" Traditionally, policymakers have approached this problem from the framework of cost-benefit analysis.[62] Given a rank ordering of medical programs and procedures, beginning with the one with the best cost-to-benefit profile and ending with the one with the least attractive profile, one might simply allocate money from the top down. Above some cutoff point, the listed interventions could be considered "worthwhile"; below that point, "wasteful." There are, however, three significant obstacles to implementing such a plan in American medicine.

The first is the unavailability of a defensible rank ordering. We have scant information about the effectiveness and costs of most clinical interventions. Moreover, we lack a firm conceptual and empirical basis for equating different kinds of medical, social, and financial benefits. In the absence of these two sorts of information, it is difficult to assign meaningful cost-benefit estimates to medical procedures.[63] The second difficulty is that the American medical care system does not operate within a fixed budget (nor do most American physicians). Without a budgetary limit, the borderline between "worthwhile" and "wasteful" simply cannot be defined. It is impossible to say which interventions would fall below a purely hypothetical cut-off. A final obstacle arises from our decentralized system of financing. We have no guarantee that cuts in "wasteful" expenditures will be compensated with shifts toward "worthwhile" expenditures. We may agree that annual mammographic screening for young women is comparatively wasteful, but we have no reason to believe that money saved by abstaining from mammography will be spent on a more worthwhile endeavor, such as universal access to prenatal care.

While rigorous cost-benefit analysis is unlikely to govern the allocation of medical services in the foreseeable future, concerns about costs and benefits will continue to have an important place in discussions of "wasteful" care. This is surely appropriate, since no medical care system can provide all possible services. But when "not cost effective" is taken to be synonymous with "wasteful," some misleading inferences can follow. One of these is the suggestion that treatments that fall below the cost-benefit cutoff point are "wasteful," and therefore do no one much good. This is certainly not true. There are many potentially lifesaving treatments that are very costly, but effective (breast-cancer screening in young women, safer diagnostic tests, and organ transplantation all fall into this category). When cutting waste on economic grounds, we inevitably eliminate some services that do some good. We should therefore not be surprised to find people fighting for access to treatments that are "not cost-effective," as did the members of the Komen Foundation for Breast Cancer in Dallas, a group of wealthy and socially prominent Republican women who successfully lobbied the Texas legislature in 1989 to require that insurance companies cover the cost of screening mammography to all women ages 35 and over.[64]

Such episodes lay bare the link between "waste cutting" and "rationing." If "waste cutting" means "trimming the fat," and "rationing" means "making rules to limit the use of beneficial services," it will necessarily be the case that in trimming fat we deny some people some beneficial services. What is particularly striking is that the perception of benefit determines the political cost of waste cutting. While the medical costs of denying young women access to screen mammography are quite small (as the analysis cited above demonstrates), the political price may be prohibitive (as the Texas legislators found out). Similarly, in the recent Oregon "rationing" movement, procedures were initially ranked according to their alleged cost-to-benefit profiles. Organ transplants were near the bottom in this initial list of services, but the political costs of cutting this form of "waste" were seen as too great, and organ transplants were moved upward on the list so that they would qualify for Medicaid reimbursement.[65] Cutting waste, when waste is either of great benefit or is perceived to be so, can be prohibitively expensive politically.

More generally, economically driven rulemaking runs counter to those American values and institutions favoring aggressive, high-technology, "do something" medicine. Opinion polls show that Americans believe, nearly unanimously, that financial considerations should not enter into life-and-death medical decisions.[66] In the legal arena, technological imperatives dovetail with our shared notions of individual rights and professional responsibilities, meaning that rulemaking could exacerbate an increasingly unacceptable malpractice environment. As people who are injured by denial of care seek restitution, several issues will be at stake: Can care be denied because it is too expensive? When harm results from denial of treatment, who is responsible? What are the responsibilities of payers and providers? Already, some interesting cases have been heard. A Washington state court recently held that a third-party payer had a duty to pay for a man's liver transplant because his life depended on it.[67] A Michigan woman with colon cancer has sued her HMO, maintaining that their cost-containment rules led to a delay in the detection of her malignancy.[68]

While commentators agree that the relationship between the malpractice standard and care cost containment is one of the most important issues confronting medical tort law in the 1990s, they are divided on how the legal system will accommodate rulemaking. Some argue that physicians who prudently adopt recommended sparer practice styles will find protection in the event of adverse outcomes.[69] Others are doubtful that the accommodation can be made so smoothly, and fear that economically based rulemaking will "create enormous confusion and, quite likely, place physicians under inappropriate and unfair economic and legal pressures"[70] as they are forced to make choices between their own professional standards and payers' rules.

Whatever the political and legal outcomes, it is clear that economically driven rulemaking could force physicians to redefine their professional roles. Many physicians find such rulemaking unacceptable,[71] and many believe that cost containment measures seriously compromise the quality of medical care.[72] Some hold that consideration of costs simply has no place in the practice of medicine. One frequently quoted passage draws a parallel between the obligations of physicians to their patients and the responsibilities of attorneys to their clients:

[P]hysicians are required to do everything that they believe may benefit each patient without regard to costs or other societal considerations. In caring for an individual patient, the doctor must act solely as that patient's advocate, against the apparent interests of society as a whole, if necessary. An analogy can be drawn with the role of a lawyer defending a client against a criminal charge. The attorney is obligated to use all ethical means to defend the client, regardless of the cost of prolonged legal proceedings or even of the possibility that a guilty person may be acquitted through skillful advocacy. Similarly, in the practice of medicine, physicians are obligated to do all that they can for their patients without regard to any costs to society.[73]

This attitude, which one might call the "professional imperative," dominates American medical practice, and it will not disappear overnight.

REALISTIC PROSPECTS FOR RULEMAKING

This brief survey of the policy to cut waste by rulemaking has revealed that it is really many policies—at least as many policies as there are kinds of waste. Three summary points should be emphasized. First, there are different senses in which treatments are "wasteful." We know that some treatments are wasteful by looking at their results; in other cases we need to examine their price tag; in still others we must make a moral judgement. While this is not a profound point, it is one that is frequently obscured in the rhetoric of waste-cutting. Medicare's rules about medical necessity (and a myriad of similarly disingenuous policies) create confusion, breed cynicism, and offer little promise as long-term strategies to guide the allocation of medical services.[74]

Second, since "waste" is diverse, policies to "cut waste" face different prospects for success. Although some forms of care can probably be prohibited with little resistance, this is not likely to be the case generally. There will be substantial professional, political, ethical, and legal obstacles to cutting waste in many cases. Although identification of wasteful practices may be conceptually straightforward, the costs of rulemaking may be high. Rules can work, but these obstacles must be faced squarely in attempts to develop coherent and realistic health policy.

Third, because the spectrum of "wasteful" care includes care that is effective, cutting waste by making rules will not always circumvent hard choices. Sometimes it may mean eliminating care that is both needed and beneficial. In other cases, it may mean cutting services that are perceived to be beneficial but are of uncertain effectiveness. In either case, we must watch out for immoderate promises about painless "waste cutting."

While doubts about rulemaking are warranted, nihilism is not. We all stand to gain from the knowledge that will flow from the outcomes movement, and rulemaking may work in some situations. As we have shown, *rulemaking is likely to be particularly successful when the treatment in question is clearly ineffective or harmful*. It is, however, far from obvious that such instances are sufficiently prevalent to justify the extravagant optimism surrounding the movement's likely impact. While the oft cited RAND study of three commonly performed procedures showed that they were performed "inappropriately" in one-third to one-sixth of the cases,[75] this figure in all likelihood overstates the prevalence of ineffective or harmful care for three reasons. First, the three procedures were apparently chosen precisely because the indications for their use are unclear. Given this uncertainty, it is not surprising that they were often used "inappropriately." Second, the RAND ratings were based on a retrospective review of medical records. It is likely that incomplete documentation produced a number of cases incorrectly rated as "inappropriate."[76] This interpretation is supported by data from two published cases in which the appropriateness criteria were used prospectively. In both cases, inappropriateness rates were simply not as impressive as might have been hoped. In the early Aetna/Value trial, only 9% of the proposed services were ultimately deemed not appropriate for reimbursement.[77] In a more recent trial of the Value software at five Blue Cross and Blue Shield plans, preauthorization review yielded a judgment of inappropriateness for 11% of the cases overall.[78]

Let us assume that 11% of all present medical practices are demonstrably ineffective or harmful. Eliminating those wasteful practices would result in substantial savings, given our present level of expenditure—an attractive prospect indeed. But are savings of that magnitude likely to be realized in the near future? It seems likely that implementation would take place over a period of years, given the AHCPR's past (and admirable) record of crafting guidelines carefully.[79] After developing guidelines, a strategy will have to be developed to change physician behavior. Whether that strategy relies on "education"—as the AHCPR would apparently prefer[80]—or on a RAND/Value-like direct linkage to reimbursement,[81] it is clear that it would begin to have its intended effect only after a period of years.

If this is the case, how can rulemaking affect our level of medical care spending over the next decade? Providing a precise answer to this question would require us to address issues of health economics that are beyond the scope of the present paper. But one can see that the possible 11% savings—particularly a savings achieved gradually—would inevitably be dwarfed by the losses exacted by the present rate of medical care inflation, which one expert has estimated to occur at a real rate of 7% per annum.[82] Unfortunately, the plan to cut waste by making rules simply does not address this cost, one of the central problems of health services allocation. Eliminating today's waste cannot help us constrain the escalation of costs attributable to the more effective and more expensive services to be developed tomorrow. Viewed from this perspective, cutting waste by making rules is, at best, an incremental reform that might produce modest gains over the medium term. Despite the claims of its more ardent supporters, it shows little promise as a solution to the so-called "health care cost crisis."

In the end, the parameters movement may founder—not because of a lack of "wasteful" medical care, but because government and business leaders want a quicker fix to the problem of rising medical care costs. With wasteful care on the public's mind, a coalition of resourceful researchers, government officials, politicians, business leaders, and professional organizations have developed a vision of a world in which scientific know-how aided by computerized wizardry will produce rules for allocating the "right" amount of medical care. But the public's "issue attention cycle" waxes and wanes quickly.[83] As it becomes clear that it would be years before hoped-for economic gains could be realized, and that cuts in "waste" entail significant social costs, the movement could lose some of its momentum and funding. As the AHCPR's director recently remarked to an audience of health-services researchers:

> We have a wonderful opportunity to make outcomes and effectiveness re-search a very important incremental chapter in the pursuit of quality and value for the health care dollar. I believe that window is only going to be open so long. The Congress indeed expects things tomorrow, and I believe that with reasonable progress reports from you, I can be a part of telling them that good work takes time. At the same time, if we say that it takes five to six years and please hold your breath, then I think we'll lose. So as I said to the [outcomes research] teams that were assembled here a few days ago, we're delighted at the progress you're making, but hurry up.[84]

IS THERE AN ALTERNATIVE TO RULEMAKING?

Nothing above is intended to imply that there is a simple solution to the problem of rising medical expenditures. The "professional imperative" that drives physicians to provide more, better, and safer services (and the desire for better health that drives patients to seek the same) will continue. If we are to curb rising costs, powerful countervailing forces must be brought to bear. Rules can certainly help in applying such forces, and the parameters movement is well underway. But is rulemaking the most promising course of action? Any an-swer must take into account two decades of frustrating failure to contain health expenditures in America. During that time, there were numerous attempts to change the way in which America delivers, pays for, and regulates medical care. None has been demonstrably successful in curbing medical care inflation or in constraining the growth in the intensity of services provided. Neither competition, managed care, prospective payment, nor numerous other purported panaceas has fulfilled its promise. Each in its day was touted as the answer to the problem of rising costs, leading to cycles of delight and disappointment[85] as expenditures resumed their seemingly inexorable rise, or costs were shifted onto other sectors of the medical care economy. To expect more of the outcomes movement would be to ignore the lessons of experience. It is worth sketching what these lessons might be.

During the same twenty-year period that costs rose in this country, other nations had substantially greater success in controlling health expenditures. Canada's and Britain's systems are most often cited, but most of Western Europe's achievements are comparable.[86] In each case, the inherently inflationary forces in medical care that Robert Evans has so eloquently described technological growth, asymmetry of information, uncertainty of evidence, and rising expectations—have been met with policy responses to counter powerful pressures for more spending. In Canada, that has meant the concentration of financial authority in single provincial payors, the use of global hospital budgets, the separate control of capital expenditures by hospitals, and the active setting of prices for physician services. In the United States, reforms failed to address those forces in a concerted fashion, and inflation has continued unabated.[87]

There are indications that America is moving toward universal health insurance. Recent public opinion polls show that a majority of Americans favor a national health insurance system over our present arrangements.[88] The appearance in the elite *New England Journal of Medicine* of an editorial[89] and an article[90] supporting some form of universal health insurance signalled that the academic wing of the medical profession is ready to consider fundamental changes in the way that medical care is financed. An entire recent issue of the *Journal of the American Medical Association* extolled the virtues of universal access,[91] suggesting that others will not be far behind. Congress appears prepared to consider such a program seriously for the first time in twenty years.[92]

Still, most of these powerful parties are unconvinced that reform should include the kind of concentrated financial and regulatory power that has repeatedly proved successful abroad. In the context of the federal budget deficit and the public's hostility toward increased taxes, it is uncertain whether reform will follow the model of direct governmental financing. Some claim that a system that preserves the present employment-based insurance scheme and maintains some role for private insurance companies is politically more feasible.[93] If such a program could be coupled with strong governmental regulatory powers, some observers believe that we might achieve universal access to medical care, while still containing costs.[94]

As the debate on major reforms heightens over the coming months, one truth will continue to be undeniable: contemporary medicine offers an astonishing array of beneficial therapies. These therapies will be sought by many patients wanting to improve their lives. They will be employed by doctors wanting to help their patients, exercise their craft, and earn their income. There is little hope that either of the intimate partners in the doctor-patient relationship will come to see most medical treatment as "wasteful."

Meanwhile, the "professional imperative" will prevail unless powerfully constrained. While many physicians will refrain from performing procedures known to be ineffective, most will not be willing to unilaterally cut other "wasteful" activities (practices of uncertain effectiveness, activities that are ethically problematic, and therapies that are not allocationally efficient). If doctors will not say "no" to their patients, then we can expect that payers will begin to say "no" to doctors. And indeed they have begun to do so. A new coalition has promised to cut health expenditures by making rules forbidding wasteful treatment. But it is doubtful that "cutting waste" is as straightforward or as painless as the most voluble members of the coalition have suggested. And it is certain that cutting waste by making rules will mean different things to different people.

Notes

The article was first published in *University of Pennsylvania Law Review* 140, no. 5 (May 1992). Dr. Jan Blustein is a physician and professor of health policy at New York University's Robert F. Wagner School. Dr. Blustein was supported by an NRSA Award from the Agency for Health Care Policy and Research. Prof. Marmor received support from the Canadian Institute for Advanced Research, of which he was a fellow. The authors wish to thank David Willis, Philip Lee, Victor Rodwin, and Colin Dayan for their helpful comments on previous drafts. The usual caveats apply.

1. *See* Katharine R. Levit et al., *National Health Expenditures, 1990*, HEALTH CARE FINANCING REV., Fall 1991, at 29, 30.
2. *See* BUREAU OF CENSUS, U.S. DEPT OF COMMERCE, STATISTICAL ABSTRACT OF THE UNITED STATES 1990, at 92 (110th ed. 1990).
3. *See id.*
4. The topic of rationing first drew widespread attention with the publication of Aaron and Schwartz's pioneering comparative study of the scale and distribution of therapeutic procedures under Britain's National Health Service and America's health care system. *See* HENRY J. AARON AND WILLIAM B. SCHWARTZ, THE PAINFUL PRESCRIPTION: RATIONING HOSPITAL CARE (1984). Their argument, that British-style rationing decisions will inevitably need to be made in this country, has subsequently been elaborated upon. *See* William B. Schwartz, *The Inevitable Failure of Current Cost-Containment Strategies: Why They Can Provide Only Temporary Relief*, 257 JAMA 220 (1987). For a critical analysis, *see* Theodore Marmor & Rudolf Klein, *Costs Versus Care: America's Health Care Dilemma Wrongly Considered*, 4 HEALTH MATRIX 19 (1986).

   A second wave of popular attention to rationing accompanied Oregon's controversial and widely noted proposal to alter the list of reimbursable services under the Medicaid program. For an evenhanded description of that program, under which reimbursement decisions would be guided by "cost-effectiveness" considerations, *see* Daniel M. Fox and Howard M. Leichter, *Rationing Health Care in Oregon: The New Accountability*, HEALTH AFF., Summer 1991, at 7; for an illuminating discussion of the politics surrounding the plan, *see* Lawrence D. Brown, *The National Politics of Oregon's Rationing Plan*, HEALTH AFF., Summer 1991, at 28; for an analysis of the ethical issues it raises, *see* Norman Daniels, *Is The Oregon Rationing Plan Fair?*, 265 JAMA 2232 (1991); and for a particularly critical review of the plan as an effort to limit services to the poor, *see* Bruce C. Vladeck, *Unhealthy Rations*, AM. PROSPECT, Summer 1991, at 101.

5. *See* Theodore R. Marmor & Jan Blustein, *Introduction to Rationing*, 140 U. PA. L. REV. 1539 (1992).

6. A reader of the popular press might well conclude that one-quarter to one-half of present medical practice is "pure waste," benefitting no one. For example, according to a *New York Times* op-ed piece of a few years ago: "[T]he evidence is now overwhelming that at least twenty-five percent of the money that Americans spend on health care is wasted. . . . There is a growing consensus that half the coronary bypasses, most Caesarean sections and a significant proportion of many other procedures . . . are unnecessary. A former editor of [JAMA] is convinced that more than half of the 40 million medical tests performed each year "do not really contribute to a patient's diagnosis or therapy." Joseph A. Califano, Jr., *Billions Blown on Health*, N.Y. TIMES, Apr. 12, 1989, at A25.

7. *See James S. Todd, M.D.: Only Parameters Will Give MDs Needed Flexibility*, AM. MED. NEWS, Jan. 6, 1989, at 23, 23 [hereinafter, *Todd Interview*] (interview with AMA Senior Deputy Executive Vice President).

8. *See* AGENCY FOR HEALTH CARE POLICY AND RESEARCH, U.S. DEPT OF HEALTH AND HUMAN SERVS., PROGRAM NOTE: CLINICAL GUIDELINE DEVELOPMENT (1990) [hereinafter AHCPR, PROGRAM NOTE]

9. *See* Mark R. Chassin, *Standards of Care in Medicine*, 25 INQUIRY 437, 437 (1988).

10. This article does not address recently developed techniques, such as "physician profiling," whereby payors examine physicians' patterns of care in order to detect tendencies toward inappropriate or wasteful use of services. *See* Robert W. Dubois, *Reducing Unnecessary Care: Different Approaches to the "Big Ticket" and the "Little Ticket" Items*, J. AMBULATORY CARE MGMT., October 1991, at 30; Milt Freudenheim, *Software Controls on Health Costs*, N.Y. TIMES, Feb. 18, 1992, at D2. Many of our comments apply equally well to these newer approaches, however.

11. Those falling into this last category are often said to be "not cost-effective," but this term is all too often used imprecisely. In the medical literature "cost-effective" has been variously taken to be synonymous with "cost saving," "effective," and "having an additional benefit worth the cost." *See* Peter Doubilet et al., *Use and Misuse of the Term "Cost-Effective" in Medicine*, 314 NEW ENG. J. MED. 253, 253–54 (1986).

12. *See* Robert H. Brook & Kathleen N. Lohr, *Will We Need to Ration Effective Health Carer*, ISSUES SCI. & TECH., Fall 1986, at 68, 72.

13. *See* Marcia Angell, *Cost Containment and the Physician*, 254 JAMA 1203, 1204 (1985).

14. *See Todd Interview, supra* note 7, at 23.

15. The rules to which we refer emanate from the Health Care Financing Administration. Although the precise content of these rules, as developed and enforced by HCFA's financial intermediaries, is confidential, a general description may be found in HEALTH CARE FIN. ADMIN., MEDICAL CARRIERS MANUAL § 7500ff. (HCFA Pub. 14) (1990).

16. *Are Guidelines, Standards or Parameters Having an Impact on the Way You Practice Medicine, and How?*, AM. MED. NEWS, Jan. 6, 1989, at 34, 34 (interviewing a private practitioner in St. Louis).

17. Glenn Kramon, *Taking a Scalpel to Health Costs*, N.Y. TIMES, Jan. 8, 1989, § 3, at 1, 9 (quoting the vice-president of a cost management company).

18. IVAN ILLICH, MEDICAL NEMESIS (1976).
19. *Id.* at 44.
20. *Id.* at 114 (emphasis omitted).
21. Edmund Faltermeyer, *Medical Care's Next Revolution*, FORTUNE, Oct. 10, 1988, at 126, 126.
22. *See* Arnold M. Epstein, *The Outcomes Movement—Will It Get Us Where We Want to Go?*, 323 NEW ENG. J. MED. 266, 268 (1990); David M. Eddy & John Billings, *The Quality of Medical Evidence: Implications for Quality of Care*, HEALTH AFF., Spring 1988, at 19, 28–29.
23. *See* Eddy & Billings, *supra* note 22, at 28.
24. These other methodologies, often subsumed under the rubric of "observational epidemiology," are clearly elucidated in J. MARK ELLWOOD, CAUSAL RELATIONSHIPS IN MEDICINE: A PRACTICAL SYSTEM OF CRITICAL APPRAISAL (1988). For a nontechnical account of the pitfalls of such studies, *see* MAX MICHAEL ET AL., BIOMEDICAL BESTIARY: AN EPIDEMIOLOGIC GUIDE TO FLAWS AND FALLACIES IN THE MEDICAL LITERATURE (1984).
25. *See* Epstein, *supra* note 22, at 268; Eddy & Billings, *supra* note 22, at 20. We do not wish to create the impression that little of value is known about effectiveness in clinical medicine. As one of our readers, Dr. Colin Dayan, has pointed out, there are numerous cases in which researchers have conclusively demonstrated the effectiveness (or lack thereof) of particular interventions. These cases notwithstanding, no one doubts that much remains to be learned about the utility of present practices.
26. *See* Robert W. Dubois & Robert H. Brook, *Assessing Clinical Decision Making: Is the Ideal System Feasible?*, 25 INQUIRY 59, 63 (1988); Eddy & Billings, *supra* note 22, at 24.
27. For a discussion of the specific methods used to develop the appropriateness ratings, *see* Rolla E. Park et al., *Physician Ratings of Appropriate Indications for Six Medical and Surgical Procedures*, 76 AM. J. PUB. HEALTH 766 (1986).
28. *See id.* at 767.
29. *See id.* at 768–69.
30. *Id.* at 767.
31. *See* Harris Meyer, *Payers to Use Protocols to Assess Treatment Plans*, AM. MED. NEWS, Dec. 9, 1988, at 1, 62–63. Actual refusal rates have increased, as early versions of the software have been replaced by more sophisticated programs. *See* telephone interview with Dr. Robert DeBois, Senior Vice President of Value Health Sciences (Mar. 2, 1992); *infra* note 78 and accompanying text.
32. *See* Epstein, *supra* note 22, at 266.
33. These differences in perception have taken several forms. Some participants have emphasized the movement's potential to cut costs; *see* Brook & Lohr, *supra* note 12, at 68; Califano, *supra* note 6, at A25; Faltermeyer, *supra* note 21, at 126; others have highlighted its promise of harnessing scientific knowledge to enhance the quality of medical care, *see* AGENCY FOR HEALTH CARE POLICY AND RESEARCH, U.S. DEPT OF HEALTH AND HUMAN SERVS., RESEARCH ACTIVITIES 4 (1992) [hereinafter AHCPR, RESEARCH]; William L. Roper et al., *Effectiveness in Health Care: An Initiative to Evaluate and Improve Medical Practice*, 319 NEW ENG. J. MED. 1197, 1197 (1988). Some members have embraced the idea of using rules to audit physicians' practice choices, *see supra* notes 27–32 and accompanying text. Others, reluctant to promote "cookbook medicine," and believing that physicians will respond to education about "appropriate" practices, appear to prefer that adherence to guidelines be kept voluntary. *See* AHCPR, RESEARCH, *supra*, at 5. *See also infra* note 80. This preference may be optimistic in light of previous studies showing that physician practice choices are relatively resistant to the "practice suggestions" of experts. *See, e.g.*, Jacqueline Kosecoff et al., *Effects of the National Institutes of Health Consensus Development Program on Physician Practice*, 258 JAMA 2708, 2712 (1987) (finding that consensus development conferences produced little change in patient care); Jonathan Lomas et al., *Do*

Jan Blustein and Theodore R. Marmor

Practice Guidelines Guide Practice? The Effect of Consensus Statements on the Practice of Physicians, 321 NEW ENG. J. MED. 1306, 1310 (1989) (concluding that while practice guidelines may affect "the perceptions of physicians," they alone are insufficient to alter physicians' behavior). Other incentives may be needed to modify practice patterns. The range of alternatives is canvassed in John M. Eisenberg, *Physician Utilization: The State of Research About Physicians' Practice Patterns*, 23 MED. CARE 461, 467–70 (1988).

Despite these differences in perception, it is undeniable that much of the enthusiasm (and funding) behind the outcomes movement has been driven by the perception that it will slow the rising cost of medical care expenditures, and it is clear that many of the key participants view the development of a link between "appropriate" practices and reimbursement as a foregone conclusion. *See infra* notes 40–42 and accompanying text. In this essay, we explore the implications of implementing such a policy.

34. Paul M. Ellwood, *Shattuck Lecture — Outcomes Management: A Technology of Patient Experience*, 318 NEW ENG. J. MED. 1549, 1551 (1988).

35. Arnold S. Relman, *Assessment and Accountability: The Third Revolution in Health Care*, 319 NEW ENG. J. MED. 1220, 1220 (1988).

36. *See* Roper et al., *supra* note 35, at 1197.

37. AHCPR, PROGRAM NOTE, *supra* note 8, at 6 (quoting the Legislative Summary to the Omnibus Budget and Reconciliation Act of 1989). Although the AHCPR has been the beneficiary of congressional enthusiasm for medical care cost savings, the Agency's leaders have recently become eager to avoid disappointment, disclaiming a connection between guideline development and cost containment. As the Agency released the first of its guidelines this spring, its director, Dr. J. Jarrett Clinton, remarked that, "[t]here are those in Congress who hoped, and still hope, that this effort would be a cost-savings device, but it has limited use for this purpose. . . . This is not about cost-cutting, but about getting the best value per dollar spent in the long run. In some cases, for instance, the guidelines may result in spending more money on some things." Warren E. Leary, *More Advice for Doctors: U.S. Guides on Treatments*, N.Y. TIMES, Apr. 15, 1992, at C14. Despite its position in the forefront of the outcomes movement, then, the Agency's perception of the movement's direction may be at odds with that of some of the movement's members and supporters, including some members of Congress, the insurance industry, the business community, and some academic researchers.

38. *See House Subcommittee Votes Level Funding for AHCPR and HCFA: Senate Likely to Increase Support (or AHCPR*, HSR REPORTS (Association for Health Services Research, Washington, D.C.), June 1991, at 1, 5.

39. *See* Epstein, *supra* note 22, at 266.

40. For example, Blue Cross and Blue Shield executive Bernard T. Tresnowski, when asked about the practice parameters approach, responded: "'Right On!'" *See* Faltermeyer, *supra* note 21, at 132. "With better data," it is believed, "business could effectively challenge proposed treatments." *Id.* at 126.

41. *See* Report of the Board of Trustees of the American Medical Association, Practice Parameters 4 (1990) [hereinafter AMA Trustees' Report] (unpublished report, on file with authors).

42. Sharon McIlrath, *AMA, Rand Corp. Plan Joint Development of Practice Guidelines*, AM. MED. NEWS, Oct. 28, 1988, at 2, 2.

43. *Todd Interview, supra* note 7, at 25.

44. For an analysis by a physician and leading researcher in the outcomes movement stressing the advantages of practice parameters, *see* Robert H. Brook, *Practice Guidelines and Practicing Medicine Are They Compatible?*, 262 JAMA 3027, 3030 (1989).

45. The relationship between practice guidelines and malpractice liability remains a point of considerable controversy among commentators. *See infra* notes 67–70 and accompanying text.

46. *See* telephone interview with Robert Isquith, Chief of Public Affairs, AHCPR (Mar. 8, 1992); telephone Interview with Stephen H. King, M.D., Chief Medical Officer, AHCPR (July 15, 1991).
47. *See* Steffie Woolhandler and David U. Himmelstein, *The Deteriorating Administrative Efficiency of the U.S. Health Care System*, 324 New Eng. J. Med. 1253, 1254–55 (1991).
48. *See* Gerald W. Grumet, *Health Care Rationing Through Inconvenience: The Third Party's Secret Weapon*, 821 New Eng. J. Med. 607, 608 (1988).
49. Faltermeyer, *supra* note 21 (quoting Dr. Paul M. Ellwood).
50. This option is discussed in detail in Brook, *supra* note 44, *at* 3029. The idea behind "of uncertain effectiveness" would seem to correspond with the RAND categorization "equivocal." *See* Park et al., *supra* note 27, at 767. Much of the popular commentary following the release of the RAND results, *see supra* text accompanying notes 31–34, conveyed the impression that half of all coronary bypass surgery had been discovered to be medically unnecessary. *See supra* note 6. Yet the RAND group's findings categorized 14% of such surgeries as "inappropriate," while 30% were classed as "equivocal"; it would thus appear that procedures falling under both of these headings were lumped together in arriving at the "one-half" estimate. *See* Constance M. Winslow et al., *The Appropriateness of Performing Coronary Artery Bypass Surgery*, 260 JAMA 505, 509 (1988). We contend that, from the perspective of health care policymaking, "inappropriate" and "equivocal" procedures are quite different, and that programs aimed at cutting these two distinct types of "waste" would for that reason meet quite different fates.
51. Meyer, *supra* note 31, at 63.
52. McIlrath, *supra* note 42, at 41.
53. A fascinating analysis of these developments can be found in David J. Rothman, Strangers at the Bedside: A History of How Law and Bioethics Transformed Medical Decision Making (1991).
54. *See generally* Daniel Callahan, Setting Limits: Medical Goals in an Aging Society (1987) (contending that medical care should be rationed based on age); Norman Daniels, Am I My Parents Keeper? An Essay on Justice Between the Young and the Old (1988) (examining the competing claims of the young and the elderly to medical resources); Norman Daniels, Just Health Care (1985) (arguing that a principle of equality of opportunity should guide distribution of health care services); A. A. Scitovsky and A. M. Capron, *Medical Care at the End of Life: The Interaction of Economics and Ethics*, 7 Ann. Rev. Pub. Health 59 (1986) (analyzing the ethical implications of devoting a disproportionate amount of medical resources to the aged); Anne A. Scitovsky, *The High Cost of Dying: What Do the Data Show?* 62 Milbank Memorial Fund Q. 591 (1984) (same).
55. *See, e.g., In re* Conroy, 486 A.2d 1209, 1220 (N.J. 1985) (citing *President's Commission for the Study of Ethical Problems, in* Medicine and Biomedical and Behavioral Research, Deciding to Forego Life-Sustaining Treatment 23 (1983) in an analysis of the question of when life-sustaining treatment may be withdrawn from legally incompetent patients).
56. *See* Callahan, *supra* note 54.
57. *See* Daniel Callahan, *Rethinking Health Care for the Aged*, N.Y. Times, Sept. 25, 1987, at A39.
58. *See Health Debate Rages over Rationing by Age*, AARP News Bull., June 1988, at 1 (quoting comments made by Nat Hentoff at a debate sponsored by the National Council on the Aging).
59. *See* David M. Eddy et al., *The Value of Mammography Screening in Women Under Age 50 Years*, 259 JAMA 1512, 1512–19 (1988). For completeness we should note that the case is more complicated than suggested above. Though the point remains that mammography is of relatively low benefit to young women, some significant health costs, such as the risk of a false positive test, are not mentioned. For example, out of one hundred women undergoing mammography, one

will be referred for a breast biopsy to investigate a radiologic abnormality that turns out not to be cancer. This raises the question of whether the health and social cost of tens of thousands of unnecessary surgeries each year outweighs the benefit of a few hundred lives saved. For an analysis that emphasizes these costs, *see* John C. Bailar, *Mammography Before Age 50 Years?*, 259 JAMA 1548–49 (1988).

60. *See* Annetta Miller et al., *Can You Afford To Get Sick?*, NEWSWEEK, Jan. 30, 1989, at 47.

61. See ROBERT H. BLANK, RATIONING MEDICINE 41 (1988).

62. Cost-benefit analysis is but one form of utilitarian program analysis. Other methods include cost-utility analysis and cost-effectiveness analysis. The application of these techniques to medical care is thoroughly discussed in MICHAEL F. DRUMMOND ET AL., METHODS FOR THE ECONOMIC EVALUATION OF HEALTH CARE PROGRAMMES 74–167 (1987). In this section, we refer to cost-benefit analysis, but many of our comments apply as well to the other related forms of analysis.

63. The theoretical difficulties involved are discussed in some detail in BLANK, *supra* note 61, at 115–16. An actual illustration arose in Oregon, where the rigorous application of cost-benefit techniques led to a rank ordering of therapies in which the treatment of crooked teeth was placed above therapy for early Hodgkin's disease, and treatment for thumb-sucking was put above hospitalization of a starving child. *See* Fox & Leichter, *supra* note 4, at 22. Although this original list was subsequently reordered, the initial result exposes the conceptual and empirical weakness of utilitarian program analysis, as it applies to medical care.

64. *See* Jane Gross, *Turning Disease Into Political Cause: First AIDS, and Now Breast Cancer*, N.Y. TIMES, Jan. 7, 1991, at A12.

65. *See* Fox & Leichter, *supra* note 4, at 23.

66. *See* Robert J. Blendon, *The Public's View of the Future of Health Care*, 259 JAMA 3587, 3590 (1987).

67. *See* BLANK, *supra* note 61, at 137.

68. *See* Harris Meyer, *Managed Care: HMOs Tighten Their Belts, Look to Hybrid Plans and Brighter Future*, AM. MED. NEWS, Jan. 6, 1989, at 12, 12.

69. *See* Troyen A. Brennan, *Practice Guidelines and Malpractice Litigation: Collision or Cohesion?*, 16 J. HEALTH POL. POLY & L. 67, 68; *see also* Mark A. Hall, *The Malpractice Standard Under Health Care Cost Containment*, 17 L. MED. & HEALTH CARE 347, 353 (1984) (arguing that the "law is fully capable . . . of recognizing the . . . emergence of cost incentives").

70. E. Haavi Morreim, *Stratified Scarcity: Redefining the Standard of Care*, 17 L. MED. & HEALTH CARE 356, 356 (1989).

71. *See* Leighton Ku and Dena Fisher, *The Attitudes of Physicians Toward Health Care Cost-Containment Policies*, 25 HEALTH SERVICES RES. 25, 25 (1990).

72. *See. e.g.*, Martin I. Broder, *The Impact of Cost Containment on Clinical Care* (Mar. 16–17, 1987), *in* THE HEALTH CARE COST CONTAINMENT MOVEMENT: A RECONSIDERATION 9 (Report of a conference sponsored by Medicine in the Public Interest, 1988) (arguing that cost-containment programs have had a "disturbing" impact on patient care).

73. Norman G. Levinsky, *The Doctor's Master*, 311 NEW ENG. J. MED. 1573, 1573 (1984).

74. The extent to which such rules can lead to bitterness, cynicism, and professional disengagement *is* well illustrated in a physician's report *of* his final 18 hospital visits to an 84-year-old woman dying *of* lung cancer, visits deemed to be "medically unnecessary." *See* Kenneth M. Prager, *Medicare Meddling*, N.Y. TIMES, Sept. 12, 1988, at A21.

75. *See* Mark R. Chassin et al., *Does Inappropriate Use Explain Geographic Variations in the Use of Health Care Services? A Study of Three Procedures*, 258 JAMA 2533, 2535 (1987).

76. *See* Epstein, *supra* note 22, at 268.

77. *See* Meyer, *supra* note 31, at 63.

78. *See* Blue Cross and Blue Shield Association, *Preauthorization Review System Finds More than 10 Percent of Medical Procedures Inappropriate*, 8 MED. BENEFITS 3, 3 (1991). In this case, inappropriate rates varied substantially by procedure, with 27% of the proposed tonsillectomies judged to be inappropriate, but none of the proposed heart bypass surgeries or carotid endarterectomies so rated. *See id.* The finding of no inappropriate operations out of the 181 bypass procedures is particularly striking in view of the voluminous commentary about the magnitude of "waste" in this category.

79. Other organizations are actively engaged in developing guidelines. For example, many of the medical specialty societies have begun working on parameter development, and by October 1990 had reportedly constructed some 1,000 different guidelines. *See* AMA Trustees' Report, *supra* note 41, at 2. While this work signals enthusiasm for the parameters approach, it also raises the question of how to coordinate the efforts of those involved in the movement to enhance appropriateness and cut waste.

80. *See* AGENCY FOR HEALTH CARE POLICY AND RESEARCH, U.S. DEPT OF HEALTH AND HUMAN SERVICES, AHCPR PUB. NO. 91–0004, REPORT TO CONGRESS: PROGRESS OF RESEARCH ON OUTCOMES OF HEALTH CARE SERVICES AND PROCEDURES 13–14 (1991) (discussing the dissemination of information about new technologies and ineffective practices). Policymakers at the agency are working to develop methods to effect change via parameter dissemination, *see id.*, since they are aware of prior studies showing that the practices of physicians are relatively resistant to the "suggestions" of experts, *see supra* note 33.

81. If rulemaking is linked to reimbursement, rules will have to be adopted by many or all payors to achieve widespread savings.

82. *See* Schwartz, *supra* note 4, at 220. It is worth stopping to consider the magnitude of potential economic gains even under the most generous assumptions. If we assume that rulemaking and waste-cutting could be implemented for all medical practices over a one-year period (i.e., with 11% of present costs instantaneously eliminated), at the end of a decade our health expenditures would total over 175% of real current expenditures, assuming that the 7% real inflation rate prevails. If we did not adopt the plan to cut waste, our medical costs at the end of a decade would be nearly 200% of their real present level, again assuming that inflation continues unabated. If the program to cut waste were adopted more gradually, the difference between the economic outcomes under the two scenarios would narrow accordingly.

83. *See generally* Anthony Downs, *Up and Down with Ecology — the "Issue Attention Cycle,"* 28 PUB. INTEREST 39, 39 (1972) (noting that "American public attention rarely remains sharply focused upon any one domestic issue for very long").

84. J. Jarrett Clinton, Address to the Tenth Anniversary Meeting of the Association for Health Services Research (July 1, 1991).

85. *See* Theodore R. Marmor, *American Health Politics 1970 to the Present: Some Comments*, Q. REV. ECON. & BUS., Winter 1990, at 32, 32–34.

86. *See* A. J. Culyer, *Cost Containment in Europe, in* ORGANISATION FOR ECONOMIC CO-OPERATION AND DEVELOPMENT, HEALTH CARE SYSTEMS IN TRANSITION: THE SEARCH FOR EFFICIENCY 29, 30 (1990).

87. An excellent technical account of these issues can be found in ROBERT G. EVANS, STRAINED MERCY: THE ECONOMICS OF CANADIAN HEALTH CARE (1984). For a more general introduction to the same material, *see* Theodore R. Marmor & Jerry Mashaw, *Northern Light: Canada's Lessons for American Health Care*, AM. PROSPECT, Fall 1990, at 18.

88. *See* Robin Toner, *Bad News for Bush as Poll Shows National Gloom*, N.Y. TIMES, Jan. 28, 1992, at A1.

89. *See* Arnold S. Reiman, *Universal Health Insurance: Its Time Has Come*, 320 NEW ENG. J. MED. 117 (1989).

90. *See* David U. Himmelstein et al., *A National Health Program for the United States*, 920 NEW ENG. J. MED. 102 (1989).

91. *See* Special Issue, *Caring for the Uninsured and Underinsured*, 265 JAMA 2491 (1991).

92. *See* Theodore R. Marmor, *U.S. Medical-Care System: Why Not the Worst?*, WALL ST. J., June 20, 1991, at A15; Theodore R. Marmor et al., *Political Handcuffs Hobble Debate*, L.A. TIMES, Oct. 3, 1991, at B7.

93. *See* HENRY J. AARON, SERIOUS AND UNSTABLE CONDITION: FINANCING AMERICA'S HEALTH CARE 130–31 (1991).

94. *See id.* at 124–28; Marmor & Mashaw, *supra* note 87, at 18–29; Ronald Pollack & Phyllis Torda, *The Pragmatic Road Toward National Health Insurance*, AM. PROSPECT, Summer 1991, at 92, 95; Paul Starr, *The Middle Class and National Health Reform*, AM. PROSPECT, Summer 1991, at 7, 11–12. *But see* Joe White, *Why Congress Should Push a National Health Plan*, WASH. POST, Sept. 15, 1991, at C3 (arguing that a Canadian style plan is more efficient and politically feasible).

The Politics of Health Care Rationing

Lessons from Oregon

Jonathan Oberlander, Lawrence Jacobs, and Theodore R. Marmor

Of all the innovations that have marked state health policy in the United States over the past decade, the Oregon Health Plan (OHP) has attracted the most controversy. The notoriety of health care reform in Oregon is a product of the state's decision to confront head-on what no other state has dared attempt: the explicit rationing of medical care services for Medicaid recipients.

Oregon's pioneering model of prioritizing funding for health care through systematically ranking medical services has been widely heralded as an important innovation in American health policy. The Oregon reforms have drawn an extraordinary amount of attention from both national and state policymakers. The state's claim to policy fame is its apparent willingness to make the hard choices and unavoidable trade-offs raised by the inflationary and technological pressures of modern medicine. From the late 1980s on, the state sought through unusual means to expand access to health insurance for uninsured Oregonians. The price for expanded coverage was to be paid by rationing medical care services provided to Oregon's low-income Medicaid population.

The rationing of services ostensibly rested on an elaborate system that merged the promise of technological progress through cost-benefit analysis and medical outcomes research with the democratic wish of public participation in policy making. The Oregon approach—budget control through explicit rationing of services—was indisputably innovative. It represented a striking contrast to the established practice of implicitly rationing medical care in the United States by income and insurance coverage, and at the time of its inception, to the conventional practice in other states that sought to control Medicaid spending by dropping coverage for low-income enrollees.

From the beginning, the OHP ignited substantial controversy. What appeared as brave innovation to some was viewed by others as a dangerous and

morally dubious experiment of federalism run amok. Positions on the Oregon
plan—whether favorable or critical—were formed early on, during the heated
debate over its enactment in the late 1980s. And those positions still largely define contemporary understandings of rationing in Oregon.

That is unfortunate because the operation and results of OHP have in crucial
respects very little to do with the original proposals, or with the debate over its
enactment. The worst fears of Oregon's critics and the tough choices promised
by its advocates both failed to materialize. Consequently, the lessons that the
Oregon experience holds for state health policymaking and medical care rationing have been widely misinterpreted.

Our aim here is to reevaluate the status of the OHP as an innovation in state
policymaking and to analyze the overlooked political dynamics of health care
rationing. In particular, we address an important puzzle: why, despite the widespread interest in the Oregon rationing experiment, has no other American
state followed the Oregon trail by adopting the OHP model? The answer, we
argue, lies in the wide gap between the expectations and perceptions of rationing in Oregon and the strikingly different reality of its implementation; misconceptions about what constitutes the real policy innovation in Oregon; and the
distinctive nature of politics and public policymaking in the state.

The chapter proceeds in three sections. First, we review the original proposals and ensuing debate over rationing in Oregon. Next, we explore how the
politics of rationing unfolded in Oregon from the enactment of the OHP to its
implementation and how its performance has defied expectations. Finally, we
consider the character of Oregon's health policy innovation and the broader
lessons it holds for reform efforts in other states. Our analysis is based predominantly on field research in Oregon, including interviews with government officials and other key participants in health politics in the state, as well as primary-
source materials, including state government documents and data.[1]

THE OREGON EXPERIMENT: CONTEXT AND CONTROVERSY

During the 1980s, Medicaid spending increased dramatically and the program consumed a growing share of state budgets. In response, many states lowered eligibility standards for Medicaid to an income level well below the federal
poverty line (FPL) and cut coverage for optional enrollee categories such as
the medically needy. By the end of the decade, the health insurance program
for poor Americans covered only 42 percent of the poor; in order to qualify for
Medicaid, AFDC recipients typically needed to live on incomes that were only
50 percent of the FPL (OTA 1992: 76–77). In addition, those who were not "cat-

egorically eligible," such as low-income adults without children, were excluded from Medicaid in most states. Eroding access to Medicaid added to the growing ranks of America's uninsured.

Oregon's reformers promised an alternative to the practice of denying coverage to the insufficiently poor. At a time when most states were ratcheting down income eligibility for medical assistance, Oregon proposed to extend Medicaid coverage to *all* persons living below the poverty line, regardless of traditional eligibility categories. Indeed, Oregon's longer-term goal was universal coverage; the expansion of Medicaid was to be followed by an employer mandate to cover all of Oregon's workers and their families.

However, it was the state's proposed financing mechanism for Medicaid expansion that drew the most attention. Put simply, Oregon said it intended to pay for enlarged Medicaid enrollment by covering fewer services. Expanded coverage for the poor would be made affordable by offering recipients "a basic set of health benefits more limited than those currently offered by Medicaid" (OMAP 1991: ES3). Services would be explicitly prioritized according to their medical benefit and contribution to the population's overall health status. The state legislature could not respond to funding shortfalls, as it had done in the past—and as was common practice in other states—by cutting eligibility for Medicaid. Instead, they would have to reduce program coverage of services according to guidelines established in the prioritization process. In other words, expanded access to health insurance for the poor was to be purchased by rationing their medical care, though advocates understandably preferred the less incendiary language of "prioritization" and "resource allocation."

In its requests for waivers from the federal government's Health Care Financing Administration (HCFA), Oregon argued its plan "would make the rationing of care—a phenomenon that already exists—more explicit and reasoned" (OMAP 1991: ES4). The stated aim of the "prioritization" process was to allocate Medicaid-covered funds in a more sensible, systematic, and utilitarian manner—benefiting the greatest number of recipients possible within limited resources—than existing program policies and federal regulations allowed. Systematic prioritization would enable the state to identify less valuable and effective services where funding could be cut, thereby making expanded coverage affordable. In the eyes of the plan's advocates, rationing meant not simply limiting services, but also rationalizing medical care priorities.

Oregon's rationing plan rested on an elaborate technical analysis that merged cost-benefit data and medical outcomes research with public preferences. A Health Services Commission (HSC) was given the job of scientifically compiling clinical information from physicians, treatment cost and benefit data, and community values from the public. Their task was to reduce over 10,000 medical services to a prioritized list that, in its first incarnation, ranked 709 so-called "condition and treatment pairs" that matched particular medical conditions with a range of likely treatments by physicians. The legislature's decision on how much to fund Medicaid literally "drew a line" in this list, with beneficiaries provided all services for conditions ranked above the line and denied all services below it. Advocates of Oregon's plan, such as senior administrator Jean Thorne, trumpeted the state's "painful and explicit choices" as necessary to "allow government to buy more health for the health care dollar" (Wiener 1992). Oregon justified its rationing scheme to HCFA as "recognizing that society cannot afford to pay for everything that is medically possible" (OTA 1992: 76–7).

Oregon's case for denying coverage to low-ranked services for Medicaid recipients touched off a firestorm of protest from outside the state. Since the OHP reforms required changes in the basic Medicaid package mandated by federal law, under Section 1115 of the Social Security Act the state was compelled to obtain a demonstration waiver from the federal government before implementing the plan. The waiver process nationalized the politics of health care reform in Oregon, turning what had been a relatively uncontroversial and quiescent story within the state into a visceral national debate over rationing. The vicissitudes of the Medicaid waiver process required not only HCFA approval, but also the support of the Bush administration. In addition, influential Congressional health policy makers and consumer advocates—including Representative Henry Waxman, Senator Al Gore, and Sara Rosenbaum of the Children's Defense Fund—set their sights on Oregon, with the intention of preventing the OHP's implementation (Brown 1991a).

Critics assailed the plan as unfair for singling out the poor, and especially women and children, for rationing. Services for the most vulnerable would be cut, it was charged, while the benefits enjoyed by those more able to absorb reductions—the insured middle-class—would be left intact. Sara Rosenbaum alleged that the "Oregon plan is not an experiment that can be justified legally, scientifically, programmatically or ethically"; it is "only one more in a long series of proposals to reduce benefits to the very poor" (Rosenbaum 1992, 103–4). Fears that the state was unjustly singling out the poor for rationing were fueled by reports that low-income Oregonians were underrepresented among attendees at community meetings to discuss the priorities of the OHP (OTA 1992: 76–77).

Critics maintained that the OHP's promise to ration care was not only unfair, but unnecessary. Eliminating administrative waste, squeezing drug companies and providers, and spending more represented, they claimed, proven alternatives. Brookings Institution economist Joshua Wiener argued, for instance, that it was "troubling to ration medically effective procedures before we have truly exhausted other routes to cost containment" (Wiener 1992: 110). The methodology of Oregon's rationing plan drew fire. The attempt to conflate thousands of complex diagnoses and treatment scenarios into 709 homogenous categories appeared to defy human and organizational ability—and common sense. Even proponents of the inevitability of rationing, such as Henry Aaron, contended that the OHP was problematic. Oregon's approach of covering all services above the line and no services below the line regardless of an individual patient's medical condition or treatment prognosis meant that "patients who stood to benefit greatly were denied care, while others, who benefited slightly, received it" (Aaron 1992: 110).[2] In the eyes of outside critics, OHP confirmed the worst dangers of administrative science. Moral and professional judgment would be replaced by the detached logic of cost-benefit analysis and a flawed methodology (Brown 1991a; Garland, Levit, and DiPrete 1991; Fox and Leichter 1993; Rosenbaum 1992).

Medicaid advocates also worried about the so-called "Mississippi" problem. Even if the Oregon reforms turned out to be benign, what would happen to Medicaid recipients in a rationing system unleashed in a state with fewer fiscal resources and more hostile attitudes toward the poor? Moreover, Oregon's reformers asked for their waiver at precisely the moment when key Congressional policymakers, such as Henry Waxman, were attempting to nationalize Medicaid policy. Their goal was to ensure generous and equitable Medicaid standards across all states. Oregon's radical departure from standard Medicaid policy implied a precedent of decentralization that ran directly against that trend, and thus provoked the opposition of lawmakers and consumer advocates who favored nationalizing Medicaid.

The firestorm of protest against rationing stalled the introduction of the OHP and in the midst of a presidential election campaign in 1991, the Bush administration turned down the state's controversial waiver application. In rejecting Oregon's request, Secretary of Health and Human Services Louis Sullivan cited potential conflicts between the criterion for ranking medical procedures in the OHP—which were partly based on citizens' perceptions of how medical care would impact quality of life—and the newly enacted Americans with Disabilities Act. However, Bill Clinton's victory in the 1992 campaign changed Oregon's fortunes. After Oregon administrators revised their list to meet the concerns that had been raised concerning the ADA, and compromised the initial rankings to satisfy HCFA officials, the Clinton administration approved the Oregon Health Plan Medicaid demonstration project in 1993 (Leichter 1997).

Yet approval of the waiver did not end the controversy over Oregon's reforms. Most observers outside the state have not followed the implementation of the plan since 1994 and the health policy community remains bitterly divided over the desirability of the Oregon rationing experiment. Depending on one's perspective, the initial debate still defines either the serious limitations or the courageous virtue of the OHP. Largely missed, however, in the decade since controversy first enveloped the Oregon plan is how the plan has actually operated. The reality is that developments during the implementation of OHP were nearly opposite of those feared by critics and yet were less than what was promised by advocates.

THE MYTHS AND REALITY OF THE OREGON HEALTH PLAN

Critics and defenders of the OHP from outside Oregon would both be surprised by four developments during its implementation. These developments reveal a persistent gap between conventional understandings of OHP—that amount, we argue, to myths—and the realities of OHP's operation.

THE RATIONING THAT NEVER WAS

OHP did not generate substantial savings—as its initial rhetoric promised— by rationing Medicaid services. Setting priorities and drawing a "line" were never implemented as a formulaic mechanism. Some savings were realized by limiting services and using managed care. But the legislature financed the expansion of Medicaid enrollment and subsidies to those above the poverty line largely through general revenues and the imposition of a tobacco tax. In 1993, the initial expansion of Medicaid coverage was funded primarily through a 17 percent increase in state general funds, and a ten-cent cigarette tax (OMAP 1997). OHP saved additional funds by pushing more Medicaid recipients into managed care plans. By 1997, 87 percent of all Medicaid recipients were in managed care plans as compared with 33 percent before enactment of the OHP (OMAP 1997). Administrators estimate that the increased reliance on managed care accounts for 6 percent of savings off the total costs of the program (OMAP 1997).

In striking contrast to their initial claim that prioritization would finance Medicaid expansion, OHP administrators estimate that the list saved the state only 2 percent on total costs for the program over its first five years of operation (OMAP 1997: ES3). The failure to cut costs through prioritization resulted from the rules imposed by the federal government and HCFA, as well as the political dynamics within the state, which we discuss later in the chapter. During the budget crisis in 1996, for instance, HCFA pared back the state's attempt to reduce the number of covered benefits, though it did fully approve Oregon's reduction the previous year.

Far from representing a radical new step toward systematic rationing of medical care, the OHP has been funded the old-fashioned and familiar way: by raising revenues and contracting with managed care plans in the hope of lowering per capita spending for Medicaid recipients. Oregon, no doubt, was well positioned to use these familiar approaches because of its growing economy and its comparatively low level of expenditures on Medicaid. For example, prior to OHP's enactment, Oregon ranked forty-sixth among all states in spending on Medicaid as a proportion of the state budget.

Not only did rationing fail to produce significant reductions in services, but the process of drawing up the "list" actually generated a more generous package of benefits than what Medicaid or even the private sector had offered prior to OHP's implementation. Mental health services, for instance, which government and private insurers have resisted covering, are not only included but are subject to no limitations on the duration of care. HIV carriers—an especially expensive, vulnerable, and stigmatized set of patients—have found that legislators are unwilling to cut off their coverage, which extends far beyond basic services (Conviser, Retondo, and Loveless 1994, 1995). Despite the fears of national critics, then, the rationing did not prove to be a significant cost containment device. Indeed, the list has functioned much more as a mechanism for defining a benefits package than as a strict rationing instrument.

In a further departure from the paradigm of strict rationing, doctors, hospitals, and private insurance companies delivering health services to OHP beneficiaries have not consistently "rationed" care, as anticipated in the original presentation of the Oregon reform. Doctors and hospitals regularly provide (and insurers pay for) services "below the line" that they consider appropriate or medically necessary. One major health plan contracting with the state found that 5 percent of its total costs for OHP were actually "below the line." Below-the-line treatment is in fact inevitable. Many OHP patients are diagnosed not with one condition on the list, but with co-morbidities that are difficult to treat separately. In addition, all diagnostic services are above the line and are often required to diagnose conditions not covered by the list. The point is that OHP's "list" has not been strictly enforced by medical providers—nor is it possible to do so.

OHP's limited rationing and external misunderstandings of that are vividly illustrated by the case of organ transplantation. OHP caught national attention when the media focused in 1987 on the death of Coby Howard, a seven-year-old

boy with leukemia who had been denied a bone marrow transplant. The Howard case seemed to confirm fears that rationing in Oregon would literally kill
patients who were denied high-cost, low-benefit services. Indeed, some transplants are understandable targets for rationing because they may require high
costs for a few patients and deliver uncertain benefits. In fact, the main propo-
nent of OHP—John Kitzhaber—targeted cuts in transplant coverage during
the initial debate as a means to generate the savings to expand access. Oregon,
he argued, should "save as many people as we can, because we can't save them
all" (Fox and Leichter 1991: 15).

    The rhetoric about rationing transplants during the debate over the enact-
ment of the Oregon plan, however, stands in stark contrast to the program's
reality. Coverage of transplants actually became more generous under OHP
than under the previous Oregon Medicaid system or under many commercial
plans. In part, the expanded coverage resulted from new federal guidelines in
the 1988 catastrophic health insurance legislation that required states to cover
transplants for children. Yet OHP exceeds the new federal requirements. The
state voluntarily expanded coverage of transplants for a number of conditions,
including bone marrow, heart, and lung transplants, from children (as mandated by the federal government) to include adults. Moreover, in contrast to
the initial rhetoric, the state's internal process for ranking health services consistently ranked transplants high on the list.

EXPANDING ACCESS

    OHP's architects promised from the outset to expand access to Medicaid to
all the poor as the payoff from rationing. On that count, OHP has more than
delivered. Oregon's Medicaid program now covers all residents below the poverty line. The number of beneficiaries has increased by almost 50 percent, with
a total of 320,000 new beneficiaries covered over the plan's first four years. At
any given time, over 100,000 newly eligible Oregonians enroll in the expanded
Medicaid program.

    National and international attention has focused mostly on the techniques of
OHP's Medicaid reform. Oregon's reformers, on the other hand, actually saw
Medicaid expansion as but one step toward their broader goal of universal access.
They proposed to reduce the number of uninsured by pursuing a self-described
"pincer movement" that combined expansion of Medicaid with a range of policies to help those above the poverty line. These policies included requiring an
employer mandate, establishing insurance pools for high-risk groups, reforming
insurance practices to allow portability and to prohibit exclusions based on preexisting conditions, and offering subsidies to individuals above the poverty line

to purchase commercial health insurance. Reforms for those above the poverty line have produced significant but mixed results. The effort to implement an employer mandate and to move toward universal coverage were blocked by opposition from segments of the business community and by federal reluctance to grant exemption from the Employee Retirement Income Security Act (ERISA). On the other hand, Oregon did establish insurance pools for small businesses and high risk groups. By 1998, there was also no evidence that the expansion of Medicaid had "crowded out" employer-based coverage, a concern raised by critics early on. Work-related health insurance coverage rates have remained essentially stable since 1994.

In 1996, 340,000 Oregon residents remained uninsured as a result of the failure of the employer mandate and other reform proposals (OHP 1997). Nonetheless, the number of uninsured Oregonians fell dramatically after OHP's implementation in 1994. In 1993, for instance, 17 percent lacked health insurance; the proportion dropped to 11 percent in 1996 (OHP 1997). In the same year, 1996, the national rate of non-coverage for health insurance was 15 percent. The percentage of Oregonian children without health insurance fell from 21 percent in 1990 to 8 percent in 1996. Nationally it rose from 14 percent to 15 percent during that period (OHP 1997).

FROM TECHNOCRATIC ANALYSIS TO ADMINISTRATIVE REALITY

Oregon did not implement the purely scientific model of rationing health care it seemed to have promised. Resource allocation decisions remained largely adaptations to political and administrative realities. This is nicely illustrated by how the prioritization list was revised. Originally, planners envisioned that medical treatments would be moved up or down (or in the case of new procedures, onto) the list on the basis of a cost-benefit formula that yielded precise quantitative values for specific medical procedures. Scientific and objective methodologies, not political pressures or other considerations, were to determine the state's health spending priorities.

In practice, however, this technocratic vision failed. Adjustments to the list have been determined not by scientific formula, but "by hand" on the basis of the judgments by the Health Services Commission. Federal requirements and opposition within Oregon over the rankings in the initial list also compromised the original rationing methodology. In fact, an analysis by the Office of Technology Assessment (OTA) found that quantitative cost-benefit data, when compared to the considerable influence of subjective judgments by the Health Service Commissioners, had "surprisingly little effect" on the ordering of health services in the list (OTA 1992: 76–77). Once the list of medical treatments was altered to reflect political pressures and administrative judgments, it became much harder if not impossible to base future ranking of services on a formulaic basis.

Many analysts predicted that OHP would be swept away (or at least stalled) by a tidal wave of opposition within the state (Fox and Leichter 1993; Aaron 1992). After all, health reform efforts in Massachusetts, Vermont, Kentucky, Washington State, and elsewhere had collapsed. In the 1990s, the added burden of an untested, and inherently controversial, rationing plan only seemed to increase the odds against the program's survival. Denying services, critics reasoned, could only spark anger and counter-mobilization by advocates of the poor and other vulnerable populations, as well as by providers resenting interference in their clinical judgments. Commentators warned that adopting OHP would touch off explosive media stories of patients going without care and predicted an unraveling of support by legislators (Aaron 1992).

However, the predictions of imminent doom turned out to be unfounded. OHP became what some observers inside the state now term the "third rail" of state politics. By the time its founding legislation passed in 1989, OHP had ample support from the general public, the Oregon Medical Association, large business organizations, and the AFL-CIO. Members of the Oregon house and senate gave the legislation nearly unanimous approval. Despite intense tobacco industry opposition, there was a 54–46 percent vote in favor of a 1994 referendum to impose a thirty-cent cigarette tax to finance OHP. Nor did the national Republican electoral tidal wave of 1994 undermine this popular support within Oregon.

Perhaps most telling, advocacy groups for the aged and disabled converted from skeptics to supporters. Their initial fears that OHP would systematically deny necessary medical care to vulnerable populations were calmed. They came to appreciate that OHP offered better benefits (especially for mental illness and disability) than many private insurers. The same advocates who once denounced OHP later supported expanding the program to encompass an even larger share of the state's population.

Years after authorizing the program, the legislature continued to reward OHP with new infusions of funds. For example, attempts to divert funds from the cigarette tax earmarked for the program in 1994 were defeated and the expansion of coverage has consistently won popular support and broad, bipartisan majorities in the legislature. Politicians from both parties frequently claim credit for the success of OHP. The program emerged relatively unscathed from a 1995 state budget crisis, which did result in the imposition of an assets test, a slight reduction in benefits, and a sliding-scale premium for those eligible for OHP as a result of the Medicaid demonstration project.

THE POLITICAL SOURCES OF OREGON'S SURPRISE

National and international observers of OHP seem to have missed the story of its increased political support, its generous benefits, and the absence of systematic rationing.[3] In part, they misjudged the Oregon case because of the initial rationing rhetoric used by OHP advocates and critics alike. Reformers now concede that they overemphasized the scientific grounding of rationing, repeatedly compromised what was presented as a scientific process, and oversold the extent to which services would be cut. These facts about OHP are only reluctantly (and quietly) acknowledged by program architects and have not reached outside observers whose impressions of the Oregon plan were seared by the original rationing rhetoric.

Yet the main reason the Oregon story has been misread, we believe, is that most analysts have overlooked or misunderstood the political dynamics of rationing in Oregon. As we have argued, rationing did not function as a key technical instrument for reallocating resources. The focus on the technical dimension of rationing has obscured its political value: namely, the extent to which the *rhetoric and process* of rationing (as opposed to its programmatic application) were crucial in mobilizing support for OHP.

MOBILIZING SUPPORT IN AN INHOSPITABLE ENVIRONMENT

The policy entrepreneurs who formulated and promoted OHP shared an unwavering devotion to expanding health insurance, a commitment that would sustain them through a decade of setbacks and harsh external criticism. Their motto was, "we keep coming back." Priority setting was never the ultimate objective of Oregon's reformers; it was celebrated as the pragmatic means to widen access to health insurance.

Oregon's policy entrepreneurs possessed a talent for interacting with a multiplicity of players and for adjusting to changes in the political environment. John Kitzhaber, who led the reform effort and is currently governor, combined the political sensitivity of a veteran state legislator with both considerable rhetorical skills and a strong commitment to fighting for health reform. Others committed to reform (within and outside government) possessed similar blends of policy expertise and broad political experience in working with legislators and the executive branch in the health policy arena.

From the beginning, reformers drew on these political skills in tailoring policy proposals to what they saw as significant political challenges, though they did not appreciate just how daunting these would be. The political situation during the second half of the 1980s was hardly propitious for health reforms. Republicans hostile to government activism had controlled the White House for three consecutive terms. They had significant influence in Oregon's government—controlling the governor's seat during 1981–1985 and cutting Democratic majorities in the state house to razor-thin margins.

Reformers designed their proposal on the premise that OHP needed bipartisan support to carry it through the natural vagaries of electoral politics. They also worried about state business interests. In the end, they were successful in winning the backing of Oregon's larger firms, or at least neutralizing them, while tempering the damage from the expected opposition of small business.

In short, the process of implementing OHP arose less from a technocratic vision than from a realistic assessment of the obvious political barriers to reform.

THE POLITICAL STRATEGY OF OREGON'S POLICY ENTREPRENEURS

Oregon's health leaders designed their strategy to mitigate the anticipated resistance of interest groups and to mobilize the state's potentially fractious political community behind a broad vision of health reform. They latched onto the language and procedures of policy science and rationing as the centerpiece of a strategy to build and "manage political momentum." Their strategy had four central components.

The first was to capitalize on Oregon's participatory culture. As noted earlier, the prioritized list was to be shaped by cost-benefit analysis and by public judgments about basic values solicited through professionally conducted town hall meetings and public opinion surveys. These meetings, and the activities of the Health Services Commission, attracted sustained media coverage and public attention.

While external critics mostly focused on the final priority list produced by the commission and its alleged shortcomings, Oregonians championed the process that produced it. Within the state, the process of discussing and prioritizing health services was viewed as a welcomed continuation of Oregon's participatory political culture. Land use planning and other policy issues in Oregon have long generated community involvement and corporatist bargaining through commissions, Oregon's traditional way of bringing together government, interest groups, and citizens in the "democratic wish" (Morone 1990).

The state's political culture thus offered reformers a political opportunity. Instead of experts designing OHP in a closed room, policy entrepreneurs chose a process that methodically sought out the attention of everyday Oregonians and sparked a very public debate across the state. Reformers solicited public participation as a part of a genuine effort to incorporate the public's "substantive input on the relative importance of health care services." But they also recognized the political benefits of public participation.

Oregon's reformers and their external critics (Brown 1991b) appreciated the technical limitations of obtaining a representative measure of public preferences (Daniels 1992: 70). They hoped that soliciting some public discussion would induce what was termed a "public buy-in" into OHP and a sense that it was "their" process.

Reformers welcomed public debate partly to avert two damaging reactions to Oregon's efforts to help the uninsured. First, in the conservative, anti-welfare national political environment of the 1980s, they worried about a backlash against creating a new health program for the poor. Proposals to expand benefits to poor residents ran the real risk of alienating Oregonians.[4] The second fear of reformers was that apathy, disinterest, and rampant public distrust of government would undermine OHP. Pursuing reform without considerable public support, OHP advocates believed, would set the process up to fail.

Inviting debate in public forums was a carefully designed tactic, its advocates explained, to "break out of the alienation from government" and to avert a welfare backlash. Indeed, OHP administrators look back and credit public participation and the prioritization discussion for restoring some confidence in Oregon government and for creating a higher level of "trust" and a "reservoir of good will." As one administrator explained to us, "the public input process was effective at building . . . consensus . . . precisely because [policy makers] said that [the public's views were] being taken seriously and reflected in policy decisions."

Critics of the design of the public forums and their admittedly skewed representation miss their political significance.[5] The primary value of public discussions was not in accurately representing or measuring citizen attitudes, but in building support for controversial reform by opening up the consultative process to them. By contrast, the Clinton administration's closed health reform process in 1993 invited mistrust and fueled damaging speculation about secret deals.

The second strategy was to transform the legislative politics that had previously dominated health policy. In particular, reformers organized the process of prioritization to change the "political paradigm" and make legislators politically accountable for explicit decisions to cut benefits. Although the stated purpose of rationing was to cut unnecessary services, the architects of OHP viewed it as largely a mechanism to "put legislators on the hook and force them to make the commitment to expanding access." They astutely calculated that explicit discussion of rationing particular services would be politically difficult. In fact, they believed it would pressure legislators to expand access without significantly reducing covered services.

Following the script of reformers, independent actuaries are first to estimate the cost of each treatment ranked by the Health Services Commission and to present the legislature with the list carrying a price tag assigned to each of the ranked services. Legislators then decide how much of the list Oregon can afford. "The idea," a longtime administrator explained, was to replace "quiet decisions" over cutting the number of people eligible for Medicaid with "very public decisions to change the benefit package according to very explicit guidelines." John Kitzhaber put it bluntly: "Let legislators make explicit decisions so that they can be held accountable for them" (Mahar 1993: 24).

The result was to put legislators in the position of reaching decisions on funding that have direct and visible cause-and-effect consequences for reducing (or expanding) the number of services offered. Under OHP, withholding treatment for specific services would be easily traceable to a specific legislative decision not to provide funding. Legislators are therefore in the politically uncomfortable position of facing voters' scrutiny over very public, explicit decisions to deny payment for specific health services to program beneficiaries. Legislators in both political parties face the clear prospect that constituents may recoil at such cuts in actual coverage and punish them in the next election.

Paradoxically, then, the use of rationing rhetoric made the actual rationing of medical care for poor Oregonians *less*, not more likely—just as reformers hoped.

The third strategy was to define their target population expansively to encompass a broad rather than restricted set of beneficiaries. National observers riveted their attention on Oregon's changes in Medicaid, but the state's reformers persistently presented their proposals within Oregon as encompassing a population much broader than Medicaid recipients. Their specific proposals for an employer mandate, insurance pools, and private insurance reforms were all aimed at dispelling the perception that health reform was a poor people's program providing "handouts" to a stigmatized target population.

In addition to supporting programs reaching beyond the poor, Oregon's reformers explicitly presented rationing as an effort to define the care of the entire population. Participants in its design were warned against singling out the Medicaid population. "The concept of OHP," one longtime OHP administrator emphasized, rested on "making the prioritized benefit package the floor for all Oregonians' coverage, not just Medicaid."

Reformers also used the process of prioritization to transcend formal boundaries between government and private individuals and groups in order to organize continuous negotiations among doctors, hospitals, insurance companies, employers, and labor. This was the fourth strategic element. As one administrator explained, "[Rationing] provided a nexus for the discussions about how limited resources would be allocated" and kept the different stakeholders "directly engaged" for a protracted period.

Hospitals supported reform from the start as a means to reduce the financial drain of handling uncompensated care and inappropriate visits to the emergency room. More telling, though, was the conversion of physicians from initial skeptics to loyal supporters. According to administrators, doctors "didn't particularly take to the idea of public input about what is important in health and health care." They were persuaded of its political importance as a tactic to induce Oregonians' support in a period when the public was in no mood to defer to experts. Physicians had a second concern: the "absence of sound, scientific, longitudinal studies" on the costs and benefits of health services prevented the Health Services Commission from devising a list based on objective as opposed to subjective evaluations. But physicians working on the commission and reformers led by fellow physician Kitzhaber persuaded doctors that they would in fact continue to make "medical decisions every day based on their best clinical judgment." After the implementation of OHP, physicians indeed continued to exercise their judgment, providing services that were at times not covered by the list. Physician support for OHP was also cultivated with the promise that Oregon would provide generous payments for covered services. That promise has held; Oregon's capitation payments for OHP enrollees are comparatively high (Bodenheimer 1997). After physicians' reservations were addressed, they rallied behind OHP's goal of expanding access to the uninsured and funding more of the cost of treating Medicaid patients.

Organizing ongoing bargaining over OHP's priorities was especially important in managing political relations with business representatives. Large and small business concerns, for example, were sharply divided over OHP reforms and the employer mandate. Small businesses were steadfast opponents; larger firms favored the mandate because it would compel small firms to contribute to their employees' health costs and thereby reduce the costs shifted to large employers. While large business initially backed an employer mandate, the election of a Republican state legislature in 1994, vociferous small business opposition, and the near certainty that the Gingrich-controlled Congress would not grant an exemption from ERISA weakened their support for the employer mandate. The result—as some reformers anticipated—was the excision of the employer mandate from OHP reforms in 1995. The prioritization process, though, kept big business "engaged" in the coalition that supported OHP as a whole even as some of OHP's components—like the employer mandate—became targets of vocal opposition and were dropped.

CONCLUSION

INTENDED AND UNANTICIPATED CONSEQUENCES

The operational Oregon Health Plan bears little resemblance to the program envisioned either by promoters or by critics during the national debate over its adoption. The political strategies of reformers were crucial in shaping the Oregon surprises. Reformers used the rhetoric and public discussion of rationing to mobilize citizen support, involve medical providers and other interest groups in the process, and establish a new mechanism for political accountability. Ultimately, this helped maintain a broad political coalition that has paradoxically made it harder for politicians to ration medical care and easier to raise funds for the state's poor.

Much of what has happened in Oregon, then, was intended but simply not well understood outside the state. Still, political strategy alone cannot explain what has transpired in Oregon. Unanticipated developments and fortuitous conditions also played a critical role in the development of OHP.

Clearly, Oregon's reformers never fully controlled or anticipated their destiny. They were blindsided by unexpected political troubles—especially the protracted battle for a Medicaid waiver and the chorus of national criticism. Ironically, the same political strategies and processes crafted to produce consensus within the state produced controversy outside it. These largely unanticipated developments had important feedback effects on the formulation of OHP. For instance, the national outcry over the Howard case, and incongruities in the initial list, intensified HCFA's scrutiny and constrained the state's ability to place services such as transplants lower on the list and cut funding for other services (ironically aiding forces both within and outside Oregon government who sought to ensure a generous benefit package). Similarly, federal opposition to the plan helped erode the scientific foundation of the prioritization process and guarantee that subsequent reordering of the list could not be done on a formulaic basis.

Paradoxically, these external challenges may have enhanced the public appeal, operational success, and perhaps, the political longevity, of the OHP. As a result of pressure from federal agencies and officials, Congress, and citizens groups, Oregon's reformers were forced to compromise their initial plan. That compromise produced a plan, while sacrificing the technical integrity mentioned above, that made more sense in its rankings of medical procedures and thereby created a politically more defensible product. External pressures also forced Oregon's reformers to satisfy a broad spectrum of national critics, an unanticipated but ultimately beneficial process that may have contributed to their subsequent success in shielding the OHP from political attacks within the state.

Oregon's health reformers also benefited from several favorable contingencies that raised the probability of success but could not have been predicted. The program was implemented during a period when the state economy prospered, national medical inflation moderated, and OHP's most prominent sponsor was elected governor. Indeed, it is hard to imagine a more favorable environment for implementing the OHP. Absent these favorable conditions, the politics of rationing in the state may have had (and may well have in future years) a much different character. With higher rates of health care inflation and a slower economy, fiscal pressures might have forced Oregon to make harder choices about spending priorities, including stronger pressures to implement strong doses of rationing. And without the critical patronage of John Kitzhaber, who played a unique role as legislator, architect, and defender of the OHP, it is unclear if the plan would have survived pressures for cutbacks from the legislature as relatively unscathed as it did.

OREGON'S INNOVATION

The formal appeal of the Oregon plan was largely technocratic. The state promised to develop a rational, scientific instrument—the list—to define medical care priorities. The reputed technical power of this administrative instrument has drawn many visitors from other states to Oregon eager to learn its precise formulas and acquire an innovative rationing tool to negotiate the technological, political, and financial dilemmas of modern medicine. Indeed, Medicaid administrators in other states have called the OHP administration asking for the state's famous list in the hope that it could be used to constrain health spending in their own Medicaid programs. Yet, the technical power of Oregon's innovation has proven largely to be an illusion.

Systematic rationing simply has not arrived in Oregon. Based on the rather small and relatively insignificant set of medical services now excluded from

OHP (as well as its generous benefit package), observers will be hard pressed to discover any evidence in Oregon of the "tough decisions" reformers promised. Nor has OHP operated as an objective, scientific vessel of resource prioritization, as the process of updating the list "by hand" has vividly demonstrated. Reformers have, in fact, repeatedly compromised the much heralded scientific rigor of their rationing decisions in order to gain political support.

In short, the actual implementation of rationing in Oregon has failed to demonstrate the successful application of quantitative cost-benefit analysis to resource allocation in medicine. Instead, OHP's operation confirms the prediction of the OTA that Oregon's "outcome and cost-effectiveness data . . . are inadequate for use as the building blocks of a ranking system for all services" (OTA 1992: 76–77).

The innovation in Oregon is consequently more political than technical. State reformers used the rhetoric of priorities to build a durable political coalition in favor of expanded access for the uninsured. Remarkably, Oregon used a method—rationing—thought to be dangerous to the uninsured in a successful effort to help them. The real innovation in Oregon, then, was developing a coherent political strategy to accomplish reform in a national environment hostile to social reform and Medicaid expansion. The political success of the OHP is all the more noteworthy given its troubled beginnings. Ironically the Oregon plan, which started under a cloud of national controversy and predictions of imminent demise, has proven far more politically durable than health reform efforts by other states that were heralded as promising alternative routes to change.

LESSONS FOR OTHER STATES

Given this durability, why, then have other states not emulated the Oregon model? The answer is that what other policymakers had thought to be the key to Oregon's success—the technical prowess of the prioritization list—had, in actuality, nothing to do with the success of the OHP. And the real key to Oregon's success—the political strategies of coalition building for Medicaid expansion—was not exportable, for it rested not on technical formulas that could simply be duplicated by health service researchers in other states, but on the singular political talents of Oregon's reformers and the liberal, participatory political culture of the state. In short, what other states thought could be copied from Oregon—a system of cost-benefit rankings that would produce large savings and a scientific cover to avoid tough political decisions about Medicaid funding—could not be exported because it did not exist. And what really made the Oregon experiment work—political innovation and a deliberative policymaking process that was inherently controversial and largely a by-product of a unique environment—could not be exported.

It is therefore not surprising that other states have failed to followed Oregon's lead. Oregon's experience does, though, offer some basis for reconsidering the traditional reticence of health reformers to publicly discuss rationing. In Oregon, the rhetoric of rationing pulled into the open the decisions that privately occur every day and that deny services to uninsured or underinsured Americans. OHP's experience points to an unanticipated but possible political benefit of rationing rhetoric: it reconfigured debate toward openly acknowledging, as a society, what medical services Americans—even the politically eviscerated poor—should receive or go without. And it put politicians in the vulnerable position of pulling the plug on particular medical services. Paradoxically, a process ostensibly aimed at saying no might force the voters and politicians—as it did in Oregon—to recoil in horror and say yes.

But in other states, the political dynamics of rationing rhetoric could produce quite different—and less benign—results. In a less liberal state, without Oregon's tradition of public involvement in policymaking, history of progressive health care reform, and strong involvement from consumer groups, it is easy to envision a system that would produce stringent rationing of needed health care services and abet a political coalition that would have a new and powerful tool ("the list") for justifying even more draconian cutbacks in Medicaid. In these states, politicians and voters might not recoil in horror as Oregonians did and instead say no, with devastating results for the health of Medicaid recipients. Put simply, what has turned out to be a virtue of federalism in Oregon—the freedom to innovate—could quickly become a vice in a different state. Indeed, given the favorable conditions mentioned above, we cannot confidently generalize the politics of (non) rationing in the OHP from 1994–1998 to future years in Oregon, let alone another state.

Ultimately, then, it is not simply a question of can other states follow the Oregon model, but do we *want* other states to try to emulate Oregon? The OHP has succeeded as a consequence of the political talents of its sponsors, unexpected favorable contingencies, and the welcome political environment of Oregon, where there was widespread support for expanding access to health insurance, a tradition of citizen participation in policy making, and a somewhat less hostile posture towards the poor. These conditions simply do not exist, nor can they be easily replicated in other state laboratories; few, if any states, are in a position to copy Oregon's politics and policymaking process.

In the end, there are two major lessons from the Oregon experience for state policy making and health care reform. The first is that with the right combination of political skill, fiscal resources, and administrative commitment, states can adopt reforms that dramatically enhance—as Oregon has—coverage for their uninsured and vulnerable populations. The second, and more sobering lesson, is that Oregon offers no magic formula for controlling Medicaid costs while simultaneously expanding access, and therefore its experience cannot be generalized to other states. Far from representing a radical new innovation in systematic rationing of medical care, Oregon's Medicaid expansion was in fact funded the old-fashioned and familiar way: by raising revenues and implementing cost-saving contracts with medical providers.

Without the fiscal and political commitments mentioned above, states will not be able to emulate Oregon's progress in funding coverage for the uninsured. The experience of health care rationing in Oregon, then, highlights at once the remarkable achievements and innovation of that state, as well as the formidable barriers to interstate borrowing of health care reform.

Notes

This article was first published in Robert Hackey and David Rochefort, eds., *The New Politics of State Health Policy—As State Policymaking and The Politics of Health Care Rationing: Lessons from Oregon* (Lawrence: University of Kansas Press, 2001).

1. Unless otherwise indicated all uncited quotes are from interviews conducted during 1996–97 with OHP administrators and elected officials in Salem, Oregon. We gratefully acknowledge the support of the Harvard Innovations in Government Project, the research assistance of Laura Sutton and Eric Ostermeier, and the cooperation of all our interviewees, especially Bob DePrete.

2. Here as elsewhere we do not deal with the validity of specific criticisms of OHP's conception of rationing or its methodology for doing so. But one should note that its moral posture did in fact seem undermined by the restriction of rationing to the poor. And one should note as well that its method was indeed flawed in quite obvious ways. For example, if a procedure was hugely helpful in just 5 percent of cases and had *on average* a lower ratio of benefits to costs than the procedure one line higher on the list, that gave no reasonable grounds for funding the latter but not the former. Critics rightly ridiculed the proposal on such grounds, but we cannot separate our own recognition of this problem from those cited by others.

3. Thomas Bodenheimer (1997) and Howard Leichter's work (1999) are notable exceptions. However, while we are largely in agreement with then on the empirical outcomes of the Oregon case, our analysis focuses on the political explanations for these outcomes.

4. After all, it was precisely this fear of the politically damaging consequences of targeting the uninsured that prompted President Clinton to frame his health reform plan as offering "security for all."

5. Misunderstanding the political significance of these public meetings does not mean that critics were mistaken about their representatives. There is no question that civic participation in Oregon's great rationing debate was dominated numerically by those working in medical care. On the other hand, the views of Oregonians were solicited in a variety of ways, which meant within the state that the external critics seemed like nitpickers.

References

Aaron, H. J. 1992. The Oregon Experiment. Pp. 107–114 in *Rationing America's Medical Care: The Oregon Plan and Beyond*, ed. M. Strosberg, J. Wiener, and R. Baker, with I. A. Fein. Washington, D.C.: Brookings Institution.

Bodenheimer, T. 1997. The Oregon Health Plan—Lessons for the Nation. *New England Journal of Medicine* 337(9):651–655.

Brown, L. D. 1991a. The National Politics of Oregon's Rationing Plan. *Health Affairs* 10(2):28–51.

——. 1991b. Letter: Settling the Score on Oregon. *Health Affairs* 10(4):310–312.

Conviser, R., M. J. Retondo, and M. O. Loveless. 1994. Predicting the Effect of the Oregon Health Plan on Medicaid Coverage for Outpatients with HIV. *American Journal of Public Health* 84(2):1994–1996.

——. 1995. Universal Health Coverage, Rationing, and HIV Care: Lessons from the Oregon Health Plan Medicaid Reform. *AIDS and Public Policy Journal* 10(2):75–82.

Daniels, N. 1992. Justice and Health Care Rationing: Lessons from Oregon. In *Rationing America's Medical Care: The Oregon Plan and Beyond*, ed. M. Strosberg, J. Wiener, and R. Baker, with I. A. Fein. Washington, D.C.: Brookings Institution.

Fox, D., and H. Leichter. 1991. Rationing Care in Oregon: The New Accountability. *Health Affairs* 10(2):7–27.

——. 1993. The Ups and Downs of Oregon's Rationing Plan. *Health Affairs* 12(2):66–70.

Garland, M., H. Levit, and R. DiPrete. 1991. Letter: Policy Analysis or Polemic on Oregon's Rationing Plan? *Health Affairs* 10(4):307–311.

Klein, R., P. Day, and S. Redmayne. 1996. *Managing Scarcity*. Philadelphia: Open University Press.

Leichter, H. 1997. *Health Policy Reform in America, 2nd ed.* (New York: M.E. Sharpe).

Mahar, M. 1993. Memo to Hillary: Here's How to Cure What Ails Our Health Care System. *Barron's*, March 1, pp. 8–11, 22–26.

Morone, J. A. 1990. *The Democratic Wish*. New York: Basic Books.

Office of Medical Assistance Programs (OMAP). 1991. The Oregon Medicaid Demonstration: Waiver Cost Estimate. Prepared for HCFA and submitted by the Office of Medical Assistance Programs. Salem: Oregon Department of Human Resources (15 April).

——. 1997. Unpublished data provided to authors, July. Salem: Oregon Department of Human Resources, 15 April.

Office of Technology Assessment (OTA). 1992. Evaluation of the Oregon Medicaid Proposal. Washington, D.C.: U. S. Government Printing Office.

Oregon Health Plan. *The Uninsured in Oregon, 1997*. Salem: Office for Oregon Health Plan Research.

Rosenbaum, S. 1992. Poor Women, Poor Children, Poor Policy: The Oregon Medicaid Experiment. In *Rationing America's Medical Care: The Oregon Plan and Beyond*, ed. M. Strosberg, J. Wiener, and R. Baker, with I. A. Fein. Washington, D.C.: Brookings Institution.

Wiener, Joshua. 1992. Rationing in America: Overt and Covert. In *Rationing America's Medical Care: The Oregon Plan and Beyond*, ed. M. Strosberg, J. Wiener, and R. Baker, with I. A. Fein. Washington, D.C.: Brookings Institution.

Rationing Health Care

The Dilemma of Choice

Rudolf Klein and Patricia Day

Health care delivery everywhere is being haunted by the spectre of rationing. Across countries, across different healthcare systems, there is anxious debate about whether rationing is necessary and, if so, how rationing decisions should be taken, by whom, and according to what criteria.

The increasing pressure on healthcare systems to curb rising costs has given new salience to the question of how resources should be allocated. But if the current preoccupation with the word is new, the underlying phenomenon is not. The problem of reconciling finite resources with the seemingly infinite capacity of medicine to create new demands as the scope for intervention increases in line with changing technology, has characterized all healthcare systems from the beginning.

Rationing is a chameleon word that lends itself to many interpretations, with many different emotional overtones. It can be used, as in the case of distributing scarce food during times of war or famine, to evoke a sense of justice being done: of making sure that everyone has a fair share of whatever is available. Alternatively, it can be used pejoratively, as in the case of people refused expensive drugs or medical procedures, to suggest that justice is not being done: that those concerned are being denied adequate treatment and are thus being discriminated against. The common element in these very different uses of the word is the assumption that there is a gap between what is available and what can be done. Rationing, whether we use the word positively or pejoratively, is about how to use and distribute resources in circumstances when we cannot do the best for all the people all the time.

THE DENIAL OF SCARCITY

Central to the healthcare rationing debate is, thus, the assumption that there is such a gap between the available and the feasible. If this assumption is mistaken, then we need not worry any further about the fine print of the concept or its implementation. Before exploring the forms and dimensions of rationing, we must address the arguments of those who deny the fact of scarcity. Such denial takes two forms.

The first argument is that scarcity is the result of political decisions about the resources to be allocated to healthcare. Rationing, seen from this perspective, is simply the consequence of political parsimony. If governments were prepared to spend more, or were willing to harness the readiness of individuals to pay more for their own healthcare, then the need for rationing would disappear.

In countries like the United Kingdom, which devotes a relatively small proportion of its national income to healthcare, this argument may seem to have a certain plausibility: rationing (in one form or another) has certainly been a feature of the National Health Service since its inception in 1948. But it becomes very much less persuasive when we look at the international picture. Concern about rationing is not correlated with the proportion of the national income devoted to healthcare. It is just as intense in the United States as in the United Kingdom, although the former spends almost twice as much of its national income on healthcare as the latter.

The second line of argument is that scarcity is self-inflicted, reflecting the wastefulness with which available resources are used; from this perspective, rationing is the symptom of a failure in healthcare management. If only waste were squeezed out, if only ineffective procedures and treatments were eliminated, scarcity would be transformed into plenty.

This argument is particularly plausible in the case of the United States, where evidence of over-treatment is abundant and where the costs of managing the system are very high. But it applies to all countries: no system can claim to be using its resources as efficiently and effectively as possible. The scope for squeezing out waste is universal, even if it differs in degree: witness the current enthusiasm, across all systems, for using "evidence-based medicine' as a vehicle for legitimizing curbs on what are seen as unnecessary or over-costly forms of intervention.

It is very doubtful, however, whether this strategy—desirable though it may be in its own right—can exorcise the spectre of rationing. Evidence-based medicine may reduce uncertainty about what works, but is unlikely to eliminate it. The concept of "effectiveness" may not prove as discriminating a tool for cutting out "waste" as the optimists claim. Most forms of intervention work for some patients in specific situations: the notion of appropriateness is contingent on individual circumstances. So there is reason for scepticism about the size of the dividends to be expected from political or managerial attempts to impose the practice of evidence-based medicine on clinicians: the evidence will always be too little and the patients too heterogeneous.

There is a still more fundamental reason for questioning the case of the optimists. Much of the debate about "waste" (and about rationing) revolves around technological interventions. The assumption is that *if* we can slow down — or, better still, halt — the juggernaut of technological innovation, all will be well. But the ever-increasing scope for medical intervention is only one of many claims on resources.

Healthcare is concerned not only with treatments, but also with care of the chronically ill, such as the elderly in nursing homes. It is also about providing a reassuring and comforting environment in which technical services can be delivered. There is no reason to suppose that demands for improvements in the standards of care can be further constrained and every reason to expect that, as populations age and expectations about acceptable conditions in healthcare rise, they will increase.

Therefore, it seems reasonable to predict that healthcare will continue to grapple with the challenge of reconciling constrained budgets with expanding demands. In any case, rationing is not confined to the distribution of limited financial resources. The issue of who should get what arises, too, when there is a limited supply of scarce goods — notably organs for transplant operations.

DIMENSIONS OF RATIONING

Healthcare rationing takes many forms. Of these, the denial of treatment to specific individuals — the refusal to carry out a particular operation or to prescribe an expensive drug — is most apt to feature in the headlines, most controversial and most debated, but not necessarily the most important. In the United States, there is rationing by exclusion: access to healthcare is difficult for the 40 million or so Americans not covered by insurance. In other countries, where coverage is universal, there may be rationing by delay, by deterrence or by dilution. Patients may be kept on waiting lists; copayments may be used to discourage use; the level and type of treatment may be sub-optimal. The repertory of rationing strategies does not end there: healthcare systems may also deflect demands to other services, redefining medical problems as social ones.

Of these approaches, rationing by dilution may be the most significant and pervasive, precisely because it is the least visible. So, for example, clinicians may opt for less expensive forms of intervention, even though the more costly alternative has advantages: they may use ionic rather than *non-ionic* contrast dyes, order a CT rather than a MRI scan, prescribe a less expensive, though also less effective, drug. They may limit the number of tests they perform. They will, above all, ration the time they give to individual patients. Similarly, hospitals will ration the number of nurses, so perhaps diluting the quality of care. They may, too, impose limits on lengths of stay: for example, some American managed care plans have aroused much ire by stipulating how long mothers may stay in hospital after childbirth.

In all such cases, patients might well benefit from the extra expenditure. But the assumption is that the resources used to achieve what may be only marginal benefits would be better used in other ways to the advantage of others. And, of course, the scope for dilution is even greater in the case of the chronically ill: it can always be argued that those in long-stay hospitals or homes (the most neglected sector of healthcare in many systems) would benefit from having more care support, better food and a more attractive environment. In this case, it is tempting to add one more category to our repertory of strategies: rationing by neglect.

The strategies are universal. The extent to which they are used depends on the characteristics of individual healthcare systems. In systems where the income of physicians and hospitals depends on how much they do, the incentives are to maximize activity rather than to ration: if budgets are open-ended, there is little reason to limit what is done. Which is precisely why, of course, the trend everywhere has been to move towards capped budgets, capitation payments and different forms of managed care: to *force* those responsible for delivering healthcare to internalize resource constraints.

It is this trend that largely explains the rising interest in the question of who should make the decisions about the allocation of limited resources and what principles or criteria should be followed. Rationing has always been with us, but the new direction of public policies has given it greater visibility and urgency.

PRINCIPLES OF DECISION MAKING

There are two distinct, if related, strands in the debate about the principles that should guide rationing. The starting point of the first is the healthcare system taken as a whole. Here, the problem of rationing is seen as one of defining more strictly and precisely the limits of the system's responsibilities. Can we devise criteria that would allow us to determine which products, procedures and services should be available and which should not? Decisions flowing from such criteria might, in turn, exclude specific groups. The starting point of the second is how to allocate resources within any given system. Can we devise criteria for determining who should be given what within the agreed menu?

While the first approach is concerned to devise criteria for limiting the reach or scope of any given healthcare system, the second is concerned to devise criteria for allocating resources to individuals.

In line with the universal nature of the rationing dilemma, and the fact that it is common to countries with very different healthcare systems and different levels of expenditure, the interest in defining a limited package or menu of healthcare is international. A series of committees and commissions in the state of Oregon in the United States, the Netherlands, Spain, Sweden, Norway, Canada and New Zealand have sought to define such a package. No consensus about the criteria to be used, let alone about the package itself, has emerged.

In the Netherlands, the Dunning Committee suggested that value for money—the ratio between costs and benefits—should be one of the criteria to be used; in Sweden, a Parliamentary Commission rejected this principle. There seems to be widespread agreement that first priority should be given to life-threatening acute conditions, but thereafter a cacophony of often incompatible criteria have been invoked.

However, the reports of these various committees and commissions have one common feature. And it is a highly significant one. This is that they baulk at listing what should be excluded. The only exception to this is the Oregon scheme, which ranked interventions in order of priority (according to their estimated healthcare value for money), with a cut-off point below which they would not be provided. But even this much-discussed scheme excludes very little and in any case was designed only for the poor. So, for example, the New Zealand Commission explicitly rejected the notion of listing a catalogue of exclusions on the grounds that almost every procedure benefits someone. And it is precisely this consideration that has persuaded health authorities in the United Kingdom to abandon the attempt—made in the early 1990s—to commit themselves to lists of exclusions. Instead, they list specific procedures or services that will be provided only if there is a demonstrable clinical need in individual cases.

Here, again, there is international convergence: the trend from outright denial to conditional inclusion is international. And, once again, there is considerable agreement about the list itself. Cosmetic surgery, in vitro fertilization, the reversal of vasectomies and sterilizations appear again and again. And there seems to be a near-consensus that dentistry can safely be excluded. Countries that have tried to be bolder have tended to retreat under political pressure: so, for example, the Netherlands abandoned a proposal to exclude contraception from its package of healthcare. Overall, then, even conditional inclusion tends to be very much at the margins of healthcare: at the blurred boundary between medical need and social demand.

But if defining an agreed package is difficult—perhaps not even desirable, given the rapidity of technological change—is it possible to achieve agreement about the criteria for allocating resources to individuals? If there is competition for constrained resources—or if, say, there is only one liver available and two patients are waiting for a transplant—how should choices be made? Again, there is a cacophony of criteria. Economists tend to favor a cost-benefit approach. This argues that, if a choice has to be made, it should favor the patient who can benefit most from treatment, as measured by gains in both the length of life and its quality consequent on intervention (quality adjusted life years, or QALYs).

This approach raises technical problems: QALYs have been much criticized on methodological grounds and raise a large question about whose judgment of "quality" should prevail. It also runs contrary to one of the guiding principles of medicine: the rule of rescue. This principle puts the emphasis not on the benefits to be gained from a particular intervention but on the seriousness of the prospective patient's condition and the urgency of his or her need for treatment.

Further, other criteria may be invoked. There is some evidence that age is often used, if only implicitly, to discriminate between patients: this is certainly the case when assessing candidates for renal dialysis or transplants in the United Kingdom. Similarly, it is often argued that the characteristics of individuals are a relevant factor: that account should be taken, for instance, of their family circumstances and their contributions to society. In practice, clinicians appear to use the capacity to benefit as a test for discriminating patients: they choose the patient who will respond best to treatment. Once more, there is no sign of a consensus, no agreed calculus that would allow difficult—sometimes agonizing—choices to be made.

WHO SHOULD DECIDE

So, we face a dilemma. In the absence of a consensus, how should rationing decisions be made and who should make them? Some decisions are, inevitably and inescapably, the province of national policy makers. Whether governments provide health services directly or regulate health plans, they decide the overall level of resources to be made available, either by fixing budgets or by influencing the level of insurance contributions. Further, in the case of countries like Britain or Sweden, where the state is directly responsible for the provision of health services, governments will also determine the distribution of funds between different services: the relative priority to be given, for instance, to acute as opposed to chronic care services. So, in the large sense, rationing decisions are political decisions and, as such, can be debated and challenged.

The real difficulties arise at the next stage, when global budgets are translated into myriad, largely invisible decisions about what services to provide, at what depth or intensity, to which patients. Here the clinician emerges as the central figure. It is the clinician who determines how many tests to perform, what drugs to prescribe and which patients should have priority for treatment or be eligible (on grounds of "need") for certain procedures. So, as the debate about rationing has intensified, the role of the clinician has become increasingly contentious. The recognition that rationing is a universal—and almost certainly inescapable—feature of healthcare has, in turn, raised questions about the autonomy and accountability of those deciding whom to treat and how.

In different ways, many countries have already limited the traditional freedom of clinicians, if only at the fringes of practice. Their ability to prescribe drugs of their choice has been curtailed and, in the United States, managed healthcare plans use guidelines and protocols to shape physician behavior. Will greater public awareness of the fact of rationing—dramatized when the media seize on examples of treatment denied to individual patients—lead to demands for further curbs on the autonomy of medical practitioners?

Equity provides one argument for doing so; efficiency provides another. Equity would suggest that the same criteria of clinical need and urgency should apply to all patients. This is much more easily stipulated than implemented, given the elasticity of the concepts of need and urgency. However, New Zealand has gone quite some way to developing such national criteria, albeit largely in areas where the clinicians can use them to argue for more resources. Efficiency would suggest that clinicians could be steered towards adopting the most cost-effective treatments for their patients. Indeed, there is a moral case for doing so, since wasteful practices deprive their patients of the opportunities for treatment, thereby aggravating the problems of rationing.

On the other hand, the concept of "waste" is, as already argued, highly contestable. Patient heterogeneity and medical uncertainty about what works in particular situations inevitably mean that as soon as attempts are made to limit clinical autonomy, discretion in interpretation rules or guidelines creeps in the back door. It may therefore be more sensible to accept that clinicians will continue to play a major role in rationing at the point of service delivery.

There may well be a case for the medical profession to develop criteria for assessing need and urgency. There may, too, be a case for making more explicit the consequences of national decisions about rationing of resources. But given the lack of social consensus about the principles that should be used in determining who gets what, it may be better to accept that responsibility for decision making should continue to be diffused.

Note
This article was first published in *Odyssey* 4, No. 2 (1998): 8–13.

Viagra

A Success Story for Rationing? A Possible Blueprint for Coverage of Other New, Much-Promoted Drugs

Rudolf Klein and Heidrun Sturm

The launch of Viagra in 1998, with a fanfare of publicity orchestrated by its maker Pfizer, prompted both consternation and perplexity among policymakers worldwide. Here was a new drug for the treatment of erectile dysfunction (ED) which threatened the budgets of health care systems and insurers. Initial estimates of the likely cost of making Viagra's cost reimbursable tended to be alarmingly and, in retrospect, excessively high. In part, this reflected uncertainty about the prevalence of the condition: estimates of the number of males suffering from ED in the United States ranged from twenty million to thirty million, depending on the definition.[1] More fundamentally, it was difficult to draw a clear line between prescribing Viagra to treat a defined medical condition and prescribing it to enhance normal sexual performance, a difficulty compounded by the fact that ED is a self-reported condition and that the notion of normal sexual performance is itself ambiguous.

These worries were all the more acute because Viagra was, if not the first, certainly the highest-profile example of a new generation of drugs—so-called lifestyle drugs—that raised these kinds of issues. If consumers could define their own medical necessity for, say, drugs to reduce their weight then, it was argued, the floodgates of drug spending would open, with dire consequences for the finances of insurers and health care systems if they chose to reimburse such prescriptions. Viagra thus posed a more general challenge and opened up a wider debate. If the distinction between drugs prescribed by doctors to deal with medical necessities and those demanded by consumers to enhance their lifestyles was often blurred—since the same drugs could serve either purpose—then how could their use be controlled or rationed?[2] And how, in any case, should medical necessity be defined, and by whom?

These questions cut across health care systems. The case of Viagra therefore offers an opportunity to compare how various countries reacted to the same specific, concrete challenge: whether or not to make Viagra a reimbursable drug by including it in the standard benefit package. In what follows, we analyze the policy responses—that is, rationing strategies—adopted in a variety of countries, drawing on the material publicly available either in print or on the Web, supplemented by some telephone interviews. Our aim in this is, first, to draw out a taxonomy of rationing strategies and, second, to relate those strategies to the characteristics of national health care systems. Accordingly, we have been selective rather than comprehensive in our choice of countries; we chose them to provide a sufficiently wide range of policy responses and types of health care systems. In all cases, we report on the immediate reaction to the introduction of Viagra and subsequent adaptations. This field is still evolving, however, so some of our information may have been overtaken by events since the completion of this study at the end of 2001.

BACKGROUND

Before turning to the policy responses, however, it is worth noting some of the relevant background information about Viagra available to decisionmakers. First, it is an effective form of treatment for ED. Soon after the launch of the drug, twenty-one randomized controlled trials concluded that about 75–80 percent of men show a statistically significant improvement after taking Viagra.[3] This eliminated the option of arguing that Viagra is an ineffective drug. Second, although ED is associated with a variety of diseases (and consequential surgical or pharmaceutical interventions), the most important correlation is with age. So the condition is not one that is self-inflicted—that is, the result of personal behavior. It cannot therefore be blamed on the patient. Third, the evidence suggests that Viagra is cost-effective when compared with other forms of treatment for ED.[4] Attempts to push the analysis further and calculate costs per quality-adjusted life year (QALY) gained run into methodological problems, and any results must be treated with caution.[5] In any case, the relative cost-effectiveness or cost-utility of using Viagra for the treatment of ED is only one consideration—and not the most important one—when considering the economics of making it a reimbursable drug. Much more important are the assumptions made about the likely increase in the demand for treatment of ED that is likely to follow such a decision. For policymakers everywhere the crucial consideration was how best to avoid an upsurge in the total volume of demand. Fourth, although in theory Viagra is a prescription-only drug, in practice it can be obtained quite easily over the Web.[6] Whatever reimbursement policies are adopted, it is therefore in effect an over-the-counter (or, strictly speaking, over-the-Web) drug, largely outside the control of the medical profession.

TYPOLOGY OF NATIONAL RATIONING STRATEGIES

In this section we set out the various strategies for rationing Viagra adopted in the countries we studied. However, before doing so, we need to put the specific case of Viagra into the wider context of health care rationing more generally, to see whether it conforms to a standard pattern or has any special features.[7]

FORMS OF RATIONING

Rationing—decisions to deliver less than the optimum amount of effective health care as a result of setting priorities among competing demands on the system—pervades across all health care systems, regardless of spending levels. It takes many forms, of which the explicit denial of a service is the most dramatic but not necessarily the most important. Other forms of rationing are exclusion (sections of the population not covered), dilution (fewer tests ordered, fewer nurses on the ward), deterrence (making access to care difficult), and delay (waiting lists). But not only do the forms of rationing differ. So, too, does the decision-making mode involved. Thus, decisions can be either made centrally or diffused among the professional service deliverers. Similarly, they can be made either explicitly (setting out the criteria for allocating resources to individual patients) or implicitly (fixing global budgets that force choice between competing demands on resources at the point of delivery). Generally speaking, diffused and implicit rationing by professionals has been the dominant mode cross-nationally, a strategy that diffuses not only responsibility but also blame. Presenting decisions about whom to treat and in what way as reflecting professional judgments—and scientific evidence, rather than budgetary limitations, is clearly in the interests of politicians and insurance managers. It also may be a rational approach, given uncertainty about which medical intervention works for whom.[8]

Various attempts have been made to devise limited menus of entitlements with explicit exclusions; Oregon's Medicaid waiver is the best-known example. But these have invariably run into trouble.[9] Not only has there been menu creep (a combination of consumer pressure and professional ingenuity in reclassifying conditions has meant that the menu of services tends to be elastic), but also attempts to exclude specific interventions immediately raise the objection that almost every procedure or drug can be medically necessary for someone. Even cosmetic surgery, a standard item in most exclusion lists, may be crucial for someone contemplating a future career as a ballet dancer, for example. So explicit exclusion policies quickly develop holes as exceptions are allowed, as the case of Viagra illustrates.

In many respects, the case of Viagra follows the standard rationing pattern. When the drug was first launched worldwide, the overwhelming, although not entirely unanimous, response of decision-makers was to exclude it from the reimbursable health care menu. Subsequently, however, policies have been modified to accommodate arguments of medical necessity. Total bans in practice turned out to be leaking colanders. However, it was mainly at this stage that differences in rationing modes emerged between countries. For the sake of simplicity, we present these differences as four models derived from the experience of specific countries. These, we must stress, are very much "ideal-type models"; that is, in practice there are overlaps between countries and modes, if only at the edges. However, they provide a useful analytic framework for analyzing policy responses across nations.

DIFFUSION BY INACTION

As so often in comparative health policy studies, the United States emerges as an outlier, unique unto itself. A nonsystem made a nondecision about Viagra. Absent a national decision, even U.S. federal programs adopted divergent positions. The Department of Veterans Affairs (VA) refused to add Viagra to its formulary on the grounds that the costs of providing the drug would add 20 percent to its pharmaceutical budget (although the ban was not complete; an escape clause allowed doctors to argue for its prescription as exceptions).[10] In contrast, the Medicaid program automatically included Viagra for the treatment of ED following its approval by the Food and Drug Administration (FDA), as required by legislation, although the agency feared clinical and financial abuse.[11] Of course, the financial implications of this were relatively modest compared with those faced by the VA health system, given that only about 10 percent of Medicaid beneficiaries are adult males. In any case, the decision was variously implemented by the states. Some resisted outright (among them, New York, Wisconsin, and Nevada).[12] Others followed the recommendations of the Centers for Medicare and Medicaid Services (CMS) designed to minimize misuse and rationed the amount prescribed: from four pills per month (for example, in Alabama and Florida) to ten (in Utah).[13] Health insurers and plans showed a similarly mixed picture. A very few plans included Viagra in their formulary from the start; one such was Tufts, which put it in its highest copayment category.[14] The great majority resisted. "Simply put, having sexual relations is not a medical necessity," one Aetna official argued to the New York

Department of Insurance. However, under the challenge of both court rulings and state regulators, many of the insurers were forced to abandon or modify the blanket exclusion of Viagra.[15] Overall, then, the consequence is that access to reimbursable Viagra prescriptions for American men—the conditions under which it is prescribed, the number of pills deemed appropriate, and the level of copayments—depends on where they live and with whom they are insured. In this respect, of course, Viagra does not represent so much a deviant case as an illustration of the U.S. health care condition.

JURIDIFICATION

Although Germany's health care system could not be more different from that of the United States, there is one shared characteristic: The courts have played a major role in shaping decisions. Germany's system is based on social insurance—that is, a network of sickness funds—and it has a corporatist style of governance. Within the broad framework set by the federal government, policy decisions are negotiated by the representatives of the medical profession and the sickness funds—the Bundesausschuss der Arzte and Krankenkassen. It was this body that decided that Viagra should not be included in the standard package of reimbursable drugs. However, the decision was appealed. The Federal Social Court decided that the Bundesausschuss did not have the constitutional right to issue an unconditional ban on any drug.[16] This left matters in limbo, and the court has yet to give a more detailed ruling about the specific issues raised by the case of Viagra and other "lifestyle" drugs. At first eager to secure such a ruling, the insurers have stopped pressing for a decision, fearing that the Federal Social Court would take its cue from the lower courts, which have consistently ruled in favor of patients appealing against refusals to reimburse Viagra.[17]

In a series of cases, the lower courts have decided in favor of reimbursing the cost of Viagra prescriptions wholly or partially. Among successful arguments have been that patients should be reimbursed when ED is the consequence of medical intervention or condition (for example, a bladder cancer operation, dialysis and kidney transplantation, diabetes, or multiple sclerosis) and when ED causes depression and psychosocial problems. In one case, the court sought to draw a distinction—central to the debate about lifestyle drugs—between using Viagra to enhance potency and prescribing it for the restitution of normal bodily function. Only in the latter case, the court determined, should Viagra be reimbursable (although normal may not be simple to define). "Intact erectile function is part of the image of a healthy man, including the elderly," the Hanover Social Court ruled.[18]

These individual, case-by-case decisions have not been generalized into any kind of applicable guidelines. Rationing in Germany continues to take the form of scattergun juridical decisions. Indeed, muddling through is in the interests of the insurers; if the Federal Social Court were to generalize the generosity of the lower courts, the result would be much more expenditure. For the time being, the original ruling of the Bundesausschuss therefore determines the policy of insurers—that is, no reimbursement, absent a specific court decision. For the longer term, it is worth noting that sickness funds and physicians share a common interest in limiting demands on their collective drug budgets: If individual physicians are overly generous in prescribing Viagra or any other lifestyle drugs, they not only limit the resources available to their colleagues but can be held personally responsible for the cost. Whether this shared interest in self-restraint will survive if the government implements its decision to remove the cap on the drug budget is another matter.

CENTRALIZATION-POLITICIZATION

In contrast to both the United States and Germany, policy in Britain for rationing Viagra in the National Health Service (NHS) was centrally determined by government ministers. Given the highly centralized nature of the NHS, this might at first appear to be a highly predictable outcome—an illustration of path dependency. In fact, this would be a misleading conclusion. The paradox of the NHS is that rationing has always been implicit. Traditionally, ministers have set budgets but have allowed the medical profession to translate financial constraints into clinical decisions—a highly effective blame-diffusion strategy.[19] The oddity of the decision about Viagra was thus that it represented not so much the logic of the NHS as a new departure. It was a reluctant departure. The first instinct of ministers was to depoliticize the issue by asking for expert advice.[20] But the Government's Standing Medical Advisory Committee refused to oblige. It concluded that there was no medical reason for refusing to make Viagra available by prescription in the NHS—"in common with many treatments available under the NHS this improves quality of life, but does not save or prolong it"—but that it was for ministers to make the final decision in light of the "availability of resources." The decision of the secretary of state for health was that since "impotence is in itself neither life threatening, nor does it cause physical pain," and since Viagra threatened to increase the cost of treating impotence tenfold, general practitioners (GPs) would be restricted in their ability to issue NHS prescriptions for Viagra. Availability would be limited to groups of men whose disabilities were linked to specific medical conditions: for example, those treated for prostate cancer or kidney failure and those suffering from Parkinson's disease and multiple sclerosis (MS). The official ration, furthermore, was to be one tablet a week. Exceptional cases not falling into the official categories would be referred to hospital specialists.

The logic of this decision was far from self-evident, as the leader of Britain's GPs was quick to point out: Its only justification appeared to be that it promised to constrain demand and spending.[21] Also, in apparently limiting the NHS's treatment responsibilities to dealing with conditions that either threatened life or caused physical pain, the secretary of state appeared to be expounding a new restrictive, unsustainable doctrine. However, subsequent correspondence in the *British Medical Journal* suggested general support among doctors for rationing. "Viagra: Nobody needs an erection at public expense" was the heading of one letter.[22] Furthermore, British GPs have a shared interest with government in controlling demands. The creation of Primary Care Trusts, with responsibility for purchasing health care for given populations, has given them responsibility for controlling their own (capped) drug budgets.

BUREAUCRATIZATION

Sweden is an interesting, because exceptional, case of a policy reversal. Although in many respects a first cousin to Britain's NHS—inasmuch as it is funded through taxes—Sweden's health care system is a far more decentralized one. County councils are responsible for running health care services and, since January 1998, for pharmaceutical budgets. However, decisions about drugs remain firmly national. As in Britain, policy is driven by the assumption that the same package of health care services should be available regardless of where people live. The result has been tension between the budget holders (the county councils) and the central decision makers. At the time of Viagra's launch on the market, the rule was that any pharmaceutical product accepted as a prescription drug in Sweden automatically had to be included in the drug benefit package. Accordingly, Viagra was included.

However, conscious of the financial implications of automatically endorsing all new products and under pressure from the county councils, the Swedish government subsequently appointed a commission of inquiry. Its report, published in 2000, recommended that drugs be divided into two categories.[23] The first, involving treatment for disease and injury, would continue to be part of the standard package. The second, which included not only Viagra but also drugs for the treatment of obesity, smoking cessation, and hair loss, would be available only in exceptional circumstances. Detailed criteria were to be defined by a governmental committee, whose report was overdue at the time of this writing, to replace present procedures.

At present, decisions are made case by case by the Ministry of Health, in consultation with the Medical Products Agency (MPA), the Lakemedelsverket, which is the regulatory agency for medical products. In effect, there is bureaucratic rationing. Applications have to be made by the individual patients concerned, with support from their doctors. In making the determinations, the criterion appears to be different from that used in Britain (and other countries). The emphasis is on the consequences of ED, not the cause or associated morbidities. Treatment is sanctioned in those exceptional cases where ED aggravates an existing condition. In practice, this means psychiatric conditions. The system appears to have been effective in containing demand and expenditure. By the end of 2001 there had been roughly 3,000 applications, of which fewer than 10 percent had been approved.[24] Given the low success rate, it is perhaps not surprising that the number of applications has been diminishing over time. A further deterrent may well be the lack of privacy: Under the Swedish system of open government, applications are in the public domain.

RATIONING BY EXPERTISE

There is an emergent fifth model of rationing, relevant to the introduction of lifestyle drugs more generally, that overlaps with those already discussed but is worth noting. This is rationing by expertise. Since 1999 Britain has had the National Institute for Clinical Evidence (NICE), an agency charged with reviewing the evidence about new health technologies and producing guidelines about their use in the NHS. Had NICE been in existence in 1998, ministers would no doubt have referred the case of Viagra to it with a profound sense of relief. And, as noted above in the case of Sweden, bureaucratic rationing is seen as a temporary expedient until effective guidelines can be devised. In both instances, the hope is that rationing decisions can be depoliticized by invoking the expertise of a neutral, authoritative agency or committee. The experience of NICE so far suggests that this may be an overly optimistic view.[25] Many of NICE's decisions have proved controversial, and some have been modified following lobbying by the pharmaceutical industry or consumer groups representing patients with specific diseases. Although it is relatively easy to determine which interventions are effective, deciding on priorities within constrained budgets is a different matter. It is far from clear that the expertise of agencies such as NICE carries legitimacy in determining this much larger question.

DO THE CHARACTERISTICS OF HEALTH
CARE SYSTEMS MATTER?

Can policy makers choose a la carte from the menu of rationing strategies outlined in the previous section? Or are their options contingent on the characteristics of specific health care systems? In the case of the four countries so far considered, different systems are matched with different rationing strategies. But if we are to draw any general conclusions from this finding, we have to test it by asking whether similar systems yield similar rationing strategies.

The United States and Britain are, in their contrasting ways, unique systems. No other country is as chaotic as the former or as centralized as the latter. But Sweden and Germany exemplify larger classes of systems. Sweden is an example of the "Nordic model" of health care: universal, tax-funded, but decentralized. Germany is an example of a social insurance–based system—with a plurality of insurers and providers and with a corporatist style of governance. In both there is a group of similar countries. Accordingly, we compare the rationing strategies of other countries within each group. In this exercise we adopt a "black swan" approach.[26] If it turns out that each group is consistent in adopting the same strategies, then there is a strong case for assuming that system characteristics influence (and perhaps determine) rationing strategies. If there is a deviant case (or black swan) within a group, however, any relationship must be more complicated.

THE NORDIC MODEL

Here Sweden started as a deviant case when it automatically included Viagra in the standard benefit package but has since moved closer to practice in other Scandinavian countries. Finland has a three-tier system of refunding drug costs, with varying criteria and copayments.[27] In the top category, refunds are automatic. In the bottom category, "significant and expensive" drugs are reimbursed only if there are "sufficient therapeutic indications." Decisions about the classification of new drugs are made by the Council of State, which also sets out the conditions under which prescriptions may be eligible for a refund. Viagra, like certain drugs to treat MS and obesity, falls into the bottom category. It can be reimbursed only if ED is caused by "serious disease," such as total prostatectomy or vertebral trauma. Unlike in Sweden, psychological indications are not included. Patients have to apply for reimbursement to the Social Insurance Institution, with the support of their doctor. In Denmark, similarly, Viagra is not automatically reimbursed.[28] Decisions are made one at a time by the Danish Medicines Agency. Once again, the criteria favor ED consequent on or associated with medical interventions. Norway, too, controls the reimbursement of Viagra strictly, a policy introduced to avoid the cost explosion that took place in Sweden before its change of policy. Patients have to apply for reimbursement to a national insurance scheme, where officials then decide on the individual cases based on agreed-upon criteria.

In the case of the Nordic countries, there is therefore no "black swan." However, some swans have gray feathers. While there may be convergence on the bureaucratic model of rationing Viagra, there are variations in both criteria and procedures. Moreover, it cannot necessarily be concluded that convergence reflects only the shared characteristics of the health care systems. Two other, more general explanations could account for this phenomenon. The first is policy learning. The Scandinavian countries may have learned from each other's experience (a point that applies strongly to Sweden and Norway). The second is that convergence may have nothing to do with the characteristics of the health care systems but may reflect a shared Nordic political and institutional culture.

CORPORATIST SOCIAL INSURANCE

Here we have only two cases to compare with Germany, those of Austria and the Netherlands. Many other countries have health care systems based on the social insurance principle (France, for example), but only Austria and the Netherlands share Germany's corporatist model of governance. The similarities in the style of health care governance between Germany and Austria are particularly striking.[29] It is the insurers (Versicherungstrager), not the government, in both countries that determine the basket of reimbursable drugs. And in the case of Viagra, the medical superintendents of the Austrian insurers decided that treatment for ED would be limited to defined conditions—again, a familiar list, including spinal cord lesions, pelvic surgery, and so forth. However, in contrast to Germany, the courts have not intervened. This may be because of a difference in political culture, or, more plausibly, because the Austrian insurers were more flexible than their German counterparts were. Instead of imposing a total ban on Viagra reimbursement, they allowed some exceptions from the start, thus making their policies more acceptable and a legal challenge less likely. So Austria is the most "pure" example of corporatist rationing—that is, government delegating the task to insurers and providers.

The Netherlands, however, provides a black swan. Here the minister of health decided to exclude Viagra from the standard package.[30] Following the standard Dutch practice of carrying out medical and economic evaluations, the insurers' College voor Zorgverzekeringen had recommended that Viagra should be reimbursed for the usual medical conditions and in strictly limited doses.[31] However, the minister of health, Else Borst, overruled the recommendation. As in Britain, this was a political decision—not, as in Germany and Austria, the product of a corporatist-style consensus-engineering exercise involving insurers and the medical profession. So, in this group, there appears to be a deviant case.

However, it may be a deviant case not because it is a black swan but because it should never have been put into this group in the first place. The Netherlands has always presented difficulties to political taxonomists, and its labeling as a corporatist state is not universally accepted.[32]

Overall, then, the relationship between systems' characteristics and modes of rationing remains an open question. Some policy decisions are indeed pre-empted by systems characteristics; a central government decision of the kind found in Britain and the Netherlands is unimaginable in the United States. But beyond that, our evidence shows that the relationship between system characteristics and rationing strategies is not direct—and that if there is a relationship at all, it is a complex one, mediated by other factors.

IMPLICATIONS FOR THE FUTURE

INTERNATIONAL NORM

So far our analysis has concentrated on analyzing differences in both the rationing strategies adopted and the characteristics of health care systems. But this is to risk overlooking something far more important: that all of the health care systems analyzed have succeeded, in their various ways, in rigorously rationing the availability of Viagra as part of the standard package of reimbursable or free health care. Contrary to what might have been expected from the general experience of rationing reviewed above, governments or insurers have decided explicitly either to exclude Viagra from the basic benefit package or to make its availability contingent on specific medical conditions. This conclusion would hold if our analysis were extended to cover other advanced, postindustrial countries, such as Italy and Switzerland. Successful rationing is the international norm, thus making nonsense of apocalyptic speculations that Viagra would cause financial havoc.

ARBITRARY DISTINCTIONS?

Is Viagra a one-off case of successful rationing, or does it point to more general conclusions? How far is Viagra representative of the wider class of lifestyle drugs and interventions? In answering these questions, the difficulty is that the whole concept of lifestyle drugs is problematic. The distinction between medically necessary and lifestyle interventions is, as has been forcefully argued, largely arbitrary.[33] If the aim of medicine is to improve the quality of life—to allow men and women to function to their maximum potential—then it is not self-evident that improving sexual performance is any different from improving the ability to carry out the activities of daily living. And in the latter case, it is accepted that medicine will intervene, often expensively, as in the repair or replacement of joints. If, further, psychological distress is put on a par with physical pain—as in practice it is—then the dividing line between medically necessary and lifestyle interventions becomes further blurred. For example, should psychotherapy be put into the lifestyle category? The problem is compounded when we consider drugs or procedures that enhance peoples ability to conform to the social norms of their society, ranging from having children (in vitro fertilization) or not having them (contraception) to having bodies of an acceptable shape and appearance (cosmetic surgery, treatment for obesity). In short, the lifestyle category turns out to be an overelastic hold-all. It covers a heterogeneous lot of drugs and interventions whose inclusion in the standard benefit package can be argued on grounds of promoting normal physical, psychological, or social functioning and for which notions of what is normal may well be contestable, vary over time, and differ between countries.

There is, however, one common element amid all this heterogeneity: that necessity is defined not by the doctor but by the consumer, not according to technical medical criteria but in light of social and cultural norms. Needs are equated with demands. A working, non-pejorative definition of lifestyle drugs or interventions might therefore be those for which the patient rather than the doctor not only diagnoses the condition but can also demand a specific remedy. It is in this respect that Viagra can be seen as representative of a wider class. To return to the starting point of this paper, the reason why the launch of Viagra prompted so much alarm among policymakers, was precisely that need appeared to be determined subjectively, bypassing the filter of medical necessity. The spectre of moral hazard haunted policymakers everywhere: How could abuse and the consequent cost explosion be prevented if a drug for a self-reported condition were made reimbursable? To the degree that other drugs or interventions raise the same question, and however different they may be in other respects, the story of Viagra has general relevance.

LITTLE PUBLIC SYMPATHY

We can concede straight away that in some respects the case of Viagra is indeed special, if only because there remain considerable inhibitions and prejudices about treatments involving sexual performance and potency. Sufferers from ED are unlikely to take to the streets carrying protest banners. Impotence is more likely to be suffered in private than paraded in public. Further, there is no concentrated constituency to campaign for a more generous policy. In contrast to homogeneous, organized pressure groups acting for patients with conditions such as MS, those suffering from ED are a scattered, heterogeneous lot without any organizational base. This limits the scope for a campaign designed to apply political pressure on governments and insurers. Moreover, any such campaign would be unlikely to enlist much public sympathy. Arguments about rationing Viagra prompt more jokes than indignation. Insofar as ED is correlated with age, it is often seen as somehow "natural" and inevitable. Private grief in such cases is not seen as calling for collective action—an argument that, however, is not applied to other degenerative conditions of old age for which treatment is automatically included in the basic package of health care benefits everywhere. Overall, there is a widespread view that treatment of ED should rank low in any system of priorities. As a leading British political commentator put it: "A nation which spends taxpayers' money on better erections, while leaving old ladies to soil themselves and starve in under-staffed wards, is sick indeed."[34]

EASE OF PURCHASE

The case of Viagra has another feature that, while not unique to it, serves to distinguish it. As already noted, it can be bought relatively easily and cheaply on the open market despite being classified as a prescription drug. If exit into the market is relatively cheap, if over-the-Web drugs are available, then it is unlikely that much voice will be raised in protest against rationing by price or that there will be serious worries about equity. Perhaps the public perception is that willingness to pay is a good measure of subjectively defined need. And, as far as equity is concerned, in the case of Viagra it can be argued that money has always bought ways of boosting sexual performance, from call girls to rhinoceros horns. No new inequity is therefore involved.

A POLICY BLUEPRINT

To the extent that other new drugs or interventions (whether or not labeled "lifestyle") share some or all of these characteristics, so policy outcomes are likely to mirror the story of Viagra. If the patient group involved is heterogeneous and unorganized, if there is little public sympathy for the specific condition involved, if demands can be met in the market place, then policymakers should be able to adopt rigorously restrictive policies without much difficulty. The converse, of course, also follows: If there is an organized constituency, if public sympathy can be evoked, and if heavy expense is involved, then policymakers are likely to encounter strong resistance when trying to restrict reimbursement for new drugs or interventions (whether or not labeled "lifestyle"). However, our analysis also suggests two more general conclusions, less contingent on the specific character of the innovation in question.

First, a common thread runs through the rationing strategies of different countries: All of the systems in our sample have allowed exceptions from a general ban on refunding, although some have done so only after regulatory or judicial rulings (as in Germany). Furthermore, the exceptions tend to follow a common pattern: Except in Sweden, reimbursement of Viagra is contingent on previous medical conditions or interventions. If there is any ethical logic in this, it appears to be a compensatory one: Somehow the men in this group are perceived to deserve special treatment as victims of unmerited, disproportionate misfortune. However, the real logic is surely economic and political. On the one hand, the criteria represent a sorting mechanism that is both reasonably objective and financially restrictive, distinguishing between need that can be defined by the medical profession and by patients' demands. The formula provides a tool for the exclusion of pure lifestyle drugs—that is, those where the patient both diagnoses the condition and can demand a specific remedy. On the other hand, the strategy leaves scope for medical discretion by leaving some judgments to doctors. It is therefore more respectful of medical autonomy than an outright ban would be. While an outright ban challenges the medical profession to devise ways of gaming the system, allowing exceptions invites the cooperation of the profession, particularly if doctors have been involved in devising the criteria.

Second, the rationing strategies adopted have, by and large, obtained at least the passive support of the medical profession. There have been criticisms of the criteria adopted but no sustained campaign of opposition. Further, doctors working in health care systems with capped budgets, as in Britain and Germany as well as in some U.S. managed care plans, have an interest in restraining demand. To the extent that such capped budgets become the norm, so governments may find the medical profession a powerful ally in resisting any kind of open-ended commitment to lifestyle drugs as they come onto the market. Indeed, such drugs can be seen as representing as much of a threat to the medical profession as to budgets, to the extent that they undermine physicians' monopoly of judgment about what is medically necessary—and, more generally, raise doubts as to what that hallowed phrase actually means.

While Viagra does have specific features that have made its rationing socially acceptable and politically feasible, the case history suggests that the same set of rationing strategies can be used successfully as other new, much-promoted drugs come onto the market. Two conditions seem necessary. First, rationing is an instance where the leaky bucket may be preferable to a water-tight one: Factoring in exceptions, based on some reasonably objective criteria, helps to make rationing strategy acceptable. Second, the acquiescence of the medical profession is essential, and including the profession in the design of rationing strategies is one way of achieving this. If these conditions are met, the new generation of drugs are unlikely to break the bank.

Notes

Heidrum Sturm is a health care researcher at the department of Clinical Pharmacology of the University of Groningen, The Nederlands.

1. A. E. Benet and A. Melman, "The Epidemiology of Erectile Dysfunction," *Urology Clinics of North America* (November 1995): 699–709.
2. A. Keith, "The Economics of Viagra," *Health Affairs* (Mar/Apr 2000): 147–157.
3. A. Burls et al., "Sildenafil," Report no. 12 (Department of Public Health and Epidemiology, University of Birmingham, September 1998).
4. E. A. Stolk et al., "Cost Utility Analysis of Sildenafil Compared with Papaverine-Phentolamine Injections," *British Medical Journal* (29 April 2000): 1168–1173.
5. N. Freemantle, "Valuing the Effects of Sildenafil in Erectile Dysfunction" (Editorial), *British Medical Journal* (29 April 2000): 1156–1157.
6. A Lycos search for "Penispill" on 12 June 1998 produced seven Web sites on how to get prescriptions or how to order Viagra via phone or on the Internet
7. R. Klein, S. Redmayne, and P. Day, *Managing Scarcity* (Buckingham: Open University Press, 1996).
8. D. Mechanic, "Muddling through Elegantly: Finding the Proper Balance in Rationing," *Health Affairs* (Sep/Oct 1997): 83–92.
9. On Oregon, see J. Oberlander, T. Marmor, and L. Jacobs, "Rationing Medical Care: Rhetoric and Reality in the Oregon Health Plan," *Canadian Medical Association Journal* (29 May 2000): 1583–1587. For another example, see D. Chinitz et al., "Israel's Basic Basket of Health Services: The Importance of Being Explicitly Implicit," in *The Global Challenge of Health Care Rationing*, ed. A. Coulter and C. Ham (Buckingham: Open University Press, 2000), 44–52.
10. Department of Veterans Affairs, "VA Reaches Decision on Viagra," Press Release (in *Mealey's Impotency Drug Watch*, 23 July 1998).
11. Centers for Medicare and Medicaid Services, *Drug Policy: Medicaid Coverage of Viagra*, www.hcfa.gov/medicaid/drpolicy.htm (5 January 2000).
12. "Managed Care Monitor—Viagra: Two HMOs, Two States Say 'No' to Coverage," *American Health Line* (6 July 1998).
13. "USA Today: States Draw Line for Viagra," *Mealey's Impotency Drug Watch* (20 August 1998).
14. Tufts Health Plan, "Pharmacy Information," www.tufts-healthplan.com/members/pharmacy-3-tier.html (19 October 1999).
15. "Viagra Coverage," *Mealey's Insurance Law Weekly* (1 March 1999).
16. "BSG-Urteil zur erektilen Dysfunktion," *Deutsches Ärzteblatt*, 15 October 1999, C-1895.
17. "Erneut Novellierung der Arzneimittelrichtlinien?" (Revised supplemental medical directive), Ärztezeitung, 9 November 2001.
18. Court decision Az: S2 KR 485/99.
19. H. J. Aaron and W. B. Schwartz, *The Painful Prescription* (Washington: Brookings Institution, 1984).
20. S. Dewar, "Viagra," in *Health Care UK, 1999/2000*, ed. J. Appleby and A. Harrison (London: King's Fund, 1999), 139–151.
21. J. Chisholm, "Viagra: A Botched Test Case for Rationing," *British Medical Journal* (30 January 1999): 273–274.
22. "Rationing of Sildenafil" (Letters), *British Medical Journal* (12 June 1999): 1620–1621.

23. Staten offentlich utredening (SOU) 2000:86, del 3 (2000) (Report of Swedish Investigation Committee); and Vanja Gavellin, Socialdepartementet, personal communication, 3 December 2001.

24. Lotta Eriksson, Socialdepartementet, and Jane Ahlquist-Rastat, Läkemedelsverket/MPA, personal communication, 3 December 2001; and Läkemedelsverket, "Aktuellt/Observanda," 6 December 2001, www.mpa.se/observanda/obso1/dispens_hokostnadsskydd.shtml (6 August 2002).

25. For a searing attack on NICE, see R. Smith, "The Failings of NICE," *British Medical Journal* (2 December 2000): 1363–1364. For the reply by the chairman of NICE and comments from a variety of sources, see the letters column of the *British Medical Journal* (24 February 2001): 489–491. For a neutral survey of NICE's work, see J. Raftery, "NICE: Faster Access to Modern Treatments? Analysis of Guidance on Health Technologies," *British Medical Journal* (1 December 2001): 1300–1303.

26. K. Popper, *The Logic of Scientific Discovery* (London: Hutchinson, 1959). However many white swans we count, Popper argues, we cannot with certainty say that all swans are white. But if we see one black swan, we can confidently say that "not all swans are white."

27. Rajaniemi Rajaniemi, Institute for Social Insurance, SII, Helsinki, personal communication, 31 March 2002.

28. For Denmark, Karen Kolenda, Department of Drug Economics, Danish Medicines Agency, personal communication, 1 February 2002. For Norway, John Anderson, Health Ministry, Oslo, personal communication, 4 February 2002.

29. Anna Buscics, Hauptverband der Sozial-versicherungsträger, personal communication, 29 November 2001.

30. E. A. Stolk, W. B. F. Brouwer, and J. J. V. Busschbach, "Vergoeding van Viagra stuit op waarden en normen" [Reimbursement of Viagra is based on values and norms], *Medisch Contact* (28 April 2000): 626–629.

31. College voor Zorgverzekeringen (CvZ) Doc. no. CUH00378 (23 March 2000), Beordeling wachtkamermiddel Sildenafil (Original letter from the CvZ to the minister of health).

32. G. H. Okma, *Studies on Dutch Health Politics, Policies, and Law* (Utrecht: Medical Faculty of the University of Utrecht, 1997).

33. See Keith, "The Economics of Viagra." Keith is former director of economic policy analysis at Pfizer.

34. A. Marr, "Viagra: A Hard Choice," *Observer*, 24 January 1999.

PATIENTS, CONSUMERS, AND CITIZENS

Over time, issues in health care tend to be recycled in new ways and in new terms. In this chapter we deal with issues of governance: how to satisfy the claims of patients, consumers, and citizens to take, or at any rate influence, decisions. The two articles here included were published in the early 1980s and analyze policy initiatives taken in the United States and Britain in the mid-1970s. The common element in these initiatives was an emphasis on giving voice to consumer concerns as a counterweight to the power of professionals, providers, and bureaucrats. The organizational products of this policy—new local representative bodies in each country—have long since disappeared from the scene. The emphasis on recalibrating the power structure within health care that drove policy in the 1970s has, however, intensified even while taking a different turn. The conceptual and analytic questions raised in the two articles therefore remain, we would argue, relevant even though they were prompted by what is now history.

First, what has changed since the two articles were written? The most obvious change is that public policy and rhetoric in both the United States and Britain now stress exit more than voice, to use Albert Hirschman's terminology. The language of the shopping mall place has dominated the language of the political market place. Faith in patient choice has driven policy. Professionals and producers will respond to the consumer preferences, it is regularly assumed, because they will lose custom (and income) if they fail to do so. Choice will put patients in the driving seat, in the words of the policy document introducing Britain's new model NHS.

The repudiation of voice in favor of exit has gone further in the United States than in Britain. Choice rules supreme in American political rhetoric and policy practice; the 1970s experiment in creating representative bodies has not been repeated. The choice of insurance plan has supplanted the more familiar emphasis on choice of doctor or hospital. "Consumer-driven health care" is the slogan for high-deductible health coverage.

In Britain, voice is still seen to have a role. While the representative bodies of the 1970s have been abolished, new ones have been invented. Foundation Trusts (a new, more independent status for provider organizations) now have "governing" bodies elected by patient, public, and employee constituencies: a symbolic nod in the direction of local accountability, given that the role of the governors is mainly ceremonial, rather than an attempt to change the balance of power in health care.

So why do the two articles in this chapter still have any claim on the reader's attention? One reason is their insistence on precision in the use of words. It is all too easy to conflate the interests of patients, consumers, and citizens. In fact, they may differ, or even conflict. A patient's interest is primarily in the services actually being used. A consumer's interest may be contingent on his or her future health care needs. A citizen's interest may lie in limiting the tax burden or expanding access to services. In short, depending on whether the focus is on improving existing services or changing the configuration of services, different interests (and different institutional ways of articulating them) will be relevant. Choice of physicians and hospitals may well be an effective way of making them more responsive to patient or consumer preferences; it is less clear that it is the best mechanism for determining the choice sets—that is, the options between different service mixes or configurations—that are available.

There are other issues raised in the two articles that remain relevant and that may be made more relevant still if the cycle of history throws up a new wave of enthusiasm for voice. They are, furthermore, issues that straddle the differences in institutional structure in the two countries. There is the tension between accountability to local communities and to national governments. There are the different ways of conceptualizing the notion of "representativeness": does it mean that any representative body should be a demographic microcosm of the community or that it should reflect communities of interest? Should a representative body be a cross-section of the population at large, or should it reflect the special requirements of specific patient or age groups? And given an imbalance between the capacity of different sections of the population to articulate their interests, is there not a danger that strengthening voice might reinforce the bias of health services against the most vulnerable? How do we account for the gap between the enthusiasm for participation among many academics (and some policy makers in Britain) and the lack of enthusiasm shown by patients, consumers, and citizens when asked to vote in elections to health boards?

Some of the changes of the past twenty years in the larger environment of health care mean that the analysis offered in this chapter's two articles need qualification. First, new interest groups have entered an expanding health care policy arena with the rise of organized patient groups and the recognition of the "expert patient." Second, the asymmetry in information as between professionals and the public (whether as patients, consumers, or citizens) has shifted in favor of the latter with the explosion of data now available on the Web. The explosion of data has created its own problems of overload and interpretative ambiguity. But there is no doubt that those engaged in either choice or voice can now draw on more resources than they could twenty years ago: they can, in other words, mount a stronger challenge to professionals and providers. Equally, though, there is little doubt that the policy debate about the competing claims of choice and voice, and the best way of giving expression to them, will continue. So, too, therefore, will the policy dilemmas identified in this chapter.

The Politics of Participation

Rudolf Klein

INTRODUCTION: FROM PATERNALISM TO PARTICIPATION?

At the heart of the debate about participation, and about the relationship between the providers and consumers of health care, there lies a profound contradiction. This is that while the National Health Service was set up in order to democratise access to health care, it is also a monument to the values of enlightened paternalism. If the overriding policy aim in designing the NHS was to make sure that everyone should have equal access to the wonders of medical science, the institutional means reflected the belief that this could only be brought about by creating more scope for professional expertise and bureaucratic rationality.[1] Indeed this flowed ineluctably from the underlying philosophy of the founders of the NHS: to create a health service where the only criterion of access would be need, and where people with equal need would have the same opportunities of receiving equal care irrespective of their financial resources or their geographical location. For who but the professional experts—that is, the medical profession—could define and identify need? And who but the bureaucratic rationalisers could ensure that health care resources were distributed equitably?

Moreover, the philosophy that shaped the NHS had a further ingredient. This was faith in the ability of medical science to deliver the goods. Improving the people's health was seen, essentially, as the problem of creating a framework in which medical science could continue to advance and yield its benefits to the whole population. Only provide a rational framework in which it could operate to the limits of its potentials, so it was assumed, and everything else would follow. If the 1948 model institutionalised the "voice of the expert"—the medical profession—this reflected not just the trade union power of the doctors but a wider social consensus about their crucial role as social engineers.

Given this approach, it was not surprising that the design of the NHS—as it emerged in 1948—put the emphasis on expertise and centralisation. The option of a locally controlled health service was explicitly rejected. Central control was essential, Bevan argued, in order to ensure the rational and equitable distribution of resources. If the aim was to universalise the best, as he optimistically put it, then it followed that there would have to be national standards. In turn, national standards implied a national service. Despite the changes brought about by the next three and a half decades, this remains—in essence—the public philosophy of the NHS. The 1974 reorganisation represented an attempt to bring the organisational reality of the NHS nearer to its original aspirations: it marked the triumph of the faith in expertise and bureaucratic rationality. The 1982 reorganisation represented, in turn, a shift in the opposite direction: a rhetorical retreat, at any rate, from centralisation and bureaucratic rationality (though not from the belief in the technical expertise of the medical profession). The subsequent Griffiths proposals imply a shift of a different kind—from professional paternalism to managerial dominance. However, despite this latest change of emphasis, it would be difficult to argue that the underlying ideology of the NHS has changed—as yet.

If this point is accepted, then it follows that the debate about participation raises fundamental issues about the nature of the NHS. In part at least, it reflects the decay of the 1948 consensus: disillusionment with some of the underlying beliefs that shaped the NHS. No longer is the professional expert's monopoly of need-definition and identification accepted uncritically. No longer does the authority of bureaucratic rationalisers go unchallenged. No longer do we believe in the infinite capacity of medical science to deliver miracles. No longer do we assume that the policy aims of the NHS can be defined in exclusively technical terms.

The debate about participation is therefore a debate about the role of politics—defined as competition between different interest groups to decide who gets what—in the NHS. To see the organisation and delivery of health care in terms of the rational development of expert-defined policy aims is, by implication, to argue for the insulation of the health care arena from politics. From this perspective politics is at best an irrelevance, at worst a damaging interference with rational planning. Conversely, to question the role of the professional expert and the bureaucrat—to suggest that they may be defining, in all good faith, the public interest in terms of their own special interests—is to argue also for the introduction of politics into the paternalistic Eden of the NHS. From this perspective, participation is all about bringing politics into the health care arena and, consequently, about changing the balance of power by challenging the decision-making monopoly of the providers. Essentially the assumption is that the logic of democratising access to health care is also to democratise access to the decisions about the organisation and distribution of health care:[2] that is, those decisions which actually determine what people have access to, how and by whom their needs are defined and the way in which they are met.

Moreover, reinforcing the case for participation is the fact of scarcity. Given that the NHS—like all other health care systems[3]—inevitably and inescapably has to ration scarce resources, then clearly the issue of who determines the criteria of making such judgments becomes central. Once again, we have become aware that this is not just a matter of applying the right techniques: such tools of analysis as cost benefit studies and health status indicators can certainly help us to clarify the options, but they do not tell us what we should be doing. If it is accepted that the criteria for rationing—like the criteria for defining needs—are essentially contested notions, then the issue of power becomes central: that is, the question of who has a voice in the process of deciding on the criteria being used in policy making and implementation. While the assumption that the aims of health care policy can be shaped by a technical consensus leads to the acceptance of paternalism, the growing realisation that the aims of health care policy involve weighing up competing (and sometimes conflicting) claims to scarce resources leads to the demand for participation.

The point can be simply illustrated. If it is generally accepted that decisions about who gets what (for example, who gets renal dialysis or a heart transplant) involve only technical criteria, then there will probably also be agreement that decisions should be left to the experts: that is, doctors. But once we acknowledge that such decisions may also involve judgments about ethics, or about the economic value to society of different lives, then it is no longer self-evident that they can be left to the experts. Indeed, there may well be no expertise when it comes to determining what weight should be attached to different, and perhaps conflicting, criteria: technocracy has to yield to a debate about the desirable or tolerable trade-offs between competing social values. And the question of who is entitled to participate in such a debate becomes crucial. In what follows, this chapter will seek to provide a political analysis of participation: to examine the NHS as a political system. In doing so, the assumption will be that—whatever one's view of the desirability or otherwise of participation—it is important to be clear about the scope for changing the existing distribution of power within the health care arena and the feasibility of different policy options. The aim of the exercise is therefore not to provide a cook-book recipe for more participation but to analyse the trade-offs involved and the implications of different options.

CONSUMERISM: A CONCEPTUAL MUDDLE

Participation is about politics: the involvement of citizens in the process of making decisions on issues of public policy. The point is obvious enough, yet all too often forgotten in the debate about participation. For when we examine the arguments for more participation, we frequently find these being put in terms of giving more power to the consumer. Yet the difference between citizens and consumers is all important.

In the first place, the consumers of health care are only a minority of those affected at any one time by the policies and practices of the NHS. As a citizen, I may have an interest in the NHS even though I am not a consumer. My interest may be that of a contingent user: someone who wants to be sure that there will be the appropriate facilities should I ever want to use them. Or my interest may be that of a taxpayer: someone who wants to make sure that my money is not being wasted. From this it follows that participation by citizens and participation by consumers do not necessarily point in the same direction. As a citizen I may well wish to minimise the investment in a particular form of health care, while as a consumer I may want to maximise it. In short, we have to be clear whether we are concerned about strengthening the responsiveness and accountability of the NHS to a wider body of citizens, or of strengthening consumers as an interest group within the NHS. Both may be legitimate aims of policy, but they are not the same or necessarily congruent.

In the second place, the language of consumerism is that of the economic market place rather than that of the political market place. Consumerism (despite its rather paradoxical adoption by the Left) is about the individual getting his money's worth. The consumer movement in health care makes much the same sort of demands as the consumer movement in other markets. It generates demands for more information about the goods being sold, for minimum standards, against poor quality, and so on. It is all about creating more scope for informed choice; for allowing the consumer to satisfy his or her demands. It concentrates attention on the individual consumer's experience of health care. Indeed the logic of consumerism is a market-based health care system, as the Institute of Economic Affairs quite rightly argues.[4] If our priority is to ensure a health care system organised around the principle of responding to individual consumer demands, then clearly there is no better machinery than the market. The simplest way of transferring power to the individual consumer is to make him or her the paymaster of the health care providers. (A policy option which is certainly feasible if we are prepared to make heroic assumptions about the willingness of governments to redistribute incomes sufficiently drastically to give all individual consumers the necessary purchasing power.) As we all know, however, the health care market is a peculiar one. In particular, it is characterised by an imbalance of knowledge between consumers and providers. The consumer does not necessarily know best (though he or she may do so more often than is assumed by the professionals). Similarly, mistakes—once made—may often be irreversible. A defective car can be returned to the garage; a defective operation poses rather more difficult and perhaps permanent problems.

So we come back to the central tension within the NHS. The whole justification for its existence lies in the rejection of the market principle as inappropriate for the organisation of health care. It is this which, in a sense, gives moral legitimacy to the paternalism of the providers: if the NHS does not exist to meet professionally determined needs, as distinct from consumer demands, why have it in the first place? Yet, at the same time, there is pressure to accommodate within the system the kind of consumer demands that would be appropriate in a market system but which go against the grain of the NHS's own ethos.

Moreover, there is a further reason why the consumer model fits rather badly into the specific context of the NHS. In the economic market place, a consumer seeking the best buy for himself or herself is not damaging the interests of anyone else. The language of equity is irrelevant. In the case of the NHS, however, it is central. What may be the best buy for the individual may not necessarily be the best buy for the community collectively: maximising the health of the community as a whole may actually involve giving individuals less than the optimum possible treatment, and possibly even denying them treatment (as, for instance, in the case of renal dialysis).

Nor is there a necessary or logical link between consumerism and participation seen as involvement in the decision-making processes. After all, the management of a firm which finds that the consumers of its products are dissatisfied does not invite them into the board room. Instead, it is likely to carry out some market research and adapt its products to meet consumer preferences. In the case of the NHS, too, management has this option. Indeed, the Griffiths report[5] takes the view that good management requires a sensitivity to consumer views. "Businessmen have a keen sense of how well they are looking after their customers," it points out and argues for a similar approach in the NHS. Thus it should be the responsibility of NHS management, the report suggests, to "ascertain how well the service is being delivered at local level by obtaining the experience and perceptions of patients and the community" using a variety of methods, including market research.

The trouble is that while a business firm which ignores consumer preferences long enough will eventually go bankrupt, there is no equivalent sanction in the case of the NHS. For the NHS, losing customers is a bonus: exit by patients (whether into self-care or the private sector) simply relieves the burden on the organisation.[6] The incentives to change organisational routines and practices, in response to information about patient preferences, are weak. Thus, for example, the survey of hospital patients carried out on behalf of the Royal Commission on the NHS[7] showed that 43 per cent of those interviewed were aggrieved about being woken up too early. This entirely predictable finding illustrates the difficulties of overcoming organisational resistance to changes designed to meet consumer preferences. The organisational bias favours maintaining those routines and practices perceived to be desirable by the producers.

If we adopt a consumerist perspective, therefore, the problem becomes one of devising ways of making the NHS more responsive: of introducing incentives to the managers and producers not only to seek information about patient preferences but to act on the signals received. But, once again, it is worth stressing the limitations imposed on such an approach by the very nature of the NHS. Given that the NHS is an instrument for rationing scarce resources equitably, there may be good reasons for refusing to respond to patient preferences if meeting these reduces the overall capacity of the service to meet the needs of the community as a whole. The real difficulty is to know when this argument is being invoked because of organisational self-interest or conservatism, and when it is a genuine reason for refusing to meet consumer preferences.

Further, there is the problem that consumer preferences tend to be shaped by what is available. Overall, the evidence of successive surveys over the decades—confirmed by the Royal Commission survey—is that most people are satisfied with the services they receive. This somewhat passive acceptance of the status quo may be changing, perhaps influenced by the increasing coverage of health care issues by the media. Certainly there is evidence that the better educated and the younger consumers tend to be more critical. But, in general, the paradox of the NHS would seem to be that it is the providers that are more aware of what could be done—the gap between existing provision and the potential scope for improving scope and quality—than the consumers.

Lastly, it is worth noting that consumer preferences—where they are expressed—tend to be biased in a particular direction: that is, towards the acute services. If we assume that the use of the private sector measures consumer dissatisfaction with the NHS (at least for those consumers who can afford to opt out), then it is clear that the repressed demand is largely for better facilities for elective surgery for people of working age (as well as for choice of timing and of consultant). In short, there would appear to be a clash between the paternalistic values that have shaped policy making in the NHS—as reflected in the priority given to the elderly and other vulnerable groups—and consumer preferences. To reject paternalism, while embracing consumerism, might therefore have profound implications for the distribution of the NHS's resources.

THE POLITICAL MARKET

So far the argument has identified two rather different reasons for worrying about the political context of policy-making in the NHS. The first, discussed in the introductory section of this chapter, puts the emphasis on wider participation in policy-making: the challenge is to the paternalistic assumption that needs can only be defined by professional experts. The second, discussed in the preceding section, puts the emphasis on making the NHS more responsive: the challenge is to the organisational assumption that the perceptions of the providers must inevitably censor consumer preferences.

Both points raise questions about the nature of the political market in the health care arena. This section therefore addresses itself to analysing this market. If we want to encourage greater participation and involvement by citizens in the formation and implementation of policy—if we want to see decisions being taken not exclusively by experts but as the outcome of a wider debate— what are the problems and options? But before discussing issues specific to the health care arena, it is important to note the central irony of the whole debate about participation. While the advocacy of more participation tends to be made in the name of anti-elitism, participation itself tends to be something of an elite activity. In other words, we cannot start with the assumption that there is a dammed-up demand for greater participation, only waiting for the institutional changes needed to open the floodgates of public involvement. Thus a survey carried out on behalf of the Commission on the Constitution in the early 1970s found only a "fairly low level of interest and involvement in political and community affairs."[8] Moreover, those rated as "very involved"—because they were active in political or community affairs, as distinct from being passive members of such organisations as trade-unions or local voluntary associations—tended to speak with an upper-class accent. While 44 per cent of professionals and managers came into the "very involved" category, only 10 per cent of unskilled workers did so (while the figure for skilled workers was 21 per cent). Interestingly, too, the survey showed an age bias: involvement tends to rise with age until people are in their 40s, declining thereafter. Not surprisingly, involvement is also linked to education: while 48 per cent of those who had gone on to higher education were rated as "very involved," only 19 per cent of those who had left school before 15 came into this category. And much the same pattern emerged when the survey examined people's knowledge of how the public services are run: again, social class and education turned out to be important factors.

At first sight this evidence would seem to be at odds with the much cited phenomenon of a boom in a wide variety of action groups: ranging from tenants' associations to self-help voluntary groups. But, in fact, a rapid growth in such groups is perfectly compatible with public involvement remaining very much a minority interest: if we assume 100 members per group (a fairly generous assumption probably) then even the birth of 1000 new groups does not amount to a large proportion of the population. And, indeed, the 1977 General Household Survey confirmed the findings of the earlier investigation: it found that only about 10 per cent of the adult population participated in social and voluntary work.[9]

All this is not to decry the extent of the commitment to participation in public affairs in Britain. In my own view, 10 per cent is an impressively high figure. It is to suggest, however, two cautioning conclusions—both with important implications for policy (and not just in the health care arena). The first is that we should not take the willingness to participate for granted: that we should examine carefully both the enabling conditions and the barriers which either encourage or discourage people from participating. The second is that we should avoid the easy rhetoric which opposes participation to elitism: the case for widening participation, it is tempting to argue, is simply that it offers opportunities for new elites to involve themselves in the policy process: to create more competition among elites (which may, in itself, be a very desirable objective—but should not be confused with populist rhetoric).

To elaborate the first point, participation involves—self-evidently—both costs and benefits. It requires time, knowledge, social skills and self-confidence: an investment of effort, in short. Conversely, participation can bring rewards. Some of these may be psychic: an intrinsic sense of satisfaction at doing one's social duty or of asserting one's rights as a citizen. Others may be more directly material. The incentive to participate is obviously greater if, as a result, one increases one's chances of getting some specific return: a motorway rerouted, a local hospital kept open, and so on.

Following on from this point, it is not surprising that, as we have already noted, the participating population is in no sense an accurate mirror of the community as a whole. It is a biased sample—because the resources required to make the most of any opportunities to participate are not equally distributed in the population at large. The less educated, less articulate and less confident are likely to lose out. Indeed it is tempting to suggest that there is an inverse law of participation—that those with the greatest need to push their own interests have the least capacity to do so effectively. Conversely, it would seem to follow that extending the opportunities to participate would favour precisely those who already have the most resources, whether social and economic.

However, this is to assume that the costs and benefits of participation are set in concrete for all time. In fact, of course, if the objective of public policy is to encourage participation, it is possible to create conditions which lower the costs and increase the benefits. Specifically, three propositions would seem to flow from the arguments put so far.

PROPOSITION 1

The costs of participation can be lowered by diffusing free information and providing organisational support. Thus it is possible to make it easier for people to participate (particularly the least knowledgeable) by deliberately setting out to provide them with information. Equally, it is possible to lower the organisational costs of participation by providing support, for example, from community workers.

PROPOSITION 2

The greater the scope for local diversity, the greater also are the incentives to participate. In other words, the benefits yielded by participation can be increased by accepting the right of local communities to be different: that is, to make their own decisions about the level and pattern of services.

PROPOSITION 3

The smaller the size of the political universe, the lower will be the costs and the higher will be the benefits of participation. To the extent that the universe is small, so information is more accessible and the organisational effort involved is lower. Conversely, the benefits will be more direct and immediate to the individuals concerned.

Each of these can now be translated into the specific context of the NHS. If the aim is to encourage participation, then clearly there has to be a greater willingness to provide free information. Similarly, from this perspective the role of community health councils can be seen—in part at least—as being to lower the organisational costs of participation: they provide a ready-made (and free) machinery which can be used by citizens to express their views.

Again, greater participation would seem to imply accepting greater local diversity in the NHS. For why should people take an interest in their local NHS services if these are determined exclusively by national decisions about the level and pattern of provision? So here we come to a trade-off between the conditions required to encourage participation and other aims of policy, such as the achievement of national priorities and geographical equity. For example, we might well wish to encourage participation by giving communities the right to levy extra rates in order to keep local hospitals open. But this might well mean that richer communities would have more by way of health care provision than poorer parts of the country, so defeating one of the objectives which the NHS was set up to bring about.

Lastly, if small size encourages participation and vice versa, then we might well have to revise our ideas about what are the appropriate administrative units for the NHS. The definition of democracy as direct participation in decision-making was born in the circumstances of the Greek city states and the Swiss cantons. And it may be that the population of a general practice is the largest compatible with this kind of definition: anything larger would certainly not have been recognised by Aristotle or Rousseau as a suitable setting for participatory democracy. Certainly even the post-1982 districts—with populations of up to half a million—would seem to be much too large administrative units for encouraging participation. Again there would appear to be a trade-off between creating what are efficient and effective units of administration and the demands of participation. If we were to give overriding priority to the latter, we might well end up with designing an NHS of local cottage hospitals: the ideal constituency for participation (to judge by the enthusiasm with which citizens mobilise to defend these much-cherished institutions).

All this suggests that while, in theory, it is perfectly possible to create a different kind of political market within the NHS, there is a price to be paid. Participation cannot be seen as icing on the cake: something extraneous to the structure and organisation of the NHS. It represents, rather, an entirely different approach, involving at least some sacrifice of other valued aims. Moreover, it presents a number of other problems as well: the subject of the next section.

PROFESSIONALS AND CITIZENS

So far the case for participation has been examined on the assumption that greater citizen involvement is desirable in its own right. And, indeed, this may well be so: there is a long tradition of political theory which argues for more participation as a way of educating the citizen to his full capacities. But, as we suggested at the start of this chapter, the case for greater participation in the NHS is usually argued in somewhat different terms: as a means towards changing the balance of power within the NHS and opening up the debate about policy aims and instruments. In other words, the concern is about effective participation — not just about token involvement by the citizen.

Once we adopt this focus, we immediately come up against the imbalance between producer and citizen interests:[10] an imbalance of both knowledge and organisational resources. By definition, NHS producers know more about the health service than citizens, have a permanent stake in defending their own interests and are organised in trade unions and professional bodies. In contrast, citizens have only a contingent interest in the NHS, as already argued, and lack both the information and organisational resources of the producers. While the producers are a concentrated interest group, the citizens are a diffuse interest group. They may well have incentives to mobilise on particular occasions and for specific causes, but they have little reason to take the kind of long-term interest which is so crucial in a service where policy making is inevitably incremental, building on past history, and where there is a complex interdependence between decisions taken at different times, in different circumstances and at different levels of the administrative hierarchy.[11] Moreover, decisions in the NHS tend to be the outcome of complex bargains between different groups of producers: untying the package may be both difficult and counter-productive. It is therefore not surprising, perhaps, that successive studies of local policy making in the NHS have all come to the conclusion that the influence of lay authority members tends to be ineffective and marginal. Much the same conclusion flows from such inquiries as the Normansfield report,[12] which seem to indicate that lay members are also ineffective when it comes to looking after the interests of consumers (although in this particular instance the members of the relevant AHA were fully alerted to the conditions at Normansfield by the CHC). This would indeed seem to follow from the imbalance in knowledge as between service providers and citizens.

Once again, however, it is important to ask whether such an asymmetry is inevitable, or whether it would be possible to create institutional devices designed to change the balance. If we see citizen participation not necessarily as direct involvement by individuals in decision-making, but more broadly as widening the interests represented in the running of the NHS, what can be done to make the representation of such interests more effective?

One obvious option would be to move towards directly elected health authorities. The argument for doing so would appear to be twofold. First, election would give the authority members a legitimacy which at present they do not have: it would strengthen their authority vis-à-vis the NHS providers. Second, and more central to the present discussion, election would give authority members a direct incentive to be responsive to the wishes of the local community: there would be a direct channel for the articulation of local interests and preferences. If the aim of policy is to democratise access to decision-making then, surely, there could be no better way of doing so than by having elected authorities.

The theory is neat but practice might be rather less so. Indeed there would seem to be reason for considerable scepticism as to whether elected authorities would be more effective — in terms of widening the debate about policies and ensuring responsiveness — than the present ones. In the case of existing local authorities, we have got considerable evidence which suggests that elections are decided not by performance but by national swings of opinion. Similarly, the problems faced by local police authorities in controlling their experts would seem to indicate that the mere fact of election does little to ensure an effective lay voice in what are perceived to be "professional" issues. Lastly, there is little evidence that local authorities are regarded by citizens as more responsive than the NHS. On the contrary, the survey conducted for the Commission on the Constitution — cited earlier — suggested that the public rate the NHS more highly than local authorities in this respect: 59 per cent of those interviewed thought that the NHS would be good at dealing with complaints from members of the public, as against 49 per cent who thought the same about the local council office. Moreover, it may be significant that many of the demands for greater citizen participation have come precisely in those areas and services controlled by local authorities: town planning, education and housing.

There is a further problem about the direct election option. Can we be really sure that the local citizens would participate in the elections? Once more, the available evidence suggests cause for scepticism. If we look at the experience of New Zealand[13] where health authorities were directly elected, there would appear to be a risk of massive apathy. Nor is this surprising. For we come back to the central dilemma, discussed earlier, of how to reconcile incentives to citizens to participate with the central aim of the NHS, which is to maintain national standards. If there is little scope for deviating from national standards, there is little incentive for citizens to participate in elections or anything else. If there is a lot of scope, then it is difficult to see the point of having a national health service — as distinct from a conglomerate of local health authorities.

The nature of the dilemma involved is reflected in the curious twists and turns of successive Conservative Secretaries of State since 1979. The aim of the 1982 reorganisation of the NHS, as expressed by Mr. Patrick Jenkin, was precisely to devolve responsibility to the districts: implicit in much of the Ministerial rhetoric was a vision of the NHS as a loose federation of local health services.[14] But no sooner had Mr. Jenkins left office than his successor, Mr. Norman Fowler, changed the emphasis. In response to criticisms from the Parliamentary Public Accounts and Social Services Committees, the new Secretary of State introduced an elaborate system of annual reviews designed to make sure that local health authorities are following national priorities and national policies. The logic of a national service, financed out of central funds, runs counter to the logic of decentralisation—which is to accept and tolerate local decisions about priorities and policies.

So if we are really serious about devolving decision-making, and encouraging local participation, we have to face up to some very hard questions about the limits of tolerable diversity. Would we be really happy if an elected health authority were to decide, in response to local community demands, to put all its money into improving the acute services at the expense of the provision for, say, the mentally handicapped or the elderly demented?

The question is not merely rhetorical. For, to return to our earlier discussion about the differential ability and desire of different groups in the community to participate, there would seem to be good reason to expect a bias towards the acute services in response to local demands. If there is an imbalance as between providers and citizens, there is also an imbalance among citizens. The most vulnerable groups are precisely those least likely to participate in any political market, and least able to assert their own interests. The example of the mentally handicapped is self-evident. But the same point applies, if with less force, in the case of the elderly. In this respect, the NHS's much-criticised bias in its budget towards acute services would seem to mirror accurately the bias of power not just within the medical profession but within the community. It is also worth noting that those social groups identified as most deprived in terms of health care by the Black report,[15] among other similar studies, are precisely the same groups who, as noted earlier, are least likely to participate: notably, the unskilled and poorly educated.

The constitution of community health councils is instructive in this respect.[16] It represents a deliberate attempt to rig the political market in favour of those with the least resources for participation. By ensuring the presence of members representing pressure groups for the mentally ill and handicapped, among others, the constitution of CHCs gives a voice to those citizens least able to participate in political processes: that is, the most vulnerable. Similarly, at the national level, successive governments have deliberately sought to encourage such pressure groups as MIND, in an attempt to load the dice in favour of the weakest—that is, those who carry least weight in the political market. For it would seem that just as we are not prepared to leave the provision of health care to the free play of the economic market place, so we are not prepared to leave it to the free play of the political market place. Paternalism, it would seem, creeps in by the back door even when it has been thrown out by the front-door in favour of participation.

So the argument of this chapter has come full circle. To the extent that the NHS embodies a vision of what society ought to be like—that it represents an attempt not just to provide services but also to embody a particular set of values[17]—so it may be that a certain degree of paternalism may be inevitable. Certainly, as the analysis of this chapter has tried to demonstrate, giving priority to the value of participation may mean sacrificing other values embodied in the structure and policies of the NHS: a reason not for preserving the status quo but for being quite clear about the nature of the trade-offs being faced.

Moreover, in conclusion, a final irony must be noted. The NHS is, in a sense, an instrument of collective altruism: a machine for redistributing resources to the most vulnerable sections of the population. But such collective altruism is particularly fragile in an era of economic crisis, when the allocation of resources becomes a zero-sum game and giving more to the vulnerable means giving less to the rest of the population. There is indeed evidence that altruism declines in hard times, when redistributing resources can no longer be financed out of the dividends of growth.[18] In such circumstances paternalism—the insulation of the health care arena from politics—could be the NHS's best protection against what might otherwise be a hostile climate.

Notes

This article was first published in Robert Maxwell and Nigel Weaver, eds., *Public Participation in Health*, published by King Edward's Hospital Fund for London, 1984.

1. Klein, Rudolf. *The politics of the National Health Service.* London, Longman, 1983.
2. Smith, Brian. *Access and the reorganisation of local government.* Brussels, European Group of Public Administration, 1982.
3. Fuchs, Victor R. *Who shall live? health, economics and social choice.* New York, Basic Books, 1974.
4. Harris, Ralph, and Seldon, Arthur. *Over-ruled on welfare.* London, Institute of Economic Affairs, 1979. Hobart paperback no. 13.
5. Great Britain, Department of Health and Social Security. *NHS management inquiry.* (Leader of inquiry: Roy Griffiths). London, DHSS, 1983.
6. Klein, Rudolf. Models of man and models of policy. *Milbank Memorial Fund Quarterly/Health and Society*, 58, no. 3, summer 1980, pp. 416–429.
7. Gregory, Janet. *Patients' attitudes to the hospital service.* A survey carried out for the Royal Commission on the National Health Service. London, HMSO, 1978. Research paper no. 5.
8. Royal Commission on the Constitution. *Devolution and other aspects of government: an attitudes survey.* London, HMSO, 1973. Research paper no. 7.
9. Ramprakash, Deo, ed. *Social trends no. 11: A publication of the Government Statistical Service.* London, HMSO, 1980.

10. Marmor, T. R., and Morone, J. A. Representing consumer interests. *Milbank Memorial Fund Quarterly/Health and Society*, 58, no. 1, winter 1980, pp. 125–165.
11. Hunter, David J. *Coping with uncertainty: Policy and politics in the National Health Service.* Chichester, John Wiley Research Studies Press, 1980. Social policy research monographs series 2.
12. Klein, Rudolf. Normansfield: Vacuum of management in the NHS. *British Medical Journal*, no. 6154, 23/30 December 1978, pp. 1802–1804.
13. Minister of Health. *A health service for New Zealand.* Wellington, Government Printer, 1974.
14. Klein, Rudolf. *Health services.* In Jackson, P. M., ed. *Government policy initiatives 1979–80.* London, Royal Institute of Public Administration, 1981, pp. 161–180.
15. Great Britain, Department of Health and Social Security. *Inequalities in health: report of a research working group* (Chairman, Sir Douglas Black). London, DHSS, 1980. Townsend, Peter, and Davidson, Nick, eds. *Inequalities in health: The Black report.* Harmondsworth, Penguin, 1982.
16. Klein, Rudolf, and Lewis, Janet. *The politics of consumer representation: A study of community health councils.* London, Centre for Studies in Social Policy, 1976.
17. Titmuss, Richard M. *The gift relationship: From human blood to social policy.* London, George Allen and Unwin, 1970.
18. Alt, James E. *The politics of economic decline.* Cambridge, Cambridge University Press, 1979.

Representing Consumer Interests

The Case of American Health Planning

James A. Morone and Theodore R. Marmor

INTRODUCTION

The National Health Planning and Resources Development Act of 1974 authorized a national network of local health planning institutions. The statute, Public Law 93–641, called for more than two hundred planning bodies — health systems agencies (HSAs) — which consumers were to dominate. The law required a consumer majority on each HSA governing board. These consumers were to be "broadly representative of the social, economic, linguistic and racial populations of the area."[1] Consumer majorities, the program's framers assumed, would be powerful forces in shaping local health plans and thus in directing American medicine toward the wants, concerns, and interests of consumers.

The institutionalization of consumer participation accompanied an ambitious conception of health planning itself. The new program was to produce "scientific planning with teeth," cut medical care costs, improve access to medical care, and assure its high quality. The HSA plans would select local health priorities and identify proposals that satisfied community goals for medical care. Their way of working was envisaged as follows: hospitals or nursing homes intent on expanding would submit to the HSA detailed proposals taking into account the official HSA plan. The HSA decisions would be serial, one after the other, each expansion measured against the planning vision of the consumer-dominated agency. In theory, each proposal would either advance the pursuit of community health aims or be rejected.

In practice, however, the HSAs' regulatory authority is severely restricted, almost wholly negative in character, and almost certainly insufficient to reshape the local politics of medicine. The HSAs do review institutional proposals for capital expenditures over $150,000, but their role is in fact advisory to the state governments which are legally empowered to issue required certificates of need. The HSAs are also supposed to review the appropriateness of all medical facilities in their area, but they have neither the positive authority to make improvements nor clear sanctions by which to constrain present operations. Overall, HSAs exhibit a curious structure: decentralized planning bodies with consumer majorities, a highly rationalistic planning mission, and limited regulatory authority to deal with the pluralistic financing and delivery features of the American medical arrangements they are to reshape.

This is not a conception of governance likely to generate confidence among the skeptical. But it is precisely what one would have expected in the context of American health politics of the mid-1970s. At that time, there was widespread alarm about rising health expenditures. Whereas in the 1950s Americans spent 5 percent of GNP on medical care, a quarter of a century later expenditures had risen 50 percent, to some 7.5 percent of GNP by 1975. These increases, heightened in the wake of Medicare and Medicaid legislation in 1965, prompted near-panic in the early 1970s. The Economic Stabilization Program (1971–74) retained controls in medical care longer than other goods and services, but by 1974 and the end of price controls, it was clear another spurt of medical inflation was in progress. Prompted by inflationary fears, the Congress that year debated the broader question of national health insurance but was stalemated by the contending proposals of a Republican administration and a Democratic Congress. Watergate deflected congressional attention from forging new coalitions, so committees with newly expanded responsibilities for health confined their actions to reshaping health *planning* institutions amid intense but narrow political scrutiny.

What emerged as the new health planning program, then, was a compound of stalemate, a commitment to scientific planning, and a faith in democratic participation. That latter faith was central, as the law's words make plain. If consumers dominated and were broadly representative, how could health planning fail to reflect consumer interests? A microcosm of the community would act on the community's behalf. Making sure the HSA board is a microcosm was the rationale for the original insistence that racial, economic, social, geographic, and linguistic categories of constituencies be explicitly represented.

Whatever the intentions of the health planning legislation, the structure of HSAs promised operational problems. What the framers never considered were the implications of the jury model of representation that the microcosm idea expressed. They had no ready answers about how diverse consumer interests in health were to be either articulated or balanced. They presumed that the *representativeness* of HSA governing bodies was the crucial feature of their legitimacy. They failed to link the board's functional task — making choices about health resources—to the representational requirements. Set against the jury notion is what one might call the instrumental view of representation. How well, one asks in this connection, do given institutional practices express the interests of constituencies? What means do constituents have to hold their representatives to account? How well do representative institutions settle the policy problems they were designed to confront? Such questions are precisely what the descriptive model of representation—the model of the jury—neglects. The central HSA dilemma is that it employs a jury model of representativeness to assure the representation of consumer interests. As we will argue, the result is conceptual confusion and practical disappointment.

The next section briefly discusses the terms of the law with regard to consumer representation and the legal cases that have practically illustrated the program's conceptual difficulties. The core of the paper sketches the competing notions of representation—and the associated ideas of participation and accountability. We think of this part as a philosophical map that analysts of consumer involvement in public policymaking should want to consider. In the particular case of health planning, we go on to discuss the kind of unbalanced political arena that promoters of policy change confront. Thus, when we turn at the close to prescriptions for improving the representation of consumer interests, it is in the light of practical constraints as well as philosophical considerations. The epilogue suggests what problems would remain with health planning even if the difficulties of its provisions for consumer representation were adequately worked out.

CONCEPTUAL MUDDLES, CONSUMER REPRESENTATION, AND HSAS

The health planning law was plain enough about consumer majorities on HSAs. Indeed, the statute required no less than 51 and no more than 60 percent of every board to be broadly representative of consumers. But the law and its regulations were silent on the details of implementing this microcosmic conception of representation. How representatives were to be chosen, for instance, was ignored. Which demographic groups should dominate under the broad headings of social, linguistic, and economic representation was not addressed. The clearest representational requirement was that metropolitan and nonmetropolitan representatives precisely mirror their proportions in the population at large.

What was explicitly addressed was the openness in which HSAs should conduct their business. Thus, there was a substitution of participatory conditions for clarity about consumer representation. Agencies, for example, were required to hold public meetings, with agendas widely available beforehand and the minutes available afterward. There were to be opportunities for public comment on almost every phase of HSA activity. All of these provisions—central to the acceptability of a legitimate substitute for representative government—failed to make the crucial connections between consumer interests and consumer representation.

Disputes over consumer roles in health planning reached the courts almost immediately and there exposed the conceptual difficulties of health planning's model of representation. Several suits claimed inadequate means for selecting consumer representatives. But a New York court ruled, in *Aldamuy v. Pirro*, that there were no criteria by which it could choose between two competing minority representatives even if one had been selected by election.[2] As long as the requisite *number* of a particular minority were board members, the law's representation requirements were satisfied. A district court in Texas determined that requisite number by referring to the census tract.[3]

In *Rakestraw v. Califano* and other cases, various social groups sued, demanding seats on the local board; the law and its regulations incorporated no principles for differentiating those with valid objections from those with merely frivolous ones.[4] Across the nation, HSAs scrambled to find poor, even uneducated consumers in a legally mandated but conceptually misguided effort to mirror the demographic characteristics of their area. And after selection, the problems of effective consumer representation continued to bedevil the HSA boards. The technical details of health planning bewildered inexperienced board members. Many had no idea whom they spoke for and, in places, were unwilling to attend meetings. There were reports, particularly in the South, of HSA meetings attended only by provider representatives.[5]

REPRESENTATION'S CONCEPTUAL PUZZLES

Establishing representative institutions requires fundamental choices. Decisions must be made about the selection of representatives, what those representatives should be like, and the expectations that should govern their behavior. Whom to represent—the constituencies—is a central puzzle where geographic representation is abandoned. In addition, the organizational structures within which representatives operate must be specified. Do these structures enhance or impede effective representation? Is the tendency toward political imbalance redressed?

The character of consumer involvement in HSAs is contingent on the answers to these general questions. Indeed, many of the difficulties that plague the health planning act follow from a failure to consider most of them.

We consider these questions in this section through discussion of three topics: the distinction between participation and representation, several conceptions of representation, and their implications for democratic accountability.

PARTICIPATION

Self-government can mean direct citizen participation in public decisions. But the conditions which make such participation feasible are largely absent in modern industrial societies. As a consequence, political representation often replaces direct participation as an operational expression of the principle that "every man has the right to have a say in what happens to him."[6] The rhetoric of the 1974 planning law emphasized consumer representation. The law itself, by contrast, concentrated on guidelines for direct public participation. Direct participation provisions tend to reinforce the political dominance of medical providers over consumers. Hospital administrators, state medical association officials, and other employed medical personnel are far more likely to pay the costs of participating in HSA meetings. The general public is not likely to do so.

Furthermore, the difficulties of fostering direct consumer participation are aggravated by the nature of most health issues. Health concerns, through important, are intermittent for most people.[7] They are not as clearly or regularly salient as the condition of housing or children's schools—situations that citizens confront daily. Consequently, it is far more difficult to establish public participation in HSAs than in renters' associations or school districts.[8]

The point is not that participation is objectionable in health planning. Rather, we argue that, without being tied to accountability and the representation of consumer health interests, the provisions for participation are at best marginally useful to consumers. They are more likely to be utilized by aroused provider institutions.

DESCRIPTIVE REPRESENTATION

Descriptive representation—the type of representation required in PL 93–641—emphasizes the characteristics of representatives. Where constituencies cannot be present themselves for public choice, the descriptive model calls for a representative "body which [is] an exact portrait, in miniature, of the people at large." The argument is straightforward. Since all the people cannot be present to make decisions, representative bodies ought to be miniature versions—microcosms of the public they represent.

The similarity of composition is expected to result in similarity of outcomes; the assembly will "think, feel, reason and [therefore] act" as the public would have.[9] A number of difficulties make this formulation problematic. First, "the public" is a broad category. What aspect of it ought to be reflected in a representative body? John Stuart Mill argued that opinions should be represented; Bentham and James Mill emphasized subjective interests; Sterne, a more ambiguous "opinions, aspirations and wishes"; Burke, broad fixed interest. Swabey suggested that citizens were equivalent units, that if all had roughly equal political opportunities, representatives would be a proper random selection and, consequently, descriptively representative. Whichever may be the case, a failure to specify precisely what characteristics are represented renders microcosm theories unworkable.

Even when the relevant criteria for selecting representatives are properly specified, mirroring an entire nation is impossible. Mill's "every shade of opinion," for example, cannot be reconstructed in the assembly hall on one issue, much less on every issue. One cannot construct a microcosm of a million consumers no matter which sixteen, seventeen, or eighteen consumers represent them on the HSA governing board. Competing opinions or interest can, of course, be represented. But the chief aim of microcosmic representation is mirroring the full spectrum of constituencies. Pitkin notes that the language in which these theories are presented indicates the difficulty of actually implementing them. The theorists constantly resort to metaphor: the assembly as map, minor, portrait. They are all difficult to express in more practical terms.

Mirroring the community may be as undesirable a criterion for selecting decision makers as it is an infeasible one. The merriment that followed Senator Hruska's proposal that the mediocre deserved representation on the U.S. Supreme Court suggests a common understanding of the limits of simplistic views of descriptive representation.[10]

In addition, if representatives are asked merely to reflect the populace, they have no standards regarding their actions as representatives. Descriptive representation prescribes who representatives should be, not what they should do.[11] Opinion polls measure public views more accurately than does descriptive representation.

Though exacting microcosm theories are not realistic, descriptive standards are relevant to the operation of modern legislatures. Legislators are commonly criticized for not mirroring their constituents' views or interests. In fact, John Adams's formulation might be recast as one guideline to selecting representatives—the public votes, essentially, for candidates who appear to "think, feel, reason and act" as its members do. But this broad conception of descriptive representation is sharply different from the utopian endeavor of forming a microcosm of the population in the HSA.

One contemporary version of the microcosm theory is what Greenstone and Peterson term "socially descriptive representation."[12] Rather than mirroring opinions or interests, this conception proposes mirroring of the social and demographic characteristics of a community's population. This amends Adams's syllogism: if people (a) share demographic characteristics, (b) they will "think, feel [and) reason" like one another, and (c) consequently, act like one another. Shared demographic characteristics, in this view, ensure like policy sentiments.

The problems with mirror theories, enumerated above, are all relevant to this version. Demographically mirroring a populace in an assembly is as unlikely as mirroring its opinions. Obviously, not all social characteristics can or ought to be represented. The problem of discriminating among them is particularly vexing. Common sense rebels against representing left-handers or redheads. What of Lithuanians? Italians? Jews? The uneducated? Mirror views provide few guidelines for selecting which social characteristics merit representation.

Even when the characteristics to be mirrored are specified, as regulations to PL 93–641 eventually did, problems remain. All individual members of a social group will not, in fact, "think, feel [and] reason" alike. And all will not represent their fellows with equal efficacy. Yet, by itself, mirror representation does not distinguish among members of a population group—one low-income representative is, for example, interchangeable with any other. As long as the requisite number of a population group is seated, the society is represented—mirrored—in the appropriate aspect. Such actors are not so much representatives as instances of population groups.

Socially descriptive representation is pernicious because it makes recourse to constituencies unnecessary. Attention to means of selection and accountability is reduced by emphasizing broad representativeness. Skin color or income, for example, mark a representative acceptable or unacceptable, regardless of what the constituency thinks. The result is that any member of the group is as qualified a representative as any other. It is a situation that invites tokenism. If the health planning law's only requirement is that a fixed percentage of a board be drawn from a specific group, there is nothing to recommend a black elected by fellow blacks or selected by the NAACP, or a woman elected by women or selected by NOW, over blacks and women drafted onto a board because they will not "rock the boat." *Aldamuy v. Pirro*, cited earlier, illustrates the application of the theory of mirror representation. The court found no criteria in either the law or the regulations by which to appraise the representativeness of the HSA board except for descriptive characteristics. Since both the representatives of the board and their challengers satisfied the criterion of minority status, there was no way to choose between them. It was not possible to select one as any better or more representative than another.

It has been suggested that socially descriptive representation might be effective if representatives were tied to their constituencies by some mechanism of oversight. That stipulation, however, changes the theory of socially descriptive representation. Selected agents are then representatives not because they share a group's features but because they are acceptable to that group. As it has been interpreted in several of the cited court cases, PL 93–641 includes no such view. It requires only that the composition of the board be a statistical microcosm of the area's racial, social, linguistic, and income distribution. Still, for all its inadequacies, there is a kernel of truth in theories of socially descriptive representation. Obviously, social characteristics are sometimes related to interests, and, as the following section argues, interests are precisely what ought to be represented. Thus, religious affiliations bespeak clear interests in Northern Ireland, race affects interests in America, and poverty relates to interests everywhere.

SUBSTANTIVE REPRESENTATION

The key issue in substantive representation is not what representatives look like but whom they look after, whose interests they pursue. Put simply, substantive representation means acting in the interests of constituencies. Doing so involves both properly apprehending those interests and effectively pursuing them.

The classic problem of ascertaining interests is immediately apparent. Are interests objective facts that intelligent leaders can best discern? Or are they more like subjective preferences that must be conveyed to representatives? The latter require a delegatory view where representatives follow constituent wishes. A more objective view of interests supports a trustee role, representatives acting in the constituency's best interest regardless of constituent desires.

In practice, substantive representation involves neither of these extremes. Representatives are neither unabashed messengers nor unfettered guardians, for interests are not completely objective or merely subjective. Various principles of representation are defensible within these broad limits—substantive representation is a general category rather than a particular principle. What we wish to stress is the change from the descriptive conception to a substantive one structured around the pursuit of consumer interests.

The nature of interests is easily caricatured in health politics. Health policy is often technical and complex. The guardian role is most often assumed not by the consumer representatives but by health professionals, accountable to professional norms rather than consumers' desires. The claim that they know the consumer's best interest is accurate, but only within the confines of the physician's office. For the issues that HSAs confront—such as the distribution of limited resources among competing, needy claimants—trusteeship on the basis of medical knowledge is inappropriate.

In practical politics, representatives regularly consider claims for which the interests of specified constituencies are no guide. Bringing the wants of various groups to the bargaining arenas of politics is insufficient; the consideration of ideal-regarding interests—for which there may be no organized constituency—is no less important in policy areas like the distribution and costs of medical care. Our emphasis on constituency interest—in contrast to socially descriptive representativeness—should not be taken as indifference to the questions for which the representation of different interests is insufficient. The intellectual failings of descriptive representation, in short, are one subject; the proper design of institutions for resolving politically charged issues of medical care is another and one beyond our capacities here. But, for that design, attention to the representation of substantive interests is a crucial requisite.

The effectiveness of representatives is crucial to substantive representation. An eloquent speaker or a skillful political operator can be said to provide better substantive representation than another with an equal understanding of constituent interests but without the same skills. And representatives in influential positions—chairs of congressional committees, officers of HSA boards—may well be more effective than less well placed representatives. The reverse, representatives in positions of little influence, can provide only minimal substantive representation. A largely submerged issue for HSAs pertains to precisely this point. If HSAs are powerless and inconsequential bodies, the furor over representation is misplaced—consumer interests are substantively represented within the HSAs but not in matters of important health policy.

The drafters of the health planning act confused representativeness with substantive representation, mistakenly believing that socially descriptive representation would lead to effective representation of interests. They presumed that a local agency with a jury-like board would adequately represent the interests of consumers and legitimate their regulatory interventions in the medical care market. Although jury-like bodies serve a representative and legitimating function in some governmental contexts—notably determinations of guilt in criminal trials—their capacity for substantive representation of interests in circumstances requiring problem solving and complex conflict resolution is limited.

ACCOUNTABILITY

Jurors have no constituencies to answer to. Substantive representation introduces constituencies and the necessity of means of making their representatives accountable. That link is the crux of accountability.

Put simply, accountability means "having to answer to." One is accountable to agents who control scarce resources one desires. In the classic electoral example, officials are accountable to voters whose votes are desired. Health officials may be accountable to legislatures that control funds, pressure groups that can extend or withdraw support, or even medical care providers who can choose whether or not to cooperate with health planning officials.

The crucial element in each case is that accountability stems from some resource valued by the accountable actor. Accountability is not merely an ideal, like honesty, that public actors ought to strive to achieve. Rather, the disposition of valued, scarce resources is manipulable by the relevant constituency.

We term the means by which actors are held accountable "mechanisms of accountability." These mechanisms can vary enormously in character and in the extent of control they impose. Voters occasionally exert some control with a yes or no decision, whereas work supervisors regularly monitor their subordinates' work, enforcing compliance with specific demands.

There is often, to be sure, a give-and-take process in which actors try to maximize their freedom of action and minimize accountability. And those indifferent to the scarce resources in question, such as officials with no desire to be reelected, are not, strictly speaking, accountable. But this illustrates the central point in speaking of accountability. One must be able to point to specific scarce resources, particular mechanisms holding representatives to account.

Many of the HSA requirements expected to enhance accountability to the public are, in fact, necessary but not sufficient conditions for constraining HSA representatives. The emphasis on public participation and openness both legitimates HSAs and eases the task of reviewing HSA performance, as the following HSA requirements illustrate: a public record of court proceedings;[13] open meetings, with notice of meetings published in two newspapers and an address given where a proposed agenda may be obtained;[14] and an opportunity to comment, either in writing or in public meeting, about designation,[15] or health system plans,[16] or annual implementation plans.[17]

Yet these requirements facilitate public accounting, not direct accountability. Since requirements for public participation and disclosure incorporate no formal mechanisms forcing boards to answer to consumers, there is little direct public accountability. Well-defined mechanisms of accountability are central to a strong conception of accountability. Propositions which substitute relationships described as "winning over" or "working with" the community for an identifiable mechanism are much weaker, conflating one common language usage of accounting for action with a stronger view of accountability to a constituency.[18]

Suggesting that HSAs would be ineffective without public support reflects an equally weak conception of accountability to consumers. The "say" of the citizenry is not expressed by "inhospitality" or "lack of trust" or "written protests" but by an authoritative decision institutionalized as a mechanism of accountability.

Accountability can be to more than one constituency. As health planning is now structured, the Department of Health and Human Services (HHS), state government, local government, consumers, providers, and numerous other groups can all attempt to hold the HSA accountable. These competing claims introduce significant tensions. One especially problematic tension lies between accountability to local communities and to national government. Since the rules of HSA operations are decided locally, the potential for local accountability is present. Yet insofar as the law takes up the issue explicitly, it presses accountability to HRS.[19]

The department is responsible for reviewing the plans, structure, and operation of every agency at least once every twelve months.[20] Renewal of designation is annually at stake. This is accountability in every important sense. But it can be traced to the public only by the long theoretical strand leading through the presidency. From this perspective, HSA boards are no more accountable to the public than any other federal executive agency, certainly a far cry from the rhetoric that accompanied PL 93–641's enactment. As the law now stands, public accountability (either directly to constituents or indirectly through states and localities) is not prohibited or rendered impossible. But neither is accountability to the public institutionalized or even significantly facilitated.

The success of instituting accountability relates in large measure to the formal means of selecting representatives. But PL 93–641 and its regulations say little about selection. In the *Rakestraw* case, HHS was sued not only regarding the composition but also the selection of HSA boards. The plaintiffs demanded not the mere specification of formal selection procedures but a means that guaranteed accountability to the public. They were even willing to waive socially descriptive representation in favor of accountability through explicit selection provisions.

WHO IS TO BE REPRESENTED: A PRESCRIPTION?

Only one representational category is precisely delineated in the planning act—the public in nonmetropolitan areas must be represented on the board in proportion to their population. Otherwise, the National Health Planning and Resources Development Act cuts representation loose from geography; representatives stand for social groups rather than precincts, and difficult choices are avoided by entitling all groups to representation. However, the liberalism which provides the theoretical foundation of the act incorporates a vision of shifting, crosscutting interests that makes it impossible to name functional categories that enfranchise everyone equally. No matter what the representational categories, some groups will gain, others lose.

Considerable HSA litigation followed from insufficiently specified representational categories. It can be halted by changing the sweeping grant of representation that flows from the microcosm view to an enumeration of the interests to be represented. Rather than boards that are broadly representative of the population, we would suggest boards that represent specified interests in that population. The specification of interests that we urge must be made on the national level, either in amendments to the act or—as is more likely—in its implementing regulations. Decisions at the national level are crucial since Congress sought to bypass the local political process in the establishment of HSAs.[21]

The next obvious question is, which consumer health interests should be represented on the HSA board? There are groups that, while part of the population and therefore potentially included on a board constituted on the microcosm principle, do not have distinctive health care interests. For example, it is not clear that those with little formal education have the distinguishable health needs that characterize the low-income or aged populations.

Interests with claims to be heard vary by health issue. Regarding access, there are different problems for rural and urban populations, or for the chronically, as opposed to the intermittently, ill. The infirm could claim representation for each of their diseases whenever the issue of new facilities arises. So could every ethnic group regarding specific genetic diseases that disproportionately or exclusively afflict its members. The list of health interests is theoretically very long. However, Congress (or its delegate) must make these difficult choices and specify the various health interests that merit representation on HSA boards.[22]

Selecting the interests to be represented requires an assessment of the purpose of consumer involvement. Presumably, it is to facilitate the articulation and satisfaction of health needs now underrepresented in American communities. As an illustration of interest selection furthering this purpose, we suggest certain representational categories for the HSAs. Although there is no inherent symmetry or formal relationship between any two categories, there is a plausible, a priori justification for representation of the following interests:

a. Payers. The most pressing issue in health politics is rising costs. The interests with the clearest stake in controlling them are the aggregated health care payers—unions, large employers, insurance companies. In traditional markets, consumers are payers, but the dominance of direct or third-party health payers has necessitated the distinction between payer and patient. Excluding the former is likely to result in biased boards, for payers have a clearly articulated financial interest that conflicts directly with that of most health care providers.

b. The poor. Reducing health services to control expenditures threatens groups that now receive insufficient care, most obviously the poor. Their interests—more and better care—conflict with those of the payers. Providing board positions for advocates of the poor may activate group interests that are difficult to organize and thus often overlooked.

c. Racial minorities. Many racial minorities have the same difficulty receiving adequate medical care as the poor because of poverty or discrimination or both.

d. The elderly. The old rely on health services more than any other age group. Despite a clear interest in medical care, their concerns about access, quality, and cost are easily overlooked in local politics.

e. Women. Women require a different mix of health care services from men. They too have clear health care interests that are not represented because of their near-exclusion from local political processes.

f. Catchment areas. Most health planning issues are, at bottom, issues of geography—where to introduce a new service or shut down an old hospital. With the exception of the criteria for metropolitan and rural representation the planning act attempts to replace a real with functional representation. But the two are not incompatible. Indeed, the empirical evidence suggests that geographic categories are emerging on many boards as counties, towns, and neighborhoods win representatives. To carry the process further, each HSA area could be broken into large catchment areas corresponding to the distribution of hospitals and health services. Representatives could be drawn from the various areas in approximate proportion to the population.

g. Special interests. There should also be a miscellaneous category for interests that form a significant segment of the HSA's population—for example migrant workers, black-lung victims, or other persons exposed to special occupational hazards. These interests would be specified by the secretary of HHS, either on the recommendation of the state or by appeal of the special interest. However, it is crucial that this be recognized as a residual category, filled by discretion of the secretary, not as a sweeping grant of representation to interests that count themselves a significant segment of some population.

Numerous objections can be raised to this specification of health interests that deserve representation on HSA boards.[23] People representing these interests may not value health in the same way as those having the same objective characteristics—whether they be related to sex, income, or minority status. They may also be members of a wide variety of groups, each with partially conflicting interests. This leads to two distinct problems: first, the temptation to multiply the number of interest groups represented until the board becomes unmanageable; and second, the tendency for representatives to neglect to speak for those interests which might be shared.

Admittedly, the notion of consumer interests in health is crude. And while we can state that some provider interests work against the interests of all consumers, we cannot unambiguously specify consumer interests because of their diversity. But this diversity of consumer interests is itself the strongest argument for interest-based representation as a necessary, if not sufficient, condition for substantive representation of consumers. Without the quasi-corporatist amalgamations that interest representation can engender, consumer interests will simply not be pursued.

Naming specific representational categories will resolve some political and legal confusion. However, it suggests a deeper dilemma. As the categories we propose illustrate, the public is not neatly divisible into broad, roughly equivalent functional categories. How can the HSA claim legitimacy to act as a public body when it does not equally enfranchise the entire population?

Following Charles Anderson, we suggest two criteria for assessing the legitimacy of such quasi-corporatist boards in a liberal setting.[24] First, the criteria for representation must be embedded in the board's function. Who is seated depends on what the body is expected to accomplish. Policy goals guide the selection of representational categories and constituencies. Interests are granted representation because it is reasonable to include them given the nature and goals of the program. Within this rubric, particular attention might be paid to interests that past politics have subordinated despite the importance of health programs to them.

More important, however, legitimacy does not flow from elaborate representational schemes. The HSAs are administrative agencies established by Congress. Their legitimacy to act as public bodies lies in that legislative mandate. Functional representation schemes may stave off provider dominance, promote sensitivity to previously overlooked interests, or engender some accountability to local groups; but such achievements make HSAs no more or less legitimate than other congressional initiatives. Ultimately, geographic majoritarianism is supplemented, not supplanted.

Of course, designation of interests deserving representation is only one part of the resolution of representational difficulties in HSAs. Another part relates to the mechanisms that will guarantee substantive and accountable representation. The treatment of such policies follows our discussion of political imbalance and health issues.

IMBALANCED POLITICAL ARENAS

The puzzles of representation are exacerbated in circumstances that stimulate representation without explicitly structuring it—where there are no elections, no clearly defined channels of influence, or only vague conceptions of constituency. The politics of regulatory agencies or regional authorities provides examples of these circumstances. Though representatives of groups commonly press their interests within such contexts, there are no systematic canvasses of relevant interests such as are provided by geographically based elections. It is unclear who legitimately merits representation or how representation should be organized and operated.[25]

Interest-group theorists address the problems of representation in precisely such political settings. In their view, unrepresented interests that are harmed coalesce and seek redress through the political system. Despite the absence of electoral mechanisms of representation, the theorists' conception of representation is central to their view of legitimate governance; every interest that is strongly felt can organize a group to speak for it. And, at their most sanguine, group theorists suggest that "all legitimate groups can make themselves heard at some crucial stage in the decision-making process."[26] Politics itself, in this view, is characterized by legions of groups bargaining at every level of government about policies that affect them. Government is viewed as the bargaining broker, policy choices as the consequences of mutual adjustment among the bargaining groups.

The group model is now partially in eclipse among political scientists.[27] One criticism is relevant here: groups that organize themselves for political action form a highly biased sample of affected interests.[28] Furthermore, that bias is predictable and recurs on almost every level of the political process. We refer to it as a tendency toward imbalanced political arenas, the unequal representation of equally legitimate but differently affected interests.

Imbalance is present in part because organizing for political action is difficult and costly. Even if considerable benefits are at stake, potential beneficiaries may choose not to pursue them. If collective goods are involved (i.e., if they are shared among members of a group regardless of the costs any one member paid to attain them), potential beneficiaries often let other members of the collectivity pay the costs and simply enjoy the benefits—the classic free-rider problem.

Free riders aside, the probability of political action generally varies with the material incentives. If either the benefits or costs of political action are concentrated, political action is more likely. A tax or a tariff on tea, for example, clearly and significantly affects the tea industry. To tea consumers, the tax is of marginal importance, a few dollars a year perhaps. The tea producers, with their livelihood at stake, are more likely to organize for political action, though even they are most likely to act if expected benefits outweigh costs. "The clearer the material incentives of the organization's members, the more prompt, focused and vigorous the action."[29]

The most common stimulant to group organization is threat to occupational status, as observers of American politics from de Tocqueville to David Truman have argued. If the group model overstated the facility and extent of group organization, some of its proponents isolated the most significant factor: narrow, concentrated producer interests are more likely to pay the costs of political action than broad, diffuse consumer interests.

Not only do concentrated interests have a larger incentive to engage in political action; they also act with two notable advantages. First, they typically have ongoing organizations with staff and other resources available. This dramatically lowers the marginal cost of political action. Second, most organizations have an expertise that rivals or exceeds that of any other political interest, even government agencies. Their superior grasp, and sometimes monopoly, of relevant information translates into political influence. The more technical an area, the more powerful the advantage, but it is almost always present to some extent.

In sum, two phenomena work to unbalance political arenas: unequal interests and disproportionate resources. The two are interrelated—groups with more at stake will invest more to secure an outcome. However, the distinction warrants emphasis, for it has important policy implications. Attempts to stimulate countervailing powers by making resources available to subordinate groups will fail if they do not account for differing incentives in their employment. For example, even a resource such as equal access to policymakers (now the goal of considerable political effort) is meaningless if the incentives to utilize it over time are grossly unequal. The reverse case—equal interests, unequal resources—is too obvious to require comment. But that clarity should not obscure the fact that the dilemma of imbalance is deeper than the obvious inequality of group resources suggests.

Naturally, diffuse consumer interests are not always somnolent. There are purposive as well as material incentives to political action. A revolt against a sales tax might necessitate cuts in programs that benefit specific groups— diffuse payers defeating concentrated beneficiaries. Tea drinkers may be swept into political action, even to the point of dumping tea into Boston Harbor. Both are examples of diffuse interests uniting for political action. Such coalitions tend to have a grass-roots style of organization. Since sustained, long-term political action requires careful organization, they tend to be temporary. With the end of political deliberation, the group disbands or sets out in search of new issues. Concentrated interests, however, carry on, motivated by the same material incentives that first prompted political action.

The advantages of organized groups increase after a policy's inception. Such groups can be expected to pursue the policy through the stages of implementation and administration. Administrative politics are far less visible than legislative ones. They are not bounded by discrete decisions, and they are cluttered with technical detail rather than the emotive symbols likely to arouse diffuse constituencies. The policy focus of program administration is dispersed— temporally, conceptually, even geographically. Concentrated groups are much more likely to sustain a commitment to participate.

Administrative processes may even grow biased to the point that other affected parties are shut out from deliberations that concern them. Important decisions are made in agencies and bureaus that define, qualify, or even subvert original legislative intent. For example, Congress included a consumer participation provision in the Hill-Burton Act, but the implementing agency never wrote the regulations for it. When consumers overcame the imbalance of interests and sued for participation, they were denied standing. Since the regulations had never been written, consumer representatives had no entry into the policymaking process.[30]

The major question for HSAs is how to overcome these tendencies and balance the politics of health or even promote consumer control. The law's emphasis on participation, its naive conception of representation, and the political economy of health all point to a continuation of imbalanced health planning arenas. The HSAs were created to exert control over health providers, yet the major issue concerning their governing boards is how to avoid provider domination.

REPRESENTING CONSUMER INTERESTS:
OVERCOMING THE POLITICAL OBSTACLES

The task is overcoming political imbalance rather than just getting consumers on health planning boards. This section suggests how more effective representation of and accountability to local health interests might be established.

The HSA staffs could help consumers achieve political parity. Staffs have considerable expertise in issues of medical care and health. Occupying full-time positions in health planning, they have a concentrated interest in the industry. If they ally with providers or fail to take consumers seriously, they will surely undermine consumer representatives who cannot match the combined expertise of providers and staff. The support of the staff is essential to an active consumer role on HSA boards. The problem is systematically harnessing the market-balancing potential of the staff to consumer interests.

The most direct approach is to restructure the HSAs so that part of the professional staff is placed under consumer control—to be selected and accountable to the consumers. The tasks of these staff members could be specified in any number of ways, but the critical function would be providing professional (i.e., expert, full-time) support to the consumer effort.

Another potential for balancing the health planning market lies in organizations that already exist within the consumer population.[31] The very existence of these groups attests to a commitment to enhance the life circumstances of some part of the population. Furthermore, they have already paid the costs of organizing. We can expect them to devote attention to issues in a relatively sustained manner; and they can often overcome low expertise by redeploying their staffs. Representatives from these groups will have clearly defined constituencies, experience in organizational politics, and resources at their disposal. These attributes will help them both in identifying group interests and in pursuing them, regardless of their other characteristics. Even minorities suing for representation in Texas, for example, were willing to accept whites representing blacks if the NAACP selected them. It is telling that much of the litigation challenging HSA boards comes from organizations formed to further the rights or general circumstances of disadvantaged groups within the consumer population.

The empirical evidence that exists supports our contention. The poverty boards of the 1960s (particularly the War on Poverty's Community Action Projects) tended to be most capable when their members were selected by organizations. Impressionistic evidence from some HSAs in which organizations have been involved in selection suggests similar experiences.

Ideally, then, the imbalanced political features of health planning will be tempered by two mechanisms—one internal to the HSA (staff assigned to the consumer representatives), the other external (selection of representatives by groups). We expect the former to facilitate organization and expertise among the consumer representatives, the latter to improve substantive representation and heighten their accountability.

Various reform groups have called for election of consumer representatives in a model roughly based on the selection of school boards. The surface plausibility of the proposal should not be permitted to obscure its difficulties. One problem with direct election of representatives to HSA boards stems from the failure of most Americans to consider themselves part of an ongoing health care community. They typically seek care sporadically and do not conceive of health care in terms of local systems. Both factors distinguish health planning from education or housing issues, where specific elections may be more effective.

Evidence from other programs supports the view that elections are problematic; less than 3 percent of the eligible population voted for local poverty boards in Philadelphia, less than 1 percent in Los Angeles. Those who did vote were moved to do so by personal, not policy, considerations. Overwhelmingly, they voted for neighbors and personal acquaintances. The policy formulated by these representatives was, predictably, particularistic. It helped their friends, not the community or the interests they ostensibly represented. Representatives generated little community interest or support. They tended to be ineffective advocates.

The evidence from HSAs that have held elections is strikingly similar—low turnout at the polls and high turnover among representatives. Representatives are uncertain of their task and their constituency. Furthermore, direct elections have facilitated the takeover of entire boards by single organizations. In northeastern Illinois, for example, abortion foes captured the HSA, linking every health concern to their own preoccupation; in Illinois, Arkansas, and Massachusetts, provider institutions chartered buses and flooded the polling places with hospital workers who voted for docile consumer representatives.[32]

Elections are appealing to reformers because they permit the public to choose health planning representatives directly; theoretically, the representatives can be held accountable with relative ease. In practice, the predictable electoral apathy of diffuse interests undermines direct elections as the mechanism of accountability to consumer constituencies.

HEALTH POLICY AND THE HSAS

The National Health Planning and Resources Development Act's vision of representation is impossibly flawed, but not irretrievably so. We have suggested one plan for achieving reasonably effective consumer representation and balancing provider dominance. But representing consumers, overcoming imbalance, even discerning the public interest in HSAs will not alter the American health system in any profound fashion. The HSA mandate—limiting costs, expanding access, and improving the quality of health—reaches far beyond the agencies' capabilities. Measured by these standards, the act's program is trivial—more symbol and rhetoric than significant potential.

Because the HSAs' planning functions are largely isolated from the process of health resource allocation, planning becomes too often a smoke screen, an empty symbol, or simply wheel spinning. The agencies' difficulties of limited authority are compounded by the uncertain relationship between HSAs and the rest of government. In their reliance on "scientific planning," HSAs are yet another manifestation of the effort to find objective solutions to political choices. But scientific planning cannot relieve the tensions between national demands and local desires or between representing community interests and programmatic efficiency.[33]

Despite these problems, the health planning law does have significance, and that significance lies in its stimulation of a broad range of consumer interests. Viewed as an effort to organize communities into caring about their own health systems, it is the largest program of its kind. And one that could influence health politics long after its particular institutional manifestation—HSA planning boards—has been forgotten.

Notes

This article is taken from *Ethics* 91(1981):431–450.Other versions have been published as "Representing Consumer Interests: Imbalanced Markets, Health Planning, and the HSAs," *Milbank Memorial Fund Quarterly/Health and Society* 58, no. 1 (1980):125–165, and in T. R. Marmor and J. B. Christianson, eds., *Health Care Policy: A Political Economy Approach* (Beverly Hills, Calif.: Sage, 1982), Chap. 8.

Our thinking, particularly at the outset, was greatly helped by the writings and comments of Charles Anderson. Our friend Rudolf Klein's *Politics of Consumer Representation*, written with Janet Lewis (London: Centre for Social Policy, 1976), which focused on Britain, fast directed our concern to thinking about issues of consumer participation and representation in an American context. We want to thank as well colleagues at the Institution for Social and Policy Studies, Yale University, and the Center for Health Administration Studies, University of Chicago, for their helpful criticism, most particularly Charles E. Lindblom and Brian Barry. The written comments of Adina Schwartz, Owen Fiss, Peter Steinfels, Arthur Caplan, Albert Weale, and Eugene Bardach were particularly useful to us in revising this essay.

1. PL 93–641 § 1512(b)(3)(c)(iii)(2).

2. *Aldamuy et al. v. Pirro et al.*, C.A. No. 76 CV-204 (N.D.N.Y., April 7, 1977).
3. *Texas Association of Community Organizations for Reform Now (ACORN) et al. v. Texas Area V Health Systems Agency et al.*, C.A. No. S-76–102-CA (ED. Texas, Sherman Div., March 1, 1977).
4. *Rakestraw et al. v. Califano et al.*, C.A. No. C77–635A (N.D.Ga., Atlanta Div., filed April 22, 1977); *The Louisiana Association of Community Organizations for Reform Now (ACORN) et al. v. New Orleans Area/Bayou Rivers Health Systems Agency et al.*, C.A. No. 17–361 (ED. La., filed March 15, 1977); *Amos et al. v. Central California Health Systems Agency et al.*, C.A. No. 76–174 (E.D. Calif., filed Sept. 10, 1976).
5. See Wayne Clark, "Placebo or Cure? State and Local Health Planning Agencies in the South," photocopied (Atlanta: Southern Governmental Monitoring Project, Southern Regional Council, 1977), for examples of such reports.
6. H. F. Pitkin, *The Concept of Representation* (Berkeley and Los Angeles: University of California Press, 1967), p. 3.
7. This is not so for certain groups — e.g., the parents of children with special diseases — as our colleague Owen Fiss points out.
8. T. R. Marmor, "Consumer Representation: Beneath the Consensus, Many Difficulties," *Trustee* 30 (1977): 37–40.
9. John Adams, cited in Pitkin, *Concept of Representation*, p. 60.
10. For notable formulations of this common idea, see Edmund Burke, "The English Constitutional System," in *Representation*, ed. H. F. Pitkin (New York: Atherton Press, 1969); or Alexander Hamilton et al., *Federalist Papers*, no. 10, by James Madison (New York: Modern Library, Inc., 1937).
11. Judged by the model of a jury, such standards are unnecessary; representativeness is the condition for legitimacy. We want to thank Owen Fiss for stressing this competing model of representation.
12. J. D. Greenstone and P. E. Peterson, *Race and Authority in Urban Politics: Consumer Participation and the War on Poverty* (Chicago: University of Chicago Press, 1973), chap. 6. We have profited immensely from this analysis.
13. 41 Federal Register 12812 (March 26, 1976), § 122.114.
14. Ibid., §§ 122.104(b)(I)(viii) and 122.109(e)(3).
15. Ibid., §§ 122.104(a)(8) and 122.104(b)(7).
16. Ibid., § 122.107(c)(2).
17. Ibid., § 122.107(c)(3).
18. We are grateful to our colleague Douglas Yates for pointing out this distinction.
19. There are indications that precisely this tension is asserting itself as HHS, e.g., drafts guidelines and local communities protest that they do not apply in their specific situations.
20. PL 93–641 § 1515(c)(1).
21. Allowing local politics to define constituencies is fraught with trouble. Note the cycle: Congress, claiming that many interests were shut out of local politics, established entirely new governmental structures for health planning and mandated that they be "broadly representative." That requirement is itself so broad that it is unclear what interests qualify: the decision is left to the local political process which Congress sought to bypass in the first place. The vagaries of congressional consistency aside, local selection of the interests to be represented will not break the cycle of litigation. Interests that are shunned will sue, arguing that the local process which excluded them does not conform to the federal mandate to broadly represent.
22. As Owen Fiss has pointed out to us, the impossibility of mirroring a community's demography is equally true for specifying its health interests. But treating the selection of interests as a political choice need not reach the impossibility test of mirroring all interests.
23. We have profited particularly from Albert Weale's incisive comments on the topic of interests.

24. Charles Anderson, "Political Design and the Representation of Interests," *Comparative Political Studies* 10(1977):127–52.

25. The problem is less nettlesome in legislatures. On a practical level, lobbying legislatures appears only marginally effective: analysts have generally found that politicians are most likely to follow their own opinions or apparent constituency desires. More important, there is at least a formal representation of every voting citizen. Of course, this does not minimize the complexities of electoral representation. But elective systems do afford a systematic canvas of community sentiment, however vague a guide it may be to policy formulation.

26. Robert Dahl, *A Preface to Democratic Theory* (Chicago: University of Chicago Press, 1964), p. 137.

27. See Andrew McFarland, "Recent Social Movements and Theories of Power in America," microfilmed (paper delivered at the American Political Science Association Convention, Washington, D.C., August 1979).

28. Recall the epigram, "The flaw in the pluralist heaven is that the heavenly chorus sings with a strong upper class accent." E. E. Schattschneider, *The Semisovereign People* (Hinsdale: Ill.: Dryden Press, 1960), p. 34.

29. James Q. Wilson, *Political Organizations* (New York: Basic Books, 1973), p. 318.

30. Rand Rosenblatt, "Health Care Reform and Administrative Law, a Structural Approach," *Yale Law Journal* (1978):243–336.

31. P. C. Schmitter, "An Inventory of Analytical Pluralist Propositions" (monograph, University of Chicago, Department of Political Science, Autumn 1975).

32. See Mark Kleiman, "What's in It for Us: A Consumer Analysis of the 1979 Health Planning Amendments," *Health Law Project Library Bulletin* 4(1979):329–36; and Barry Checkoway, "Citizens on Local Health Planning Boards: What Are the Obstacles?" *Journal of the Community Development Society* 10(1979):101–16.

33. For a fuller discussion of these issues, see the version of this paper published in *Health and Society* 58(1980):125–65.

11

THE POLITICS OF PANICS

Fear and panics go together. Panics are about fearful threats accompanied by uncertainty about the causes, scale, and consequences of the threat. The political response to health panics is the subject matter of this chapter.

We begin the chapter with articles addressing HIV/AIDS as illustrations, but in two different, but related contexts. The broad, comparative article on the disease, written in the late 1980s, discusses the responses of governments in the United Kingdom, the United States, and Sweden. The narrower article on contaminated blood—one carrier of the virus—takes on a wider set of eight national responses and was written long after the hemophiliac community was devastated by the disease. In these articles, we see combinations of common and divergent responses.

The centrality of uncertainty in cases of panics is one source of political commonality. Panics are about threats that in one way or another are not well understood. This is as true about hurricanes as mad cow disease, bird flu, or floods, though the sources of uncertainty differ. With natural disasters, the greatest uncertainty is about the scale and location of damage. With public health threats, it is more about causation and the distribution of the threat. In all panics, there are concerns about how the victims will be treated and whether traditional constraints on the use of coercion will be set aside in the name of reducing the uncertainty of the scale of the threat.

As the articles make clear, health panics call forth standard operating procedures from organizations. In our illustrations, the response of governments was slow and cautious as long as scientists were uncertain about the causes and character of the disease. Moreover, governments relied on public health professionals to take the lead in both characterizing the problems and advocating remedial approaches. The interplay of scientific and governmental elites across borders was also a feature in these cases and marks panics generally, whether health-related or not. Cross-border transfers of expertise and experience were at work in these cases, aided of course by the speed of transport and communication in the modern era.

The illustrations we provide include some other commonalities. Though health panics prompt interest in compulsion, the response to AIDS among industrial democracies generally protected citizens from unwanted intrusions. Educational campaigns, professionally led guidance, and pressures from groups especially victimized dominated the scene. Finally, a common paradox emerged in all these instances: namely, that the governmental actors most concerned who had to dramatize the threat to prompt remedial action faced the prospect that treating the disease as an ordinary public health matter meant losing fear as a source of public cooperation with the campaign.

Once these common elements are noted, however, one can see sources of differentiation that illuminate as well. Institutional differences among the countries investigated emerged as important, especially in the allocation of blame. In the case of contaminated blood, the differences were stark. Some government leaders went to jail where blameworthy behavior could be clearly identified. In some cases, the Red Cross was relieved of its role in distributing blood products; in others, courts sorted out wrongs and distributed compensation. In still others, governments became dispensers of compensation for harm without using fault as the operative premise. In short, both institutional arrangements and firmly held beliefs came into play in what otherwise seemed like a common source of panic.

This category of political analysis and policy analysis highlights other features of our approach to the world of health and health care. In the panics described, the victims became insistent and durable players in the policy process. They highlight the growing role of victims and their families as interested parties and represent one thread of what we have loosely called "consumerism" in health policy. The transmission of evidence and influence across borders applies both to patient groups and to the scientific and medical leaders whose standard approaches play such an important role in situations of panic. As noted, the articles suggest in their portraits how configurations of ideas, interests, and institutions account for the panics we investigated. In these particular sources of panic, it might well have turned into moral crusades about the sexual and drug transmission of the virus. That by and large did not take place, which distinguishes our discussion here from what we will address in the next chapter on the politics of health crusades.

The Comparative Politics of Contaminated Blood

From Hesitancy to Scandal

Theodore R. Marmor, Patricia A. Dillon, and Stephen Scher

INTRODUCTION

The story of blood and AIDS is one of genuine tragedy.[1] By the time scientific and regulatory authorities understood the sources of infection from contaminated blood, thousands of blood transfusion recipients and a substantial proportion of hemophiliacs in advanced industrial nations had already been infected with HIV. The period from 1981 to 1985 was one of uneven but profound change: from hesitancy to understanding, and from skepticism to heat treatment of blood products. It was a period of coping with confusion, of conflicting organizational priorities, and of variously channeled demands for what seemed like costly preventive actions. After these actions were taken—by the mid-1980s—the source of controversy shifted, first to restitution and later to retribution. From initial offers of victim compensation to full-scale reviews of official (mis)conduct and professional (mis)judgments, the stories have involved everything from tawdry commercialism to high scandal, from substantial punishment to diffuse regret.[2]

The patterns of the countries studied reveal that the post-1985 responses to the tragedy of HIV-contaminated blood are far more varied than the initial reactions. The central puzzle this chapter addresses is what accounts—in probabilistic terms—for both the similarities in the initial reactions and for the variations that emerge thereafter. The chapter proceeds in three parts. The first sets the stage by sketching the assumptive world regarding blood products and hemophilia that was largely taken for granted at the outset of the 1980s. Our contention is that those widely shared assumptions help to account for much of the hesitancy in responding to signs of contaminated blood in the early 1980s. The second part sets out to portray what in retrospect appears to be the compressed differences in national responses to contaminated blood in the 1982–85 period.[3]

445

The third and most extensive part explores the variation in national responses that began to take shape in the mid-1980s.

The variations from country to country in the post-1985 period fall into three broad categories: high, moderate, and low-intensity scandal politics. Despite its limitations, this categorization helps to understand the particular mix of institutional arrangements, cultural beliefs, and feelings of bitterness and betrayal that account for the variation the national stories reveal. In a larger context, these different national responses provide a lens through which to view the capacity of each country's institutions to assess and respond to risk under conditions of uncertainty. This is a complicated, cross-national story, however, and comparative analysis can play only a partial role in illuminating why and how such a tragedy took place and what followed from it. Nonetheless, the recurrent themes in this story—which lies at the intersection of science and policy—are hardly restricted to the AIDS crisis or to the distribution and use of blood and blood products for medical purposes.

PART I: INSTITUTIONAL LEGACIES AND THE TRAGEDY OF CONTAMINATED BLOOD

In 1981, after the report of the sentinel cases of *Pneumocystis carinii* pneumonia in Los Angeles,[4] and in 1982, after AIDS was reported in a patient with hemophilia,[5] the nature of this new syndrome was unclear. HIV had not been isolated. The latency period and rate of progression to AIDS were unknown. The dominant scientific and regulatory actors, uncertain about the scientific features of this new threat, and lacking clear direction within their own institutions,[6] fell back on their familiar understandings about blood safety and the risks to health in dealing with new blood-related threats. As a result, one cannot understand the unfolding tragedy of infected blood without first taking into account the institutional and belief legacy concerning blood and blood products, the regulation thereof, and responses to hepatitis B in the 1970s.

The entry of HIV into the blood supply in the late 1970s took place at a time of extraordinary technological attainment and rising expectations in the community of hemophiliacs and their specialist physicians. The development of blood products that promised to reduce spontaneous bleeding—the wonder of the drug treatment known as factor VIII—meant that young men with hemophilia, who had faced limited mobility, crippling pain, disability, and early death[7] from intracranial and joint bleeding, could suddenly look forward to normal family life and strenuous sports. Moreover, the life expectancy for hemophiliacs was rising sharply, to sixty years by 1980.[8,9,10] These dramatic improvements required pharmaceutical preparations that were expensive and dependent on a large, reliable supply of blood plasma. Paralleling these developments, blood banks, donor groups, and the Red Cross directed their attention toward ensuring the availability of blood products and to maintaining a blood supply that was adequate and reliable. These factors set the stage for the "iatrogenic tragedy" of blood and AIDS.[11]

Although the reader may already be familiar with the beliefs associated with maintaining an adequate, reliable, and safe blood supply, a brief summary here will prove helpful. While a commercially driven, pharmaceutically based system was central to the production of clotting factors for hemophiliacs, the institutional framework for whole blood was based on voluntarism. Commercial blood was presumed less safe than blood drawn from voluntary sources. Since the stability of the blood supply in a voluntary system depended on willing donors, appeals to altruism and reassurances about safety had become standard procedures. Some risks—like that of hepatitis B—came to be regarded as "acceptable" and manageable for hemophiliacs, most of whom were known to have been already exposed. When balanced against the blessings of the new blood products the threat of hepatitis B seemed remote to both blood professionals and patients. The emphasis was on increasing the supply and availability of "convenience products."

This assumptive world, tragically, would prove disastrous for both hemophiliacs and blood transfusion recipients. Altruism was no safeguard against the HIV infection. Nor would assumptions about "acceptable risks" hold true for the deadly HIV virus. The gap between institutional claims about blood and blood products, on the one hand, and the realities of practice, on the other, would later shape the politics of retribution. The extent to which transfusion recipients and hemophiliacs had depended upon trusted medical and political elites would contribute greatly to the sense of betrayal and the search for the guilty in the aftermath of the tragedy of HIV-contaminated blood.

PART II: THE PATTERN OF HESITANCY, 1982–85

Despite differences in financing and institutional arrangements in the eight nations investigated, broadly similar patterns emerged in their initial, hesitant response to the emergence of AIDS among transfusion recipients and hemophiliacs. First, physicians underestimated the extent to which those exposed to potentially contaminated blood would suffer irreparable injury. Second was the importance everywhere of blood-community elites in setting policy, with the role of other interest groups more varied. Third was delay at critical points because of difficulties in balancing industrial policy and goals against uncertain scientific information. Fourth was the reluctance to screen donors, because such efforts might have undercut public perceptions of a safe blood supply and potentially stigmatized high-risk groups. Last was the marginal political position of the hemophiliac population, a patient group that had not yet developed a political identity, and the absence of political identity among those who shared nothing but the fact that they had been patients in need of blood transfusions.

In country after country, the tragedy of underestimating the risk of the deadly new virus had a profound impact. Just as they had previously accepted the tradeoff between hepatitis infection and the benefits to hemophiliacs of reduced disability, the major institutional actors were reluctant to disrupt the supply of blood and blood products by measures that promised but could not assure a measure of security against AIDS (Although, ironically, those who feared that AIDS might spread like hepatitis were the first to sound the tocsin). Perceptions about risk were also influenced by a common reluctance to take on the cost of screening and, later, heat treatment, and by beliefs about the groups first infected with AIDS. Since it was "the American disease" and a disease of homosexuals, drug users, and Haitians, familiar national policies were thought adequate to protect hemophiliacs. These perceptions of risk, coupled with the patterns discussed above, bred resistance to safety measures that would have protected the blood supply and, consequently, hemophiliacs in the 1982–85 period. The results of this common pattern of hesitancy would turn out to be tragic.

A common pattern does not, of course, mean an identical one. There surely were variations in the timing of heat treatment, of taking untreated blood out of distribution, and of excluding high-risk groups from blood donation.[12] And small differences—even of months—in the introduction of safety measures had deadly consequences. Nonetheless, by 1986, the nations *Blood Feuds* portrayed had broadly similar policies. The differences among nations that would emerge in response to policies were much greater, ranging from scandal to quiet adjustment, from punishing attacks on public officials to what was largely business as usual.

PART III: VARIETIES OF SCANDAL IN THE AFTERMATH OF UNDENIABLE TRAGEDY

In contrast to the hesitancy and relatively narrow range of institutional responses to the appearance of HIV, the aftermath of actual infection exhibited considerable cross-national variation. Each of the countries experienced some elements of a blood scandal, and there were important similarities in their experiences. Most obvious was the emergence of organizations of hemophiliacs and their growing independence from (and anger at) former allies in medicine. There was a common sense of violation of deeply held social beliefs about responsible medical practice. Among other similarities were the limited role played by transfusion recipients and a pattern of initially settling for compensation in the 1980s. In the 1990s, the search for guilty parties became widespread. That search included extensive use of the media, more frequent reliance on the courts, and the demonstration of greater political influence by hemophiliacs than their numbers alone would have predicted. These common elements were nonetheless shaped by organizational and cultural differences, channeled through distinctive legal and political institutions. In the end, the results were very different.

Accounting for the variation among countries does not require a taxonomy of scandal itself. Nonetheless, some conceptual preliminaries are justified. First of all, measuring the intensity of scandal is not the same as measuring wrongdoing. Scandal is by accepted usage a public matter. It is not the world of closed meetings but rather the exposure of wrongdoing at such meetings. Even when wrongdoing becomes known, the intensity of the scandal it prompts need not be proportionate to the wrongdoing. Second, policy scandals typically involve the disclosure not of wrongdoing (or alleged wrongdoing) in general, but wrongdoing of particular kinds: the abuse of institutional power or the violation of some important community norm. Third, exposing scandalous conduct does not, in itself, generate a scandal. Whether a scandal emerges in any particular case depends in large part upon the degree to which those disclosing or investigating the wrongdoing are successful in capturing and maintaining public attention as the investigation and disclosures continue. Fourth, scandals generally, though not necessarily, lead to adverse consequences for the wrongdoers. Typical outcomes include criminal punishment, civil liability, loss of office or position, and damage to one's reputation. Fifth, unless scandals are very quickly contained, they tend to cast a broad net of wrongdoing and wrongdoers. Just how broad depends on how the issues are framed, on the intensity of the scandal, and on how long the public's interest is sustained. These factors will depend, in turn, not just on the social, political, and legal setting in each country, but also upon the precise role that the protagonists—in our case, hemophiliacs—come to define for themselves and how aggressively and effectively they act in pursuit of their goals.

Central to the development of the blood scandals was the transformation of hemophiliacs into a cohesive group with a core identity and political goals.

What is remarkable is that this transformation—a very difficult one, as David Kirp has noted—took place at all.[13] Prior to the advent of hemophilia (AHF) products, hemophiliacs had often suffered in isolation while they coped, as best they could, with their disease. Then, thanks to AHF products, they had come to lead mainstream lives. Though no longer in isolation and no longer suffering, they had little incentive to band together around their disease for political purposes. After exposure to HIV, they were forced into their private worlds again, to face the personal calamities of physical deterioration, financial ruin, the disease or death of family members, and even violence from frightened neighbors. Even so, despite their previously apolitical history and the personal desperation and private nightmares that resulted from being infected with HIV, hemophiliacs banded together, found identity in a group, and mobilized into social movements.

Once organized, the social movements of hemophiliacs generated the conflicts—and ultimately the scandals—we see in each of the countries we have studied. The intensity of each scandal lies on a continuum having three broad categories: high scandal; moderate scandal; and low scandal. Any such grouping of countries will necessarily be imperfect; each country has a distinctive configuration of government, health care arrangements, and political culture. The categories nonetheless are helpful in analyzing how industrial democracies confronted the tragedy of transmitting HIV through blood and blood products.

INSTANCES OF HIGH SCANDAL

Canada, France, and Japan experienced the most prolonged and bitter public debate about wrongdoing in connection with HIV infection through contaminated blood and blood products. They all punished major figures and made substantial changes in their institutional arrangements for the supply and regulation of blood.[14] Their scandals, in short, demonstrated intensity, durability, and stability. The best predictors of such high scandal are a unified group of hemophiliacs with a political identity, a compelling narrative appealing to the larger population, a paternalistic political culture, and a centralized decision-making regime.

POLITICAL ORGANIZATION, HEMOPHILIACS, AND SCANDAL

The Japanese story is a clear example of the role that interest groups played in the shaping of blood scandals. Japanese hemophiliacs, as Eric Feldman explains, had adopted a rights-based strategy by 1987 in response to proposed legislation (the AIDS Prevention Law) targeted at people with AIDS.[15] Moreover, unlike what happened in other countries, Japanese hemophiliacs expanded their coalition to include students and others who were not hemophiliacs.[16] They sued the government and the pharmaceutical industry in 1989, stressing that litigation was not merely a plea for financial relief (which had already been offered in 1985),[17] but a demand for dignity. They sought an apology from a government that had failed to protect them.[18] The persistence of the Japanese hemophiliac community, coupled with further disclosures of both public and corporate wrongdoing, ultimately led to the long-sought apologies. Key figures in the formation of policy during the early 1980s subsequently faced criminal prosecution.[19]

Unlike those in Japan, hemophiliacs in Canada did not organize themselves effectively until the 1990s. Canada, like many other countries, had established in 1989 a compensation scheme without admitting fault. But the details of the program angered many hemophiliacs. Families were compelled to forfeit rights to file separate legal actions, and to accept compensation by a certain date or forfeit it forever. Moreover, payments were limited to four years and excluded surviving spouses. But there was no organized political action that resulted. Even the severe criticism of the Canadian Red Cross, deriving from its role as protector of the voluntary blood supply and from its control (along with the Canadian Blood Commission) of blood collection and fractionation, failed to motivate hemophiliacs to consolidate as a political force. What finally triggered organized national action was the persistence of a small, new provincial group that brought its cause to Ottawa after its lobbying success in Nova Scotia. In that province, advocates forced compensation for the victims of contaminated blood.[20]

In 1990, many provinces jointly decided to provide no additional compensation to supplement what had already been provided in the national compensation program.[21] It was in this particular context—facing a 1993 expiration date for his benefits—that Randy Conners, an infected hemophiliac, and his wife, Janet, formed the group Infected Spouses. They convinced Nova Scotia to break with the other provinces, establish its own compensation scheme, and extend the scheme to spouses.[22] They then took their cause to the Canadian capital, where the House of Commons held hearings that led to the establishment of the Krever Commission on Canada's blood system. That commission's hearings, discussed by Norbert Gillmore and Margaret Somerville, were to draw the nation's attention to the plight of hemophiliacs and their families.[23] The Conners' lobbying tactics were subsequently adopted by other provincial groups, leading some provincial ministers to abandon the 1990 interprovincial pact and establish their own compensation schemes. The confidence of Canadians in their blood system has been indisputably shaken, and the Red Cross compelled to withdraw from blood collection and distribution.[24]

French hemophiliacs had the most limited political organization of those in the three high-scandal countries. In 1989, they, too, had accepted a lump-sum compensation plan offered by the national government. But Peter Garvanoff, the lawyer for the nation's hemophilia society, proved central to mobilizing French opinion. Garvanoff, an infected hemophiliac who had lost two brothers, rejected compensation and persisted with litigation. A journalist following the plight of hemophiliacs proceeded to publish a sensational series of disclosures, which kept the issues before the public, galvanized the hemophiliac community, and made further investigations inevitable.[25] Jean Marie Le Pen's right-wing National Front provided some hemophiliacs with counsel and used the legal cases and ongoing disclosures to excoriate the Socialist Party, which had been in control of the government since the initial outbreak of AIDS in the early 1980s. In addition to contributing to the Socialists' loss at the next election, Monica Steffen notes that the growing sentiment on behalf of hemophiliacs led to the revision of the French Constitution itself, which now limits the immunities available to public officials for acts committed in office.[26]

COMPELLING NARRATIVE

Consistent with the formation of a group identity, groups of hemophiliacs constructed narratives of betrayal, suffering, and stigmatization in every country. Those in the high-scandal group, however, broadened the agenda beyond their own claims for justice concerning a past injury. They engaged the public through champions and were persuasive in arguing that everyone's security was threatened.

In Canada, Randy and Janet Conners emerged as sympathetic symbols. They highlighted the debate about infection of the blood supply while engaging the media and broader community of Canadians. Anxious for the financial security of their son after Randy's impending death, they pressed the case for additional compensation.[27] Later that year the Canadian weekly news magazine *Maclean* recognized their courage and achievements by naming them to its 1993 Honor Roll. Randy Conners's accusation before the Krever Commission was powerful: knowingly distributing unsafe products was "murder." This charge was supported by evidence that the Red Cross had kept a "Schindler's List" of hemophiliacs who were to receive safer, heat-treated products. Such charges led the press, in turn, to describe the Krever Commission hearings as "a damning portrait of the Canadian Red Cross . . . and of government officials."[28] After Randy's widely reported death, Janet Conners became the avenging angel of Canada's blood-supply victims,[29] a vocal and highly visible public presence, commenting on key testimony and arguments presented before the Commission, and conducting interviews on the yearly anniversaries of her husband's death.

An articulate, appealing woman, Janet Conners gave a human face to the tragedy and opened a window into the homes of infected families. Hemophiliacs' surviving spouses—almost always women and often infected with HIV themselves—had no life insurance. They owed medical bills beyond the limits of Canada's universal health insurance, and coped with their own infection and their anxiety about the children who would be orphaned after their deaths. A 1997 interview on Canadian television about the Red Cross effort to limit the Krever inquiry highlighted Janet Conners's ability to go beyond appeals to pity for hemophiliacs and their families, and to address the concerns and values of the broader Canadian community: "This [limit] would set a precedent," Conners claimed. "If anyone in government is unhappy with the findings of any commission, they can just run off to the Supreme Court and have the truth hidden. If Justice Krever is not allowed to write his report, more Canadians will die."[30]

In Japan it was only after years of demonstrations, litigation, and settlement offers that the transmission of HIV through blood products came to be seen as involving broad social and political issues that concerned not just hemophiliacs, but the entire nation. Instead of being viewed as a devastating problem for a small fraction of the populace, the plight of hemophiliacs and their families was reframed in terms of an ongoing civic battle against secrecy, corruption, and betrayal of public trust by elected officials and career bureaucrats. That battle, later known as the "The Kan-Kan War" was instigated not by a hemophiliac, but by a new, ambitious Minister of Health and Welfare, Kan Naoto, who took on the Japanese bureaucracy.[31] In this context, the picture of the President of the blood supply firm Green Cross, down on his knees with his forehead to the floor, was striking. It represented, to be sure, the humiliation of Japan's political and industrial elites.[32] But for hemophiliacs and their families, it also signaled a new era in which their concerns were not isolated and separate from those of the Japanese mainstream.

In France, the compelling narrative with broad public appeal was constructed by neither a hemophiliac nor an ambitious government minister. Instead, the narrator was a tenacious medical reporter, Anne-Marie Casteret, whose story, as in Japan, involved secrecy, betrayal, and money.[33] Among other things, she proved that Dr. Michel Garretta, director of the national transfusion center, had consciously decided to keep his contaminated factor VIII on the market.[34]

She published the minutes and also covered subsequent court proceedings at which the hemophiliac association's lawyer (Peter Garvanoff) called out "Assassins!" during the defendants' testimony. The stark contrast between the legal immunity of public officials and the deterioration and death of hemophiliacs undermined the French public's trust both in their blood-supply system and in their government.[35]

PATERNALISM AND SCANDAL INTENSITY

The media tactics of hemophiliacs in high-scandal countries exploited the shock value of public disclosures, especially in political cultures like those of Japan and France, which are marked by the tight control of information and presumptions of governmental paternalism. This tactic, revealing the seeming wrongdoing of elites who were supposed "to govern," in itself heightened the drama associated with the disclosures. The prospect of disclosure engendered, in turn, efforts to prevent disclosure—efforts that when known, only further heightened the drama associated with the blood scandal.

The hierarchical structure of French and Japanese[36] government is highly visible, and the prevailing view of their governing elites is that they should attend to the public's business without too much interference from ordinary citizens. French and Japanese citizens have no legal right, for example, to see government documents; in France, even documents introduced in court proceedings can be obtained only by consent of the Justice Ministry.[37] It is no surprise, then, that after Casteret published the minutes of the Garretta meeting, the media, especially TV stations, took up the story with abandon. The credibility of France's medical establishment was severely shaken by the accusation that a respected physician and researcher, Dr. Jean-Pierre Allain, had knowingly given contaminated blood products to hemophiliacs.[38] The Japanese medical establishment was shaken in much the same way when the well known physician Dr. Takeshi Abe was accused of accepting money from manufacturers, and of delaying clinical trials of heat-treated products so that Green Cross could catch up with US and European manufacturers.[39] More revelations followed, ones that undermined the credibility of both nations' revered "political class";[40] the opening segment of the nightly news often featured a new disclosure, complete with a visual of a document stamped "Confidential." Most damaging of all were the accusations that government officials in France and Japan had, in order to promote domestic industry, refused to import heat-treated products.

The connections among paternalism, governmental hierarchy, and the intensity of scandal require further elaboration. The major claim is that both French and Japanese bureaucrats have traditionally been expected to do their public jobs with confidence, competence, and little interference. Entrance into the elite ranks of these bureaucracies is reserved for those who have demonstrated high intelligence, gone through established channels of socialization, and successfully competed with other talented contenders. They are expected to take care of the public policy issues in their separate domains and are, in that sense, paternalistic. Moreover, they are expected to do so with high levels of skill and reliability. It is because high-ranking bureaucrats had earned, and been entrusted with, such paternalistic authority that citizens came to feel betrayed by their failure to protect the public. Added to this mix was the rage that came from knowing that the policy of governmental secrecy, which was taken for granted, both protected the bureaucrats from disclosure and prevented citizens from knowing the truth. Put another way, expectations determine evaluations of behavior; in the case of Japan and France, those expectations of protective security were high, and, once disappointed, all the more angering.

The Canadian case does not fit easily into this portrait of the public's disappointed expectations for paternalistic elites. In Canada, citizens have easier access to government information than in France and Japan. Moreover, while governmental officials in Canada have traditionally had higher status than in, for example, the United States, Canadian political culture is not strongly hierarchical and paternalistic. So why did the level of scandal there come to rival that of France and Japan?

As the blood scandal evolved in Canada, the Canadian Red Cross—a nongovernmental organization—received increasingly prominent attention because of its central, paternalistic involvement in the world of Canadian blood donation, distribution, and regulation. The Red Cross was also presumed by most Canadians to be utterly reliable. In these respects, there is a limited parallel between the Red Cross in Canada and the governmental elites of France and Japan. An additional factor is that the Red Cross, as a private, nonprofit organization, enjoyed more protection for its internal documents than did Canadian governmental organizations, and that it attempted to block blood investigations by public officials. Indeed, many questions about the role of the Red Cross are still unanswered; for example, whether, as alleged, the Red Cross maintained secret lists of donors for heat-treated blood.[41] In this respect, too, there is a parallel with France and Japan; the sustained scandal of Canada hinged, in part, on the rage that elites provoke when they have disappointed public expectations and have shown themselves to be protecting themselves from scrutiny when challenged.

The cases we have characterized as instances of high-intensity scandal are a mix of features, some present in those countries alone, some present in other countries where similar features produced less conflict. For instance, the physician who violated his or her trust was a source of anger in many countries, and discredited physicians played a prominent role in moderate and low intensity countries as well. It is important to distinguish, however, between the generalized anger many hemophiliacs felt towards formerly trusted physicians, and the scandal created when physicians in high office are charged with misconduct. Rather than being individual physicians who disappointed their professional clients, actors in France and Japan, and the Canadian Red Cross had official capacities—and positions of special trust—within the blood-regulation context.

The argument, then, is that configurations of culture and institutions distinguish the cases of high scandal, not distinctive levels of real or alleged misdeeds. To see that more clearly, we turn to national instances of iatrogenic tragedy that did not produce the same level of scandal experienced by France, Japan, and Canada.

MODERATE-INTENSITY CONFLICT

The countries with scandals of moderate intensity included, among our cases, the United States, Denmark, Germany, Australia, and Italy. In each, the discovery of infection led to episodes of panic or spasms of intense anger, but there was a limited quality to the conflicts. To be sure, disputes over compensation and broader policy options persisted from the late 1980s until the late 1990s. But, for present purposes, the important point is that in these cases the public's attention to scandal was either brief or intermittent, in large part because of the role hemophiliacs played politically. In Germany and Australia hemophiliacs scored early political victories that helped to defuse the momentum for later collective action.[42,43] In Denmark initial victories on compensation were also important.[44] Hemophiliacs in Italy and the United States were more divided than they were in Germany and Australia, making sustained collective action of any kind difficult. The roads to intermittent conflict are therefore understandable, but not identical.

Germany, like the other countries under study, experienced a panic. It was not sustained over time, however, and it neither broadly eroded confidence in the government nor resulted in major reform. German hemophiliacs were treated early with the Bonn cure (using extremely high doses of factor VIII). This treatment was envied and much sought after by hemophiliacs in other countries. They did not develop a strong political identity as victims unjustly treated or make powerful demands beyond that of compensation. The German Hemophilia Society, physician dominated as in most countries, appears to have taken little initiative to shape the response to the aftermath of infection.[45]

No splinter group of hemophiliacs emerged.[46] Nor did infected victims or any champion from the press step forward to engage and sustain public attention.

There were, however, raw materials for a sustained German scandal involving the fear of AIDS, the safety of the public, and malfeasance by a corporation. This story involved an ambitious—and impetuous—federal health minister who caused an international panic by issuing an alert that German transfusion recipients might have AIDS.[47] The short-run political result in Germany was to blame the government for disclosure, not for secrecy. This relatively benign framing of the incident all but guaranteed that it would not expand into broader areas of civic trust (which it did not). Individuals were arrested at the companies involved, and there was minimal change in German blood regulation.[48]

Hemophiliacs in Australia were better organized politically than they were in Germany. They had been included in policy making for some time, a status and position of influence that had eluded even their politically alert and aggressive counterparts in Denmark. In view of the hemophiliac community's strong political organization, Australia may well have turned into a high-scandal country had the government responded ineffectively to their concerns, or had there been disclosures of serious malfeasance, either governmental or corporate. The issue of wrongdoing, however, was moot; the country has responded very early on with blood safety measures. Though the government was initially resistant to compensating hemophiliacs infected with HIV, pressure from the hemophiliac community, parliament, and the courts led, in halting stages, to a generous compensation scheme for all citizens with medically acquired HIV. As in Germany, the issues remained narrowly defined throughout the process, and no major crisis resulted.

The United States experience was marked by litigation, high emotions, and occasionally heated conflict, but also by deep divisions within the hemophiliac community about how to understand and address their situation.[49] The National Hemophilia Foundation (NHF) itself became a political target of militants who had broken from that organization to form the Committee of Ten Thousand (COTT) and the Hemophilia/HIV Peer Association. These splinter groups charged that, beginning in the 1970s with its failure to heat-treat for hepatitis B and continuing through the early years of the HIV epidemic, the fractionation industry had placed profit over safety. But perhaps more important, they believed that the NHF had failed to alert the hemophiliac community about the changes in treatment methods that produced the HIV scandal in the 1980s.[50] They picketed NHF meetings, accusing the NHF and medical elites of "genocide"[51] (a charge that echoed the claims of gay-rights groups). They lobbied for public compensation and for congressional hearings, and initiated a class-action suit against the pharmaceutical industry. The results were emotional public hearings, a stinging 1995 report of institutional failures within the blood industry and public-health sector,[52] increased FDA surveillance of the blood industry (including the Red Cross), and settlement of their class-action suit. Other compensation was left to the courts, although legislation to establish a compensation fund, called the Ricky Ray Hemophilia Relief Fund Act,[53] was as of mid-1998 still pending in Congress. There was no crisis, either governmental or nongovernmental, however, perhaps because of the dispersion of authority and therefore of blame in the US, and because divisions within the hemophiliac community prevented the development of a more powerful and unified public movement. The results in the United States were relatively modest institutional reforms.

In Italy, as in the United States, differences within the hemophiliac community diffused efforts for redress. The national organization, the Italian Hemophilia Foundation (IHF), was closely tied to the medical profession and formally represented the interests of hemophiliacs. Cultural differences between the northern and southern regions of the country[54] had always meant that organizational unity was a great challenge. But whatever unity there was dissolved after the first data on HIV infection in Italy became available in 1988. With IHF's ties to the medical community, the organization preferred a course of accommodation (a "dialogue line") with authorities,[55] and the legislative redress they sought followed a social-insurance model. In contrast, Turin's regional association, more highly developed organizationally,[56] was considerably more aggressive, preferred a media-based strategy, and ultimately formed a new organization of transfusion recipients, the Italian Multi-Transfused Association (API). The legislation this group sponsored in 1990 called for recoverable damages—a radical divergence from the approach of IHF. The executive, not the legislative, branch ultimately took action, in part to avoid potential embarrassment during the soon to be held international conference on AIDS in Florence, and in part to close the door on new claims arising from a recent Supreme Court decision that approved just compensation for mandatory vaccination.[57]

Reflecting both the failure of the Italian hemophiliac community to present a unified position and the associated failure to galvanize public support, not only was the compensation fund modest, but there were administrative barriers to filing a claim. The victory was, as Umberto Izzo suggests, more symbolic than real.[58]

The Danish case sits at the borderline between the high- and moderate-intensity scandal politics. It involved the most protracted judicial sequel in Danish political/administrative history. Danish hemophiliacs were, in a number of respects, successful in having their demands met. They organized in the early 1980s to obtain the "Bonn cure" and resisted the political fragmentation that had undercut hemophiliacs' efforts in Italy and the United States. They forced the resignation of a health minister (later known as "Blood Britta"), helped ensure that heat-treated blood products were introduced and that all donated blood was screened for HIV antibody, gained institutional representation on the governmental body responsible for blood products, and received the highest compensation award ever granted by the nation's health system.[59] Within a broader social and political perspective, Danish hemophiliacs were also successful in publicizing the existence of danger to the entire Danish blood supply, and in highlighting gaps between government pronouncements and practice. All of these achievements, coming in bursts of public attention, were notable. But it was the very success of Danish hemophiliacs, coupled with the intermittent rather than continual attention they received, that defused the sustained resentment underlying the high-intensity scandals we have seen elsewhere.[60]

In the countries that experienced moderate-intensity conflict, the road from angry criticism to sustained, high-intensity scandal was blocked for one reason or another. The explanation for the difference cannot be found, however, in the relative number of infected hemophiliacs or in the relative degree of neglect or wrongdoing by organizations and individual actors in the world of blood. The fact that the United States, for example, had a greater proportion of infected hemophiliacs than any other nation was not expressed in a substantial and sustained public debate over who was responsible and what should be done. The fragmentation of American political institutions meant that many channels of criticism were open and that it was difficult to focus on the specific failures of particular individuals or governmental organizations. Attention to the safety and stability of the blood supply was dispersed among many actors—from the FDA to blood banks, from the fractionators to the hematologists. And the review of their behavior was split among Congress, bodies like the Institute of Medicine, and the courts. That disputes continue to this day surprises no one familiar with the litigiousness of American society.

The American experience is but one illustration of how culture, politics, and science come together to produce outcomes, in this case an example of what we have called moderate-intensity scandal politics. To put that level of scandal in better perspective, it is helpful to consider very briefly nations where the distribution of contaminated blood led to compensation for hemophiliacs, but little scandal or political impact.

CONTAMINATED BLOOD PRODUCTS AND LOW-INTENSITY POLITICS

The experience of the Netherlands represents an example of a country that escaped divisive social and political scandal. Some brief observations are in order despite the fact that Holland was not one of the eight countries initially investigated.

The aftermath of infection in Holland was not one of confrontation. As was true with other areas of AIDS policy, there emerged a consensual effort both to provide a remedy for the victims of contaminated blood and blood products, and to work out acceptable ways of securing the blood supply. Consensus building had begun early. For example, in discussions that included the various interest groups involved, Holland had instituted a system of voluntary, but not mandatory, measures (such as self-exclusion) to protect the blood supply. But beyond that direct preventive goal, the process of consensus building also had the effect of reducing the likelihood of later rage. In 1992, for example, the Dutch Society of Hemophiliacs (NVHP) requested an investigation into cases of HIV contamination and then filed a formal complaint against the Dutch authorities. While these developments may have reflected a breakdown of the consensus model (or even just an instance of cross-national learning in the politics of hemophilia activism), the governmental response demonstrated its continuing commitment to pursue consensus in lieu of open political and legal conflict. The complaint was handled not by the courts—an inherently adversarial and confrontational forum—but through the National Ombudsman. The result was an official admission of liability from the government, accompanied by an increase in the compensation to victims to approximately the average level in other countries.

PART IV. CONCLUSION

The tragic stories presented in this chapter continue to be troubling. Across the world, nations still struggle with the impact and meaning of the experience with contaminated blood and blood products. That experience bears not only on questions of political accountability, legal liability, and compensation, but also on issues of prudent prevention in the future. Contemporary discussions about risk, decision making under conditions of uncertainty, and the application of science to policymaking all involve lessons drawn (and overdrawn) from the experiences this writing has reviewed. Heightened awareness of the exposure of vulnerable groups, indeed of the whole community, to new pathways of infection has led to various policy changes, some that may threaten the pace of innovation, others that rank safety over cost in ways that will no doubt prove problematic. The excitement associated with earlier advances that improved the lives of hemophiliacs has in many contexts been replaced by grief, anger, and ambivalence about science and government.

The scandal politics we have analyzed raise a broad issue concerning the media. Contemporary media has the ability to accelerate cross-national learning in ways that would have been hard to imagine in a world without the fax, email, and institutions like CNN and Sky Television. It can transmit information (and myths) beyond traditional elites to ordinary citizens and in so doing fuel the possibility of scandal. To be sure, scandal politics may help to balance systems where power is distributed unequally. In the countries under study, the level of scandal, remedies, and punishments depended significantly on the level of organization of the hemophiliacs themselves, the institutional channeling of protest, and the tenacity of the press. The actual levels of infection or timing of responses explained far less than one might have expected.

As the national cases demonstrate, there is a highly uncertain relation between the realities of risk and the reactions of nations to them. The complex mix of factors that produce reactions are unlikely to yield simple prediction or lessons. There is the danger that, given the tragic experience of HIV-tainted blood, governmental regulators will be excessively cautious and restrictive in reacting to future threats—real or imagined—to the safety of medical products. There is also the likelihood that excessive caution will in turn yield to more relaxed regulation. Either way, the uncertainty that characterized battles over HIV and blood will reappear in an ever-changing array of disguises. As in the conflict over hepatitis C, once again the legal, political, and social systems of the industrialized democracies will respond to common threats, and to the burdens that result from unforeseen dangers, in the most uncommon of ways.

Notes

1. This article was first published in *Blood Feuds, Aids, Blood, and the Politics of Medical Disaster* (New York: Oxford University Press, 1999). The article was the concluding chapter. This essay draws extensively from the case studies that make up the chapters of *Blood Feuds*.

   Each chapter of that book took up the story of how contaminated blood and its devastating impact on hemophiliacs were coped with by the following countries: England, Germany, Denmark, France, Japan, Italy, Canada, Australia, and the United States. This comparative analysis constituted the closing chapter of the book and is reprinted here with minor revisions and editing, all directed at making the article clear to the new reader.

2. Feldman, E., and Bayer, R., *Blood Feuds*, "Introduction: Understanding the blood feuds," pp. 13ff.

3. Although it has been argued that there was wide variation in initial responses (see, for example, Trebilcock, M. J., Howse, R., and Daniels, R., "Do institutions matter? A comparative pathology of the HIV-infected blood tragedy," *Va. L. Rev.* 82(8): 1407–92 (1996)) and that differences in

institutional arrangements account for this variation, what is most striking about the countries under study is the similarity of institutional responses during this period, especially in view of the obvious differences in their institutional arrangements—legal, political, and medical.

4. CDC, *Morbidity and Mortality Weekly Report* (MMWR) 30: 250–52 (5 June 1981).
5. *MMWR* 31: 644–52 (10 December 1982).
6. Leveton, L. B., Sox, H.C., Jr., and Stoto, M., eds., *HIV and the Blood Supply: An Analysis of Crisis Decisionmaking* (Washington, D.C.: National Academy Press, 1995), p. 212.
7. Izzo, U., in Feldman and Bayer, *Blood Feuds*, quoting Rizzo et al., "Emofilia e lavoro," in *Difesa Sociale* 6:151 (1992), to the effect that 90 percent of Italian hemophiliacs died before entering their twenties.
8. Leveton, Sox, and Stoto, eds., *HIV and the Blood Supply*, p. 171.
9. Larsson, S. A., "Life expectancy of Swedish hemophiliacs, 1831–1980," in *Br. J. Haematol.* 59(4): 593–602.
10. Triemstra, M., et al., "Mortality in patients with hemophilia: Changes in a Dutch population from 1986 to 1992 and 1973 to 1986." *Ann. Int. Med.* 123(11): 823–27 (1995).
11. *Blood Feuds*, p. 2.
12. Trebilcock, M. J., Howse, R., and Daniels, R., "Do institutions matter?"
13. Kirp, D., "The politics of blood: Hemophilia activism in the AIDS crisis," p. 293ff. in Feldman and Bayer, *Blood Feuds*.
14. For detailed descriptions of the changes see the individual country studies in Feldman and Bayer, *Blood Feuds*.
15. Japanese hemophiliacs came to be almost entirely identified with AIDS, not the gay community, as was the case in other countries. Feldman interprets this as the result of the largely silent and unorganized gay community in Japan. Feldman, R., "HIV and blood in Japan: Transforming private conflict into public scandal," in *Blood Feuds*, p. 65.
16. Feldman and Bayer, *Blood Feuds*, p. 9.
17. Ibid., p. 14.
18. Importantly, they chose not to sue the Japanese Red Cross; because the family of its honorary chair had been included in the Japanese royal family since the Meiji period, such an act would not only have been culturally unthinkable, but have alienated public support for their position. Feldman and Bayer, *Blood Feuds*, p. 16.
19. Ibid., p. 82.
20. Gilmore, N., and Somerville, M., "From trust to tragedy: HIV/AIDS and the Canadian blood system," in Feldman and Bayer, *Blood Feuds*, pp. 141ff.
21. Blassing, R., "Nova Scotia to compensate people who contracted AIDS virus from tainted blood," *Buffalo News*, 18 April 1993.
22. Ibid.
23. Gilmore and Somerville, "From trust to tragedy," p. 146.
24. Ibid., p. 150.
25. Kramer, J., "Bad blood," *The New Yorker*, 11 October 1993, p. 80.
26. Steffen, M., "The nation's blood: Medicine, justice, and the state in France," in *Blood Feuds*, p. 121.
27. Blassing, R., "*Nova Scotia*," p. 174.
28. Fennell, T., "Voices of the victims: An inquiry reveals how the blood system failed," *Maclean's*, 19 September 1994, p. 28.
29. CBC-TV *National Magazine*, "Janet Conners: Private pain, public battle: Why she turned personal tragedy into political action," 5 June 1997 (follow-up on 26 September 1997, with related stories on 10 October 1996 and on 17 January and 25 June 1997).
30. Evening news, CBC-TV, 26 September 1997.
31. Ibid., p. 78.

32. Ibid., p. 36.
33. Kramer, J., "Bad blood," p. 94.
34. Steffen, M., "The nation's blood," p. 108. The details of the French scandal proved truly startling. In June 1985, according to minutes discovered by Casteret, Garretta insisted that untreated blood products should remain the standard prescription; in August of 1985 he encouraged two Parisian hospitals to distribute again.
35. Ibid.
36. Feldman and Bayer, *Blood Feuds*, p. 11.
37. Kramer, J., "Bad blood," p. 94.
38. Ibid., p. 75.
39. "AIDS advisors disagree over events in HIV blood scandal," *Nature*, 25 April 1996.
40. Kramer, J., "Bad blood," p. 93.
41. Nor has it been possible to determine whether, as alleged, the Canadian Blood Commission shredded public documents in order to frustrate investigations into individual liability. Kennedy, M., "Files destroyed to hide facts: Information czar targets federal official," *Ottawa Citizen*, 23 January 1997. Though not directly involving the Red Cross, this continuing uncertainty concerning the Canadian Blood Commission added to public frustrations about the lack of access to information central to the investigation of the Canadian blood scandal.
42. Ballard, J., "HIV contaminated blood and Australian policy: The limits of success," in *Blood Feuds*, p. 265ff.
43. Dressler, S., "Blood 'scandal' and AIDS in Germany," in Feldman and Bayer, *Blood Feuds*, p. 201ff.
44. The Danish compensation was the largest ever granted to a patient group. But another important political outcome was the establishment of a medical injury insurance making it easier for future patients to obtain compensation for injury sustained in the Danish health care system. Albaek, E., "The never ending story? The political and legal controversies over HIV and the blood supply in Denmark," in *Blood Feuds*, p. 185.
45. Dressler, "Blood 'scandal,'" p. 195. The dominance of physicians is important because they continued to support the use of the Bonn cure.
46. Ibid., p. 19.
47. Groom, B., "A case of bloody madness," *Scotland on Sunday*, 7 Nov 1993.
48. Dressler, "Blood 'scandal," pp. 207ff.
49. Bayer, R., "Blood and AIDS in America: Science, politics, and the making of an iatrogenic catastrophe," in Feldman and Bayer, *Blood Feuds*, pp. 38ff.
50. Ibid., p. 39.
51. Ibid., p. 43.
52. The report was published as *HIV and the Blood Supply, supra.*
53. The Ray fund is targeted to hemophiliacs alone and excludes transfusion recipients. The Act was named in honor of Ricky Ray, a Florida boy with hemophilia, who died from HIV/AIDS in 1992 at the age of 15.
54. Izzo, U., in Feldman and Bayer, *Blood Feuds*, pp. 7, 11, 17. Although Italy officially promotes the "gift" culture of donation, regions vary in their acceptance. Turin has a high collection rate, but the South is more tribal and less collective; loyalty is tied to family. The sale of "red gold" and charges of usury are not unusual.
55. Ibid., p. 32.
56. Ibid., pp. 5–6.
57. Ibid., p. 36.
58. Ibid,, p. 233.
59. Albaek, E., p. 185.
60. Ibid.

The Power of Professionalism

Policies for AIDS in Britain, Sweden, and the United States

Daniel M. Fox, Patricia Day, and Rudolf Klein

The response to the epidemic of human immunodeficiency virus infection and related diseases reveals similarities as well as differences in the policy systems of the three countries we examined for this article—Britain, Sweden, and the United States.[1] Both the incidence and therefore the financial and emotional impact of the HIV epidemic have been considerably greater in the United States than in either Britain or Sweden. Moreover, familiar differences in the political cultures of the three countries influence the making of health policy. The politics of health, for instance, is considerably more acrimonious in the United States than in Britain or Sweden.[2] Nevertheless, in late 1988, the health policies of all three countries defined AIDS primarily as a professional problem in the management of what was increasingly seen as a chronic condition.

As a professional issue, the epidemic was mainly a problem for experts in clinical medicine, research, and public health and was, by and large, an unseemly subject for partisan debate. In each country, some people emphasized moral and emotional issues in the epidemic.

But even in the United States, where these groups have been loudest and occasionally effective, policies have been made mainly in response to the opinions of the customary actors in health affairs. Policy for the AIDS epidemic was no more an issue in the American presidential campaign in the fall of 1988 than it was in the Swedish election campaign in the summer or in the rhetoric of the British political parties during their annual conferences. Moreover, in all three countries, despite their very different approaches to balancing individual rights and social obligations, protecting the right to privacy of individuals with HIV infection was, for both practical and ideological reasons, assumed to be a central purpose of policy. The protection of confidentiality, even anonymity, had become a technical aspect of public-health practice.

This interpretation of how three countries have responded to the epidemic may appear to be naive about the wisdom of experts and insensitive to the profound tensions and conflicts about what is proper policy. Two limitations on our story must therefore be noted. First, we do not attempt to evaluate the effectiveness of the policy responses in each country, either compared with each other or against some idealized standard. Second, we are not presenting a social history of the reaction to the epidemic in the three countries but concentrating exclusively on the policy responses.

Our story has three themes:

1. The initial government reaction to AIDS in all three countries was slow and cautious, even dilatory in the eyes of some.

2. Once government (national government in Britain, both the federal government and that of some states in the U.S.A., and the central government, the county governments, and municipal governments in Sweden) decided to take strong initiative, it quickly established the terms of debate. Governments pursued AIDS policies modeled on historical responses to outbreaks of plague and other virulent infections.

3. Policy in the three countries has, in the main, been based on consensus, both professional and political: a consensus that has ruled out certain options (like widespread mandated screening for infection) but that has also generated considerable support for the course pursued. In particular, policy has rested on agreement that the epidemic, whatever its unique features and however menacing it might appear, is a disease like any other as far as research and treatment is concerned. The consensus has evoked dissent in all three countries. But in all three, governments have employed their standard procedures for hearing, acknowledging, and to a very limited extent, accommodating the dissenters.

First we summarize central issues in the history of policy responses to the epidemic in Britain, Sweden, and the United States. Then we draw some conclusions about what this history suggests about the adequacy of the three policy systems for dealing with unexpected epidemiological threats.

BRITAIN

AIDS was first diagnosed in Britain toward the end of 1981. The scale of the epidemic remained small for some time. By the end of 1983, 29 cases had been reported, and by the end of 1985, 271. Mid-1988 statistics show a cumulative total of 1,800 cases. Cases are reported on a voluntary and confidential basis to the Communicable Disease Surveillance Centre. At last count, some 9,000 positive tests had also been reported to the organization, although estimates of the total number infected range from 19,250 to 48,200.[3]

AIDS in Britain is largely a phenomenon of London and Edinburgh and their hinterlands. Over half of all reported AIDS cases have been concentrated in three inner London health districts. The distribution of cases by patients' characteristics is also skewed. A full 83 percent involves homosexual or bisexual men. The second largest category, 8 percent, involves recipients of blood products. Among those with HIV positive tests, the distribution is the same, with one important exception—Scotland, where intravenous drug abusers are the largest category of all. Moreover, women and children account for 28 percent of seropositives in Scotland but for only 6 percent of known AIDS cases in the rest of the country.

The turning point in public policy toward AIDS came in 1986. Before then, the Department of Health relied on established services and existing public-health routines. Circulars were sent out to the medical profession. The discovery that infection could be transmitted through blood led, first, to an appeal to high-risk groups not to become donors and, following the availability of the ELISA test, to the screening of all blood donations. The provisions of the 1984 Public Health (Control of Disease) Act were extended to cover AIDS—including a provision that permits patients to be compulsorily hospitalized—but were never activated following an unsuccessful test case. The task was left, however, to the civil servants and technicians of the department, in particular to Sir Donald Acheson, the chief medical officer, who was required, in the words of one of his colleagues, to "batter his head against a brick wall" of indifference among ministers who "tended to have complicated feelings about homosexuality."

Then came 1986 and a rush of activity. Ministers set up a cabinet committee and initiated parliamentary discussions of AIDS. Generous funding for research and the management of persons with AIDS by health authorities started to flow. The government launched a public-education campaign, unprecedented in its scale and its frankness about sexual habits.

Why 1986? A number of complementary explanations offer themselves. First, there was increasing evidence that an epidemic previously confined to deviant minorities might be spilling over into the population at large. Second, there was the visit of Britain's secretary of state for health, Norman Fowler, to the United States, where he saw the impact of the epidemic for himself. Third, there was the fact that within the department there was a strong public-health lobby, headed by Acheson, pressing for action. Fourth, a series of lurid AIDS stories in the tabloids prodded ministers into taking an interest. Fifth, the Government's dawning interest in turn presented an opportunity for a variety of lobbies to press their case to the ministers—for example, the research community and the medical staffs of the Clinics for Sexually Transmitted Diseases. The gay lobby was less visible in Britain than in the United States, perhaps because it had fairly easy access to the department. Lastly, the secretary of state may have seen, in the rising salience of AIDS, an opportunity to wring extra cash for the National Health Service out of the Treasury.

In all this, the Government was intent on creating and maintaining political consensus. In November 1986, it initiated the first House of Commons debate on AIDS. The debate provided an impressive picture of Britain's politicians establishing a consensus within which future policy was to be made. This consensus rested on the repudiation of the view that AIDS could be seen as a "gay plague," a belief that the solution lay in changing the entire population's sexual behavior through public education and a rejection of measures such as compulsory testing, which might threaten civil liberties as well as be ineffective.

The consensus was sealed by the 1987 report of the all-party Social Services Committee of the House of Commons. Just as Government policy itself was shaped by the public-health model, articulated within the Department of Health by Acheson, so the committee's report was shaped by three doctors it recruited as its advisory staff for the inquiry. While giving its blessing to the consensual professional approach of public policy, the committee added a quasi-theological gloss: AIDS, its report concluded, had "highlighted things that are wrong with our society" and provided a "focus to try to remedy such problems." In short, the problems of AIDS had become opportunities for those seeking new arguments for pushing old causes, whether the advocacy of chastity or the pressure for more research funding.[4]

The Government's subsequent strategies reflect the consensus forged in 1986 and 1987. The most conspicuous of these—unique to Britain perhaps in its scale and outspokenness—has been the education drive. For the first time, a British government launched a national media campaign to change the sexual behavior of the population. Its message was: if you cannot cut down the number of your partners, use condoms. The strategy has been as much to raise general awareness as to target the message exclusively to high-risk groups, although drug users were picked out for special attention. This strategy avoided stigmatizing the homosexual community, the education of which was largely left to voluntary organizations like the Terrence Higgins Trust. But it is not known as yet whether public education has changed heterosexual behavior. There is a strong case for the community as a whole to change sexual behavior in order to limit the future spread of AIDS; however, the incentives for heterosexual individuals to change their behavior are weaker given the risk factors known at present.

From the start of the epidemic, policy for the treatment of AIDS has been shaped by the assumption that the existing services of the National Health Service provide the means for managing the disease, that there is nothing special about AIDS except for the extra demands on resources. In practice, therefore, the management of care has been left to clinicians. But the Department of Health has made large-scale extra grants to health authorities in the worst affected parts of the country. Such disease-specific grants are against precedent. To some extent, Britain has joined Sweden and parts of the United States in making AIDS an exception to established rules about financing health care.

The same pattern is evident in the case of research—reliance, at first, on normal organizations' routines followed by an injection of extra funds. Until 1986, AIDS research had to compete against other fields at a time of much complaint in Britain's scientific community about dwindling funds. By 1987, the Medical Research Council had made just eight special grants for AIDS research. But in 1986 the cabinet committee sanctioned spending on an ambitious program of AIDS research submitted by the MRC and designed to develop a vaccine and antiviral drugs. AIDS then became a source of extra money for the scientific community.

The only instance of AIDS overriding established policy objectives has been in the field of drugs. The risk that AIDS might spread into the heterosexual population through drug takers led, early on, to the Department of Health providing funds for drug-misuse agencies to expand their activities. Experimental needle-exchange schemes were extended and made permanent in 1988. The Government had abandoned its previous stance of augmenting its restrictive and punitive policies on drugs now that AIDS had come to be seen as the greater danger.

Nevertheless, AIDS has not been seen as justifying any dilution of traditional libertarian or professional values in Britain. Ministers, the medical profession, and the homosexual communities appear to be united in resisting demands for compulsory screening programs and in insisting on both confidentiality in testing and on making testing conditional on the availability of counseling. The position of the medical profession—as articulated both by the General Medical Council (the regulatory body) and the British Medical Association—has been a key factor in giving priority to the doctor-patient relationship rather than to epidemiological information. Even the announcement of the anonymous testing of routine blood samples in the autumn of 1988 caused rumbles and, in contrast to Sweden, there is no systematic contact tracing of the kind used to control other sexually transmitted diseases.

The combined weight of Government and professional pronouncements—backed by all political parties—has thus made overt discrimination socially unacceptable. This is not to claim that there is no discrimination. Because it is defined as unacceptable, its occurrence is not monitored systematically. For example, the Department of Employment condemns discriminatory practices at work, but there are no legal provisions (except suit for wrongful dismissal) to back its exhortations. Similarly, people at high risk of illness, whether AIDS or high blood pressure, have difficulty in getting life insurance and therefore home mortgages. Overall, AIDS in Britain is emerging as a long-term health policy problem rather than a dramatic moral or social crisis. From being seen primarily as a condition to be treated in the acute medical services, AIDS is being perceived as requiring care mainly outside hospitals. The disease will be testing Britain's health services at their weakest point, which is coping with chronic disease in the community.

Increasingly too, it is being realized that any spread in the heterosexual population may be slower than had been anticipated.[5] The latest predictions suggest that the future may be less scarifying than expected. There is a paradox at the heart of Britain's consensus. In order to mobilize support for their policies, in particular policy designed to change sexual mores, politicians have dramatized the epidemic. If AIDS comes to be seen as just another routine killer disease like cancer or coronary disease, professionals and Government will lose one of the few weapons they have for the mobilization of support: fear.

SWEDEN

The first cases of AIDS in Sweden were diagnosed late in 1982. The annual incidence grew slowly; 6 cases in 1983; 10 in 1984; 30 in 1985; 49 in 1986; 64 in 1987. By mid-1988, just under 200 cases had been reported, 80 percent of them in gay and bisexual men. Approximately 2,000 people had been diagnosed as infected with HIV (of almost half a million tested) though some independent estimates put the number as high as 5,000 or even 10,000.[6] As the number of cases grew, medical and lay leaders of a few gay organizations and a handful of other doctors and epidemiologists called attention to the threat posed by the disease. Responding to their concerns, the national press regularly covered the growth of the epidemic, particularly in the United States.

There was, however, disagreement about the extent of the threat to Sweden. In 1983, when a leading Stockholm academic specialist in infectious disease wrote a newspaper article about the spreading epidemic, he was criticized for exaggeration by a group of gay doctors.[7] The doctors who have treated most of the persons with AIDS in Stockholm since 1983 recalled in 1988 that as late as 1985 their chiefs denied their requests for additional staff and space for treatment. A gay physician who is now the president of a prominent voluntary organization providing services to persons with HIV infection said that in the early years of the epidemic, "authorities here as in the United States . . . tried to cover big needs but without great generosity."

Since 1985, the central government has asserted its considerable authority in making AIDS policy. In September of that year, the cabinet classified AIDS as a venereal disease under the Prevention of Infectious Diseases Act. Under this act a "person who suspects that he may be suffering from a venereal disease is bound to seek medical attention." Patients are tested anonymously. Anyone who is infected must, however, be identified in the medical record, though names are not submitted to public-health authorities. Doctors initiate contact tracing, which is conducted mainly by social workers. The act also provides sanctions against patients who refuse to cooperate, but to date the sanctions have been used in only a few cases.[8]

Provision for treating persons with AIDS also increased rapidly after 1985. Doctors at Roslagstull Hospital, the infectious disease division of the Karolinska Institute, were authorized to open a unit for outpatient treatment in June of that year. At that time two and a half doctors, three nurses, and a secretary provided treatment for 500 outpatients and inpatients with HIV infection and related diseases. By 1988, seven doctors, six nurses, three social workers, and two secretaries were serving 600 patients.

The rapid expansion of treatment programs after 1985 was a result of the pressure of officials in the central government on county authorities and reluctant members of the academic medical hierarchy. A change of leadership in the hierarchy of academic internal medicine, particularly in the specialty of infectious disease in Stockholm in about 1985, appears to have been both a cause and an effect of this pressure. Another ingredient was the growing consensus among leaders of both the ruling Social Democratic Party and the opposition parties that the epidemic required more active policy, especially to prevent heterosexual transmission of the virus. A few leaders of the opposition considered using AIDS as an example of the deficiencies of Prime Minister Eric Carlsson and of Minister of Health and Social Affairs Gertrud Sigurdsen. Attacks on Sigurdsen began in 1985 and accelerated in 1987. She was accused of underestimating the number of seropositives and being overoptimistic about controlling the epidemic. Opposition leaders wrote newspaper columns or gave interviews attacking government policy for not giving HIV infection sufficient priority. The doctor in charge of the AIDS treatment unit at Roslagstull wrote a newspaper article advocating more resources for treatment; he recalls that his budget was quickly increased.

The prime minister and the minister for health and social affairs responded to this political threat by creating a formal body of about twenty members to advise the government on policy. The members included Social Democratic and opposition politicians, civil servants and interest-group leaders. The Swedish name of this body, the AIDS-delegationen, is usually translated into English as National Commission on AIDS. But Swedish officials insist that it has never behaved as a typical government commission, which customarily meets in closed sessions and then issues a report. The AIDS-delegation (as we will translate it) is, according to a senior official, "unique . . . [and] its constitutional role unclear." Even the principal secretary of the AIDS-delegation agreed that it was "not a very typical way" of making policy in Sweden. Similarly, the chairman of the parliamentary committee on health and social affairs, when asked for a parallel to the AIDS-delegation, of which he is a prominent member, said "probably something like it was created during a cholera epidemic in the last century."

The conventional Swedish system for achieving consensus on policy was in disarray as officials, politicians, doctors, and interest group leaders grappled with AIDS in 1985. The debate over amending the Prevention of Infectious Diseases Act had been uncommonly divisive. Gay organizations bitterly opposed classifying AIDS as a sexually transmitted disease. Feminist groups were troubled by what they regarded as threats to the civil liberties of prostitutes in the amendments. Moreover, there was criticism in the press of the government's public information policy—its emphasis on the risk of heterosexual spread and its relative blandness in comparison with campaigns in Britain and some cities in the United States. AIDS was also causing increasing debate about the government's policy for controlling drug use. Members of county councils were worrying about the costs of treating persons with AIDS. National politicians in the opposition parties were testing the viability of challenging the government on AIDS policy.

The AIDS-delegation was a forum for reestablishing consensus. Its original members represented the National Board of Health and Social Welfare, the national bacteriological laboratory, the association of county councils, the national federation of local authorities, the two largest of the five political parties, and medical experts. "When you have these, you have everybody in Swedish so-ciety," its principal secretary said. A few months later, the government redefined everybody to include the other three parties.

The AIDS-delegation moved quickly to shape consensus. The members agreed unanimously that AIDS should be regulated as a sexually transmitted disease. They agreed on the necessity of contact tracing and that routine test-ing, with informed consent, was a good policy for clinics treating infectious and venereal disease and pregnant women. Although "every member of the delega-tion knows" that doctors are illegally preserving the anonymity of some people who test positive, there was consensus to ignore the problem because "we're trying to encourage people to be tested."

Consensus has been difficult to achieve on two subjects: the intensity of public-education campaigns and policy to control the transmission of HIV in-fection among intravenous drug users. Some members of the delegation believe that AIDS education has exceeded the attention span of most members of the general public, that "people are tired of hearing about it."[9] Others sympathized with a staff member who quit in December 1987 because the delegation's infor-mation campaigns were insufficiently aggressive.

Considerable conflict remains about policy for controlling HIV infection among intravenous drug users and their sexual partners. The reason for the conflict, according to a senior civil servant, is that the policy dilemmas in this area are "too difficult politically" to engage. When the conflict became public in 1985, Sweden had vigorous policies to control the supply of narcotic drugs and provide drug-free treatment. In 1985, ministry officials proposed, and the AIDS-delegation endorsed, a policy goal of treating all intravenous drug us-ers. Over the next two years, local government expenditures for drug treatment more than doubled. "AIDS meant that now local government was taking the official goal seriously," the civil servant recalled.

There is still controversy over methadone maintenance and needle-exchange programs, but consensus is emerging. Under pressure from doctors and volun-tary association leaders whose primary concern is AIDS, the ministry has reluc-tantly agreed to double Sweden's modest methadone maintenance program to 300 places. Similarly, officials opposed establishing needle exchanges because the "message will be too schizophrenic." Nevertheless, a doctor at a university clinic in Lund established a program that has had favorable publicity, con-siderable local support, and the endorsement of the chairman of the all-party parliamentary committee on health and social welfare. Officials of the National Board of Health and Social Welfare reluctantly admit that exchanges "will be hard to resist."

Many gay leaders who have been critical of government policy are active in the quasi-official Noah's Ark Red Cross Foundation. Noah's Ark mounts programs of education, offers counseling and support services, and is establishing a guest-house, hospice, hot-line, and reception service.[10] Its budget, guaranteed by the Swedish Red Cross, is being financed this year by grants from the national government and from the Stockholm municipal and county authorities. Its president, a prominent gay doctor, supports, with reservations, government policies for controlling the epidemic. In the last year, he says, "powerful people have stopped doing as little as they could." But he worries that there is still considerable denial of the extent of the epidemic, reflected in official underestimation of the number of people who are infected and resist needle exchanges.[11]

Some muted dissent remains. A few academic doctors have worried in public that AIDS is deflecting funds from other priorities. When Astra, the largest Swedish drug manufacturer, withdrew from research related to HN earlier this year, the prime minister embarrassed its managers by telling the International Congress on AIDS in Stockholm that pharmaceutical companies have moral as well as commercial responsibilities.

During the first few years of the epidemic, Swedish officials were cautious, like their counterparts in Britain and the United States. A few critics accused them of ignoring a potentially devastating problem, others of being unnecessarily alarmist. Beginning in 1985, the central government organized a coalition to establish the epidemic as a classic public-health problem requiring case finding, education, and treatment. Achieving consensus became an important goal, both because consensus is central to Swedish political culture and because less dissent is tolerable in a classic public-health response to an epidemic than during political business as usual. The AIDS-delegation, a new political device, was the instrument for achieving the symbolism and much of the substance of consensus. Only in the area of policy for drug treatment was there disarray; but in mid-1988 there was evidence that a consensus was emerging.

UNITED STATES

The scale of the epidemic is greater in the United States than in either Britain or Sweden. As this article was being written, almost 70,000 cases had been reported in the United States since 1981, whereas in Britain 1,700 had been reported and in Sweden only 200. Estimates of the number of people infected ranged from 500,000 to 1.5 million.[12] The cumulative incidence in the United States (237.7 per million) was an order of magnitude greater than in Britain (which had an incidence of 25.2 per million) and in Sweden (21.5).

Most accounts of the epidemic in the United States create a superficial impression that AIDS policy in the United States has been characterized more by conflict than by consensus. These accounts emphasize disputes about screening, testing, needle exchanges, drug research, and treatment.[13] Since about 1985, however, policy for the epidemic has been made mainly by the same professionals, supported by the same coalitions, nationally and in the states, that have dominated health affairs for half a century. The disagreements about policy that remain appear to be more intense than similar controversies in Britain or Sweden do, in large part because the public rhetorical dramas of symbolic politics are a mechanism for coping with the fragmentation of political authority in the United States.

When the AIDS epidemic began, the American health polity was changing more rapidly than it had in a generation. The individuals and institutions that had dominated health affairs were poorly prepared to take aggressive action against an infectious disease that was linked in the majority of cases to individual behavior, was expensive to study and treat, and required a coordinated array of public and personal health services. The epidemic of HIV infection began in a political climate characterized by what appeared to be a fundamental shift in the locus of authority for health policy from the federal government to state governments and the private sector and in the willingness of public officials to let doctors and scientists continue to control spending with minimal oversight. Moreover, the strength of right-wing pressure groups seemed to preclude sympathetic policies for a disease that was most prevalent among homosexual men and intravenous drug users and that afflicted a disproportionate number of blacks and Hispanics.

In the early 1980s, many people criticized the Reagan administration for not mounting a conventional public-health attack on the epidemic. The critics included some officials of state and local government, a few influential members of Congress, leaders of gay-rights organizations, and several high-ranking officials of the agencies that compose the United States Public Health Service.[14]

These critics had considerable evidence. The Reagan administration was, until 1986, reluctant to request funds from Congress for research on and services for dealing with the epidemic. Right-wing members of Congress blocked proposals to spend federal funds for education to prevent AIDS on the ground that abstinence, from both sexual relations and drug use, was the only appropriate message. Leaders of major gay-rights organizations criticized the surveillance guidelines of the federal Centers for Disease Control (CDC), which coordinated data collection nationally and strongly influenced policies in the states. They feared that policies that promised confidentiality rather than anonymity, or that required contact tracing (euphemized as partner notification), would drive underground many persons at risk and generate resistance to pleas to practice safer sex and use clean needles. Health-insurance executives and hospital administrators complained to the press and to legislative committees that the cost of treating persons with AIDS was a heavy burden that was made worse by the absence of federal subsidies.

Although there is still considerable dispute about priorities in the United States, as there is in Britain and Sweden, policy for the epidemic is being made mainly by experts in clinical medicine, research, and public health. The triumph of professionalism at the federal level was symbolized by the advocacy, from 1986 on, of vigorous federal action to combat the epidemic by C. Everett Koop, surgeon general of the Public Health Service. Koop had been appointed in 1981 on the basis of right-wing credentials. Now he insisted that his responsibilities as a doctor and a public-health official took precedence over his religious beliefs about sexuality. He has been warmly supported by officials of the Public Health Service, by members and staffs of key congressional committees, and in general by the press.

The same experts who dominate other arenas of health policy are now leading the response to AIDS. Two reports by the Institute of Medicine of the National Academy of Sciences gave advice that is often cited as guidance for proper policy by officials of the federal government and most of the states. The President's Commission on the HIV Epidemic, after a politicized false start, submitted a report that was widely praised by the media and by leaders of clinical medicine, research, and public health.

After an acrimonious beginning, biomedical scientists have resumed their conventional public stance of international cooperation and pride in the rapidity of the advance of knowledge. Robert Gallo of the National Institutes of Health and Luc Montagnier of the Pasteur Institute publicly resolved their acrimonious conflict over who had first discovered the virus responsible for AIDS. Clinical trials of potential drug treatments for HIV-related diseases are proceeding at more than thirty institutions, funded by the NIH and supervised by a committee of principal investigators. The Food and Drug Administration has promised to expedite approval of new drugs.

Controversies over surveillance policy have been contained. A few states (nine by early 1988) mandate confidential reporting of the names of seropositive individuals. Partner-notification programs of varying types are in place in every state.[15] Officials of state and local government and leaders of gay-rights organizations less frequently question CDC recommendations and policies in public. A bitter debate between CDC staff and social scientists in other agencies and outside government over how to measure the incidence of HIV infection—indeed about whether accurate research is even possible—has largely been conducted in private.

The content of mass education campaigns is increasingly left to experts. At the urging of Surgeon General Koop, the federal government mailed an informational pamphlet to every household. In the summer of 1988, conservative senators and representatives ended their resistance to using federal funds for education about avoiding infection.

Disputes about how much it costs to treat persons with AIDS have subsided. By 1986, there was evidence that the early estimates of the cost of treatment were unnecessarily alarmist.[16] In 1987, Congress responded to testimony about the high cost of AZT, the first moderately effective therapy for some persons with AIDS, with an appropriation to the states to subsidize purchase of the drug. Federal officials encouraged states to seek waivers of Medicaid regulations to permit them to pay for noninstitutional services for persons with AIDS. In the fall of 1988, Congress authorized additional funds to treat AIDS.

Physicians became increasingly prominent advocates for making out-of-hospital services available for persons with HIV infection. A few physicians began specializing in managing HIV infection, especially in the metropolitan areas with the highest incidence of the disease and growing numbers of infected persons. Many of these specialists direct hospital units for persons with AIDS and coordinate out-of-hospital services through case managers who are paid by public and by insurance and foundation funds. These physicians collaborate with public-health officials and with leaders of voluntary organizations that provide support services for persons with HIV infection to press for more resources for testing, laboratory work, nursing homes, and hospice care.

In 1988, federal funds for programs to treat and study intravenous drug addicts were substantially increased for the first time in a decade. The politics of drug treatment and of law enforcement are now in conflict, however. Needle exchanges have been proposed in several states, but most police officials and prosecutors oppose them. The history of the AIDS Institute of the New York State Department of Health exemplifies the reassertion of the authority of conventional medical and public-health leaders in policy-making for HIV infection. After its creation by legislative initiative in 1984, the institute was led by a social worker who had previously directed the New York City voluntary organization the Gay Men's Health Crisis. His principal associates were planners, social scientists, and health administrators—some of them gay, none of them physicians. Both the budget of the institute and its dominance by medicine have grown in the past two years. Although that budget continues to finance a network of community-based organizations that provide support services and to sponsor educational programs, the main activities of the AIDS Institute are financing and coordinating testing programs and hospital-based AIDS treatment centers.

In the United States, particularly in New York City and San Francisco, the crisis of authority in health affairs in the early 1980s and the concern about AIDS among gay men, many of whom were politically sophisticated, permitted new players to have considerable influence for a time on health policy. This influence appears to be waning, in part as a result of the death of some leaders from AIDS and the exhaustion of others, partly as a result of increasing incidence of the disease among drug users, but mainly because of the restoration of the traditional sources of authority in health affairs however fragmented they may be in the United States in comparison with those in Britain and Sweden.

Neither presidential candidate made AIDS an issue in 1988, perhaps because sex, homosexuality, and drug abuse were divisive issues in a campaign that already involved uncommon hostility. But both candidates committed themselves to maintaining the surveillance, research, and financing policies now in place: there was little new for them to say—certainly no sound bites for television.

The national political consensus also reflected broad agreement about policy (and who was in charge of it) in the states with the highest incidence of the disease. For example, an initiative on the 1988 ballot in California that would have sanctioned considerable discrimination against persons with HIV infection was defeated by more than two to one after being opposed by public-health officials and the leading organizations of health professionals.

Despite the vastly different scale of the epidemic, the history of policy in the United States resembles, in broad outline, events in Britain and Sweden. The federal government and most of the states acted cautiously (too slowly, critics said) during the early years of the epidemic. Since 1985 and especially 1986, however, the federal government and many of the states have become more active in setting policy for the epidemic, relying on experts for advice. At the same time, the fragmentation of American government—by jurisdiction, by competing interests and experts—and the strong impact of moral and emotional issues—especially in local and state affairs have added tension to the consensus.

CONCLUSIONS

In all three countries, policy has been made mainly on the basis of the advice of experts after political leaders in central government (and in several American states) have decided to take the initiative. Moreover, especially since 1985 and 1986, policy in each country has been based on a broad consensus from which there is, as yet, politically ineffective dissent. In all three, interest groups in health affairs have used the epidemic as an opportunity to press for additional resources for AIDS research and prevention and for treatment of drug addiction. Moreover, in all three countries, though with considerably more acrimony in the United States, the institutions that finance health services have accepted the obligation to pay the unanticipated costs of caring for persons with AIDS.

Leaders of organizations of homosexual men have behaved with similar ambivalence in all three countries. On the one hand, they have insisted on positive discrimination: the allocation of additional resources to prevent, treat, and study AIDS. On the other, they have sought to avoid discrimination that could enhance stigmatization. As a result, they have at times emphasized the extent of the danger of HIV to gay men and, at other times, either minimized the threat to their own communities or universalized the epidemic as a threat to heterosexuals.

There are also important differences in the politics of the epidemic and therefore the policy responses to it among the three countries. In the United States, alone of the three, the epidemic is strongly linked to poverty and race. The British have given priority to education and innovative drug programs. The Swedes have emphasized traditional forms of prevention-testing and contact tracing and have greater confidence than the British or Americans that the people handling data about seropositivity will maintain the privacy of individuals. Americans, as they have since the 1940s, find it easier to reach consensus on policy for research than on financing health care.

The policies of all three countries in 1988 are evidence of the authority that medical, scientific, and public-health professionals have acquired during this century, especially since the 1940s. In all three countries, AIDS has been defined as a classic public-health crisis, a temporary threat requiring special policies selected from the repertoire of professionals. As AIDS becomes a chronic problem, however—as it comes to resemble tuberculosis in the nineteenth century or any of the many chronic diseases today—the classic public-health policy model may become less appropriate. If AIDS turns out to be just another killer disease, governments may no longer be able to use fear to justify the allocation of additional resources to study, prevent, and treat it. AIDS already resembles a chronic disease or a severe disability because of its claims on long-term care as well as acute services and its relatively high cost per case. New treatments that increase survival time after infection would make it even more obviously a chronic problem; so would a slowing in the rate of incidence.

Yet AIDS is unlike the leading chronic diseases that provide the epidemiological context for contemporary health policy. It is not a disease of the middle and later years of life. The behaviors that lead to most of the cases evoke little sympathy, much less than overeating, drinking alcoholic beverages, and even smoking do. In the absence of the fear of rapid heterosexual transmission that currently sustains the classic public-health model of response to this epidemic, it may be difficult for experts to continue to make policy by consensus. And if the consensus breaks up because the sense of urgency that has sustained it evaporates, persons with HIV infection may be more at risk of being stigmatized under a chronic-disease model of policy than they are at present.

AIDS raises questions about fundamental values, most of which have, up to now, been transposed into debates among professionals about how to allocate scarce resources. During the past century, experts and public officials devised highly effective methods for restating questions about values as problems of technology and information. To date, policies for AIDS in the three countries we have studied offer many examples of the triumph of the ethic of professionalism over the confused and conflicting claims of morality and ideology. Given uncertainty, it has suited everyone to leave AIDS, like most areas of policy, to the professionals.

Notes

This article was first published in *Daedalus* 118, no. 2 (1989).

Daniel Fox is Professor of Humanities in Medicine and Director of the Center for Assessing Health Services at the State University of New York at Stony Brook. Patricia Day is Senior Research Officer at the Center for the Analysis of Social Policy at the University of Bath in Bath, England.

1. We are grateful to many people in the three countries who spoke with us both on and off the record. Our generalizations are based on these conversations as well as a review of newspapers, magazines, pamphlets, and public documents, which we do not cite here.

2. Our generalizations about political culture and the politics of health care are amplified in Daniel M. Fox, *Health Policies, Health Politics: The British and American Experience, 1911–1965* (Princeton: Princeton University Press, 1986), and in Rudolf Klein, *The Politics of the National Health Service* (London: Longman, 1983 and 1989). For a recent comparative analysis of Sweden, see Christopher Ham, "Governing the Health Sector: Power and Policy Making in the English and Swedish Health Services," *Milbank Quarterly* 66 (2) (1988): 389–414.

3. Sir David Cox, chairman, *Short-term Prediction of HIV Infection and AIDS in England and Wales: Report of a Working Group* (London: Her Majesty's Stationery Office, 1988).

4. House of Commons Social Services Committee, *Problems Associated with AIDS, Session 1986–87* (London: Her Majesty's Stationery Office, 1987), House of Commons, 182–1. See also the Government's response: Department of Health and Social Security, *Problems Associated with AIDS* (London: Her Majesty's Stationery Office, 1988), Cm. 297.

5. Cox.

6. National Swedish Board of Health and Welfare, *HIV and AIDS in Care: An Analytical Survey for the Health Care and Medical Services* (Stockholm: Social-styrelsen, 1988). See also David Finer, "The HIV/AIDS Situation in Sweden," *Current Sweden*, no. 364 (June 1988).

7. National Swedish Board of Health and Welfare, *This Is What the Law Says about HIV and AIDS* (Stockholm: Socialstyrelsen, 1987).

8. *Stockholms Tidningen*, 17 April 1983, 32.

9. Bengt Brorsson and Claes Herlitz, in "The AIDS Epidemic in Sweden: Changes in Awareness, Attitudes and Behavior," unpublished paper, Swedish Medical Research Council, July 1987, reporting results of three mail surveys, conclude that "changes in awareness, attitudes and beliefs have accelerated since the start in March, 1987 of the Swedish AIDS information campaign."

10. Noah's Ark Red Cross Foundation, *An Organization Against HIV and AIDS* (Stockholm: Stiftelsen Noaks Ark-Roeda korset, 1988).

11. For a dissenting view, see Benny Henriksson, *Social Democracy or Societal Control: A Critical Analysis of Swedish AIDS Policy* (Stockholm: Institute for Social Policy-Glacio Bokfoerlag, 1988).

12. For a recent summary, see William L. Heyward and James W. Curran, "The Epidemiology of AIDS in the U.S.," *Scientific American* 259 (4) (1988): 72–81.

13. For a bibliography of leading accounts to 1988 as well as sources for much of what follows, see Daniel M. Fox, "AIDS and the American Health Polity: The History and Prospects of a Crisis of Authority," in Elizabeth Fee and Daniel M. Fox, eds., *AIDS: The Burdens of History* (Berkeley: University of California Press, 1988), a revised version of an article published in *Milbank Quarterly* 64 (suppl. 1) (1986): 7–33.

14. The best account of events within CDC and the Public Health Service in the early 1980s is Elizabeth W. Etheridge, "The Believers: A History of the CDC," unpublished manuscript, Centers for Disease Control, 1988.

15. Various publications of the Intergovernmental Health Project of George Washington University report state law and regulation concerning AIDS. On contact tracing, see Centers for Disease Control, "Partner Notification for Preventing Human Immunodeficiency Virus Infection-Colorado, Idaho, South Carolina, Virginia," *Morbidity and Mortality Weekly Report* 37 (25) (1988), reprinted in the *Journal of the American Medical Association* 260 (5) (1988): 613–15.

16. Daniel M. Fox and Emily H. Thomas, "AIDS Cost Analysis and Social Policy," *Law, Medicine and Health Care* 15 (4) (1987–1988): 186–211. For papers on the cost of the epidemic, see Daniel M. Fox and Emily H. Thomas, *Financing Care for Persons with AIDS: The First Studies, 1985–1988* (Frederick, Md.: University Publishing Group, 1989).

THE POLITICS OF HEALTH CRUSADES

A crusade is one way to describe a campaign for a cause or against an abuse. When the cause is about improving the health of a population, the emphasis is on the positive, the gains available if we exercise more, eat less fat, find employment more quickly, or help our neighbors when they need support. That is part of all public health movements. Framed negatively, the public health position is one of attack. The curbing of abuse requires excising—or at least reducing—bad (unhealthy) conduct or bad (harmful) policy. The history of health promotion provides many instances of crusades. The earlier efforts to reduce or ban drinking alcohol has parallels with the tobacco controls of the late twentieth century; the recent campaigns against obesity and its ill effects on health recall the assault on polluters in the name of health during the early years of the environmental movement. Protecting the population's health provides a powerful justification—the rhetoric of harm reduction—for taking remedial action is common to public health campaigns. Damming the perpetrators of ill health offers a quite different, additional basis for mobilizing support in such initiatives.

There are features of crusades, however, that set them apart and call for attention to their distinctive role in influencing public policy. Consider, for example, tobacco control, the topic of the comparative article that follows. On one side of such policy campaigns are those with substantial stakes at risk if smoking, for example, is banned in pubs, restaurants, and most office buildings. In the language we have used to describe interests, these parties fear substantial material losses. The financial stakeholders—including government monopolies, tobacco companies and farmers, and the other businesses that profit from smoking—have a concentrated, material interest in resisting antismoking policies, whether bans, increased taxes, or more diffuse constraints like ad campaigns. Smokers themselves have obvious (nonmaterial) interest in avoiding control. They can also appeal to libertarian ideas about freedom from the restraints of others where the separation of smokers from nonsmokers is possible.

This was the nature of the struggle over tobacco control through much of the twentieth century: public health campaigners in and outside of government, with their allies in the scientific community set against well-organized financial stakeholders and their anti-paternalistic allies. For most of the twentieth century and across the globe, the tobacco interests were not only protected by public policy, but often subsidized. So, what accounts for the broad demands for increased control that became evident in the 1960s and over the next forty years became the norm across the industrial democracies? And, equally, what explains the great differences in tone, timing, and content of antismoking policies adopted by the countries we studied?

Public health campaigners against smoking have always had difficulties with the traditional liberal claim that citizens should be free to choose their habits provided their behavior did not harm others. Endless appeals to the harm smoking does to the smokers did not so much fall on deaf ears as fail to respond to the libertarian counterargument and mobilize latent interests in tobacco control. An important rhetorical answer—as with campaigns to prohibit drinking, prostitution, and all such ills—was to associate the health harm with sin, with wrongful conduct. Put differently, public health campaigns have regularly insisted that we not only give up habits that are *bad* for one's health, but also accept that it is *wrong* to do harm to innocent others. The appeal—to moral language as against the reduction of harm—is only one approach to balancing concentrated material interests with compelling nonmaterial stakeholders. Advocates of right conduct have a chance to redress the balance of interests if and only if they give nonsmokers good grounds for helping their cause. After all, even those who would prefer a nonsmoking environment, or one without fat people, have no selective incentive to help the campaign. (By selective we mean that there is no way those who don't support the campaign can be denied the benefits of its success.) The politics of reform in these areas, then, takes on the element of moralistic campaigning. And moral sentiment, if more widely shared, further empowers the public health reformers against their organized and financially better placed opposition. This is precisely the story outlined in the discussion of the roads to increased tobacco control in eight democracies over the last four decades of the twentieth century. The direction of change was toward increased control everywhere, while the pace and character of the policy responses varied considerably. Indeed, moralistic campaigning, it is clear, was far more prominent in the United States and Canada than, for instance, in Great Britain.

The analysis of interest representation and its impact on the strategy of reform is not, however, restricted to the tobacco story. The standard analysis of political influence begins with the importance of organized, intense interests. What the politics of crusades illustrates is the need—evident in tobacco control—to supply an intense opposition that goes beyond the ideals of public health reformers. And that additional element is identifying wrong behavior, not just unhealthy behavior.

This brings us back to the importance of how interest groups can reframe what is at issue to change the balance of power. The public health community has many more causes than successful crusades. The benefits the public health campaigns celebrate are typically distant in time or likelihood: greater longevity, lesser chances of diabetes, or less likelihood of injury. The costs it promotes are almost always immediate, material, and significant. No wonder then that we see in public health the elements of crusading, the celebration of a positive cause, and the demonization of those associated with the threat to health.

Health crusades are not the only area where appeals to moral rightness and decent conduct are found. All the efforts to change how health care is financed, delivered, and regulated have principled sources. But the language of good and bad is especially salient in many public health campaigns, transforming scientific appeals about harmful consequences into a more complicated rhetorical mix of improvement and punishment. The tobacco wars provide a particularly clear illustration of this process. The scientific frauds the tobacco companies committed in how they used and abused medical research gave the public health reformers villains to attack. That in turn gave credence to a posture of moral outrage and strengthened the argument that tobacco should be more severely controlled. But how and when that argument prevailed varied substantially, as our article shows. (What is equally fascinating, but not elaborated here, is how social norms have transformed who smokes rather than where. What was once fashionable to the middle and upper classes has increasingly become a pariah status, leaving smoking more and more to the less privileged members of society.)

Tobacco Control in Comparative Perspective

Eight Nations in Search of an Explanation

Theodore R. Marmor and Evan S. Lieberman

Since the 1960s, governments in economically advanced democratic nations have significantly increased their regulatory control of tobacco. The prevalence of cigarette smoking has diminished in these countries. Factors other than government policy—especially shifts in social norms—have influenced that decline, but those norms have themselves been directly and indirectly influenced by government policies. In short, tobacco consumption has become, in part, a political outcome. Governments have been sites of great conflict over the use of tobacco, with reform regularly taking on a moralistic tone in all the country experience reviewed in this writing: Japan, France, Germany, Denmark, The United Kingdom, Australia, Canada and The United States.[1]

There are solid grounds for believing that the contemporary efforts of industrial democracies to control smoking reflect some common causes and, as a consequence, similar control policies. After all, the scientific evidence about the effects of smoking has substantiated long-standing, widespread health concerns about tobacco. Moreover, the international dissemination of scientific knowledge has undeniably helped to legitimate reform efforts across the nations. In addition, by the end of the twentieth century, diverse modern democracies had come to use very similar instruments in the effort to discourage smoking in their populations. Available to the advanced industrialized democracies, at least from the late 1950s, the widely published information emerged in summary form in the U.S. Surgeon General's report of 1964[2] (British and Canadian counterparts were published earlier). By the 1960s, elites in all the industrial democracies had substantial information about, and overwhelming scientific support, for claims that tobacco use harmed their citizens generally and was a major contributor to lung cancer and heart disease. Moreover, since health expenditures constituted a large share of the national budgets of all the industrial democracies, the costs of treating tobacco-related diseases were (and are) plain to informed health policy actors. Concerns about the costs of smoking-related illness thus provided another common source of pressure to reduce tobacco consumption. Of course, governmental revenues from taxation on tobacco have provided an obvious countervailing force—since budget officials gained revenues from the consumption of tobacco.[3]

Policymakers faced a relatively common and well-understood menu of possible control policies. In Australia, Canada, Denmark, France, Germany, Japan, the United Kingdom, and the United States, tobacco products are taxed above and beyond ordinary taxation on most goods. In most democracies, government policy makes some effort to limit tobacco-company advertising, to control tobacco sales and distribution, and to apply warning labels on cigarettes and other tobacco products in order to prevent or to limit the use of tobacco. Paternalistic constraints on sales to non-adults have long been regarded as consistent with liberal democratic values. Moreover, certain public places came to be protected by every government as smoke-free zones. Airlines are now the most commonly restricted site.[4] But the range of restricted sites varies from hospitals (common) to workplaces (increasingly common) to public parks (rare). The last two decades of the twentieth century were years of convergence in the tobacco-control agendas in most industrial democracies.

The convergence of policy calls for explanation. Indeed, one of the most important findings of this comparative study is the active and successful dissemination of evidence, argument, and program examples across the borders of quite different nations. Identifying the reasons for convergence in these respects is an explanatory task that we address later. First we want to address differences in the pace and paths taken in the tobacco-control efforts of the eight countries investigated in depth.

It is much less clear exactly how to represent and interpret the magnitude of these comparative differences. Each of the eight countries, from the perspective of detailed policies and practices, employs what could be considered a unique configuration of tobacco controls. So, for instance, it is obvious that Denmark came to rely on heavy tobacco taxes long before Canada and the United States and did so less in order to control use than to increase tax revenues. Likewise, modest French efforts (as of 1999) to control where smoking is permitted shows how much more vigorous such constraints were in Australia, Canada, and the United States. When we turn to the intensity of implementation, the differences appear to be matters more of degree than of kind. Nonetheless, there is a serious problem in characterizing the level of implemented controls, and explaining why varied patterns of control may have emerged across the advanced, industrialized countries.

One way of thinking about such national differences is to raise the following hypothetical question. If a foreign visitor, innocent of the prevailing national norms and customs, were to travel to each of these countries and wanted to smoke, how would that person's experiences vary in terms of government prohibitions and controls? If we had a common measure of restriction, we would be better able to arrange the nations on a spectrum of tobacco control intensity. With a more refined comparative measure of control, we would be able to more precisely analyze similarities and differences in the regulation of smoking in particular settings, whether bars, hospital waiting rooms, public parks, or public libraries. With broad strokes, we seek to describe *tobacco-control regimes*, by which we mean the aggregated set of policies and practices that governments use to control tobacco.

Our further aim is to identify the extent to which these differences in tobacco-control regimes are predictable or unexpected from the perspective of well-known political, economic, and institutional features of these countries. For our purposes, the historical characterizations of tobacco control introduce more complexity than we can handle for our cross-national comparison. We therefore focus on explaining patterns of cross-national variation in tobacco-control regimes at the end of the twentieth century, and do not attempt to account for patterns of continuity and change within the respective country histories. Even this more modest task is neither straightforward nor easy. Detailed, "thick" descriptions of national control policies are not easily compared or explained.[5] Precisely because these country histories avoid simplistic characterizations of national policies, grouping countries into clusters that suggest explanatory patterns is a significant challenge. So, for example, legal traditions (common law versus civil code) do not seem to illuminate these policy histories. Nor does an easy division between Catholic and Protestant nations — and our sample was suitable for testing that hypothesis. Taking into account the structure and dynamics of states with unitary, rather than federal, political institutions proved a more promising approach, as Nathanson has argued in a probing essay on comparative tobacco politics.[6] The respective tobacco control regimes emerge as largely consistent with broader public attitudes about the importance of health and "well-being," but we have less confidence about whether such attitudes influence the development of control legislation, or if the direction of causation is reversed.

VARIATION IN TOBACCO-CONTROL REGIMES

We can begin to understand the range of variation in tobacco-control regimes by considering five logically possible outcomes:

- *Hands-off tobacco regimes.* Governments in these countries have no policies restricting tobacco use or distribution, and any taxation associated with tobacco is indistinguishable from taxes on other products.
- *Low-control regimes.* Such countries are defined by minimal efforts to control the use of tobacco. Policies to make the public aware of the dangers of smoking and to prevent minors from having easy access to cigarettes characterize such regimes. Tobacco taxes are low in these regimes.
- *Moderate-control regimes.* These countries are defined by a significant set of tobacco-control policies across the broad spectrum of policy targets, including the promotion, distribution, and consumption of tobacco. What differentiates moderate- from high-control regimes is the degree of restrictiveness: the enforcement of some or all of the control policies may be more lax in the moderate regimes; taxation may not be particularly high; and restrictions on tobacco may be more measured.
- *High-control regimes.* These countries are characterized by high levels of taxation on tobacco products and by across-the-board policies that tightly restrict the promotion and consumption of tobacco.
- *Prohibitionist regimes.* Tobacco use is banned completely, and people are seriously punished for selling or consuming tobacco.

In practice, none of the countries investigated is an example of either of the two extremes. The eight nations vary across the range of what we have described as low to high control. To classify the countries by degree of policy restraint, we distinguish sharply between taxation and other forms of tobacco control. One reason for doing so concerns the countervailing fiscal imperative of tobacco taxation. After all, for much of the history of tobacco use, governments regarded tobacco taxation exclusively as a means of generating revenue, not as an instrument of health promotion. It makes sense, then, to separate taxation levels from the other types of restrictions placed on the tobacco industry and cigarette consumers. The problem is not that taxation levels are less important in influencing smoking behavior. In fact, the scientific consensus is that the price elasticity of tobacco consumption is relatively high.[7] Rather, the problem is that taxation is a more complex policy matter than, for example, regulating where smoking is permitted. With taxation, finance and health ministries can agree on higher prices for opposite reasons: increasing revenues in the first instance and reducing smoking in the second. Whether this tax measure correlates well with regulatory restrictions is something to be discovered rather than assumed. And as we have discovered, there is room for doubt.

In the case of taxation, it is relatively easy to compare the tax that each country levied per pack of cigarettes during any given time period. We gathered data from the World Bank Economics of Tobacco Control Project, which reported

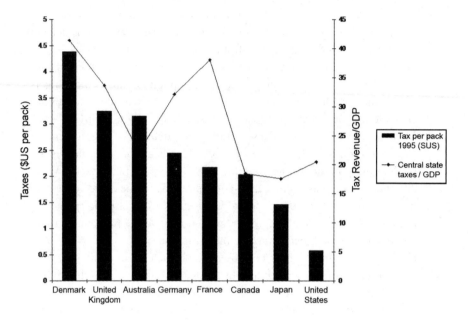

Figure 1. Tobacco Taxes and Total Taxation in
Eight Advanced Industrialized Countries

cigarette taxes per pack for 1995 in U.S. dollars. In 1995, the average taxes for the
eight countries were $2.43 per pack, and ranged from a low of $.58 per pack in
the United States to a high of $4.38 per pack in Denmark.[8]

In examining the results in Figure 1, we found ourselves wondering whether
in trying to control tobacco consumption, countries use tax and non-tax policy
instruments in tandem. As it turns out, there is clearly some correlation between
these two components of tobacco-control regimes as we have defined them. But
the connection is quite mixed, with Canada and the United States providing
contradictory evidence. Tax competition under federalism may well be part of
the explanation for the low level of tobacco taxation in the United States; the
fear is that wide variations in tax levels among states would encourage interstate
smuggling. But Canada's federal regime provides evidence of high national levels of taxation along with significant variations in provincial taxes. The instability of the high-tax Canadian regime may well make the North American experience less problematic, but we are still left with the puzzle of the Australian
federal example of very high tax levels as shown in Figure 1.

There is clearly a strong relationship between levels of tobacco taxation and
overall levels of taxation in the countries studied. Although a cohort of eight

countries is not a powerful sample for statistical analysis, the correlation coefficient estimating the relationship between tobacco taxes per pack and the ratio of central state taxation to gross domestic product is .67—implying that almost 50 percent of the variance in tobacco taxes can be explained by the country's tax regime. (If taxes from all levels of government are included, the statistical relationship is weaker.) Of course, there are several possible causal explanations for this correlation. One hypothesis is that in high-tax countries, it is easier to pass high taxes of any kind. A second is that levels of taxation reflect the size and authority of the state within society, and that in countries with higher levels of taxation, we should expect higher levels of tobacco control, of which tobacco taxation is one component. Where substantial welfare states are involved, any substantial luxury tax that is legitimate commands attention.

Regarding non-tax policies designed to restrict smoking, it was necessary to aggregate the instruments used to change smoking behavior and those used to limit the available options for where people may smoke. Given the difficulties of measuring such policies comparatively with any precision, we opted for a rough-and-ready three-point scale, ranging from low (1), to medium (2), to high (3). Applying this scale required that we categorize countries in terms of both the scope and the (apparent) intensity of their tobacco-control policies. (We could not confidently categorize the enforcement of those policies, for which reliable data are much harder to obtain.) That is to say, we considered both the sheer quantity of restrictions on tobacco use, as well as the degree to which they appear to have been implemented through voluntary agreements, legal guidelines, or bans on smoking in particular places.

Without a shared standard for measuring non-tax policies for restricting smoking, we deployed two main sources of data and several alternative specifications for interpreting those data. First, we used Feldman and Bayer's detailed country portraits as the initial source of data.[9] On that basis we initially scored each country on the three-point scale. Second, we surveyed the authors of those studies and asked them to reduce their detailed characterizations of the contemporary tobacco-control regimes and provide us answers using the same metric. We received responses from most of the authors and found that our readings were somewhat at odds with how the authors themselves characterized their respective national portraits. In the cases of Canada and Japan, there was agreement that the evidence pointed to cases of high and low control, respectively. Denmark, the United Kingdom, and the United States produced only small discrepancies, with all three countries scoring as high or medium-high for at least the contemporary period.[10] But in France and Germany, important differences in interpretation emerged. Both of us interpreted Germany as an

Table 1: Comparing Country Scorings of National Tobacco Control

| Source: | Tobacco Control Scores | | | Tax/Pack |
	Readers	Author	American Cancer Society	Bank World
Australia	3 (3,3)	N/A	3	$3.15
Canada	3 (3,3)	3	3	$2.04
Denmark	2.5 (3,2)	2.5	3	$4.38
France	2 (3,1)	3	3	$2.17
Germany	1 (1,1)	2	2	$2.44
Japan	1 (1,1)	1	1	$1.46
United Kingdom	2.5 (3,2)	3	3	$3.24
United States	2.75 (2.5, 3)	3	2	$0.58

Sources: Country chapters, World Bank Economics of Tobacco Control Website

instance of low control, while the author scored it as one of medium control. The two of us initially interpreted the chapter on France differently—one as involving high control, and the other, low control—while the author scored it as a case of high control. How strongly the antismoking policies were implemented and/or enforced proved to be the source of our different interpretations. Ultimately, we concluded that France was best classified as a case of "low-medium" control. Legal rules and their enforcement are separable dimensions of such restrictions. Simply knowing what the "law" is does not enable us to say which particular practices dominate.

Finally, we considered the very extensive American Cancer Society report on tobacco control around the world, which included country profiles of national policies.[11] In investigating four of the report's policy categories (advertising and sponsorship, sales and distribution restrictions, tobacco product regulations, and smoke-free indoor air restrictions), we developed a numerical index for the state of legislation in each area, assigning more weight to policies that involved outright bans, and less weight to policies encouraging voluntary cooperation. We then took a straight average of the scores of those four policy areas, each of which had been assigned a numerical score of 1 for low control, 2 for medium control, and 3 for high control, in order to arrive at an overall index of the extent of non-tax tobacco control in each country.

The results of the above exercise largely confirmed the findings from the interpretations set forth in the country chapters—with modest, but not trivial, discrepancies. The American Cancer Society's data suggested, for example, that the United States had a less intensive control regime than what is reported in Alan Brandt's report. The society's score for Denmark was slightly higher, and its scores for France and Germany were a full point higher than ours (as were the scores by the respective authors). These differences illustrate the general problem in cross-national studies of identifying which phenomena are equivalent and therefore need to be similarly explained. With these qualifications in mind, we compare the eight cases in an exploratory mode.

In Figure 2, we plotted each of the eight countries by what we take to be their tax and non-tax control policies during the late 1990s. We found several interesting patterns of convergence and divergence in the scoring of national policies. These patterns bring into clearer relief some of the more interesting puzzles apparent in the countries' distinctive trajectories of tobacco control. No country is a more obvious example of a low-control tobacco regime than Japan, where both tax and non-tax control policies were slack. But that does not mean that Japan is free of antismoking influences. Indeed, there have been important changes in the world of Japanese smoking; for example, as Eric Feldman notes, the level of smoking has fallen substantially in recent decades, and the range of places where it is thought appropriate to smoke has become much more restricted.

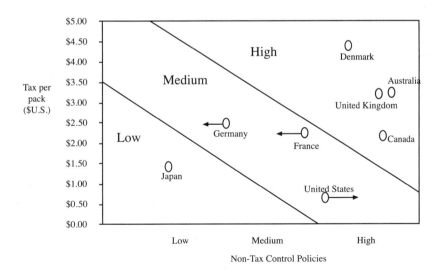

Figure 2. Tobacco Control Regimes in Eight Advanced Industrialized Countries

What is especially noteworthy, however, is that Japanese public policy does not appear to have been the main instrument of these changes.[12] The Japanese case study illustrates,[13] moreover, the cross-national transfer of tobacco-control strategies; witness the recent efforts to use litigation as a means of circumventing the inaction of the executive and legislative branches of government.

We have classified as high-control regimes Australia, Canada, Denmark, and the United Kingdom. Although in Canada, taxes per pack are lower than in the other high-control cases,[14] and most of the intensity of Canada's tobacco control arose fairly late. Nonetheless, Canada's extensive non-tax controls during the last decades of the twentieth century justify its classification as a case of high control.

In the middle of our grouping are France, Germany, and the United States, all of which are more difficult to classify. Both France and Germany—as of the late 1990s—had medium-level taxes between $2.00 and $3.00 per pack, and the United States had extremely low tobacco taxes (on average). Our interpretation of non-tax control policies suggests that France and Germany may be closer to the low-control regimes and that the United States may be closer to the high-control regimes based on levels of implementation in practice. Nathanson's overall portrait of French law and practice supports our interpretation, by emphasizing the gap between strict legal controls and restrained enforcement, especially on the issue of where one might smoke in public.[15] Likewise, Frankenberg's study of tobacco policy in Germany does not support an interpretation of vigorous control.[16] Indeed, what is striking about both the French and German cases is the degree to which the enforcement of non-tax tobacco controls remains relatively lenient. Moreover, in the United States there are wide differences in how particular states regulate and control tobacco. The interpretation of policy in these federal countries is, as a consequence, strongly mediated by how subnational variation is taken into account.

DISCUSSION AND ANALYSIS

As noted earlier, we began our investigation with a variety of hypotheses about what might explain variations in tobacco-control policies. In practice, we have mostly sought to understand the shape of those policies and to suggest, more than provide, explanations. For example, in reflecting on our scores for the eight countries' tax and non-tax control policies, we ended up highlighting puzzles for which no easy answers are immediately apparent. Some aspects of the cross-national variation seem readily explainable from what we already know about these countries. Other aspects appear explainable only in terms of historically contingent political contexts or the countries' idiosyncratic configurations of the tobacco industry, political organization, and policy responses—that is, through the "thick" descriptive accounts set forth in country case studies. In this section, we want to describe our admittedly tentative interpretation of some of the leading explanatory claims about tobacco control.

There is now a moderately large literature that purports to describe and explain tobacco politics and policies.[17] Our purpose here is not, however, to provide a definitive statement about the merits of different explanatory approaches, but simply to highlight what seem to be promising ways to make sense of the complex portraits. In particular, we address three classes of explanatory approaches—policy diffusion, political culture, and political institutions.

The *policy diffusion* literature in comparative political analysis provides accounts that link national experience through the various means by which policy-reform ideas move across borders. This approach is undoubtedly helpful in making sense of the increased control of smoking that we observe in all the national portraits (if not all of the OECD nations). It is surely the case that cross-border diffusion helps to explain the similar menu of programmatic interventions in tobacco control. The scientific information about tobacco's effects has been widely diffused. Moreover, there was also surely diffusion of information about tobacco-control modes. These approaches to control—whether tax increases, education campaigns, limits on where smoking could take place, or restrictions on advertising or sports sponsorship—were first diffused by networks of scientific and public health actors, and later by what amounted to internationally linked social movements and pressure groups.

Indeed, from a global perspective, the diffusion of these pressures has led to some degree of convergence in tobacco-control regimes. Smoking has been transformed from an accepted (and romanticized) habit in the middle of the twentieth century to a challenged, if not reviled, practice by the opening of the twenty-first century. Donley Studlar's work demonstrates the increased salience in contemporary control regimes of "denormalizing" smoking.[18] That has involved making smoking itself sinful, stupid, or both. And it can also involve demonizing those who produce, sell, or use tobacco products. By contrast, the harm-reduction principle of traditional public health is perfectly consistent with educational campaigns, but not vilification. There is considerable evidence that by the beginning of the twenty-first century, the effort to turn tobacco smokers and producers into pariahs had become crucial elements in anti-tobacco movements.[19]

However, the diffusion argument is less useful for explaining patterns of variation. Typically, diffusion arguments suggest the importance of physical proximity as a basis for policy adoption, but the comparative portrait we present in Figure 1 contradicts this view: the neighboring pairs of Germany and Denmark and the United States and Canada appear more different than similar in the overall characterizations of tobacco control. Moreover, the clustering of the United Kingdom, Australia, and Canada as largely similar types of tobacco control regimes, despite the fact that these countries are located at different corners of the globe, suggests the need to consider other approaches. Even in the face of the European Union's (EU) efforts to gain supranational control over tobacco use, the codification and implementation of policies have remained nationally distinct within Europe.

What is termed *political culture* in comparative politics is another plausible approach to explaining variation in the control measures adopted or rejected.[20] We reject the notion of a "smoking" culture as a determinant of tobacco control regime-type, because smoking has been popular in all of the countries under examination in this volume, and norms and patterns of tobacco use have changed in response to new information and especially to changes in government policy. An alternative view of the possible influence of culture would relate more general norms and customs regarding the paternalistic nature of the state and authority, and the value of liberal individualism to the propensity of a given country to adopt more or less aggressive control measures.

A classic statement of how such cultural patterns can shape other types of political and economic outcomes is Max Weber's *Protestant Ethic*,[21] which is perhaps the most well-known example of how religious orientations can shape institutions and outcomes as profound as the functioning of modern capitalism. For the more focused problem considered here, one might imagine that the more Catholic the nation, the more accepting its political culture would be of alleged "sins" like smoking, and the less onerous would be the implemented forms of control. Alternatively, one could imagine higher levels of paternalism in Catholic approaches. Yet neither the country portraits in this book nor our own interpretations provide a solid basis for this way of explaining tobacco-control policies. For instance, the varying policies over time within each country argue against using religious or cultural orientations as a cross-national explanation. As Brandt has argued, basic cultural foundations change less rapidly than smoking habits.[22] The United States, where prohibitionist zeal was vividly expressed in alcohol control, went from a nation that broadly celebrated smoking during the World War II era to one that, a few decades later, was home to some of the globe's most zealous critics of smoking behavior and of tobacco companies.[23] Similarly, Canada's widespread acceptance of smoking as late as the early 1980s gave way to an equally zealous condemnation by both public authorities and antismoking figures a decade later.

A more promising approach to culture is contained in the investigation carried out by Ronald Inglehart and his collaborators on the World Values Survey.[24] Although their view of culture is not infinitely malleable, it explicitly allows for changing norms and values over time. Reporting results from their 1990–1 surveys, they provide a mapping of countries in terms of the values emphasized by different societies—both in terms of the emphasis on "survival" versus "well-being,"[25] and "traditional authority" versus "secular-rational authority." Along these dimensions, the U.S. clusters with Canada as a "North American group," and Denmark with Germany as a "Northern Europe" group. France clusters with "Catholic Europe," Japan with China and Korea (labeled by Inglehart as the "Confucian countries"), and the United Kingdom straddles both the "Northern Europe group" and a larger cluster of "English-speaking countries," which includes Canada and the United States. Although the survey was not conducted in Australia, one would assume that it would cluster with this last group. This ordering of countries in terms of culture does a better job of predicting tobacco control regimes then would a more narrow focus on religious orientations, particularly given the high degree of religious heterogeneity in many of the countries studied.

Most importantly, Denmark and Japan are described in Inglehart's study as extreme cases in terms of the degree to which societies value "well-being" (Denmark) versus "survival" (Japan), and this maps perfectly onto our scoring of the tobacco regimes, as depicted in Figure 1. France and Germany appear as "intermediate" cases along the cultural continuum; they are intermediate cases of tobacco control. However, the cultural framework is less useful for explaining differences in tobacco control regimes among the United Kingdom, the United States, and Canada, which are depicted as having highly similar cultures. Nonetheless, Inglehart's view of culture provides a reasonable degree explanatory power, as the basic emphasis on "well-being," within societies appears to correlate, if not perfectly, with the extent of tobacco control. We still cannot be sure, however, if tobacco and other forms of social control influence these cultural attitudes or if the reverse is true.

A third explanatory framework can be drawn from a literature on *political institutions*, which relates variations in institutional rules to cross-national differences in policy outcomes.[26] The notion here is that policy outcomes depend not merely on the underlying preferences of actors within society, but on how those preferences get aggregated and adjudicated. Among the economic interests with influential concerns are tobacco farmers, those media that are dependent on tobacco advertisements, the manufacturers and distributors of tobacco products, and most importantly, local and multinational tobacco companies. They compete with ministries of health, finance, and various political groups who may desire both tax and non-tax controls. All of the countries studied face these constituency pressures (with the exception of tobacco farmers in countries where this crop is not a significant industry). What differs from country to country is the particular configuration of the institutional channels through which these interests seek expression.

In particular, the impact of a polity being organized along federal or unitary principles should be considered as an important explanatory principle. However, there are again conflicting views about how to interpret the influence of such institutional differences. One hypothesis is that unitary states, if they have the political will, have the institutional structure to implement control policies more quickly and effectively because they enjoy a more uniform sphere of influence. Holding reform pressures constant, it is plausible that unitary regimes would be able to implement more extensive controls earlier and more concertedly than non-unitary regimes. On the other hand, it appears quite plausible that the location and influence of reform pressures actually vary across countries according to institutional differences. In federal polities, political pressures for control are more likely to be pressed in those subnational units where they are most likely to meet success, providing greater opportunities for innovation. In unitary regimes, there is arguably only one key arena in which political conflict over tobacco control is likely to take place, and opponents of control can focus their power and influence at the national level. The implications for tobacco control appear to be important.

For example, Constance Nathanson argues that different types of actors will emerge as influential within different types of institutional settings. She has noted that where hierarchical and centralized political arrangements provide access for elites—especially scientific ones in the case of tobacco—a distinctive mode of tobacco-control policymaking emerges.[27] The cases of unitary states in our sample—Denmark, France, Japan, and the United Kingdom—support that claim. By contrast, the less centralized, federal states—Australia, Canada, the United States, and, to a lesser extent, Germany—show the relatively greater impact of outsiders, of nonscientific advocates willing to be more provocative in their challenge to smoking and the tobacco firms. The federal states provide ample evidence of diffusion—of evidence, argument, and tactics—across the subnational units.

In all regimes, institutional arrangements shape the strategies of the actors, as the country portraits fully document. In every case, the tobacco industry spends substantial sums defending its interests; that is no surprise. But which groups take up the banner of tobacco control does vary considerably among the cases. In federal regimes with ideological heterogeneity, one would expect control advocates to shop for venues to pursue antismoking policy reforms. Elite accommodation of organized interests is more likely to be found in the unitary states. We would expect extreme political actors to be more powerful in federal systems, and indeed, with the exception of Germany, that is precisely what we found in the country portraits.[28]

This perspective makes sense of the commonality in the high level of non-tax control policies that emerged by the end of the twentieth century in Australia, Canada, and the United States. We are not suggesting that federalism itself is the explanation. Indeed, it is surely true that federal regimes make national leadership over subnational units generally more difficult, as the case of Canada suggests. (Canada represents an instance where national institutions came to play a major role in advocating tobacco controls.) Instead, we believe that there is a crucial interaction of federalism, pressure-group strategies, and social movements in liberal regimes. That interaction makes it more likely that the most vigorous attacks on tobacco interests will arise first at the local level rather than at the level of national politics.[29]

Although most of the federal cases tend toward high-control, non-tax policies, the unitary states are more varied in their approach to tobacco control. Again, Japan and Denmark represent the important extremes along the control continuum while simultaneously being cases of unitary states. Within our small sample, this suggests that the presence of federalism provides a more consistent influence on outcomes than does the absence of this institutional feature. Although we have not systematically compared the extent of tobacco control at the subnational level, the evidence available to us indicates that some of the most extreme forms of tobacco control are enacted within particular subnational units in the federal countries. For example, California and Minnesota are antismoking leaders, even while states such as Alabama and Georgia maintain more minimal controls. Similarly, British Columbia is far more restrictive than Alberta, and New South Wales than Queensland. We believe that federalism provides more opportunities for policy innovation, and in turn, that policy diffusion tends to be easier across subnational units than across countries (as discussed earlier in the article). In unitary states, antismoking radicals are less likely to be influential if they do not have a strong, national constituency. This may explain why the unitary states demonstrate very high or very low control regimes, whereas the federal polities tend towards medium and high control. In federal countries, just a few important pockets of tobacco control advocacy can be successful in pushing for at least a modicum of legislation.

Germany is an exception to the claim that federalism will lead to more to-bacco control. As it turns out, the potential impact of "competitive federalism" has been counter-balanced by resistance to aggressive health promotion poli-cies. Günter Frankenberg's portrait of Germany[30] identifies several factors that, he hypothesizes, have contributed to relatively low levels of tobacco control. These include the revenue imperative, skillful tobacco and media industries, the popularity of smoking, a limited group of enlightened experts, and the ab-sence of a successful social movement, in the wake of resistance to state pater-nalism. Frankenburg argues that such resistance rests, in part, on the legacy of coercive, morally objectionable, Nazi-era policies directed at improving the health of the German nation. Of the plausible explanations for German ex-ceptionalism, only the last withstands comparative scrutiny.[31] The first three are present in cases of both low- and high-control regimes, and the absence of experts seems to be more a product of potential political impact than lack of information, given the widespread availability of common scientific knowledge about the effects of smoking. This is not to say that the other factors he identifies do *not* matter. Rather it is that the task of explaining the German case requires that we identify why these forces were *more* powerful as checks on efforts to control tobacco than in the other countries.

While cross-national variation in the presence or absence of federalism helps to explain some of the important differences in tobacco control regimes, clearly the relationship is not perfectly linear, nor does it trump all nationally-specific political histories and legacies. If we had characterized countries in an alterna-tive manner—for example comparing countries in terms of the most extreme local examples of control, rather than using broad national portraits that in-corporate "typical" subnational policies, the relationship between federalism and the extent of tobacco control might have appeared stronger. Other types of institutional variation, including the nature of political party systems, or the presence/absence of plebiscitary mechanisms for adopting policies could be explored in future research about the political determinants of tobacco policy.

CONCLUSIONS

Understanding the determinants of contemporary tobacco regimes requires that we understand the factors and pressures that simultaneously influenced convergence and divergence across countries. A mix of generalizable and historically contingent factors must be taken into account.

Our comparative analysis has attempted to provide a coherent synthesis of contemporary tobacco-control regimes in eight advanced, industrialized democracies. It prompted us to ask some general questions about the determinants of policy and practice. We do not pretend to provide any simple conclusions about why tobacco control regimes vary across these countries—our analyses are admittedly rudimentary. However, we have attempted to demonstrate some of the added analytic value of an expressly comparative approach, in which the possibilities for reaching general conclusions are far greater than in single-country studies.

One of the lessons from this collective exercise is simple, but important. In comparative policy analysis, the twin problems of conceptualization and measurement are, to say the least, challenging. State authority comes in many forms, and it is not always easy to describe the differences as simply "more" or "less."

Our overall conclusion is that certain factors predictably constrain the development of tobacco-control regimes, and political institutions provide an important starting point for explaining patterns of cross-national variation, even if they do not determine the control policies of a given country or the role of the state in tobacco more generally. More general cultural orientations towards "well-being" do appear to be associated with the extent of control policies, but the exact direction of causality cannot be inferred from our analysis. Because these countries are all wealthy democracies, levels of income and political regime type cannot be said to explain differences among these countries, but such factors would likely be influential in a broader comparative study.

Although we do not take a normative approach in this investigation of tobacco control, we believe that this restricted comparative analysis will be useful to others trying to understand the national histories of tobacco control in order to design and to reform policy. Simply put, it is not possible to draw lessons about tobacco reform from other countries without a baseline understanding of how countries compare, particularly in the contemporary era. The complexity of national context and national histories is important. But given the welter of experience there is value to simplification as well.

Notes

This article was originally published in Eric A. Feldman and Ronald Bayer, *Unfiltered: Conflicts over Tobacco Policy and Public Health* (Cambridge, MA: Harvard University Press, 2004). This work was supported (in part) by an Investigator Award in Health Policy Research from The Robert Wood Johnson Foundation. The views expressed are those of the authors and do not imply endorsement by The Robert Wood Johnson Foundation.

The authors gratefully acknowledge the careful attention and comments from Ron Bayer and Eric Feldman, who have commented extensively on several drafts. We thank the various authors of the chapters from *Unfiltered: Conflicts over Tobacco Policy and Public Health* for providing the basis for much of our analysis, and for responding to our repeated queries. Thanks also to members of the Robert Wood Johnson Health Policy Seminar at Yale University for their probing comments and questions.

1. This comparative analysis constituted the closing chapter of the book and is reprinted here with minor revisions and editing, all directed at making the article clear to the new reader.

2. The report was published by the Surgeon General—the federal government's principal spokesperson on matters of public health—appointed by the President with the advice and consent of the Senate. In 1964 the Surgeon General reviewed more than 7,000 scientific articles with the help of over 150 consultants. The report highlighted the deleterious health consequences of tobacco use.

3. Frank J. Chaloupka, Melanie Wakefield, and Christina Czart, "Taxing Tobacco: The Impact of Tobacco Taxes on Cigarette Smoking and Other Tobacco Use," in *Regulating Tobacco*, eds. Robert L. Rabin and Stephen D. Sugarman (New York: Oxford University Press, 2001).

4. A. Brandt, "Differences and Diffusion: Cross Cultural Perspectives on the Rise of Anti-Tobacco Policies" in *Unfiltered*, p. 268ff.

5. Our original aim was to offer explanations for the different patterns of control policies across the eight cases. We anticipated accounting for this variation on three dimensions. One was the *timing* of policy action—the dates of which differed widely in the country studies. A second dimension was variation in the extensiveness of policy interventions. We thought of that as the *scope* of tobacco control. Those controls range in principle from outright bans on smoking in all public places, to financial penalties to the smoker and restrictions on advertising to the young (and others), to limited educational campaigns about the dangers of smoking. A third potential dimension was the *intensity* of policy implementation. By that we understood the policies in practice, which would most reliably indicate the character of each tobacco-control regime. Unfortunately, this aim was impossible to satisfy in practice. The elements of policy action were differently conceptualized, and the documentation of implemented policies was not consistently available across all the cases. The different country narratives stimulated the quest for a better understanding of how tobacco control policies varied cross-nationally from a more static perspective at the end of the 20th century. For a discussion of the costs, benefits, and limits of cross-national policy research, see Theodore R. Marmor, Amy Bridges, and Wayne Hoffman, "Comparative Politics and Health Policies: Notes on Benefits, Costs, and Limits," in *Comparing Public Policies: New Concepts and Methods*, ed. Douglas E. Ashford (Beverly Hills, CA: Sage Publications, 1978). For an informed discussion of the problem of comparability in what is to be explained in, and learned from, comparative policy analysis, see Rudolf Klein, "Learning from Others: Shall the Last Be the First?" (paper presented at the Four Country Conference on Health Care Reforms in the United States, Canada, Germany and the Netherlands, Amsterdam, February 1995). Also appeared in JHPPL, Vol. 22, No. 5 (October 1997), pp. 1267–1278.

6. See Constance A. Nathanson, "Tobacco Politics: Nation-States and Collective Action" (unpublished).

7. Chaloupka, Wakefield, and Czart, "Taxing Tobacco: The Impact of Tobacco Taxes on Cigarette Smoking and Other Tobacco Use," op. cit.

8. Using alternative measures of taxation, such as tax as the proportion of cigarette price in 2000 (Judith Mackay, Michael P. Eriksen, and the World Health Organization). *The Tobacco Atlas* (Geneva: World Health Organization, 2000) provides essentially the same rank orderings, and the two measures are highly correlated (Pearson's $r = .84$). We prefer the nominal, per-pack measure because it is not influenced by the relative cost of consumer goods in each country. The persistence of the relative tax burdens across countries during the last decade of the twen-

tieth century suggests that while within-country changes may seem dramatic from the vantage point of a single nation, a comparative perspective highlights the need to distinguish between variations of degree and of kind. We are focused on the latter.

9. Eric Feldman and Ron Bayer. The specific country studies were the following:

1. "Children and Bystanders First: The Ethics and Politics of Tobacco Control in the United States," by Ronald Bayer and James Colgrove
2. "The Limits of Tolerance: Cigarettes, Politics and the Society in Japan," by Eric A. Feldman
3. "Rights and Public Health in the Balance: Tobacco Control in Canada," by Christopher P. Manfredi and Antonia Maiono.
4. "The Politics of Tobacco Control in Australia: International Template?" by John Ballard.
5. "Militants, Manufacturers, and Governments: Postwar Smoking Policy in the United Kingdom," by Virginia Berridge
6. "Libertè, Egalitè, Fumèe: Smoking and Tobacco Control in France," by Constance A Nathanson
7. "Between Paternalism and Voluntarism: Tobacco consumption and Tobacco Control in Germany," by Gunter Frankenberg
8. "Holy Smoke, No More? Tobacco Control in Denmark," by Erik Albaek

10. Had we tried to describe these three countries over time, however, they would not have constituted a consistent set of countries with medium-high controls.

11. M. A. Corrao, G. E. Guindon, N. Sharma, and D. F. Shokoohi, eds., *Tobacco Control Country Profiles*, American Cancer Society, Atlanta, GA, 2000, available at http://www5.who.int/tobacco/page.cfm?sid=57, accessed April 29, 2003. The report, *Tobacco Consumption 1970–1994 in the Member States of the EU, in Norway & Iceland*, available at http://www.globalink.org/tobacco/docs/misc-docs/tobacco.pdf, accessed April 29, 2003, attempts a similar type of classification scheme for the European countries based on similar data, but from an earlier (1994) report.

12. Eric A. Feldman, "The Landscape of Japanese Tobacco Policy: Three Perspectives," *American Journal of Comparative Law* 48 (2001):679– . More recently, Japanese legal restrictions have increased on *where* smoking is permitted in major cities, with substantial fines for smoking on the crowded streets of Tokyo, for example. The general rationale for this change is the traditional liberal argument about externalities and protection of children. The particular grounds are fascinating: cigarettes smoked outdoors in Japan are commonly held at one's side—a level that endangers both little children and the clothing of walkers.

13. See E. Feldman, pp. 8–38 in *Unfiltered*, for further explanations.

14. We are attempting to make broad characterizations, in order to distinguish general, cross-national differences. Clearly, there remain important limits to the ideal-type scores we have provided. For example, no visitor to Denmark would regard the constraints on the location of smoking as being as restrictive as those in Australia (especially New South Wales) or Canada (especially British Columbia). The chapter portraits of Australia, Canada, and Denmark support these distinctions, but they do not fit with the American Cancer Society's rankings.

15. See C. Nathanson, pp. 138–160 in *Unfiltered*.

16. See G. Frankenberg, pp. 161–189 in *Unfiltered*.

17. See, for example, Rabin and Sugarman, *Regulating Tobacco*; Donley Studlar, *Tobacco Control: Comparative Politics in the United States and Canada* (Peterborough: Broadview Press, 2001); Carrick Mollenkamp, Adam Levy, Joseph Menn, and Jeffrey Rothfeder, *The People vs. Big Tobacco: How the States Took On the Cigarette Giants* (Princeton: Bloomberg Press, 1998); David Phelps, Deborah C. Rybak, Tom Mason, and Mark Luinenburg, *Smoked: The Inside Story of the Minnesota Tobacco Trial* (Minneapolis: MSP Communications, 1998); Cassandra Tate, *Cigarette Wars: The Triumph of the "Little White Slaver"* (New York: Oxford University Press,

1999); Mike Males, *Smoked: Why Joe Camel Is Still Smiling* (Monroe, ME: Common Courage Press, 1999); Stanton A. Glantz and Ethel Balbach, *Tobacco War: Inside the California Experience* (Berkeley: University of California Press, 2000); Dan Zegart, *Civil Warriors: The Legal Siege on the Tobacco Industry* (New York: Delacorte Press, 2000); David A. Kessler, *A Question of Intent: A Great American Battle with a Deadly Industry* (New York: Public Affairs Press, 2001); and Tara Parker-Pope, *Cigarettes: Anatomy of an Industry from Seed to Smoke* (New York: New Press, 2001).

18. Studlar, *Tobacco Control: Comparative Politics in the United States and Canada.*

19. The distinction between the politics of harm reduction and the politics of "denormalization" is, we believe, an important one for further understanding of tobacco control. A number of the political analyses of tobacco regulation have used this distinction in one form or another, but not for a comparative study of the kind that has been attempted in this book. Kagan and Nelson, for example, have contrasted interest-group understandings with those emphasizing entrepreneurial politics; that dichotomy highlights the standard distinction between reducing the harm to others, on the one hand, and the social movement features of political entrepreneurs who, with moral fervor, rebuke both tobacco firms and inconsiderate smokers, on the other. In combination with an emphasis on the dispersed nature of the American polity, Kagan and Nelson use this distinction to make sense of the nation's low tobacco taxation and its typically zealous control of where tobacco can be used. But since the authors do not engage in any comparative analysis, they cannot distinguish the general from the idiosyncratic in the American case. Robert A. Kagan and William P. Nelson, "The Politics of Tobacco Regulation in the United States," in *Regulating Tobacco*, eds. Rabin and Sugarman. The emphasis on social movements and moralistic appeals is one of the themes of Nathanson's essay on tobacco politics, and most of the political analyses in this book have focused on the moralism of contemporary tobacco reformers and on how such attitudes have influenced the controls that have come into prominence. Without that emphasis, it would be impossible to understand why a California community actually proposed banning smoking in public parks. No understanding of the harm principle could justify that option, though aesthetic objections might justify suggesting keeping some physical distance between smokers and nonsmokers.

20. For an important debate about the merits of culture as an explanatory variable in comparative politics and political science more generally, see, David Laitin and Aaron Wildavsky, "Political Culture and Political Preferences," *American Political Science Review* 82 (2):589–597.

21. Max Weber, *The Protestant Ethic and the Spirit of Capitalism* (Hammersmith, London, UK: Harper Collins Academic, 1991).

22. A. Brandt, pp. 255ff in *Unfiltered.*

23. See R. Bayer and J. Colgrove, pp. 34–36 in *Unfiltered.*

24. Ronald Inglehart, and Marita Carballo, "Does Latin America Exist? (And Is There a Confucian Culture?): A Global Analysis of Cross-Cultural Differences," *PS: Political Science and Politics* (March 1997): 34–47.

25. Essentially, this dimension distinguishes societies in terms of the emphasis on basic economic needs (survival) as compared with more subjective notions of well-being that incorporate many non-economic goods.

26. See, for example, Sven Steinmo, *Taxation and Democracy* (New Haven: Yale University Press, 1993); Sven Steinmo, Kathleen Thelen, and Frank Longstreth, eds., *Structuring Politics: Historical Institutionalism in Comparative Analysis* (New York: Cambridge University Press, 1995); Markus M. L. Crepaz, "Inclusion Versus Exclusion: Political Institutions and Welfare Expenditures," *Comparative Politics* 31 (1):61–80; and Ellen M. Immergut, *Health Politics: Interests and Institutions in Western Europe*, Cambridge Studies in Comparative Politics (Cambridge : Cambridge University Press, 1992).

27. See also Constance A. Nathanson, "Tobacco Politics: Nation-States and Collective Action" (unpublished).
28. Ibid.
29. Few scholars have regarded Australia, Canada, and the United States as similar in the appeal of moralistic politics or in the spread of prohibitionist constraints on personal habits. Indeed, appeals to the frontier feature—including claims of libertarian strains from Alberta to Texas to Queensland—would be more common. But the data reported in this book support the characterization of these three federal regimes as the most restrictive on the use of tobacco—particularly the use of tobacco in public places.
30. See G. Frankenberg, pp. 161–189 in *Unfiltered*.
31. Frankenberg explain the liberal tobacco regulation after the Second World War as partially a result of the prohibitive and racist Nazi propaganda of the 1930s and 1940s. For further explanation see Frankenberg, pp. 171ff in *Unfiltered*.

NEW PARADIGMS

Health Care to Population Health

Previous chapters have touched on changes in the assumptive world of both government actors and the public that shaped discourse and policy in health care over the past decades: the challenge to the notion that organized medical care is the prime instrument for improving the health of the population. Not only has this paradigmatic shift helped to change attitudes toward, and the dominating position of, the medical profession, as we have seen. But it has been used to justify public action to change private behavior, as in the case of tobacco. The two articles in this chapter enlarge on this theme by focusing on two landmark reports in the history of the rise of the new population health model: the Lalonde Report published in Canada in 1974 and the Black Report published in Britain in 1980. The articles offer both a critique of those reports and an analysis of their policy implications. Here we also add a sketch of their subsequent impact on public policy.

The two reports are different in character, had a very different policy intent and impact, but were at one in stressing lifestyle and environment—as distinct from medical intervention—as the main determinants of population health. But while the Lalonde Report's focus was on the health of the population as a whole, that of the Black Report was on health inequalities within the population. The prescription for policy that followed differed accordingly. More than the Lalonde Report, the Black Report stressed socioeconomic factors, even while arguing for improved access to health for disadvantaged groups. Black's thesis was that differences in health outcomes between social classes reflected what it called structural factors: that is, inequalities in income, poor housing, inadequate educational opportunities, and so on. And its recommendations were accordingly wide and expensive: in effect the report proposed a major program of social engineering and income redistribution.

Black's specific recommendations were ignored. Commissioned by a Labour Government, the report was published under a Conservative Administration coping with a major economic crisis. However, government interest in population health did not die with the Black Report—if only because improving health could mean less pressure on the NHS—while the Labour Party continued to press the cause of inequalities. So on being returned to office in 1997, the Labour Government immediately appointed yet another inquiry into health inequalities, and the resulting Acheson Report appeared the following year. Significantly (and in line with the Black Report, if on a more modest scale), only three of its thirty-nine main recommendations were addressed to the NHS, while others ranged from poverty relief to strengthening support for disadvantaged families and communities.

The government accepted most of the recommendations in principle, though controversy continues about the extent to which they have been implemented. It also set targets for the reduction of various kinds of inequality: for example, one target was to reduce by at least 10 percent the gap between "the quintile of areas with the lowest life expectancy at birth and the population as a whole" by 2010. Much was made too of all government departments coordinating policies that might have any impact on the population's health. However, the government's interim evaluation showed a mixed picture in the progress toward achieving its targets: not surprisingly, perhaps, given that public policy is only one of many factors influencing health. So Britain offers an example of an institutional structure in which central government can adopt a coherent, overarching policy strategy—but also a warning that such a strategy does not necessarily guarantee successful implementation, let alone desired outcomes.

The picture in Canada is different, reflecting both the differences between the Lalonde and Black Reports and institutional factors. Lalonde's concern was to start a conceptual rather than social transformation: to offer a new way of thinking about health. It expounded a strategy rather than a program, though identifying specific issues calling for public action. These included (on the lifestyle side) the use of seat belts, reduction in cigarette and alcohol consumption, and increases in exercise level, as well as (on the environmental side) the regulation of water and air pollution. To caricature, while Black blamed social conditions for poor health—if the poor smoked it was because of the deprived conditions in which they lived—Lalonde blamed poor health on personal conduct and a polluted environment. Different ideas, as always, pointed to different policy priorities.

No surprise, then, that Canada did not adopt the kind of national program of social engineering developed in Britain. Nor could it have done so easily, given the division of responsibility and power between the federal government and the provinces. But the discourse of "population health" became pervasive in the decades following the publication of Lalonde. This was, in any case, the language of an already existing interest group: the public health profession. So, while there was no national program, many of the provincial and local initiatives had the same intellectual DNA as those in Britain, with an emphasis on health promotion programs designed to reach the most disadvantaged, on coordinating different policy strands, and on encouraging physical exercise.

The post-Lalonde story in the United States has a different twist yet again. Again, there was no national program on the British model, reflecting the dispersal of authority in America. Again, too, the decades following Lalonde marked the rise of "population health" talk and local policy initiatives—whether or not directly inspired by the report. And the Secretary of Health and Human Services has set out population health targets, though without specifying how these are to be reached. But as the article on Lalonde argues, there was something of a displacement effect: the report could also be used to disparage medical care and thus to dilute the case for financial reform. The academic concern about health "disparities," expressed in a torrent of studies, does not have the natural political and ideological constituency offered by the Labour Party in Britain.

The experience of the three countries provides two common themes. The first is that the new paradigm puts health in the driving seat of social change. Its logic assumes that if population health is to be improved (and who can be against that?), then people have to change their habits and governments have to spend more on a variety of social programs. The point applies most strongly in the British case—where health now provides a new flag for old causes—but also has application in Canada and the United States. Second, their experience underlines yet again not only the importance of ideas in shaping policy but also that the impact of those ideas will depend on the way in which they fit (or do not fit) into the structure of institutions and interests. Over time ideas may and do change perceptions, both of what is desirable and how it can be achieved. But while they modify definitions of self-interest, they also depend on self-interest for their adoption. If the new paradigm of health has appeal, it is not only because of its persuasive diagnosis but because it appears to offer a way of restraining the rising cost of health care.

A New Perspective on Health

Learning from Lalonde?

Theodore R. Marmor and Albert Weale

In 1974 the Canadian government published A *New Perspective on the Health of Canadians*, which is also known as the *Lalonde Report*, after the then Federal Health Minister, Marc Lalonde.[1] The *Lalonde Report* is the most widely read, or at least most widely purchased, government document in Canadian history, selling widely domestically and internationally. Moreover, it was something of a trend-setter, anticipating the UK's *Prevention and Health: Everybody's Business*[2] in 1976 and *Healthy People: The Surgeon General's Report on Health Promotion and Disease Prevention*,[3] published in the U.S. in 1979. It continued for some time to have influence among policymakers in many contexts; for example, the first report on Public Health under the new "post-Acheson" regime in the U.K. for the Norwich District Health Authority, published nearly 15 years later, began with a ringing restatement of the approach in *Lalonde*.[4] The fate of the ideas Lalonde set forth is a case study in how difficult it is to transform thinking in health and health care policy.

In terms of its style it is easy to see why *Lalonde* should have been so popular. It is short (only some 70 pages of generously printed text), but it manages to communicate a serious message about the reorientation needed in public policy if contemporary health problems are to be effectively tackled. Within this brief compass, *Lalonde* managed to quote from, among others, an early nineteenth century work on natural theology, Thomas McKeown's work on the modern rise in population, *Scientific American*, the *Imperial Oil Review* and the *Journal of the Canadian Medical Association*, as well as ancient Chinese proverbs and the Canadian Treasury's supply estimates—a potent brew indeed. Since it also discussed sexually transmitted diseases and sport, emphasised uncertainty and provided a "Panorama of Mortality in Canada," only a reference to royalty would have been needed to ensure that it contained the popular press's recipe of mixing sex, death, sport, mystery and aristocracy in every story.

The medium was in some ways part of the message. *Lalonde* was clearly the work of a professional, well-educated class of policymakers willing to admit how little they knew and even more willing to offer their technically competent services to remedy the defects of understanding. Its central message—that health policy should be redirected from its concern with the supply and costs of medical services towards the behavioural, environmental and biological determinants of health—also caught a rising wave of public concern. Since *Lalonde* was published, all economically developed societies have seen a massive growth in consumer attention to personal fitness, diet, product safety and environmental quality. It is plausible that this rise in concern is associated with the maturation of a generation of well-educated professionals capable of influencing national, social and political agendas. Moreover, insofar as the rise of new social movements can be identified with a preference for the values of self-development and participation over an increase in conventional standards of living, there were elements in *Lalonde*, particularly in stress on lifestyle, that would appeal to an emerging post-materialist generation.[5]

Appeal, of course, is no substitute for cogency and coherence—where the *Lalonde Report* also scores highly. For a governmental publication, even by Canadian standards, it is a sophisticated and theoretically rich document. Admittedly short on discussion of policy instruments and implementation, it is primarily devoted to achieving a conceptual change in the intellectual presuppositions of health policy. This theoretical elaboration will be the main focus of concern in this chapter. The aim is to assess the adequacy and plausibility of the theoretical argument contained in Lalonde and then to see how far it provided a framework for social learning, or the development of public policy through an improvement in knowledge and understanding. This exercise provides not only an example of the promise and pitfalls of "healthy public policy" but also illustrates the quest for "global" health policy solutions.

Many aspects of the substantive concerns of *Lalonde* clearly have not been taken up in subsequent policy developments in Canada or elsewhere. This is so for a number of reasons, including logical weaknesses in the original report, the variety of interpretations that *Lalonde* could bear and the tendency of policy systems to replace substantive concerns with the professional and bureaucratic interests of their members. The central methodological message of this chapter is that the interplay of ideas and institutions cannot be understood unless sufficient attention is paid to the cognitive and intellectual dimensions of policy developments. Reflecting on the *Lalonde Report* enables us to understand how such a methodology might be developed.

THE NEW PERSPECTIVE

The main thrust of the *Lalonde Report* is simply stated: "It is evident now that further improvements in the environment, reductions in self-imposed risks, and a greater knowledge of human biology are necessary if more Canadians are to live a full, happy, long and illness-free life."[6] This claim can best be understood by examining both what it denies and what it asserts. Implicit in the central message of the *Lalonde Report* is a denial of the claim that improvements in the quality and access to medical care, chiefly hospital-based treatment, are the best or most effective means to secure improvements in the health status of modern populations. Given this denial, the report goes on to claim that improvements in health status can only be achieved by getting at the causes of prevalent morbidity and mortality. These causes can be broken down into the environment, life-style and human biology. Together with the organisation of the medical-care system, these categories of causation determine the "health field concept" the central organising idea of the report. Since the organisation of medical care is unlikely to yield large gains in health status, the logic of the *Lalonde Report* asserts that greater public emphasis needs to be placed on the other elements in the health field concept.

To understand fully the logic of this argument, it is necessary to look at the grounds by which the *Lalonde Report* arrives at its conclusions. The negative claim, which denies the importance of organised medical care, is essentially supported by two arguments. The first is that Canadian medical care is both of high quality and secures near universal access. In 1974, it provided a system in which "close to seven billion dollars a year [was] spent on a personal health care system . . . mainly oriented to treating existing illness."[7] Moreover, when attention is turned to specific causes of morbidity and mortality, the *Lalonde Report* argues that the most prevalent conditions are not amenable to effective treatment by conventional medical procedures. The report focuses upon "early deaths," that is deaths before average life expectancy, and shows that the principal contributors, when measured by aggregate expected years of life lost, include motor-vehicle accidents, ischaemic heart disease, miscellaneous accidents, respiratory disease and lung cancer, and suicides.[8] Thus, by 1974, chronic illness and accidents had replaced infectious diseases as the major causes of premature death. The implication is that, whereas improvements in medicine could make a significant contribution to the reduction of infectious diseases, no such contribution could be expected for chronic illness, and certainly no significant contribution from medicine could be expected in the reduction of accidents. Hence, given high-quality, universal medical care, the marginal effectiveness of further increasing the resources going into medicine is low.

The second argument to support the relatively small part to be played by the medical-care system in promoting further gains in health essentially depends on an historical analogy and draws upon Thomas McKeown's work on the modern rise of population.[9] McKeown examined the decline in major infectious diseases in England and Wales from the eighteenth to the mid-twentieth centuries. He discovered that rates of prevalence declined substantially for all major infectious diseases before the introduction of therapeutic drugs, and he attributed the decline principally to limitations of family size, an increase in food supply and a healthier physical environment. McKeown's conclusion, endorsed by *Lalonde*, was that past improvements had been mainly due to modifications in behaviour and changes in the environment, and it was to those same influences that we must look for further advance.

There is, of course, an ambiguity in this conclusion. Is the claim that a further decline in the prevalence of infectious disease depends upon behavioural and environmental factors, or is it that a decline in the currently prevalent causes of mortality are likely to arise from behavioural and environmental changes? To support its overall claims about the relative lack of importance of organised medicine in securing improvements in health, the *Lalonde Report* needs to be able to sustain the second interpretation, whereas McKeown's original text only sustains the first.

The positive part of *Lalonde*'s use of the health-field concept is to draw attention to the importance of lifestyle, environment and human biology, particularly the first two, in determining future contributions to health gains. The essential argument here depends upon identifying the main underlying causes leading to premature deaths. Improvements in driving habits, including the use of seat belts; reductions in cigarette and alcohol consumption; and increases in average exercise levels are identified as relevant to the necessary changes in lifestyle, while regulation of water and air pollution to control health hazards are picked out as central to environmental improvement.

As Robert Evans pointed out, the central thrust of the *Lalonde Report* can bear a variety of interpretations.[10] There is no innocent reading of the text, and its diverse, and sometimes inconsistent, messages can be picked out and amplified

by various self-interested groups to their own advantage. Evans himself identifies three groups who could use the message of *Lalonde* to support positions
that they favoured on independent grounds. Both provincial and federal governments in Canada could interpret *Lalonde*'s scepticism about the inefficacy
of medical care to underpin their search for improved control over medical-
care costs. Providers could use the arguments about individual responsibility to
buttress their campaigns to allow physicians to bill their patients directly. And
the private sector could seize upon the lifestyle aspects for marketing purposes.
Lalonde could be invoked as governmental support for sports equipment sales,
health spas, specialised travel and vacation packages, sports clubs and obesity
programs. Indeed, all of these blossomed in the decade after *Lalonde*, as did a
whole series of nutritional spin-offs. Other, more radical critics alleged that the
way in which the lifestyles argument was taken up by health promotion professionals in Canada (and, as we shall see later, especially in the United States)
led them to neglect structural economic and social inequalities that underlay
the uneven distribution of health status: "Current health-promotion programs
focus exclusively on the narrow band of personal health behaviour and discon-
nect individual health from its social context. Likewise, social problems such
as poverty and pollution are perceived as topical political issues disconnected
from personal health."[11]

There is, however, something paradoxical in these interpretations. They
all suggest that the lifestyle message was amplified from the *Lalonde Report*.
No doubt this is true, but it is a message to which the *Lalonde Report* itself
anticipated strong resistance. Noting strongly libertarian values in Canadian
political culture, at least as far as matters of lifestyle are concerned, the report
devotes considerable rhetorical energy to persuading its readers that it is appropriate for government to encourage citizens to lead healthier lives. There
is, perhaps, an irony here. Had the crafters of *Lalonde* expected less resistance
on this score, they might have toned down their emphasis upon lifestyle factors,
thereby leaving less room for one-sided interpretations. As it was, the lifestyle
message seemed to resonate only too well in the consciousness of North American publics.

This use and misuse of the *Lalonde Report*'s "new perspective" is an important part of the story about the public debate that the report prompted and
promoted. But there is still a question to pose about the relationship between
the logic of the new perspective itself and the character of the subsequent policy
developments that it inspired. How valuable, in short, was the role of the *Lalonde Report* as an instrument of policy learning?

THE LOGIC OF CONCEPTS

Between the idea and the reality, as T. S. Eliot wrote, falls the shadow. Undoubtedly the most significant contribution *Lalonde* made was the introduction of the idea of the "health field concept." The simple act of distinguishing between health policy and the organisation of medical care was a significant contribution in itself.[12] It established clearly that medicine was only one route, and perhaps not the most important one, to health improvements. It is worth considering, however, what functions the health field concept played in the processes of policy development.

The report itself identifies one of the main functions for the health field concept, namely as a source of reorientation in the administrative mind. In performing this function, *Lalonde* asserts that the concept "provides a new perspective on health, a perspective which frees creative minds for the recognition and exploration of hitherto neglected fields."[13] Although not developed in the main body of the text, the implications of this point are considerable. The problems of selective attention and the narrowing of concerns are familiar in administrative organisations. Standard operating procedures, lines of communication and the professional composition of policy communities typically tend to narrow the attention span of policy makers. Various strategies of decision, including disjointed incrementalism, "satisficing" (accepting the satisfactory), or simply muddling through, are all responses to pressures of time and limited attention span.

The argument of *Lalonde* is that the simple incremental developments of traditionally conceived medical care will no longer meet the challenges of modern health needs, and so an expansion of the range of reference and concern among health policy makers is necessary. The health field concept is an intellectual device by which health policy makers can ensure that they are paying attention to a sufficiently wide range of considerations. In this sense the health field concept resembles a procedural device, rather like a checklist, to force policy makers to extend the limits of their conventional attention span.

It is worth stressing the procedural role of the concept because the *Lalonde Report* itself tends to present the concept in a rather different way, namely as an analytic construct having the virtues of comprehensiveness and analytic precision: "The Concept . . . is comprehensive. Any health problem can be traced to one, or a combination of the four elements . . . the Concept permits a system of analysis by which any question can be examined under the four elements to assess their relative significance and interaction."[14]

While the health field concept may play an important role in expanding attention spans narrowed by the standard operating procedures of bureaucratic organisations, it lacks the analytic virtues the *Lalonde Report* claims for it. By no means comprehensive, it is not detailed enough to perform the mapping function required. One simple way of identifying this weakness is to note that the report provides no logical space for occupational health and safety, even though it mentions occupational causes of disease in passing. Only the most banal libertarian would say that occupational risk is a matter of lifestyle and hence the outcome of personal choice, and that such risk is clearly distinct from environmental hazards. If there is an analytic concept capable of organising the issues with which *Lalonde* is concerned, it is the statistical notion of analysis of variance, which is evidenced in its distinction of within-group and between-group effects. None of *Lalonde's* analyses, however, refer to or imply that approach.

Implicit in the logic of the *Lalonde Report* approach to health is pressure towards extending attention spans provided by the health field concept is implicit in the logic of the *Lalonde Report's* approach to health. *Lalonde's* new perspective seeks to move to causes of morbidity and mortality rather than effects and patterns. Yet modern illness typically has many causes. When analysts seek to move from effect to cause, they typically discover a number of causes associated with any one effect. This is the principal difference between infectious and non-infectious diseases. With infectious disease it is possible to identify one causal agent, the pathogen, responsible for the condition. With circulatory diseases and concerns, this is usually not possible, and so a variety of causal factors are typically implicated. In seeking to address the causes of illness, rather than focusing upon treatment through conventional medical care, the *Lalonde Report* inevitably raised problems of social and economic organisation, the environment and patterns of personal preference.

In this respect the type of problem the *Lalonde Report* raised falls into a large and significant category. Environmental protection exhibits a similar logic. Protection of the atmosphere from pollution typically involves identifying a variety of sources that are dispersed in time and space. Thus, just as environmental protection requires attention to problems in transport, energy use, agriculture and industry, so preventive health measures require attention to the environment, occupational hazards and consumption patterns. Improving the environment and the health status of human populations requires a recognition that the causes of the problem are embedded in a wide range of forms of social organisation. Similar points can be made in connection with ethnic, gender or other forms of inequality. Indeed, all the topics under the heading of the "new social regulation" have the feature that the phenomena that they address are embedded in diverse points in the social structure of modern societies.

From this perspective it could be argued that the broadening function of the health field concept is only one part of the story. Just as it is necessary to alert policy makers traditionally preoccupied with medical care about the non-medical determinants of health status, so it is necessary to alert policy makers traditionally preoccupied with transport, industry or consumption about the health implications of their decisions. The task of suffusing a series of policy sectors with a concern for health is not one that emerges naturally from the *Lalonde*'s new perspective.

In this respect it is important to understand the degree of theoretical elaboration that a problem receives and the extent to which it is possible to secure consensus on what the nature and dimensions of the problem are. Environmental protection again provides a useful parallel, and a specific example will illustrate the point. Achieving successful environmental protection requires the co-operation of a wide range of policy-makers, most particularly those concerned with industry, agriculture and transport. Dutch environmental planners confronted the problem of inter-sectoral collaboration when drawing up the Netherlands National Environmental Policy Plan. The ability to generate inter-sectoral collaboration across a range of bodies and agents depended upon two factors. First, the Dutch planners sought to develop a detailed theory of the sources of environmental pollution using a general systems approach. Secondly, they could rely upon the research of the Dutch Institute of Public Health and Environmental Protection as an independent source of evidence about the extent of environmental damage and its future deterioration. Once the theoretical framework and the empirical findings were accepted, they provided a point of intellectual convergence and policy orientation for policy makers who were not part of the environmental establishment.[15] A particular problem for the project that *Lalonde* initiated is that there is not the same degree of intellectual convergence around the issues of preventive health as the Dutch planners succeeded in obtaining around the issue of environmental protection. The health field concept lacks the degree of theoretical embeddedness that the Dutch appeal to a mass balance or general systems approach had, and the data relating lifestyles or environmental hazards is notoriously imprecise and contentious.

Another way of looking at the same point is in terms of the organisation of the bureaucratic apparatus. Again a parallel with environmental protection is instructive. Because of the inter-sectoral nature of environmental protection, the design of bureaucratic organisation faces a dilemma that Müller has labelled the conflict between "concentration" and "integration."[16] In order to promote environmental policy, should specialist expertise be concentrated in one portion of the bureaucracy or should responsibility be dispersed throughout different departments? Müller shows that there is no general answer to this question, but that it all depends upon the phase of the issue attention cycle that is involved. In the case of preventive health, a similar point could be made. There are reasons for creating preventive health sections in non-health ministries, just as there is reason for the health ministry taking a broader view of the determinants of health.

The organisational implications of the *Lalonde Report* favoured concentration rather than integration. That is, the report favoured specialist units within the Health and Welfare Department rather than units within other ministries taking on responsibility for health. Thus in 1978 a new Health Promotion Directorate (HPD) was formed by amalgamating four broadly preventive departments within Health and Welfare Canada. Significantly, the focus of HPD was on public education through nation wide campaigns, with a concentration on diet, cigarettes, alcohol and drugs and with an emphasis upon target groups, including low-income groups, disabled people, native peoples, women and older individuals.[17] At the provincial level Toronto's Public Health Department developed a "health advocacy" role, in which the department worked with community groups to improve the environment and lobby for policy change.[18] Yet, whether the style be education or advocacy, the structure and functioning of these organisations make it clear that they were not integrated with the sectors of public policy most likely to have the largest impact upon health status.

On the logic of *Lalonde*, there is one further general point worth making. The move from effect to causes forces attention on the variety of contexts within which decisions on health-related matters are taken. There appears to be a logic at work here that leads to a stress upon the moralisation of citizenship. A similar phenomenon is found in the Dutch *National Environmental Policy Plan*. In part this moralisation may be seen as part of the humanistic stream of thought contained in the *Lalonde Report*. It, for instance, criticises conventional medicine for tending "to regard the body as a biological machine which can be kept in running order by removing or replacing defective parts, or by clearing its clogged lines."[19] The report's rejection of philosophical determinism as irresponsible in the face of threats to health provides further evidence of this type of moralisation.[20]

IDEAS AND INSTITUTIONS: COMPARATIVE CONTEXTS

So far we have only examined the logic of the ideas contained in the *Lalonde Report*. To understand how that logic played out in practical forms we need to look comparatively at the ways in which issues and arguments were handled in different policy systems. In this context the most striking contrast is with the way that similar ideas were received and developed in the US.

The new perspective on health illustrated and inspired by *Lalonde* implied some subordination of medical care as a source of improvement in the health status of nations. But it did not entail ridicule of medicine. In the United States that ridicule arose, as it did in some other industrial democracies, as a logical extension of earlier repudiations of authority. Such assaults were very much associated with challenges in the 1960s to university hierarchies, the political legitimacy of established office holders, and even the sway of music, art and sartorial critics. The symbol of this extended version of a new perspective was Ivan Illich, a philosopher of what became known as "medical nihilism."[21] Illich's message was twofold. Medicine could do little about the ills that actually shaped the health status of societies and, what was more, it could be dangerous itself. Talk shows, popular magazines and newspapers, and pundits took up this theme with a vengeance and, for a time at least, Americans heard a lot about "iatrogenic" illness. By that, Illich meant harm caused by medical treatment itself. He stressed the greater risk of infection within the hospital and the danger of excessive intervention where simpler approaches were appropriate: for example, caesarean section versus natural births, deliveries in hospitals rather than homes or birthing clinics, infant formulas versus nursing as sustenance to the newborn.

The dissemination of this sharpened distinction between health and medicine meant that the older public health was newly popularised. This development was evident internationally, but assumed a different significance in the United States. Unlike the rest of the industrial democracies, only the United States (and Australia until 1975) did not have universal health insurance. As a result, the claims of medicine's limits (or dangers) affected American medical debates quite distinctively; the same arguments that appeared in *Lalonde* had different implications.

The central difference was this. Where access to medical care had, broadly speaking, been assured to citizens—in Britain, Canada, France and Sweden, among others—medical nihilism directed attention to more pressing health-promotion policies. But in the United States, medical nihilism became for some a new weapon in the discrediting of universal health insurance. If medical care was limited in its impact on health status, if the cost of medical care was persistently rising above the rate of general inflation, then avoiding the controversial development of national health insurance seemed to make some sense. Why add new lifeboats to the medical Titanic when a new direction might avoid major mishaps? This implication was less stated than suggested, less a formulation than a quiet inference from all the noise about medicine's troubles, limits, and dangers.

In the U.S., then, the new scepticism about the advances to be expected from an expansion of conventional medicine had more dramatic policy implications than elsewhere. Properly understood, national health policy was a challenge to conventional aims to redistribute access, rationalise medical finance, and improve the quality of medical services and their organisation. If we had a proper *health* policy, so the argument went, we could legitimately dismiss the political enthusiasm for enacting what should be called universal *sickness* insurance.

The details of these arguments were, of course, an intellectual's delight, not the preoccupation of most Americans. Debate raged in the professional journals, but symbols of scepticism about medicine drifted into popular consciousness. That Americans consider good health vitally important was never in doubt; they have what one British observer called a "national preoccupation with health."[22] Among the social values prized by Americans, according to one Gallup poll, the two "most frequently cited were a good family life (82 per cent) and good physical health (81 per cent). Another study found that 42 per cent of the respondents 'think more about their health than just about anything else, including love, work, and money.'"[23]

What the new perspective did was challenge the "prevailing wisdom that citizens can maximise their prospects for good health through access to adequate health care."[24] This challenge—to the extent it was noted and believed—helped demystify some of medicine's special cultural status at the same time as it reinforced the national preoccupation with health. The official reports on prevention sounded the same themes. The major causes of morbidity and mortality, they commonly asserted, were automobile accidents, heart disease, respiratory ailments, lung cancer and suicide. And the sources of these threats were, in most of the formulations, self-imposed risks (that is, style of life) and environmental conditions (particularly the various forms of pollution).

The American public, while continuing to be concerned about the access, cost and quality of medical care, came to hear much more about the new perspective on health through the 1970s. Leading health professionals, policy makers, academics, corporate executives and labour officials embraced the proposition that "greater progress toward our becoming a healthy people [could] be made through reducing both environmental hazards and self-indulgent, health-endangering personal behaviour than in expanding access to health care."[25] Though there has been considerable scholarly criticism of the validity and implications of the new perspective on health, there is little doubt that a shift in health policy debates took place in America.

Where national medical care programmes were already in place, the politics of entrenched interests assured that personal medical care would not fall victim to the new emphasis on prevention. Indeed, there is a quite separate tale to be told about the difficulties of changing the priorities of health-care budgets in Canada, Britain, Sweden, and other OECD nations. But in the United States, the shift in policy attention has been, arguably, the most pronounced. Sustained discussion of national health insurance virtually disappeared in the period after 1975.[26] The realities of stagflation and budget constraints—and the shift in attention to new policies—reduced national health insurance to a subject for study in the Carter Administration, which instead highlighted cost containment proposals and the promise of health promotion and disease prevention. Only in the 1990s, when the Democrats regained control of the White House, Senate and House, was discussion about national health insurance even feasible. Even then, the utter collapse of the Clinton Administration's proposal for universal health insurance in 1994 illustrated how difficult the task of medical reform remained.

Medical scepticism contributed to a radically altered agenda in U.S. health policy. The character of that agenda was partly determined by the shear conjunction of economic travail, the absence of national insurance as an operating programme, and the timing of the widespread dissemination of the new perspective on health. The environmental and lifestyle components of the new perspective raise quite different issues for public policy. Environmental policies highlight questions of collective and, especially, corporate behaviour, while the promotion of healthy habits typically addresses individual choice. But together they call attention away from the traditional concerns about medical care, especially the championing of equality in access to medical care itself.

To the extent that costs are relevant to the new perspective on health, they are a problem of waste, a diversion of funds to the increasingly expensive system of medicine from less costly programs of preventing and reducing disease.

CONCLUSION

For those nations like Canada that had satisfactorily dealt with issues of distributive justice in medicine, the new perspective was liberating. It provided guides to promising ways to improve health without implying that equalising access to medical care was trivial. The issues remained somewhat separate, though it is fair to say that advocacy of the newer view was directed at restraining the continual pressure for more resources in medicine. As a guide to what should be emphasised at the margin of future health policy, the new perspective was genuinely that—an altered angle of vision on what to emphasise. But as a guide to how to rationalise medicine's access, quality and cost, it was largely irrelevant in most countries and somewhat perverse in America. In a world of limited attention—and constant pressures on governmental and corporate budgets—it is perfectly possible for defensible medical care reform to become for a time a victim of newfound enthusiasm for prevention. To the extent that took place in the United States, it illustrated the dangers of policy panaceas that undermine efforts at marginal improvement.

Notes

This article was first written in 1990 with Albert Weale, then of the University of East Anglia and now Professor of Government at the University of Essex. An early version of it was presented at the British Association for Canadian Studies 1991 Conference: "Politics, Culture and the Environment in Contemporary Canada." This chapter represents our joint revision of the article.

1. Lalonde, Marc, *A New Perspective on the Health of Canadians* (Ottawa: Information Canada, 1974 [hereinafter *New Perspective* or the *Lalonde Report*]).

2. Department of Health and Social Security, *Prevention and Health: Everybody's Business* (London: HMSO, 1976).

3. US Department of Health, Education and Welfare, *Healthy People: The Surgeon General's Report on Health Promotion and Disease Prevention* (Washington, D.C., 1979).

4. Walker, Paul, *Norwich and District: On the State of Its Health 1988* (Norwich: Norwich Health Authority).

5. Compare Ronald Inglehart, *The Silent Revolution* (Princeton: Princeton University Press, 1977). Inglehart, Ronald, "Value Change in Industrial Societies," *American Political Science Review* 81.4 (1987): 991–1071.

6. *New Perspective*, 6.

7. *New Perspective*, 12.

8. *New Perspective*, 20.

9. McKeown, T., *The Modern Rise of Population* (London: Edward Arnold, 1976).

10. Evans, Robert "A Retrospective on the "New Perspective," *Journal of Health Politics, Policy and Law* 7.2 (1982): 325–44.

11. Leboute, Ronald, and Susan Penfold, "Canadian Perspectives in Health Promotion: A Critique," *Health Education* (April, 1981): 8.

12. Hubert Laframboise was the major author of the *Lalonde Report*; he was a high-ranking civil servant in the federal health ministry, but remained largely unknown in the international health policy community.

13. *New Perspective*, 32.

14. *New Perspective*, 32. Environment, Life-Style, Human Biology, and the Organisation of the Medical Care System Are the Four Elements of the Health Field Concept.

15. Weale, Albert, "A Tale of Two Strategies," *Centre for Public Choice Studies Working Paper No. 8*, University of East Anglia, 1991.

16. Müller, E., *Innenwelt der Umwelt politik* (Opladen: Westdeutscher Verlag, 1986). (*Inside the World of Environmental Policy*).

17. The recent British initiative "Saving Lives: Our Healthier Nation" is similar to this.

18. Robbins, Christopher, ed., *Health Promotion in North America* (London: Health Education Council/King Edward's Hospital Fund, 1987), 22–24.

19. *New Perspective*, 25.

20. *New Perspective*, 36.

21. Starr, Paul, and Theodore Marmor, "The United States: A Social Forecast." Jean de Kervas-doue, John R. Kimberly, and Victor G. Rodwin, eds., *The End of an Illusion: The Future of Health Policy in Western Industrialized Nations* (Berkeley: University of California Press, 1984), 236. Paul Starr, "The Politics of Therapeutic Nihilism," *Working Papers for a New Society* (Summer 1976).

22. Leichter, Howard M., *Free to Be Foolish: Politics and Changing Lifestyles in Britain and the United States* (Princeton: Princeton University Press, 1991), p. 5. Citing Christopher Potter, "Show Down for Health Vigilantes," *Health and Social Sciences Journal* (22 September 1983): 1140.

23. Cited in Leichter, *Free to Be Foolish*, p. 5, citing Carin Rubenstein, "Wellness Is All," *Psychology Today* (16 Oct. 1982): 28–37.

24. Leichter, op cit., 6.

25. Ibid., 7.

26. In 1970 and 1971, for example, the *Congressional Record* noted 50 references to national health insurance; between 1981 and 1986 there were no references to national health insurance in the *Congressional Record*.

Acceptable Inequalities

Rudolf Klein

INTRODUCTION

Much is made of inequality in health and health care. Inequality, it seems, is always with us. The harder we try, the more we invest in the National Health Service and the more effort we put into health and safety at work, health promotion and all the rest of it, the worse the situation appears to become. Not only is there inequality in the use of health services, but, it is asserted, there is also widening inequality in life expectancy and the experience of ill-health. Such was the theme of the Black Report published at the beginning of the decade.[1] Such has been the message of a succession of reports since, culminating in the last will and testament of the outgoing management of the Health Education Council.[2]

Deeply engrained in the national consciousness, constantly reiterated in the medical press and the media, is the sense of another British social policy failure. From this follow demands for higher spending on the NHS, for greater investment in health education, for more generous income support for poor families and, indeed, for more urgent action to bring unemployment down. Inequalities in health are perceived, as it were, as the barometer which measures the ills of society in the largest sense as well as the failures of the NHS.

Such, at least, appears to be the consensus. It is, however, a consensus which depends on filtering out dissonant evidence and excommunicating or ignoring those who offer more optimistic interpretations. In what follows I shall briefly review the available evidence, and the various ways in which it can be read, before addressing my main theme, which is to try to break up and analyse the notion of "inequality" itself. It is a notion which, like equality itself,[3] is more complicated and more multi-dimensional than the current debate would imply. In effect, inequality is a many-threaded tapestry.[4] If (as I shall argue) there are different kinds of inequalities, and different ways of interpreting their significance, it follows that we have to consider which of them we *can* do something about and which of them we *want* to do something about. Some inequalities may be acceptable; others may be intolerable; yet others may be unavoidable. The purpose of this essay therefore is to make a start, no more, on the task of unpicking the threads.

In tackling the theme, I stand as an aesthetic egalitarian, to adopt a phrase thrown out somewhat contemptuously by Joseph and Sumption.[5] My instinctive preference is for more equality rather than less. The extreme kinds of inequality, I would argue, are like the worst kinds of pornography: they corrupt the sensibilities of society as a whole, and make us all less than fully human, by blunting our sense of sympathy (to use Adam Smith's terminology).[6] It is a position which implies that what matters is not so much the degree of inequality in itself (as measured statistically, using Gini co-efficients or whatever) as the degree of deprivation or degradation implied by being at the bottom end of any given distribution of resources. conversely, inequality may be justified to the extent that it improves the lot of the worst-off. But, equally, I would maintain that inequality does not speak for itself in terms of the policy responses that should be made. There are many kinds of inequalities that have always been tolerated, and always will be: more of that below. To pretend that we need not choose policy priorities between tackling different kinds of inequalities in health and health care is simply to invite the kind of disillusion that has followed the long campaign to eliminate poverty: the best way of ensuring a global sense of defeat, and total paralysis, is to invent a global policy target. Conversely, the best way of making some headway is to define as precisely as possible what is acceptable and what is not on different assumptions and criteria.

There is also the general question of whether, in discussing health and health care, we are dealing with something different from other spheres of inequality. Are inequalities in health and health care any different from, and less acceptable than, inequalities in income, education, housing and so on? In putting this question, we need to distinguish sharply arguments about the principles that should determine the distribution of health and those which shape the distribution of health care, and the factors that should in each case be taken into account when devising the machinery needed to give effect to any desired distribution. For there are different causes of inequality in health and health care, just as there are different arguments about what implications to draw in each case. The argument for seeing health as different rests on the contention that health is a necessary condition for the achievement of all human potentials, whether as political citizens or as participants in the economic marketplace or as family actors. It is precisely this which makes Nozick's response to

Williams—that if medical need should be the only criterion for medical treatment then the only proper criterion for the distribution of barbering services is barbering need—frivolously irrelevant: long hair is somewhat less of a barrier to being able to work than, say, an unset broken leg. It would seem, then, that the health needed to function properly (and the health care required to ensure such functioning) is a necessary enabling condition for all human activities.

HEALTH CARE—"NEEDS" AND PREFERENCES

This is, at first sight, a persuasive principle. But some general difficulties about it have to be noted, since they will haunt the subsequent discussion. One is that the argument for the primacy of health, as somehow unique and different, has been developed in the context of claims to the provision of health *care*, i.e. access to treatment. If, however, it turns out that health, seen as the ability to function adequately in different contexts, is determined largely by factors other than medical intervention—such as income, education and housing (as well as personal habits such as smoking and drinking)—then does the principle apply equally strongly to all these spheres and any other goods that may be relevant to the production of health? If so, does the argument for equal claims flowing from equal "needs" for health care inevitably lead to universal egalitarianism? Or should we conclude that inequalities in health and health care are not so uniquely different from, and not necessarily less or more acceptable than, those in other spheres? Furthermore, there is the notorious problem of giving anything like a precise, operational definition of what is meant by the "health" required to function effectively. This, inevitably, is contingent on occupation, family circumstances and environment. Even with a broken leg, I can probably function reasonably well as a university professor; however, things would be very different if I were a trapeze artist. If my hearing is bad and I am to function effectively as a citizen I probably require a deaf-aid, but do I also need a hip replacement to go to political meetings or should I be pushed there in a wheelchair? What, in any case, is the dividing line between "needs" (a dangerously abstract concept) and preferences? What distinguishes those conditions which set up a claim against society from those which simply raise a question about an individual's willingness to spend money on his or her health as against, say, opera or holidays abroad?

The other difficulty revolves around the long debate on whether health care is just one more consumer good, and should be treated as such, when it comes to designing the machinery to give effect to any desired distribution. If we examined the distribution of motor cars in a society where a computer infallibly assigned income according to need to every man, woman and child—Egalitaria, let us call it—we would expect to find wide divergences. Some people would have decided to do without a car, others would stick to their old bangers; a few might starve themselves in order to buy a Rolls. On the whole, it would seem reasonable to guess that no one would get terribly excited about, or that an academic industry would develop around, the theme of inequalities in car ownership. We would simply assume that the Egalitarians were following their own preferences. Would we have the same reaction, even in Egalitaria, if some people chose not to take out adequate health insurance policies? The answer, surely, is "No." We do not treat health care as a market good like any other, for complex reasons: partly because self-neglect may have social spill-over effects and costs, partly because of the problems posed by the imbalance of information as between the consumers and producers of health care, partly because of the contingent nature of health-care needs and the difficulties of switching from one supplier to another (changing consultants is rather more problematic than trading in cars, particularly if the first one called in botched the job).

In considering inequalities in health care provision, then, we assume that a certain degree of paternalism is justified. The problems of an unequal distribution of either health or health care cannot be tackled, as I shall argue, by moving towards a more equal distribution of incomes (highly desirable though that might be for other reasons). Such an approach will always remain inadequate as long as there is an unequal distribution of other resources: the accumulated stock of intelligence, information, social skills and the other abilities developed over time and required to manipulate any given bundle of income, claims or entitlements to the maximum effect.

Are Inequalities the Same as Differences?

A final prefatory remark. The inequalities discussed in this essay must be distinguished from what might be called mere differences. If it turns out that red-haired people have a life expectancy twice that of brown-haired people, this might well be an interesting, researchable difference. If it turns out that people living in parts of the country with hard water have a lower incidence of coronaries[7] than those living in soft-water areas, then again this is a highly significant difference for exploring the causes of cardiovascular disease. In neither case, however, would we talk about inequalities. To invoke this word is to set up the presumption of a *prima facie* case for social concern, perhaps even moral outrage, and policy action. In other words, there has to be an element of perceived social injustice: a pattern of systematic arbitrariness or unjustified discrimination. So if it turned out that red-haired people had a life expectancy twice that of brown-haired people because they were systematically given preferential treatment in the NHS, while the latter were regularly sent to the back of the queue, we might properly invoke the concept of inequality. We might well come to the same conclusion, also, if we found that the poorest people were condemned by their own poverty to living in the soft-water parts of the country, and thus to a higher rate of coronaries.

Indeed, as we shall suggest in the next section, the resurgence of interest in inequalities in health in the 1980s largely represents the semantic tactics of political mobilisation: the use of differences/ inequalities in health to mobilise opinion against perceived inequalities in other spheres—income, housing and employment—since these, in turn, are related to differences/inequalities in health.

2. THE DEBATE ABOUT INEQUALITIES

The link between low incomes, inadequate housing, a bad environment and poor health has been recognised for a long time. It was this realisation that dominated health policy in the 19th century, starting with Chadwick's 1842 report.[8] It was Chadwick who drew attention to the "comparative chances of life in different classes" and to the effects of environments on health. He did so not in order to mobilise opinion against the inequalities in social conditions that gave rise to health inequalities but to identify the specific factors amenable to action by government in order to change this situation: notably clean water, good sewers and better housing. It was a tradition of thinking about health that was to be displaced, for the most part of the 20th century, by the myth of scientific medicine as the *deus ex machina*. And while the contribution of scientific medicine has indeed been great—despite the controversy as to precisely how much it has contributed to either the quantity or quality of life (probably more to the latter than to the former)—by the 1970s it was becoming clear not only that excessive hopes had been invested in it but also that it represented an accelerating cost escalator.

The naive assumption of the founders of the NHS—that improved health services would liquidate the demand for medical attention by improving the nation's health—proved a delusion.[9] As Enoch Powell pointed out,[10] in medical care *l'appetit vient en mangeant* if there are no price barriers. Hence the revival of interest, internationally, in the social conditions and individual behaviour which promote ill-health. As the scope (and cost) of medical technology turned out to be ever-expanding, so there seemed an increasingly urgent case for moving from the provision of health care to the promotion of health itself. If the former was not delivering the hoped-for goods (and was getting ever more expensive), why not try the latter strategy? It was in this new intellectual context that the Black Working Group was appointed. Its objectives were:[11]

> To assemble available information about the differences in health status among the social classes and about factors which might contribute to these.
> To analyse available information about the differences in health status among the social classes and about factors which might contribute to these.

THE BLACK REPORT AND HEALTH INEQUALITIES

However, the reason why the Black Report continues to have political reso-nance and to be invoked in debate even today reflects the way in which mem-bers of the Working Party moved from differences to inequalities, and so trans-lated a diagnostic into a prescriptive role:

> "Present social inequalities in health in a country with substantial resources like Britain are unacceptable, and deserve so to be declared by every section of public opinion. . . . We have no doubt that greater equality of health must remain one of our foremost national objectives and that in the last two de-cades of the twentieth century a new attack upon the forces of inequality has regrettably become necessary and now needs to be concerted," they wrote in their preface. Health inequalities were seen, it would seem, as a way of gener-ating more political support in the battle against poverty: a campaign which was otherwise flagging.

At the heart of the Black Report, and of the subsequent debate about inequali-ties, was the analysis of differences both in health status and the use of health services in terms of social classes, based on the Registrar-General's occupational categories. This, of course, represents the central tradition in British sociology and social analysis, going back to Chadwick and beyond; a tradition which has generated as much intellectual fog as insight. If there is a difference between social classes (so ran the Black Report's implicit assumption), then this in it-self represents an inequality in the sense of giving cause for moral or political concern. But social class is a rubber tin opener as far as analysis is concerned. Why should we be concerned if we do not know the precise significance of any finding? And we don't. As the Black Report itself pointed out (only subse-quently to ignore its own reservations), there are serious problems about using social class as a tool of analysis: problems which range from the classification of married women under their husband's occupation to the fact that there can be wide variations in resources relevant to health (housing, education and in-come) within any given social class. If our intention is to try to relate *specific*

differences in housing, education and income to *specific* differences in health
and health-care use, then social class is much too blunt a tool. Similarly, if
our concern is to identify unacceptable inequalities—systematic patterns of discrimination against particular groups of the population, equivalent to brown-
haired people being put at the end of the queue—then, once again, social class
is far too broad a concept.

It is, therefore, not surprising that a large literature[12] has developed in the
wake of the Black Report, given the ideological overtones of the whole debate.
Its interest, for the purpose of this essay, lies as much in the style of the academic
debate as in its contents: a style which is much closer to a theological controversy than to a dispassionate scientific inquiry. Any challenge to the Black Report is seen as a betrayal: any article or paper which argues that the differences
identified by the Black Report either do not exist or do not merit the status of
inequalities brings a flood of attempted rebuttals, with a strong suggestion that
anyone who does not agree with its conclusions must be in favour of poverty,
slums and illiteracy (or, worse still, a supporter of Mrs. Thatcher!). A new industry has developed designed to demonstrate the link between deprivation and
poor health, with a not so hidden agenda of trying to prove that Conservative
policies are widening inequalities in health; particularly because of the effect
of unemployment.

Since no one since the days of Chadwick has ever attempted to deny that
there is a link between social conditions and health (the real challenge, rather,
is to identify with precision which particular aspects of deprivation are crucial),
and since the case for reducing unemployment, getting rid of poor housing and
giving everyone a decent education would be just as strong even if none of these
factors were linked to ill-health, much of this discussion seems to be redundant.
To the extent that the post-Black research industry is addressing the problem of
identifying the specific factors linked with ill-health so, ironically, it is casting
doubt on the original Black use of social class as the main analytical tool: for
example, Townsend's micro-study of health in one NHS region demonstrates
significant differences *within* social classes—which might have to do with such
environmental factors as pollution, but which are certainly not caught in the
catch-all concept of social class.[13] As yet, however, there is no debate about
inequalities *within* the working class, and about the need to re-distribute resources *within* it: a point to which we shall return.

ERRORS IN BLACK REPORT'S CONCLUSIONS

In any case, it seems reasonably clear that the Black Report was wrong in
some of its most headline-catching conclusions, which have since passed into

the conventional wisdom. Most notably, the work of Raymond Illsley and Julian Le Grand has raised very large questions indeed—to put it cautiously—against the report's conclusion of widening inequalities in health over time (for a summary, see Illsley (1987)).[14] Again, the flaw in the Black analysis is the reliance on social class. Since social classes change over time both in their composition and in their size, any comparison over time does not compare like with like. Moreover, the Black conclusion rests on an analysis of the working population. It thus excludes, by definition, that part of the population—the over-64s—which has notched up the greatest improvements in health (as measured by life expectancy) over this century.

Lastly, the Black Report brushes aside the evidence that at least some of the differences between social classes reflect selective social mobility: the healthiest move upward, the least healthy drift downward. Not surprisingly, therefore, and entirely in line with the commonsense assumption that the improvements in living standards of recent decades must have had *some* effect, the alternative analyses carried out by Illsley and Le Grand—using individual life expectancies rather than social class mortality figures—show a diminution of differences in the distribution of health over the decades.

Similarly, the Black Report's assertion that access to the NHS is biased against the working classes—once use is related to "need" as measured by the available, unsatisfactory, indicators of morbidity—has been shot down. There is little evidence of bias in access to general practice, the gateway to the rest of the NHS.[15] Perhaps the most interesting aspect of this study is that, as with Illsley's and Le Grand's work, it prompted an immediate avalanche of attempted rebuttals: inequalities were something to be cherished and defended as political ammunition, and not to be lightly surrendered to the first critic; inequalities have, in effect, become political property. In the event, the finding has been fully supported by subsequent studies.[16] And the strategy of those who continue to defend the original Black thesis has switched to arguing that while, just conceivably, quantitative equity in access to the NHS might have been achieved, this tells us nothing about the quality of care given once access had been obtained. To switch the argument from quantity to quality does, indeed, raise some important issues about what should or should not be regarded as acceptable inequalities. So, having shown just how problematic and value-laden even the ostensibly neutral exercise of measuring and interpreting differences may be, we turn next to examining which of these differences might be regarded as acceptable or unacceptable inequalities.

3. WHICH DIFFERENCES MATTER?

Let us return to Egalitaria. This is a country, to remind the reader, where a computer divides out everyone's income according to need: so, for example, someone with severe disabilities will get more money than someone who is fully mobile and active. It is a just society, as far as income distribution is concerned. If we found differences in health and health-care use in Egalitaria, we would presumably simply describe these as interesting differences—possibly relevant for research, but certainly not cause for indignation. There could, in such a society, be no beating of the political drums about inequalities in health. We would therefore be identifying acceptable inequalities, in the sense of differences which (while possibly regrettable) do not call for social and political action.

To start with, we would almost certainly find a continuing difference in life expectancy between men and women. These differences have indeed been widening:[17] in 1950 women could expect to live five years longer than men, but by 1981 this widened to 6.4 years. And this trend is in no way unique to Britain. Conversely, of course, women tend to suffer from more ill-health than men. But it would seem rather odd, certainly in Egalitaria but also in contemporary Britain, to describe this as something unjust or perverse. There would be little cause for the men to take to the streets in protest against such discrimination.

Nor is it totally clear that life expectancy, as such, should be seen as an unmitigated "good": would even the most dedicated of egalitarians want to argue for an absolutely equal share of "life expectancy" to go to everyone, irrespective of sex, irrespective of genetic inheritance, irrespective of the capacity actually to enjoy life? The question needs to be put only because the Black Report, and the literature spawned by it, continues to use mortality as its main analytical tool. This is reasonable enough to the extent that mortality statistics are the only reliable data available over time; it only becomes dangerous when the limitations of using this kind of data are forgotten.

GEOGRAPHICAL ENVIRONMENT, SOCIAL CLASS AND LIFE EXPECTANCY

Similarly, we would find continuing differences in Egalitaria between people living in different parts of the country. Strikingly, geographical differences in life expectancy—and indeed disease patterns—have persisted for more than a century, particularly between town and country. In 1842 Chadwick's researchers found that while the average age of death in Manchester was 38 for professional persons and gentry, it was only 17 for mechanics and labourers; in Rutlandshire, however, the average age of death was 38 for mechanics and labourers and 52

for professional persons and gentry.[18] In other words, the geographical environment often overrode social class in the 19th century. And the same is true today.
If we examine standardised mortality ratios, we find that men in social classes
IV and V in East Anglia have almost as good a record as those in social classes I
and II in Scotland, while women in social classes IV and V in East Anglia have
a better record than those in social classes I and II in both Scotland and the
North West. This would suggest that, even in Egalitaria and even in a society
where social class had been abolished, there might still be large regional differences, just as it suggests that the distribution of income (and all that goes with
it, such as housing and education) is only one factor determining health: East
Anglia is not the richest region in the country. Once again, then, we would
seem to have identified an acceptable kind of inequality.

We might also discover in Egalitaria differences in life expectancy related to
specific occupations as distinct from social class. Some occupations are more
dangerous than others. In Egalitaria, we probably would not get too concerned
about such differences. Given an equitable distribution of income, the choice
of occupation could be seen as unconstrained: if some people choose to risk
their lives and limbs by climbing chimneys or by working in noxious surroundings, so be it (provided they take out adequate insurance policies and do not
impose costs on others). In any other society, however, such differences might
well be thought of as unacceptable inequalities, insofar as the choice of occupation is dictated either by lack of income or by lack of alternatives.

This point is to underline the importance, and also the difficulty, of determining when a difference can be ignored because it reflects things which cannot be altered by anyone (such as one's sex or genetic inheritance), or factors
which represent personal preferences and decisions freely made (such as the
choice of job or smoking). If a difference in health or health-care use falls into
either of these categories, then it can surely be described as an acceptable inequality. And in Egalitaria, there is little problem about making this sort of cat-
egorisation. But in a country where, unlike Egalitaria, decisions about health
and health-care use are made under often severe constraints, cultural as well as
economic, the situation is more complex and more worrying. If health can be
seen as an investment good, then we have to ask whether there are unacceptable inequalities in the resources people bring to the investment decisions—
which would, in turn, produce unacceptable inequalities in health.

SMOKING AND SOCIAL CLASS

Smoking provides a classic example for analysing this particular issue. It is related to the incidence of both cancer and heart disease. In Egalitaria, we would

presumably not classify the differences in mortality between smokers and non-smokers as inequalities, even though governments might still wish to try to persuade individual smokers to give up their habits because of the discomfort and injuries imposed on others: smoking is emphatically not a self-regarding activity. But in Britain smoking is related to social class. While the middle classes have been giving up their cigarettes in recent years, the working classes and in particular working-class women have been smoking more. If these trends continue, then almost certainly the differences in life expectancy between social classes will widen in future. Should the illness and shortening of life so created be classified as an unacceptable inequality on the grounds that smoking represents pressures—poor housing or unpleasant jobs or low incomes—which make it impossible for people to take wise investment decisions about their health? Or do we regard it as an acceptable inequality on the grounds that none of these pressures robs people of their freedom of choice, and that to accept this line of reasoning would inevitably lead one into denying personal responsibility for all sorts of destructive and anti-social behaviour? Indeed, might it not be argued that the pattern of smoking reflects the fact that the rise in incomes is greater than the spread of middle-class behaviour, so that the working classes are now adopting the habits that the middle classes are giving up in pursuit of health?

The answers to these questions are not self-evident, and it may help to shift the argument onto somewhat different if related ground. Let us return to Egalitaria. This is a country, be it emphasised again, which has got an egalitarian income distribution. It need not, however, necessarily be a country with an egalitarian distribution of other kinds of resources (notably education) or other influences (notably family background) relevant to investment decisions about health. The real difference between Egalitaria and Britain lies in the fact that the former's people all have an equal chance to buy themselves a good education. If they choose not to do so, the losses they suffer as a result can be seen as morally neutral. In Britain today, however, these conditions certainly do not hold. If the wrong investment decisions are taken about smoking—or diet, come to that—because of the inegalitarian distribution of education, we probably should describe the consequent differences in health as unacceptable inequalities. In short, when talking about the distribution of life chances—including health—we should probably first consider the distribution of skills to take any chances that are going.

SOCIAL CLASS RESPONSES TO HEALTH EDUCATION

Shifting the argument from the distribution of income as an enabling condition for health to the distribution of other resources, such as education, also reveals a paradox and raises a large question. Not only are there differences in the smoking habits between different social classes, but there are also striking differences in their response to health education. The middle classes respond to such education much more readily than the working classes. The paradox, therefore, is that health promotion may eventually widen the differences in life expectancy between the social classes, and that the best way of narrowing the gap between them would have been to encourage everyone to take up smoking! There is nothing as egalitarian as universal self-indulgence.

In turn, this raises the question—to which we shall return in the conclusion— of whether narrowing differences between social classes (or any other groups) can or should ever be seen as an *overriding* policy objective. If, for example, our policy objective were to be to improve the population's health, however defined, by as much as possible, we might deliberately decide to *widen* differences by concentrating on those groups where government intervention is most feasible and cost-effective. Inequalities may be seen as acceptable, to introduce a new consideration into our analysis, if the cost of diminishing them is higher than the health improvements that could be brought about in other ways. In short, we have to consider the social and moral opportunity costs of dealing with inequalities.

Conversely, those committed to the reduction of differences might wish to argue that the distribution of health is like the distribution of income: that it does not matter if those at the top end of the distribution lose some of their health (by being encouraged to smoke or drink?), provided that the gap between them and the bottom of the distribution narrows. If there is a trade-off between social justice, seen as the reduction of inequalities, and the total sum of "health welfare," difficult choices still have to be made on either approach to the question. Even if we agree that a difference should be classified as an inequality—that is, a cause of social and moral concern—it does not automatically follow that we are obliged to give it urgency, primacy or priority in our actions regardless of other claims on our resources, energies and attention.

CRITERIA AND DETERMINATION OF "NEED"

Turning to differences in the use of health services, we again encounter a series of difficulties when we start working through the implications of applying seemingly simple principles. Let us start with the "strong" principle of equality in health care, mentioned earlier. This is the principle that everyone should have an equal chance to get equal treatment for equal "need." Not only does this raise the question as noted already, of what is meant by effective functioning. But it also raises the problem of who defines "need," according to what criteria.

The solution of this problem, in the context of the NHS, is to leave the determination of "need" to the professional providers. Present policy is to ration resources geographically in such a way as to ensure that, in theory at least and given equal efficiency, people with equal degrees of professionally defined "need" will have equal chances of getting treatment irrespective of where they live. So an unacceptable inequality is a difference which biases such chances arbitrarily and without justification: a reasonable enough definition, it would seem, and one which allows a feasible policy response in the shape of re-distribution policies (RAWP) within the NHS.

But we are still left with some difficulties. The medical profession is notoriously jealous of its autonomy and it is far from clear that there is anything like professional consensus about how to define "needs" and how to respond to them. Indeed, it is tempting to argue that what the NHS offers is not so much equal treatment for equal "need" as equal access to consultants who will then apply different criteria of "need" and different kinds of treatment. This inevitably creates differences which, however, stop short of unacceptable inequalities: if the consultants in my district pursue extremely conservative methods of treatment, and I am thereby denied an equal chance of aggressive intervention, I would be hard put to it to describe it as an unacceptable inequality. More crucially still, my chances of getting any treatment may depend as much on my own resources as on the level of NHS resources in my district: in other words, on my own abilities to manipulate the system. If there is a bias in the NHS it is as much in the distribution of the abilities required to make best use of access as in the distribution of the access itself. If I am middle-aged, middle-class, assertive and with high expectations then I will get more out of my doctor, and the NHS, than if I am elderly, working class, deferential and with low expectations. Here, quite clearly, there is a systematic difference, but does it amount to an unacceptable inequality calling for remedial action?

ARE THERE ANY UNACCEPTABLE INEQUALITIES IN HEALTH CARE?

So the argument comes back to a central question put at the beginning of this article. Are there any differences which are unacceptable simply because they happen to be found in the health-care arena? Is the differential ability to shop effectively and claim entitlements aggressively somehow more shocking or objectionable when displayed in health care than in, for example, getting the most out of the education system or exploiting every loophole in the tax system? Depending on our answers to these questions, very different strategies will follow. If differences in the ability to get *health care* are seen as unacceptable inequalities calling for action, then it would follow that more NHS resources should be devoted which discriminate actively in favour of those patients who otherwise do not assert themselves or indeed avoid the health-care system. If so, we may be back to choosing between investing our resources in the reduction of inequalities, as such, and maximising the total supply of health. If, however, we argue that it is differences in the general ability to exploit any situation which represent an unacceptable inequality, then we are left with the problem of how to tackle such inequalities—and we might perhaps conclude that education, rather than health, should have primacy in any strategy.

To emphasise the role of non-financial resources in creating differences in the use of public health care is also to stress a central irony in the debate about private health care. The case against private care, as it is usually put, is that it creates unacceptable inequalities by allowing people to buy quicker and more comfortable treatment. The assumption, in other words, is that the unacceptability derives from the fact that the preferential treatment is *bought* with hard cash: i.e. that it is wrong for health care to be distributed according to the ability to buy rather than "need." It is, of course, quite clear that if I have got a health insurance policy, I will do better than my neighbour who has not should I want to get my hernia fixed up or a new hip joint. I am, therefore, buying an advantage by jumping the NHS queue. But is there really anything to choose morally between buying an insurance policy and inviting one's GP to dinner?

There is indeed a certain paradox in the frequently put argument that private health care is undesirable because it allows the middle classes to exit from the NHS, instead of using their voices and political muscle to demand improvements for everyone within it. For, on past evidence, the result of locking the middle classes into the NHS might well be to widen inequalities within the service. By pushing for the expansion of those services, like repair surgery, from which they benefit most themselves (and which they otherwise get in the private sector), the middle classes might well divert resources from those parts of the service used by the politically least effective sections of the population—the chronically sick elderly, the mentally handicapped, and so on. Political power, like financial power, tends to be lopsided and bureaucratic, and professional biases may be just as important as market biases.

INEQUALITIES IN THE HEALTH-CARE ENVIRONMENT?

The case of services for those who cannot be cured underlines the importance of another, much debated dimension of inequality. In theory, at least, it may be possible to devise neutral, technical criteria for determining the allocation of resources according to "need" in dealing with specific medical or surgical conditions. But how do we start devising fair or just principles of allocation, which would allow us to decide whether inequalities were or were not accept-able, when it comes to the environment in which care is provided? The point applies even in the case of acute medicine. Few people would argue that being able to have a private room while being treated for, say, a broken leg or a coro-nary, represents an unacceptable inequality. But the point becomes crucial in the case of, for example, the chronically ill elderly or the mentally handicapped where the environment is, to a large extent, the care. In this case, it is difficult even to identify the groups who should be compared in the process of identify-ing differences which, in turn, might or might not be categorised as acceptable or otherwise. They raise, in a particularly strong form, a dilemma identified by Schelling, when he asked which differences should be seen as inequalities in medical care or merely another manifestation of what it means to be poor:

> The poor who are merely sick and in no need of a physician's attention, who spend the day in bed not feeling well, do it in drearier surroundings than sick people who are well-to-do. People who are lame or arthritic or fatigued who have to ride crowded buses are worse off than those who can afford taxis. The sick and injured who have to get out of bed and cook their own meals are noticeably worse off than those who can afford help. And this is truer of those who never feel well, who hurt during whatever they do, who have trouble breathing, who are partly paralysed, or who are so old that even hav-ing to remain standing is a mild form of torture. It is not easy to distinguish between those whose discomfort or fear is due to the poor surroundings in which they receive medical care and those whose discomfort or fear is due their being poor.[19]

In short, Schelling concludes, it is crucial to be clear as to whether we are arguing that the poor who are sick should be made better off compared with the sick who are not poor, or whether we are saying that they should be made better off compared with the poor who are not sick. Our definitions of what differences should be categorised as unacceptable inequalities will depend on such judgements.

4. CONCLUSION

This essay ends, as it began, with questions rather than answers. It does not provide ready-made criteria for distinguishing between acceptable differences and unacceptable inequalities. For the purpose has been to argue that there are no such set-in-concrete criteria: that inevitably the process of deciding which differences should be put on the policy agenda will depend on intellectual argument and political bargaining, with the frontiers changing over time. Even for inegalitarians, there will be some differences which are so shocking as to demand action, but *what* shocks will change over time. Even for egalitarians, there will be many differences where the opportunity costs are too high to justify action, but the nature of these costs will also change over time. And health, it would seem, is not so very different from any other policy arena; differences in health status and health-care use do not carry any privileged status, which justifies their immediate translation into unacceptable inequalities demanding remedial policies. To the extent that differences in health care reflect unacceptable inequalities in society at large, so the case for action should be argued in the larger context and in the currency of argument appropriate to it.

Notes

My thanks are due to my colleague, Patricia Day, for allowing me to draw on the stock of ideas developed in our joint research and for comments on the draft.

1. A. Weale, *Political Theory and Social Policy* (London: Macmillan, 1983); N. Daniels, *Just Health Care* (Cambridge: Cambridge University Press, 1985); R. Nozick, *Anarchy, State and Utopia* (New York: Basic Books, 1974); B. Williams (1967), "The Idea of Equality," in P. Laslett and W. G. Runciman, eds., *Philosophy, Politics and Society*, 2nd Series (Oxford: Basil Blackwell, 1967).
2. Sir Douglas Black, *Inequalities in Health: Report of a Research Working Group* (London: DHSS, 1980); Margaret Whitehead (1987), *The Health Divide* (London: Health Education Council, 1987).
3. T. C. Schelling, "Standards for Adequate Minimum Personal Health Services," *Millbank Memorial Fund Quarterly/Health and Society* 57, no. 2 (1979): 212–234.
4. D. Rae, *Equalities* (Cambridge, MA: Harvard University Press, 1981); M. O'Higgins, "Egalitarians, Equalities and Welfare Evaluation," *Journal of Social Policy* 15, part 3 (1987): 293–315.
5. L. S. Tempkin, "Inequality," *Philosophy and Public Affairs* 15, no. 2 (1986): 99–121.
6. Sir Keith Joseph and J. Sumption, *Equality* (London: John Murray, 1979); A. Sen, *On Ethics and Economics* (Oxford: Basil Blackwell, 1987); J. Rawls, *A Theory of Justice*, (Oxford: Oxford University Press, 1973).
7. N. Morris, *Uses of Epidemiology*, 3rd edn. (Edinburgh: Churchill Livingstone, 1975).
8. M.W. Flinn, ed., *Report on the Sanitary Condition of the Labouring Population of Great Britain, 1842* (Edinburgh: Edinburgh University Press, 1965).
9. R. Klein, "Models of Man and Models of Policy," *Millbank Memorial Fund Quarterly/Health and Society* 58, no. 3 (1980): 416–429.
10. E. Powell, *Medicine and Politics* (London: Pitman Medical, 1966).
11. Sir Douglas Black, *Inequalities in Health: Report of a Research Working Group* (London: DHSS, 1980).
12. M. Whitehead, *The Health Divide* (London: Health Education Council, 1987).
13. P. Townsend, P. Phillmore and A. Beattie, *Inequalities in Health in the Northern Region* (Bristol: University of Bristol, 1986).
14. R. Illsley, "Occupational Class, Selection and Inequalities in Health," *Quarterly Journal of Social Affairs* 3, no. 3 (1987): 213–223.
15. E. Collins and R. Klein, "Equity and the NHS," *British Medical Journal*, Vol. 281 (1980): 1111–1115.

16. E. Collins and R. Klein, *Self-Reported Morbidity, Socio-Economic Factors and General Practitioner Consultations*, Bath Social Policy Paper No. 5 (Bath: Centre for the Analysis of Social Policy, 1985); F. Puffer, "Access to Primary Health Care," *Journal of Social Policy* 15, Part 3 (1986): 293–315; Office of Population Censuses and Statistics, *General Household Survey for 1984* (London: HMSO, 1986).

17. M. Whitehead (1987), *The Health Divide*, London: Health Education Council. This is the source of most of the figures that follow.

18. M.W. Flinn, ed., *op. cit.*

19. R. Klein, "Models of Man and Models of Policy," *Millbank Memorial Fund Quarterly/Health and Society* 58, no. 3 (1980): 416–429.

CODA

Looking Back, Looking Forward

Looking back over the previous chapters, we are struck by, but not apologetic about, what we have left out. There is nothing about the politics of abortion, euthanasia, or genetic engineering, all of which raise moral issues that generate intense political passions. There is nothing, either, about the politics of the pharmaceutical industry and drug pricing, an example of how the encounter between the same powerful interest group and different governments can yield contrasting outcomes depending on national institutions. And the list could be extended still further. And if this book had been intended to be a comprehensive guide to all the important political struggles that take place in the field of health care, these omissions would be a serious weakness. But this was never the intention. Rather, the aim throughout has been to provide a demonstration of how our analytical framework, as outlined in Chapter 1, can be used in a variety of settings and in doing so to provide the reader with a do-it-yourself conceptual tool kit, as it were, for analyzing both those issues which are not covered and new issues as they come up in future.

There is one omission that perhaps deserves more attention. There is no chapter explicitly dedicated to regulation: the harnessing (or constraining) of private interests to the public interest by the state. Regulation is an all-pervasive phenomenon in modern societies. It can apply to individuals, professions, or giant corporations. It can be about personal conduct, quality control, or environmental planning. It can involve prohibitions, commandments, or the imposition of standards. It can be exercised in many different ways: through legislation and the courts, through inspectorates or audit bodies, and through special agencies. In policy terms, public regulation can also be a substitute for public provision and for public financing: the costs of implementing policy are imposed on the regulated—calling the tune without paying the piper, as it has been termed.

It is precisely because of the protean nature of regulation—the fact that so many different types of policy and so large a range of instruments shelter under the same label—that we have not dedicated a chapter to it. Several chapters do indeed touch on the topic, such as the regulation of the medical profession (Chapter 6) and the regulation of tobacco consumption (Chapter 12). But there is no attempt at a comprehensive treatment, and it may well be that none is possible. The regulation of standards in nursing homes raises a different set of issues from those prompted by the regulation of drug safety or the regulation of health insurance plans. What we would claim, however, is that our analytic trinity remains a helpful starting point, if no more, for any analysis of regulatory issues. In all cases, it is important to ask questions about the nature of the regulatory institutions: their history, their composition, and their relationship with the regulated. In all cases, too, it is relevant to unpick the nature of the interests that are affected, with a particular focus on their place on the concentrated to diffuse spectrum. In all cases, finally, it is essential to take account of changing ideas about what constitutes good regulatory practice, with particular attention to the cyclical nature of those ideas: the way in which enthusiasm for deregulation is in turn displaced by a new spurt of concern about tightening regulatory machinery—as vividly illustrated in the aftermath of the banking and financial crisis of 2008, but by no means limited to this dramatic example.

So much for retrospection. Looking forward, what have we ourselves learned from this exercise in selecting case studies and commenting on them? First and foremost, the exercise has sharpened our own awareness of the importance of the way in which issues are framed. We touch on this in most of the chapters, but the point deserves both more emphasis and elaboration. Our analytical trinity sets out, as it were, the basic anatomy of political analysis. But to understand the physiology of the political process, it is necessary to go one step further: to examine the way in which the parties involved in any political dispute seek to impose their definitions of what is at stake, what the relevant facts are, and what counts as good currency of argument in the debate. What matters is not so much the facts of the case, but how those facts are presented and understood. In short, the study of rhetoric (as it has been known since the days of Aristotle) or discourse analysis (as it is now fashionably termed) must be part of the analytic tool kit.

In summary, analysis of the battle of ideas must be prior to—or at a minimum an essential part of—any analysis of interests and institutions. The point is all the more important given the centrality of the notion of self-interest in policy analysis, particularly when practiced by economists. Actors in the policy process, it is axiomatically assumed, will pursue their self-interest. But this is to reify the notion of self-interest, to assume that it is somehow a given and a constant in the equation of power. But this is to ignore the possibility—indeed the likelihood—that policy actors will redefine their self-interest over time in the light of changing ideas and changing notions of what counts as good argument in any dispute.

Conventionally, books dedicated to an analysis of health care policy tend to end with prescriptions for, and predictions about, the future. We have resisted this temptation. Our intention in this book has been to promote an understanding of the politics of the policy process in the health care arena and, by so doing, to equip the reader with tools helpful for analysis. If we have succeeded in this, readers should be able to make prescriptions and predictions of their own that are all the more robust for taking the political dimension into account. The only finger-waving conclusion we would want to leave with the reader is that conceptual precision and verbal clarity are the essential foundations of any analysis: words matter and jargon is the enemy.

CREDITS

Chapter 1: Politics and Policy Analysis

Adapted from "Reflections on Policy Analysis: Putting It Together Again," in *Oxford Handbook of Public Policy*, ed. Martin Rein, Michael Moran, and Robert Goodin (Oxford: Oxford University Press, 2006). By permission of Oxford University Press.

Chapter 3: The High Politics of Systems Change over Time

Theodore R. Marmor, "American Health Care Policy and Politics: The Promise and Perils of Reform," *One Issue, Two Voices*, no. 9 (April 2008).

Theodore R. Marmor and Gary J. McKissick, "Medicare's Future: Fact, Fiction and Folly," *American Journal of Law and Medicine* 26, no. 2–3 (summer and fall 2000).

Rudolf Klein, "From Church to Garage," in Rudolf Klein, ed., *The New Politics of the NHS*, 5th ed. (Abingdon, UK: Radcliffe, 2006).

Chapter 4: High Politics, or Explanations of Great Conflict in the World of Health Care

Rudolf Klein, "The Politics of the Big Bang," in Rudolf Klein, ed., *The New Politics of the NHS*, 5th ed. (Abingdon, UK: Radcliffe, 2006).

"The Politics of Universal Health Insurance: Lessons for and from the 1990s" was also published as T. R. Marmor, M. L. Barer, and E. M. Morrison, "Health Care Reform in the United States: On the Road to Nowhere Again?" *Social Science and Medicine* 41, no. 4 (1995): 1–8. It was first published as Chapter 14 in Theodor J. Litman and Leonard S. Robins, eds., *Health Politics and Policy*, 3rd ed. Copyright 1997 Delmar Learning, a part of Cengage Learning, Inc. Reproduced by permission. www.cengage.com/permissions.

Chapter 5: Ideas

Theodore R. Marmor, "Fads in Medical Care Management and Policy," Rock Carling Lecture (London: TSO for The Nuffield Trust, 2004). Reprinted with permission from World Scientific Publishing Co. Pte. Ltd. The section in the chapter titled "A Return to Realism" has appeared in different forms in two other articles: Theodore Marmor and Jerry Mashaw, "Rhetoric and Reality," *Health Management Quarterly* 15, no. 4 (Oct.–Dec. 1993); Theodore R. Marmor, "Hope and Hyperbole:

The Rhetoric and Reality of Managerial Reform in Health Care," *Journal of Health Service Research and Policy* 3, no. 1 (January 1998).

Theodore R. Marmor, Donald A. Wittman, and Thomas C. Heagy, "The Politics of Medical Inflation," *Journal of Health Politics, Policy and Law* 1, no. 1 (1976): 69–84. Copyright 1976, Duke University Press. All rights reserved. Reprinted by permission of the publisher.

Rudolf Klein, "The Great Transformation," *Health Economics, Policy and Law* 1, no. 1 (January 2006): 91–98.

Rudolf Klein, "O'Goffe's Tale: Or What Can We Learn from the Success of the Capitalist Welfare States?" in Catherine Jones, ed., *New Perspectives on the Welfare State in Europe* (London: Routledge, 1993).

Chapter 6: Values, Policies, and Programs

An earlier version of "Values, Institutions and Health Policies" was published in *Sociology of Health and Illness (Kölner Zeitschrift für Soziologie und Sozialpsychologie)*, May 9, 2006. This version was previously published as Theodore R. Marmor, Kieke G. H. Okma, and Stephen R. Latham, "Values, Institutions and Health Policies: Comparative Perspectives," pp. 383–405 in Claus Wendt and Christof Wolf, eds., *Soziologie der Gesundheit* (Weisbaden: VS Verlag, 2006).

Rudolf Klein, "Values Talk in the (English) NHS," pp. 19–28 in Scott L. Greer and David Rowlands, eds., *Developing Policy, Diverging Values? The Values of the United Kingdom's National Health Services* (London: The Nuffield Trust, 2008).

Chapter 7: The State and the Medical Profession

Theodore R. Marmor and David Thomas, "Doctors, Politics and Pay Disputes: 'Pressure Group Politics' Revisited," in Theodore R. Marmor, *Political Analysis and American Medical Care* (Cambridge: Cambridge University Press, 1983).

Theodore R. Marmor and David Thomas, "Doctors, Politics and Pay Disputes: 'Pressure Group Politics' Revisited," *British Journal of Political Science* (October 1972).

Patricia Day and Rudolf Klein, "Constitutional and Distributional Conflict in British Medical Politics: The Case of General Practice, 1911–1991," *Political Studies* 40 (1992): 462–478.

Chapter 8: No Analysis Without Comparison

Theodore R. Marmor, Richard Freeman, and Kieke G. H. Okma, "Comparative Perspectives and Policy Learning in the World of Health Care," special issue of *Journal of Comparative Policy Analysis*, 7, no. 4 (December 2005): 331–48.

Rudolf Klein, "Learning from Others: Shall the Last Be the First?" in *Journal of Health Politics, Policy and Law* 22, no. 5 (1997): 1267–1277. Copyright 1997 Duke University Press. All rights reserved. Used by permission of the publisher.

Chapter 9: Resources and Rationing

Jan Blustein and Theodore R. Marmor, "Cutting Waste by Making Rules: Promises, Pitfalls, and Realistic Prospects," *University of Pennsylvania Law Review* 140, no. 5 (May 1992). This article was first published in Robert Hackey and David Rochefort, eds., *The New Politics of State Health Policy- -As State Policymaking and The Politics of Health Care Rationing: Lessons from Oregon* (Lawrence: University of Kansas Press, 2001).

Jonathan Oberlander, Lawrence Jacobs, and Theodore R. Marmor, "The Politics of Health Care Rationing: Lessons from Oregon," in Robert Hackey and David Rochefort, eds., *The New Politics of State Health Policy* (Lawrence: University of Kansas Press, 2001).

Rudolf Klein and Patricia Day, "Rationing Health Care: The Dilemma of Choice," *Odyssey* 4, no. 2 (1998): 8–13. Reproduced with permission from Elsevier Science.

Chapter 10: Patients, Consumers, and Citizens

Rudolf Klein, "The Politics of Participation," in Robert Maxwell and Nigel Weaver, eds., *Public Participation in Health* (London: King Edward's Hospital Fund for London, 1984).

James A. Morone and Theodore R. Marmor. "Representing Consumer Interests: The Case of American Health Planning," *Ethics*, 91 (1981): 431–450.

Chapter 11: The Politics of Panics

Theodore R. Marmor, Patricia A. Dillon, and Stephen Scher, "The Comparative Politics of Contained Blood: From Hesitancy to Scandal," pp. 349–366 in Eric A. Feldman and Ronald Bayer, *Blood Feuds (Oxford: Oxford University Press, 1999).* By permission of Oxford University Press.

Daniel M. Fox, Patricia Day, and Rudolf Klein, "The Power of Professionalism: Policies for AIDS in Britain, Sweden, and the United States," *Daedalus* 118, no. 2 (1989): 93–112. Copyright 1989 by the American Academy of Arts and Sciences.

Chapter 12: The Politics of Health Crusades

Theodore R. Marmor and Evan S. Lieberman, "Tobacco Control in Comparative Perspective: Eight Nations in Search of an Explanation," pp. 2075–2290 in Eric A. Feldman and Ronald Bayer, eds., *Unfiltered: Conflicts over Tobacco Policy and Public Health* (Cambridge, Mass.: Harvard University Press, 2004). Reprinted by permission of the publisher. Copyright 2004 by the President and Fellows of Harvard College.

Chapter 13: New Paradigms

Theodore R. Marmor and Albert Weale, "A New Perspective on Health: Learning from *Lalonde?*" Rock Carling Lecture (London: TSO for The Nuffield Trust, 2004).

Rudolf Klein, "Acceptable Inequalities," pp. 1–21 in David Green, ed., *Acceptable Inequalities* (London: Institute of Economic Affairs Health Unit, 1988). First published by the Institute of Economic Affairs.

INDEX

Aaron, Henry J., 66–74, 140, 147, 351n4,
    363, 368
Abel-Smith, Brian, 43
Abortion, 37, 42, 538
Abrahamson, 227
Academic Medical Center Consortium,
    340–41
Accidental Logics (Tuohy), 311
Accountability: and British National
    Health Service, 123; and consumers of
    health care generally, 404; definition
    of, 430; mechanisms of, 430–31; and
    U.S. health systems agencies (HSAs),
    430–32
Acheson, Sir Donald, 466, 467
Acheson Report, 505
Acquired immune deficiency syndrome.
    See AIDS/HIV
ADA (Americans with Disabilities Act),
    363
Adams, John, 426–27
Aetna insurance company, 339, 348,
    390–91
Agency, 195, 198–99
Agency for Health Care Policy and
    Research (AHCPR), 340–41, 348, 349,
    354n37, 357n80
Agriculture policy, 189n20

AHCPR (Agency for Health Care
    Policy and Research), 340–41, 348, 349,
    354n37, 357n80
AIDS/HIV: advocacy for AIDS patients,
    342; in Britain, 324, 464–69, 477–79;
    case managers for AIDS patients, 334;
    comparative perspectives on policies
    for, 443–44, 464–79; and confidentiality
    issues, 468–69, 474–75; contact tracing
    and partner-notification programs for,
    469, 470, 472, 475, 478; contaminated
    blood from, 445–61, 466; denial of
    "questionable" drugs to AIDS patients,
    342; discovery of virus responsible for,
    475; gay activism regarding, 467, 471,
    473, 475, 476–78; heterosexual spread
    of, 469, 479; in homosexual or bisexual
    men, 466, 474, 478; immediate action
    regarding, 327; initial underestima-
    tion of danger of, 447–48; and intra-
    venous drug users, 468, 472, 474, 476;
    introduction to, 31, 443–44; in Japan,
    450; media coverage on, 467; and nee-
    dle-exchange programs, 468, 472, 473,
    474; politics concerning, 41; prescription
    drugs for, 473, 474, 475, 476; public-
    education campaigns on, 466, 467–68,
    476; research on, 468, 475–76; screen-

Drive-in church model of health care, 92–94

Drugs. *See* Prescription drugs

Eckstein, Harry, 255–56, 261, 262–63, 265, 273n16, 288, 292n2

Economics and economists: and economic policy, 13, 152; and international language of policy discourse, 96; and Keynesian theory, 13, 152, 192, 196, 202, 203, 205; on medical inflation, 154, 179; and monetarism, 152, 192, 196–97; role of, in health care policy, 35, 39, 66–74, 83n112, 85n135, 96–97, 114, 121, 141, 146–47, 154; on self-interest, 197, 539–40; Titmuss on, 197

ED. *See* Erectile dysfunction (ED); Viagra

Education: in Britain, 116–17, 196, 207; compared with health care policy, 27, 116–17; expenditures on, in OECD countries, 209. *See also* Public-education campaigns

Edwards, John, 50

Elderly: as beneficiaries of welfare state, 207, 228; as consumers of health care, 27; and health systems agencies (HSAs) in U.S., 433; in nursing homes, 314n8, 382; and Oregon Health Plan, 368; public support for, 84n126, 84–85n128; rationing of medical care based on age, 343, 385. *See also* Medicare, U.S.

Eliot, T. S., 512

Elizabethan Poor Law, 218, 221

Ellwood, Paul M., Jr., 337, 339–41

Employment Retirement Income Security Act (ERISA), 143, 367, 374

England. *See* Britain

ENHS. *See* British National Health Service

Enthoven, Alain, 96, 114

Environmental policy, 32, 139, 513–15

Environmental Protection Act, 139

Epstein, Arnold M., 145–46

Equal autonomy, 196

Erectile dysfunction (ED), 387–88, 391, 392, 396, 398–99. *See also* Viagra

ERISA (Employment Retirement Income Security Act), 143, 367, 374

Esping-Andersen, G., 220, 231, 232

Eurobarometer, 233–34

Europe. *See* OECD (Organisation for Economic Cooperation and Development); Welfare state; *and specific countries*

European Commission, 304

European Court of Justice, 304

European Union (EU): formal contacts between politicians and civil servants within, 319; and immigration policy, 12; research by, 313; role of, in domestic policy making within OECD nations, 304; and tobacco control, 494; on values of health care, 246

Euthanasia, 37, 42, 538

Evans, Robert, 350, 510–11

Evidence-based medicine, 25, 381

Expenditures on health care. *See* Cost containment; Cost of/expenditures on health care

Expert patients, 26, 405. *See also* Patients

Fads. *See* Managerial fads

Falk, I. S., 145

Fallows, J., 128, 137

FDA (Food and Drug Administration), 390, 458, 459

Feder, Judith, 146

Federal Insurance Contributions Act, 46

Federation of American Health Systems, 65

Feingold, Eugene, 146

Feldman, Eric, 315n17, 450, 489, 491, 501n9

Feldstein, Martin, 179

Ferge, Zsuzsa, 203

Ferrera, 227